Deglutition and Its Disorders

Anatomy, Physiology, Clinical Diagnosis, and Management

Edited by

Adrienne L. Perlman, Ph.D.
Konrad S. Schulze-Delrieu, M.D.

THOMSON
DELMAR LEARNING

Australia Canada Mexico Singapore Spain United Kingdom United States

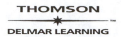

Deglutition and Its Disorders
Anatomy, Physiology, Clinical Diagnosis, and Management
Edited By:
Adrienne L. Perlman, Ph.D., Konrad S. Schulze-Delrieu, M.D.

Vice President,
Health Care Business Unit:
William Brottmiller
Editorial Director:
Cathy L. Esperti

Acquisitions Editor:
Kalen Conerly
Marketing Director:
Jennifer McAvey

Marketing Coordinator:
Chris Manion
Production Editor:
James Zayicek

Library of Congress Cataloging-in-Publication Data

Deglutition and its disorders: anatomy, physiology, clinical diagnosis, and management /
    Edited by Adrienne Perlman and Konrad Schulze-Delrieu.
        p.; cm.
    Includes bibliographical references and index.
    ISBN: 1-56593-621-3
    1. Deglutition disorders. 2. Deglutition.
    I. Perlman, Adrienne.
    II. Schulze-Delrieu, Konrad.
    (DNLM: 1. Deglutition Disorders
    2. Deglutition.   WI 250 D318   1996)
    RC815.2.D44   1996
    616.3'1---dc20
    DNLM/DLC
    for Library of Congress   96-17369
                                                CIP

Notice to the Reader

Publisher does not warrant or guarantee any of the products described herein or perform any independent analysis in connection with any of the product information contained herein. Publisher does not assume, and expressly disclaims, any obligation to obtain and include information other than that provided to it by the manufacturer.

The reader is expressly warned to consider and adopt all safety precautions that might be indicated by the activities described herein and to avoid all potential hazards. By following the instructions contained herein, the reader willingly assumes all risks in connection with such instructions.

The publisher makes no representations or warranties of any kind, including but not limited to, the warranties of fitness for particular purpose or merchantability, nor are any such representations implied with respect to the material set forth herein, and the publisher takes no responsibility with respect to such material. The publisher shall not be liable for any special, consequential, or exemplary damages resulting, in whole or part, from the readers' use of, or reliance upon, this material.

Contents

Preface

During swallowing, the nervous system integrates a myriad of functions of the oral cavity, pharynx, esophagus, airway, and other structures. Sensations trigger swallowing or modulate the swallow. Circuits at various levels of the central nervous system and in the neuronal plexuses of the esophagus orchestrate complex patterns of activity. This activity guides the bolus swiftly from its origin in the mouth to its destination in the stomach. Despite saliva or food crossing the upper airways hundreds of times in a day, they virtually never trespass into the larynx and lower airways.

Swallowing is vital to nutrition and health; it gives the pleasure and satisfaction that comes from the taste of foods, the stilling of hunger, and the quenching of thirst. Impaired swallowing is a source of misery, poor nutrition, and poor health. Impaired swallowing may result in malnutrition, dehydration, or in debilitating illness, and it can deprive individuals of the ability to care for themselves. The difficulty in finding professionals who can recognize and treat their problems often adds to the misery of swallowing-impaired patients. This difficulty is, in part, because the structures and mechanisms involved in swallowing transgress the boundaries of conventional scientific and clinical disciplines. Because of this frequent need for evaluation and treatment by health care providers from various disciplines, communication between disciplines can sometimes complicate patient care. Like anyone else, medical professionals often have difficulty understanding the conceptual, methodologic, diagnostic, and therapeutic tools of disciplines other than their own. Many of the book's authors have experienced firsthand what misunderstandings may result when different meanings are attached to certain terms. For example, in radiologic jargon, the term *aspiration* may be used to refer to a trickle of contrast material penetrating the vocal folds; in pulmonologic jargon, it may mean a massive pulmonary infiltrate following vomiting by an unconscious victim; and in neurologic jargon, it may be an indication for feeding gastrostomy.

The missions that disciplines set for themselves in patient care can also be misunderstood outside of a specific discipline: Eliminating any disease possible is the goal of some, while rehabilitation for a given deficit is the aim of others. Surgeons are held responsible for removing tumors and correcting structural problems that interfere with bolus passage. Consequently, surgeons may consider their surgical treatment a cure if the patient survives for 5 years no matter what the residual dysfunction or quality of life. Speech pathologists are challenged to devise techniques that circumvent problems from a given dysfunction. To a speech pathologist, treatment may be considered successful if it compensates for a swallowing defect, regardless whether that defect resulted from an operative resection or a relentlessly progressing neurologic disease. Such outcome criteria used by surgeons or speech pathologists may not mean much to radiologists or neurologists, let alone to the patients and their caregivers. But these are the foundations onto which additions and improvements must be built.

This book seeks to provide current information about normal and disordered swallowing in a manner that bridges the gap between various disciplines. Our hope is that it will provide the basis for a common language among disciplines. Basic information in didactic format as well as critical commentaries with references for in-depth research are provided in each chapter. Glossary terms and cross references to other chapters should allow the student of any biological or clinical discipline to follow the contents. Through the organization and writing of their chapters, contributors struggled to translate the jargon of their discipline and to explain the rationale for their discipline's undertakings to other students of swallowing and clinicians dealing with swallowing disorders.

The contributors have addressed what information is missing from the literature that would be useful in assisting the clinician in deciding one mode of diagnosis or treatment over another. This critical review of the state of the art in this field should enable professionals to judge new developments on their own rather than being overwhelmed by claims and counterclaims. Defining areas of current ignorance is vital to future progress and likely to spawn interdisciplinary research and clinical care. Improving the understanding of what various disciplines are about should also minimize the risk of turf battles.

In chapters where different perspectives strengthen the approach to problem solving, we have combined the expertise of physicians and clinicians who are well known for their contributions to the study of normal and disordered swallowing. To arrive with simple and harmless tools for the most comprehensive and specific assessment possible is a pride shared by all professions, an expediency appreciated by all patients, and a saving dear to all underwriters of health care. Most chapters make clear distinctions between information that has been tried and solidly tested and information that is based on tenuous assumptions and still being reshaped. Many commentaries identify areas in need of better data before public policies are shared, before diagnostic modalities or treatment interventions are more widely promoted, and before referral patterns are solidified. If the commentaries challenge some cherished dogmas, fine. If the book sets the tone for a critical dialogue between disciplines and professions, even better.

The need for this book occurred to the senior editor first in her work at the Veterans Administration Center in Iowa City. She had served on task forces that defined practice standards for speech pathologists dealing with dysphagic patients in the VA system. In this work she was endorsed by the farsightedness of Dr. Allen Boysen, VA Central Office. The project of the book subsequently was backed by resources largely of the Research Office of the Iowa City VA, whose Associate Chief of Research, Steve Breese, took personal interest and pride in its completion. This included specifically conferences with consultants Dr. Behar of Providence, RI, and Dr. Bieger of St. John, Newfoundland. Dr. Bieger then also became a contributor to the book. Dr. Behar was instrumental in helping to clarify what the book's aims and audiences should be and what it should contain. In the person of Beverly Goodwin the research office supported an able editorial assistant whose polite insistences kept contributors on target, at least almost. The research office also supported the work of Matthew Klan, a graduate student at the University of Illinois. Matthew put in many hours contacting people by phone or by mail, developing the index, and finalizing the product for submission to the publisher. The research office also supported Doris Walters in the Department of Medicine at the Unviersity of Iowa. Mrs.Walters kept many of the local contributors from revolting against editorial demands by treating them to her baking. Pam Cimin-

era, also in the Department of Medicine at Iowa, performed word processing for many of the chapters, some of them dozens of times. Of course, the book could not have come into being without an interested publisher. Its scope and ambition particularly pleased Dr. Sadanand Singh, and he and Marie Linvill knew exactly how to keep ailing editors and unruly contributors on task. We hope that readers will appreciate the results, not just the intentions, of these many efforts.

Adrienne L. Perlman, PhD
Konrad S. Schulze-Delrieu, M.D.

Contributors

Joan C. Arvedson, Ph.D.
Director
Speech-Language and Hearing
   Department
Children's Hospital of Buffalo
Buffalo, New York

Detlef Bieger, M.D.
Professor of Pharmacology
University of Newfoundland
Faculty of Medicine
The Health Sciences Centre
St. Johns, Canada

Bruce P. Brown, M.D.
Associate Professor
Department of Radiology
University of Iowa Hospitals and Clinics
Iowa City, Iowa

David W. Buchholz, M.D.
Associate Professor of Neurology
Johns Hopkins University School of
   Medicine
Director
The Neurologic Consultation Center
The Johns Hopkins Medical Institutions
Baltimore, Maryland

James Christensen, M.D.
Professor of Internal Medicine
University of Iowa Hospitals and Clinics
Iowa City, Iowa

Jeffrey L. Conklin, M.D.
Department of Internal Medicine
University of Iowa Hospitals and Clinics
Iowa City, Iowa

Donald S. Cooper, Ph.D.
Associate Professor of Research
Department of Otolaryngology
School of Medicine
University of Southern California
Los Angeles, California

Jeffrey L. Curtis, M.D.
Assistant Professor, Internal Medicine
University of Michigan School of
   Medicine
Chief, Pulmonary Section
Veterans Affairs Medical Center
Ann Arbor, Michigan

Gulchin A. Ergun, M.D.
Assistant Professor of Medicine
Northwestern University Medical School
Division of Gastroenterology and
   Hepatology
Chicago, Illinois

Henry T. Hoffman, M.D.
Associate Professor
Department of Otolaryngology, Head
   and Neck Surgery
University of Iowa Hospitals and Clinics
Iowa City, Iowa

Debra M. Jaffe, M.D.
Research Fellow
Department of Otolaryngology—Head
   and Neck Surgery
University of Iowa Hospitals and Clinics
Iowa City, Iowa

Bronwyn Jones, M.D.
Department of Radiology and
   Radiological Science
Johns Hopkins Hospital
Baltimore, Maryland

Peter J. Kahrilas, M.D.
Associate Professor of Medicine
Department of Medicine
Department of Communication Sciences
Northwestern University Medical School
Division of Gastroenterology and
    Hepatology
Chicago, Illinois

Susan E. Langmore, Ph.D.
Chief, Audiology and Speech Pathology
    Service
Department of Veteran's Affairs Medical
    Center
Ann Arbor, Michigan

Jeri A. Logemann, Ph.D.
Professor and Chairman
Department of Communication Sciences
    and Disorders
Northwestern University
Evanston, Illinois

Charles C. Lu, M.D.
Professor
Department of Radiology
University of Iowa Hospitals and Clinics
Iowa City, Iowa

Benson T. Massey, M.D.
Assistant Professor of Medicine
Director
GI Manometry Laboratory
MCW Dysphagia Institute
Medical College of Wisconsin
Milwaukee, Wisconsin

Timothy M. McCulloch, M.D.
Assistant Professor
Department of Otolaryngology, Head
    and Neck Surgery
University of Iowa Hospitals and Clinics
Iowa City, Iowa

Arthur J. Miller, Ph.D.
Professor
Department of Growth and Development
School of Dentistry
University of California, San Francisco
San Francisco, California

Robert M. Miller, Ph.D.
Chief, Audiology and Speech Pathology
    Service
VA Medical Center
Clinical Associate Professor
University of Washington
Seattle, Washington

Joseph A. Murray, Ph.D.
Assistant Professor
Department of Gastroenterology
University of Iowa Hospitals and Clinics
Iowa City, Iowa

Adrienne L. Perlman, Ph.D.
Associate Professor
Department of Speech and Hearing
    Science
University of Illinois at Urbana-Champaign
Champaign, Illinois

Satish S. C. Rao, M.D., Ph.D.
Assistant Professor
Department of Internal Medicine
University of Iowa Hospitals and Clinics
Iowa City, Iowa

JoAnne Robbins, Ph.D.
Associate Professor, Medicine
University of Wisconsin, Madison
Associate Director of Research
Geriatric Research , Education, and
    Clinical Center
William S. Middleton V.A. Hospital
Madison, Wisconsin

Brian T. Rogers, M.D.
Clinical Associate Professor of Pediatrics
    and Neurology

State University of New York at Buffalo
Developmental Pediatrician
Children's Hospital of Buffalo
Buffalo, New York

Reza Shaker, M.D.
Associate Professor of Medicine and
  Radiology
Director, MCW Dysphagia Institute
Medical College of Wisconsin
VA Medical Center
GI Section
Milwaukee, Wisconsin

Konrad S. Schulze-Delrieu, M.D.
Professor
Department of Internal Medicine

University of Iowa Hospitals and Clinics
Iowa City, Iowa

Edy E. Soffer, M.D.
Staff Physician
Cleveland Clinic Foundation
Cleveland, Ohio

Barbara C. Sonies, Ph.D.
Chief
Speech-Language Pathology Clinical
  Center
Department of Rehabilitation
The National Institutes of Health
Bethesda, Maryland

To Ida and Lee
Thank you for your patience and support.

1

Introduction to the Field of Deglutition and Deglutition Disorders

Benson T. Massey and Reza Shaker

In the 1990s the study and treatment of deglutition disorders have been recognized as important and growing concerns. Evidence in support of this statement is seen in Figure 1–1. Review of the MED-LINE database suggests that in the past decade publication in the area of deglutition is accelerating at a nearly exponential rate. Important associated milestones in the development of this field include the establishment of dedicated "swallowing centers" at different health care institutions throughout the country, the introduction of a scientific journal specifically devoted to the field (*Dysphagia*) in 1986, and the chartering of an organization with the goal of promoting research in this field (the Dysphagia Research Society) in 1992. All of these developments portend great promise for the field of deglutition. To understand the importance of this growing field, however, one must have an appreciation of the magnitude of the clinical problem, both for the individual patient and for society as a whole. The goal in this chapter is to allow the reader to develop this appreciation as well as an understanding about the limitations of the current fund of knowledge regarding deglutition and its

disorders. Finally, the reader should develop a grasp of the uncertainties and controversies in the cognitive and methodologic approaches to research, therapy, and training in this field.

THE DYSPHAGIC PATIENT

In working with individual patients, one comes to appreciate how problems with dysphagia affect their daily lives. First, one has to remember that the exceedingly complex process of deglutition is one that normal individuals can generally take for granted as they go about their daily routine. The fact that dysphagic patients may have to remain vigilant about such a normally subconscious act as swallowing to avoid discomfort or even death means that their deglutition disorders greatly interfere with normal living.

Swallowing begins at the lips and ends at the stomach. Hence, dysphagia can result from abnormalities in deglutition that occur anywhere along that path. Typical symptoms of dysphagia include a feeling that swallowed solids or liquids are not going down or are only partly going down,

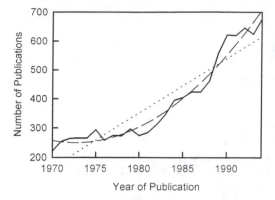

Figure 1–1. Time trend for publication on deglutition and deglutition disorders. Data are obtained from a search of the MEDLINE database, using Ovid 3.0 search software (CD Plus, Inc.). The search strategy used the subject headings *deglutition* or *deglutition disorders* and the words *deglutition, dysphagia, dysphagic, swallow,* or *choking* from titles or abstracts. The solid line represents actual data, the dotted line linear fit of data, and the dashed line exponential fit of data.

then sticking or hanging up. This sensation by itself is unusual enough to be alarming and noxious. Yet even more disturbing symptoms frequently accompany dysphagia, depending upon the underlying deglutition disorder. Patients can experience hiccups as well as pain or pressure in the throat or chest, at times severe enough to make patients concerned that their heart is the cause. Patients may have to regurgitate forcibly a stuck bolus, while at other times material regurgitates spontaneously when patients least expect it, even while they are sleeping; this can leave them with the unpleasant task of disposing of this regurgitated material somehow. Patients may not be able to swallow even their own saliva, having instead to keep spitting this into a tissue or cup. A swallow can result in coughing, sputtering, food coming out the nose, or even airway blockage with an inability to breathe. The voice can become faint and raspy, with wheezing during most breaths.

To avoid these symptoms, dysphagic patients have to modify their diets and eating habits to various and, at times,

profound degrees. Some eat so slowly that they are consistently the last at the table to finish a meal, if they finish the meal at all. Many patients come to consciously or subconsciously avoid certain foods and beverages altogether, because they have learned that these items can cause them trouble. Alternatively, patients attempt to consume troublesome foodstuffs using compensatory maneuvers. Some chew their meat to mush before swallowing it, while others artificially thicken any liquids before swallowing them, even then taking only one small swallow at a time. Yet despite their best efforts, patients frequently drop their guard, resulting in embarrassment when they must excuse themselves abruptly and dramatically from the meal or have their companions save them from asphyxiation. Incompetence at deglutition can be as socially discomfiting as incompetence at the other end of the alimentary canal, so that many individuals become recluses, rather than risk the embarrassment and have their colleagues pity them for their sick role. This can be especially true for those whose deglutition is so impaired that they must have all feedings delivered by a nasally or abdominally placed feeding tube.

Symptoms of dysphagia make patients anxious and thus prompt visits to the doctor. Patients can often come to medical attention for complications of deglutition disorders also. They may die abruptly from asphyxiation or survive this but with various cognitive sequelae from a cardiorespiratory arrest. They may develop aspiration pneumonia, which can be fatal. Their airways and lungs can become scarred, making breathing difficult and dependent upon supplemental oxygen and medication. Some develop sinus infections. Patients may tear their alimentary tract trying to regurgitate a stuck bolus, with lethal bleeding or rupture. They can develop severe weight loss and malnutrition, becoming setups for infection and poor wound healing. Finally, the underlying process causing the deglutition disturbance, such as embolic stroke or cancer, can progress, leading to further disability and demise. It is hardly surprising, then, that deglutition disorders can have such an adverse effect on the quality of life (Gustafsson & Tibbling, 1991; Gustafsson, Tibbling, & Theorell, 1992; Tibbling & Gustafsson, 1991).

In addition, the quality of life of caregivers may be affected, as they have to spend additional time helping the patient with meals or tube feedings. For many caregivers the burden becomes too great and patients are then transferred to expensive chronic care facilities, often with the mandate that gastrostomy tubes be placed for nutrition, because there are insufficient personnel to provide the considerable assistance the patient may need to maintain an oral diet. Such tube feeding raises ethical issues when the quality of the life so maintained becomes minimal (Quill, 1989).

PATIENTS AT RISK FOR DEVELOPING DEGLUTITION DISORDERS

Because deglutition disorders can have such serious consequences, it is important to identify groups of patients with conditions that predispose them to these disorders. Such identification allows for more aggressive efforts to diagnose deglutition disorders in these high-risk patients, so that treatment can be initiated before they develop complications, such as malnutrition and aspiration pneumonia. In general, patients with conditions that result in destruction or dysfunction of the neural pathways controlling deglutition—from the cortex to the brainstem swallowing centers to the peripheral nervous system—are prime candidates for developing swallowing difficulty. These conditions include, but are not limited to, dementias of varying etiologies, cerebrovascular disease, toxic or inflammatory encephalopathies, space-occupying intracranial lesions, Parkinson's disease, poliomyelitis, cerebral palsy, multiple sclerosis, amyotrophic lateral sclerosis, and esophageal achalasia. Conditions affecting striated or smooth muscle function within the swallowing axis can also give rise to dysphagia. Such conditions include poly-

myositis, myasthenia gravis, progressive systemic sclerosis, Kearns-Sayre syndrome, Eaton-Lambert syndrome, and the various muscular and myotonic dystrophies. Many diseases produce dysphagia by structural alteration of the deglutitive passageways. Neoplasms are the most obvious causes, but strictures from reflux disease or of congenital or iatrogenic origin are also frequently encountered. The above lists are by no means exhaustive, and in addition, a variety of rare systemic conditions can give rise to deglutition disturbances, frequently by more than one mechanism. These have been enumerated and reviewed in more detail elsewhere (Jones, Ravich, & Donner, 1993).

Unfortunately, for many of the above conditions, the association with disturbances in deglutition remains at best anecdotal, so that it is difficult to define precisely the risk of developing swallowing difficulty in a given patient with a disease. Even for relatively common conditions, such as stroke, the estimates for frequency of associated abnormal deglutition vary widely. In some studies over half of patients with stroke have abnormal swallowing when studied acutely or in a specialized referral setting (Barer, 1989; Chen, Ott, Peele, & Gelfand, 1990; Gordon, Hewer, & Wade, 1987; Gresham, 1990; Young & Durant-Jones, 1990). Studies of stroke patients later in their course show a prevalence of dysphagia as low as one sixth (Gresham, 1990; Kuhlemeier, Rieve, Kirby, & Siebens, 1989).

THE SOCIETAL BURDEN FROM DEGLUTITION DISORDERS

Essentially no information exists regarding the incidence and prevalence of dysphagic symptoms and disorders for the entire population. Some data are available regarding the elderly, a population felt to be at high risk for deglutition disorders by virtue of the comorbid illnesses that become more prevalent with age. This statement is supported by an examination of the 1993 United States Veterans Administration (VA) patient treatment files, which contain information on the patients' diagnoses at the time of hospital discharge for over half a million patients hospitalized in the VA system that year. Patients older than 85 years were over 18 times more likely to have a diagnosis of dysphagia than were patients under age 25. Indeed, about 1% of this hospitalized population was discharged with the diagnosis of dysphagia. United States hospital discharge rates for two esophageal disorders that frequently produce dysphagia—achalasia and peptic stricture—increase with age within the geriatric population (Sonnenberg, Massey, & Jacobsen, 1994; Sonnenberg, Massey, McCarty, & Jacobsen, 1993). Other diseases that can cause oropharyngeal dysphagia, such as head and neck cancers and stroke, are also more common in the elderly. Direct community surveys of the geriatric (older than 55 years) population indicate prevalences of dysphagic symptoms ranging from 16 to 22% (Bloem et al., 1990; Kjellen & Tibbling, 1981; Lindgren & Janzon, 1991).

These data indicate the potential for a substantial health care burden due to deglutition disorders, especially given the increasing age of the population. Despite such presumptions, there are very little hard data about the burden of dysphagia on the health care system and its economic impact on society as a whole. Certainly, dysphagic patients can undergo many expensive diagnostic and therapeutic interventions, including endoscopy, fluoroscopic swallow studies, CT and MRI scans, scintigraphy, ultrasonography, manometry, electromyography, stricture dilation, stent placement, feeding tube placement, and surgery. The chronicity of most dysphagic disorders results in ongoing health care costs. Abnormal deglutition can also complicate other comorbid conditions and prolong the hospital stay, as has been demonstrated for stroke patients (Young & Durant-Jones, 1990).

To get some idea of the potential costs of deglutition disorders to society, it may be instructive to review the costs of esophagitis, diaphragmatic hernia, and esophageal cancer, since symptoms of dysphagia are present in a substantial fraction of patients with these diseases. It has been estimated

that in 1985 the direct and indirect costs of these three diseases totaled nearly two and a half billion dollars (Brown & Everhart, 1994). Another measure of the economic burden of deglutition disorders is the costs for enteral tube feedings, which are necessary in many of these patients (Howard, Ament, Fleming, Shike, & Steiger, 1995): In 1992 Medicare covered enteral feedings for 73,000 patients at home (a 115% increase since 1989) and 133,000 patients in nursing homes, at a cost of $505 million (80% of the allowable charge). It has been estimated that, for home enteral nutrition, a nearly equal number of patients were covered by a provider other than Medicare. Neurologic swallowing disorders account for just over 30% of cases requiring home enteral nutrition and only 19% of these patients return to full oral nutrition after a year of therapy. The implication from these figures is that the economic burden from deglutition disorders is considerable.

THE DYSPHAGIA TEAM

The varied and often protean manifestations of deglutition disorders result in patients presenting or being referred to a variety of health professionals, including general practitioners, gastroenterologists, otolaryngologists, speech pathologists, neurologists, radiologists, psychiatrists, pulmonologists, dentists, and surgeons. Given the burden of disease within the population and the economic burden to society, it is imperative that these health professionals approach these disorders effectively and efficiently. Each specialty has its own biases toward approaching dysphagic patients, biases based on the expected spectrum of patients referred, and the methodologies typically employed for diagnosis and treatment. Such biases mean that not all dysphagic patients can be expected to be managed optimally by the approach of a single specialty. Hence the development of dysphagia teams, wherein different specialties communicate and collaborate, has the potential to orchestrate more expeditiously a patient's evaluation and therapy. At least one study has suggested that this team approach leads to diagnosis and treatment of conditions that had been missed previously (Ravich, Wilson, Jones, & Donner, 1989).

EDUCATION IN DEGLUTITION AND DEGLUTITION DISORDERS

Members of different health care disciplines are often not accustomed to working together in a team approach; thus, in some instances successful formation of such teams likely will require additional education for all team members about the expertise the other members possess. Along educational lines, arguments could be made for expanding the amount of teaching done on deglutition disorders in medical schools, or at least developing a multidisciplinary block of curriculum time focused on the topic. Deglutition disorders tend to get short shrift in most medical school curricula because they are not "owned" by any one department or division. Indeed, one has to wonder whether in the future postgraduate training in this field should begin to cross departmental lines, with the creation of the deglutition specialist, one who has mastered the array of skills other specialties bring on a part-time basis to the field.

The case can be made for expanding the public understanding of deglutition and its disorders, especially since the population is aging and becoming more susceptible to dysphagia from a variety of causes. Interaction with health care providers is one obvious source for this education, but methods for reaching the community at large should also be developed. It is clear from our experience that many patients do not know where to turn when they first develop symptoms of dysphagia. Most people (and many health care professionals) are also completely unaware of the iatrogenic risks for dysphagia many treatments carry, such as pill-induced esophageal injury or severe xerostomia resulting from radiation therapy.

DEGLUTITION RESEARCH

From the above discussion, it should be evident that deglutition disorders constitute an important health care problem, and as such should command a substantial research effort, both in fundamental investigations into etiopathogenesis as well as in clinical trials to improve outcomes. Certainly investigators in the field seem to be responding to this need for new understanding and treatments, if the rising number of publications is any indication. As diverse avenues of investigation begin to coalesce into a unified field of deglutition research, however, researchers need to heed and address several fundamental challenges to the advancement of this area, both within the academic and scientific community as well as within the broader health care arena.

Research and the Challenge of Cognitive Dualism

Perhaps the foremost conceptual challenge in the field is the lack of a cohesive and comprehensive cognitive framework upon which to base research and clinical practice of deglutition disorders. This lack of framework stems in part from what can be construed as a dualism in the cognitive approach to swallowing disorders. One side of this dualism is to view the swallowing disorders as being manifestations of underlying pathophysiologic conditions, rather than being pathophysiologic entities in and of themselves. The counterpart to this view is the traditional swallow therapy view, where the cognitive approach tends to be oriented toward the process and mechanics of swallowing, without primary regard of the underlying disease states that may alter the swallowing process. As an example, the neurologic orientation toward a patient with dysphagia following a cerebrovascular event centers around the afferent and efferent denervation engendered by the ischemic neuronal destruction, whereas the traditional swallow therapy orientation toward such a patient focuses on where and how transport of the swallowed bolus fails. Both cognitive approaches are valid and useful. However, research along these two different cognitive lines theoretically will lead to different end points. The deglutitive process-oriented approach ideally should lead ultimately to mechanisms that allow a stroke patient to overcome completely the bolus transport abnormalities induced by the stroke. In contrast, the pathophysiologic approach ultimately should come to a method of preventing stroke in the first place or at least limit or repair the damage resulting from stroke so that impaired bolus transport does not become a clinical issue. It is this goal of preventing or eliminating disease that gives the pathophysiologic approach its appeal. However, the process approach is more likely to provide improvements in patient well-being until the underlying disease can be eliminated or ameliorated.

Other conceptual challenges arise from this dualism because of the lack of one-to-one correspondence between abnormal deglutitive processes and associated symptoms and specific pathophysiologic processes. As an example, dysphagia associated with pharyngeal muscle weakness can be a consequence of such varied entities as post-polio syndrome, myasthenia gravis, or polymyositis. From a medical standpoint, this lack of correspondence often causes the abnormal swallow process and its associated symptoms to be viewed primarily as signs of an uncertain pathophysiology that must be diagnosed. Once the underlying pathophysiologic process is elucidated, the presenting deglutitive symptoms become cognitively subsumed under a specific pathophysiologic entity for that particular patient. Hence, the dysfunctional deglutitive mechanics may receive less directed attention, although they are actually what prompted the patient to seek medical care initially. Conversely, the swallow therapy approach may be similar for the deglutitive manifestations of diverse underlying pathophysiologic states, with this approach not having to heed the fact that the medical treatment of the underlying pathophysiologic conditions themselves may be vastly different.

An unresolved issue that stems from this dualism is what aspects of the pathophysiologic approach to a disease entity are justified in being placed under the rubric of deglutition disorders. Studies into the etiopathogenesis underlying deglutition disorders may not involve the concept of deglutition whatsoever, yet successful outcomes of such research would eliminate many causes of deglutitive disorders. For instance, esophageal cancer can cause dysphagia. Certainly, research involving the development of new stenting methods for maintaining patency of the esophageal lumen to improve dysphagia would fit under the rubric of deglutition disorder research. However, research to identify genetic abnormalities in esophageal cancer would probably not be placed under this rubric, even though such research might ultimately lead to cancer cures and thereby relieve dysphagia also. Similarly, patients with gastroesophageal reflux disease may have deglutitive problems associated with abnormal peristalsis and stenosis. Yet deglutitive problems are not always present in reflux disease, so that it is unclear which aspects of research into reflux disease should be considered deglutition-related research. An example of how uncertain the borders of the field of deglutition are is evidenced by the MEDLINE literature search that resulted in Figure 1–1. That search strategy identified only 28% of articles dealing with esophageal achalasia and only 26% of the articles dealing with esophageal stenosis, conditions in which dysphagia is a paramount feature.

The foregoing discussion should not be construed as concluding that this cognitive dualism is detrimental or that one approach is to be preferred to the other. Both approaches are valid and likely to be complementary in advancing the field of deglutition research. Nevertheless, deglutition researchers need to remain cognizant of the potential for these two approaches to become competitive also, as issues of "turf" emerge when research and health care funds are specifically earmarked for deglutition disorders.

Research and the Challenge of Determining Normalcy

A formidable challenge that deglutition researchers continue to face is the determination of the appropriate definitions and parameters for normalcy in deglutition. While it would seem obvious that one has to have a firm grasp on what is normal before trying to evaluate and treat the abnormal, there are many aspects of deglutition in which there is no gold standard for, or even overwhelming consensus about, what is normal. There are several facets to this problem. A critical difficulty in defining normalcy is that no criteria are likely to be universally acceptable and without exception. For instance, if one uses the subjective absence of deglutitive symptoms as a sign of normalcy, this definition will frequently be at odds with objective measures of what is felt to be abnormal deglutition. For example, a patient may be found to aspirate silently without having a complaint of swallowing symptoms and with no physical indicator such as coughing. Conversely, a patient may have complaints of dysphagia without any abnormality in bolus transport being identified.

If only objective deglutition parameters are to be used in defining normalcy, then additional issues emerge. For many deglutition parameters, abnormality may be a matter of degree rather than an invariant "state-change" from normal to abnormal. For a given parameter there can be considerable overlap between normal and abnormal populations, such that sensitivities and specificities of that parameter in distinguishing between these two states must be determined.

These considerations can make it difficult to identify an appropriate normal population or reference group. For instance, certain aspects of deglutitive dynamics differ in the "normal" elderly compared to younger subjects (Ekberg & Feinberg, 1991; Fulp, Dalton, Castell, & Castell, 1990; Perlman, Guthmiller Schultz, & VanDaele, 1993; Ren et al., 1993; Robbins, Hamilton, Lof, & Kempster, 1992; Shaker et al., 1993; Tracy et al., 1989; Wilson, Pryde, Macintyre, Maran, & Heading, 1990). Does this mean that the elderly should be considered abnormal or that different ranges of normalcy will need to be determined for different subgroups for some deglutition parameters? And how many subgroups?

A related issue is the appropriate sample size of the reference group for determining normalcy. Most published studies of normal deglutitive function have examined fewer than 100 subjects and at times fewer than 30. These studies can show statistically significant differences between the reference and abnormal groups for the mean values of the parameter in question; however, the sample sizes are frequently too small to ascertain reliably the degree of overlap between the two populations.

A final challenge regarding the issue of normalcy has to do with the generalizability of the normal range for a measured parameter to different study conditions. For example the normal manometric parameters for esophageal peristalsis while supine (the usual study position) are not the same for studies with a subject upright (Sears, Castell, & Castell, 1990; Wilhelm, Freiling, Enck, & Lübke, 1993). Oftentimes, subjects are studied in a constrained manner (e.g., head immobilization, standardized boluses) to reduce the variability in the recorded parameter. Data from such studies cannot necessarily be taken as normative standards for that deglutition parameter when recorded in less constrained, or differently constrained, conditions. This means that it may be very difficult to compare the normative data for the same parameter from different studies that did not use exactly the same constraining conditions.

Research and the Challenge of Methodology

A growing array of technologies is available to assess various aspects of deglutitive function and dysfunction. In general these technologies allow measurement of the movement of deglutitive structures and/or boluses or the activity of muscles involved in deglutition in temporospatial domains.

Several challenges confront the optimal use of these methodologies. An inherent difficulty with essentially all modalities is that they are more or less invasive or constraining on the natural act of deglutition. This means that some aspects of the deglutitive process can be altered or interfered with by the examining methodology and some aspects simply cannot be recorded. An obvious example would be the subject who gags on barium. A more subtle example is the increase in swallow frequency resulting from stimulation of salivary flow when a nasopharyngeal catheter is present (Helm et al., 1982; Kapila, Dodds, Helm, & Hogan, 1984). Some modalities require substantial constraints of movement to avoid movement artifacts in the recordings, such as CT and MRI. Little data are available for many such methodologies about how the imposed constraints affect natural deglutition (Lang, Dantas, Cook, & Dodds, 1991; Robbins, Hamilton, Lof, & Kempster, 1992).

Scant information exists about sources and degrees of error in making measurements for many of these methodologies. In some instances, error ascertainment may be impossible because there are no gold standard criteria for measurement. For instance, there is no ready way to assess how accurately and precisely the surface EMG signal reflects the magnitude of muscle activity in vivo. Nor, for example, is there information about how much of the variability in scintigraphic bolus clearance from swallow-to-swallow is a result of the inherent variability in the swallow process or the variability of the technique. Unpublished observations from our laboratory suggest that, for movement of hyolaryngeal structures during deglutition, the intraobserver variability of measurement is on the order of 10%. Hence, changes in any parameter felt to affect such movement will have to do so by an amount larger than this for the effects to be detectable.

For a given methodology there are significant differences in specific techniques among different practitioners. Manometry offers an obvious example: The probe

composition and position can have striking effects on the measurements obtained, making comparisons among studies difficult (Massey, 1993). Another example would be videofluoroscopically recorded swallow studies, where different institutions will use different bolus sizes and compositions. Another challenge in terms of different methodologies is to determine how they relate to each other and which is preferred. The phenomena measured by different methodologies are generally interrelated, such as manometry and EMG both recording certain aspects of muscle activity. Sophisticated models for relating information from more disparate methodologies, such as manometry and videofluoroscopy, are under development (Brasseur & Dodds, 1991). While the diverse information provided by the use of several different methodologies can at times be complementary, there can also be a wasteful redundancy in the data so obtained. Little knowledge exists for determining which is the most useful methodology in specific situations.

Research and the Challenge of Epidemiology

The epidemiology of deglutition disorders remains in its infancy. In general two different approaches are available for obtaining epidemiologic information about deglutition disorders. One is to abstract information from large health databases, such as that of the Health Care Financing Administration (HCFA) for hospitalized Medicare patients. The other is to obtain information from samples of the population by direct interrogation. Each approach has its advantages and disadvantages.

The advantages of the database approach include (a) potential access to large sample sizes with wide geographic sampling, (b) ability to determine time trends from a series of data sets, (c) lack of a priori bias regarding deglutition disorders (since such databases were not constructed specifically to examine such disorders), (d) relatively low cost for the amount of data obtained, and (e) potential for gaining insights into etiopathogenesis by studying comorbidities coded within the data set. An example of this last feature comes from data on hospitalizations in Maryland in 1989. In the hospitalized patients with a diagnosis of dysphagia, comorbity with circulatory and respiratory diseases was about twice as common as with digestive diseases. Also, the incidence of dysphagia among hospitalized patients rose over threefold in the preceding decade (Kuhlemeier, 1994).

The disadvantages of the database approach include the fact that the database population may not be representative of the population at large (e.g., only hospitalized patients in the database). Also, there may not exist a database for the target population desired (e.g., no database for urban dwellers or nursing home residents). There can be uncertainty about the accuracy and reliability of the data in the database (i.e., were the patient's diagnoses coded correctly). This latter problem in part can be a manifestation of the cognitive dualism discussed above. For instance, hospital discharge databases may underreport swallowing disorders, because the diagnosis code for the underlying pathophysiologic disorder is recorded (e.g., cerebrovascular accident, cardiospasm), rather than the code for "dysphagia" (which in the ninth revision of the International Classification of Diseases [ICD-9] is coded 787.2). Moreover, many such databases have limited numbers of diagnostic codes that can be entered, so that the code for dysphagia might be omitted simply owing to space limitations. Databases generally provide data only about the presence or absence of a condition, without providing any measure of the severity of the condition. Finally, since most databases are limited in the variety of data obtained, and were generally constructed for other purposes, commonly they don't contain important material regarding potential risk factors that would be of interest to perhaps only dysphagia researchers (e.g., dietary data includes calories but not food consistencies).

One of the advantages of interrogations of community samples is that the population to be studied can be established at the outset. Hence, the researcher can focus on an unbiased sampling of the general population or examine specific subsets of the population. Additionally, objective methods used for determining the presence of a deglutition disorder can be defined ahead of time and thus potentially avoid observer or reporting bias. Data can be gathered to examine specific hypotheses about certain risk factors a priori. Scales can be developed to determine the severity of dysfunction.

Community survey methodologies can also have several pitfalls such as response bias (patients with symptoms being more willing to participate in surveys, thus being overrepresented). If the condition being studied is rare, then the size of the population that must be sampled to obtain meaningful numbers of subjects may make the study prohibitively expensive. Areas of particular concern for deglutition research have to do with reliability and validity of the interrogation instruments. Many surveys regarding dysphagia have not been demonstrated to be reliable (i.e., good intrasubject agreement on the responses to interrogation at different times or in different settings). For example, a recently evaluated questionnaire, while demonstrating excellent reliability for the presence of dysphagia, had a test-retest agreement that was only fair to good for the duration and severity of dysphagia, as well as the type of bolus associated with dysphagia (Locke, Talley, Weaver, & Zinsmeister, 1994). Nor has the validity (i.e., does the measuring instrument really measure what is sought) of many questionnaires been established. This may prove to be an especially difficult challenge for deglutition disorders, since (a) as discussed above, a consensus about normalcy has not been reached in many instances and (b) some disorders may be silent until a complication occurs. Attempts to avoid some of these challenges by obtaining objective measures of swallowing function using any of the methodologies discussed above will be hampered by the costs of such methodologies and the acceptance of the unpleasantness and risks imposed by such methodologies upon the population sample to be so studied.

Research and the Challenge of Clinical Outcomes

The hope exists that further research into etiopathogenesis of and therapeutic modalities for deglutition disorders should eventually result in improved outcomes or at least more accurate diagnosis and prognosis for these disorders. Yet it remains to be seen how much of the explosion of new information about normal and abnormal deglutition implied by the data in Figure 1–1 will have clinical relevance. For instance, improved methodology may allow a more detailed delineation of the swallowing process and thus identify heretofore unrecognized disturbances in this process. But, it is also possible that it will not be useful in most patients to quantitate subtle disturbances in hyoid bone movement, EMG signal timing or amplitude, or scintigraphic bolus residuals. Although each of these methods might prove to be quite useful with various individuals, to date the data are insufficient for firm statements to be made.

As in many medical fields, many of the diagnostic and treatment modalities for deglutition disorders have evolved along empirical lines without rigorous testing of their efficacy. As the competition for health care funds becomes more acute, there will be greater pressure to demonstrate that use of these clinical modalities leads to improved clinical outcomes. Such demands will pose several challenges. The first is to develop a reliable, valid system for determining the extent to which deglutition disorders cause morbidity and disability in patients. An approach similar to the Sickness Impact Profile (Bergner, Bobbit, Carter, & Gilson, 1981), which has been used to assess the global impact of a variety of disorders (Drossman et al., 1991), will likely have to be developed. Such a scheme will have the particular challenge of determining the incremental disability resulting from degluti-

tion disturbance over and above the other manifestations of the underlying disease (such as hemiplegia and dysarthria from a stroke). Such a system will be necessary to demonstrate improved outcomes from a clinical intervention. For instance, the mere demonstration of decreased laryngeal bolus penetration after a specific therapeutic maneuver will be irrelevant, unless this can be shown to predict a clinically useful outcome, such as shorter hospital stays or decreased episodes of pneumonia or a return of independence in activities of daily living.

Not only will therapeutic interventions be required to demonstrate improved outcomes, they will have to demonstrate cost effectiveness. Measures for cost effectiveness often take the form of dollars spent per quality-adjusted years of life gained. This will require development of a system for quality-adjusting life with a deglutition disorder, better data on years of life gained, and improved accounting of diagnosis and treatment costs. Moreover, new or competing therapeutic modalities may have to demonstrate not only cost effectiveness but also incremental cost effectiveness. For example, the costs of evaluating stroke patients with a videofluoroscopic examination might hypothetically be $10,000 per quality-adjusted year of life saved; addition of concurrent scintigraphic studies might have an incremental cost of $250,000 per year of life saved, given that the preponderance of benefit is derived from the videofluoroscopic examination alone for most patients.

With the constraints being placed on health care expenditures, multidisciplinary teams for deglutition disorders will be challenged to demonstrate their cost-efficacy. The potential for bringing diverse skills to bear on a clinical problem so as to improve diagnosis and treatment may be offset by the increased costs of the multitude of diagnostic modalities to which the patient may be submitted in such a milieu. Dysphagia teams will be challenged to determine which aspects of their approaches are truly complementary and which are expensively redundant.

SUMMARY

This introductory chapter depicts the complications of dysphagia in individual patients, delineates the patient groups at risk for dysphagia, and suggests the magnitude of the health care burden imposed upon society by deglutition disorders. The need for further development of dysphagia teams and education in deglutition disorders is emphasized. Several conceptual challenges to continued research on deglutition and its disorders—involving cognitive dualism, normalcy, methodology, epidemiology, and clinical outcomes—are discussed. Although these challenges may appear daunting, they also indicate the need for further basic and applied research in the field of deglutition. The magnitude of the dysphagia burden for individual patients and society at large is ample reason for investigators to strive to meet these challenges.

MULTIPLE CHOICE QUESTIONS

Select all of the correct answers for the questions below.

1. Which of the following statements are true about research in deglutition and its disorders?
   a. Over the past decade publication of deglutition-related research has plateaued.
   b. Many studies have used too few subjects to identify reliably the normal range of the parameter being measured.
   c. Research studies must take account of the effect of aging on normal deglutition.
   d. Research methodologies are standardized throughout the research community.

2. The following are true about the use of existing databases for studying the epidemiology of deglutition disorders:
   a. They can provide large sample sizes for analysis.
   b. Every patient with a deglutition disorder within the database can be identified.
   c. Dysphagia has a specific International Classification of Diseases code.
   d. These databases allow one to correlate comorbid conditions with the severity of the deglutition disturbance.

3. Regarding the epidemiology of deglutition disorders, it is known that
   a. over half a million U.S. veterans are discharged from hospital with a diagnosis of dysphagia each year.
   b. the majority of elderly subjects within the community have deglutition disorders.
   c. among hospitalized patients dysphagia is diagnosed more frequently in the elderly.
   d. in Maryland the fraction of hospitalized patients having dysphagia has declined over the past decade because of improved treatment of comorbid illnesses.

4. Patients with deglutition disorders
   a. may require feeding tube placement to maintain their nutrition.
   b. can be reliably identified by their reported complaints.
   c. requiring enteral tube feedings as a result of a neurological disorder can usually be weaned to oral feedings within a year.
   d. can have similar symptoms from different underlying diseases.

REFERENCES

Barer, D. H. (1989). The natural history and functional consequences of dysphagia after hemispheric stroke. *Journal of Neurology, Neurosurgery and Psychiatry, 52,* 236–241.

Bergner, M., Bobbit, R., Carter, W., & Gilson, B. (1981). The sickness impact profile: Development and final revision of a health status measure. *Medical Care, 19,* 787–805.

Bloem, B. R., Lagaay, A. M., van Beek, W., Haan, J., Roos, R. A. C., & Wintzen, A. R. (1990). Prevalence of subjective dysphagia in community residents aged over 87. *British Medical Journal, 300,* 721–722.

Brasseur, J. G., & Dodds, W. J. (1991). Interpretation of intraluminal manometric measurements in terms of swallowing mechanics. *Dysphagia, 6,* 100–119.

Brown, D. M., & Everhart, J. E. (1994). Cost of digestive diseases in the United States. In J. E. Everhart (Ed.), *Digestive diseases in the United States: Epidemiology and impact* (pp. 57–82). Washington DC: U.S. Government Printing Office.

Chen, M. Y., Ott, D. J., Peele, V. N., & Gelfand, D. W. (1990). Oropharynx in patients with cerebrovascular disease: Evaluation with videofluoroscopy. *Radiology, 176,* 641–643.

Drossman, D. A., Leserman, J., Mitchell, C. M., Li, Z., Zagami, E. A., & Patrick, D. L. (1991). Health status and health care use in persons with inflammatory bowel disease: A national sample. *Digestive Diseases and Sciences, 36,* 1746–1755.

Ekberg, O., & Feinberg, M. J. (1991). Altered swallowing function in elderly patients without dysphagia: Radiologic findings in 56 cases. *American Journal of Roentgenology, 156,* 1181–1184.

Fulp, S. R., Dalton, C. B., Castell, J. A., & Castell, D. O. (1990). Aging–related alterations in human upper esophageal sphincter function. *American Journal of Gastroenterology, 85,* 1569–1572.

Gordon, C., Hewer, R. L., & Wade, D. T. (1987). Dysphagia in acute stroke. *British Medical Journal, 295,* 411–414.

Gresham, S. L. (1990). Clinical assessment and management of swallowing difficulties after stroke. *Medical Journal of Australia, 153,* 397–399.

Gustafsson, B., & Tibbling, L. (1991). Dysphagia, an unrecognized handicap. *Dysphagia, 6,* 193–199.

Gustafsson, B., Tibbling, L., & Theorell, T. (1992). Do physicians care about patients with dysphagia? A study on confirming communication. *Family Practice, 9,* 203–209.

Helm, J. F., Dodds, W. J., Hogan, W. J., Soergel, K. H., Egide, M. S., & Wood, C. M. (1982). Acid neutralizing capacity of human saliva. *Gastroenterology, 83,* 69–74.

Howard, L., Ament, M., Fleming, C.R., Shike, M., & Steiger, E. (1995). Current use and clinical outcome of home parenteral and enteral nutrition therapies in the United States. *Gastroenterology, 109,* 355–365.

Jones, B., Ravich, W. J., & Donner, M. W. (1993). Dysphagia in systemic disease. *Dysphagia, 8,* 368–383.

Kapila, Y. V., Dodds, W. J., Helm, J. F., & Hogan, W. J. (1984). Relationship between swallow rate and salivary flow. *Digestive Diseases and Sciences, 29,* 528–533.

Kjellen, G., & Tibbling, L. (1981). Manometric oesophageal function, acid perfusion test and symp-

tomatology in a 55-year-old general population. *Clinical Physiology, 1,* 405–415.

Kuhlemeier, K. V. (1994). Epidemiology and dysphagia. *Dysphagia, 9,* 209–217.

Kuhlemeier, K. V., Rieve, J. E., Kirby, N. A., & Siebens, A. A. (1989). Clinical correlates of dysphagia in stroke patients. *Archives of Physical Medicine and Rehabilitation, 70,* A56.

Lang, I. M., Dantas, R. O., Cook, I. J., & Dodds, W. J. (1991). Videoradiographic, manometric, and electromyographic analysis of canine upper esophageal sphincter. *American Journal of Physiology, 260,* G911–G919.

Lindgren, S., & Janzon, L. (1991). Prevalence of swallowing complaints and clinical findings among 50–79–year–old men and women in an urban population. *Dysphagia, 6,* 187–192.

Locke, G. R., Talley, N. J., Weaver, A. L., & Zinsmeister, A. R. (1994). A new questionnaire for gastroesophageal reflux disease. *Mayo Clinic Proceedings, 69,* 539–547.

Massey, B. T. (1993). The use of intraluminal manometry to assess upper esophageal sphincter function. *Dysphagia, 8,* 339–344.

Perlman, A. L., Guthmiller Schultz, G., & VanDaele, D. J. (1993). Effects of age, gender, bolus volume, and bolus viscosity on oropharyngeal pressure during swallowing. *Journal of Applied Physiology, 75,* 33–37.

Quill, T. E. (1989). Utilization of nasogastric feeding tubes in a group of chronically ill, elderly patients in a community hospital. *Archives of Internal Medicine, 149,* 1937–1941.

Ravich, W. J., Wilson, R. S., Jones, B., & Donner, M. W. (1989). Psychogenic dysphagia and globus: Reevaluation of 23 patients. *Dysphagia, 4,* 35–38.

Ren, J., Shaker, R., Zamir, Z., Dodds, W. J., Hogan, W. J., & Hoffmann, R. G. (1993). Effect of age and bolus variables on the coordination of the glottis and upper esophageal sphincter during swallowing. *American Journal of Gastroenterology, 88,* 665–669.

Robbins, J., Hamilton, J. W., Lof, G. L., & Kempster, G. B. (1992). Oropharyngeal swallowing in normal adults of different ages. *Gastroenterology, 103,* 823–829.

Sears, V. W., Castell, J. A., & Castell, D. O. (1990). Comparison of effects of upright versus supine body position and liquid versus solid bolus on esophageal pressures in normal humans. *Digestive Diseases and Sciences, 35,* 857–864.

Shaker, R., Ren, J., Podvrsan, B., Dodds, W. J., Hogan, W. J., Kern, M., Hoffmann, R., & Hintz, J. (1993). Effect of aging and bolus variables on pharyngeal and upper esophageal sphincter motor function. *American Journal of Physiology, 264,* G427–G432.

Sonnenberg, A., Massey, B. T., & Jacobsen, S. J. (1994). Hospital discharges resulting from esophagitis among Medicare beneficiaries. *Digestive Diseases and Sciences, 39,* 183–188.

Sonnenberg, A., Massey, B. T., McCarty, D. J., & Jacobsen, S. J. (1993). Epidemiology of hospitalization for achalasia in the United States. *Digestive Diseases and Sciences, 38,* 233–244.

Tibbling, L., & Gustafsson, B. (1991). Dysphagia and its consequences in the elderly. *Dysphagia, 6,* 200–202.

Tracy, J. F., Logemann, J. A., Kahrilas, P. J., Jacob, P., Kobara, M., & Krugler, C. (1989). Preliminary observations on the effects of age on oropharyngeal deglutition. *Dysphagia, 4,* 90–94.

Wilhelm, K., Freiling, T., Enck, P., & Lübke, H.-J. (1993). Body position and bolus consistency influence manometric recordings from the esophagus in healthy volunteers. *Zeitschrieft Gastroenterologie, 31,* 475–479.

Wilson, J. A., Pryde, A., Macintyre, C. C. A., Maran, A. G. D., & Heading, R. C. (1990). The effects of age, sex, and smoking on normal pharyngoesophageal motility. *American Journal of Gastroenterology, 85,* 686–691.

Young, E. C., & Durant–Jones, L. (1990). Developing a dysphagia program in an acute care hospital: A needs assessment. *Dysphagia, 5,* 159–165.

2

Topography and Functional Anatomy of the Swallowing Structures

Adrienne L. Perlman and James Christensen

Accurate diagnosis and appropriate treatment of disordered swallowing first requires understanding of the neuromuscular controls of the normal swallow. The primary objective of this chapter is to present information on the anatomy and mechanics of swallowing. The first portion of this chapter is devoted to discussion of the peripheral controls associated with the oral, laryngeal, and pharyngeal structures active during a swallow; cranial nerves, branches of nerves, and muscles that are not associated with deglutition are not discussed. The second portion of this chapter is devoted to the anatomical and neurological systems that are involved in the esophageal stage of the swallow. On completion of this chapter, the reader should recognize the importance that a careful cranial nerve examination can have in the assessment of the dysphagic patient and for treatment planning.

Traditionally, swallowing has been described as a three-stage event: oral, pharyngeal, and esophageal (Magendie, 1836); however, it has also been described as consisting of four stages: oral preparatory, oral transport, pharyngeal, and esophageal (Logemann, 1983). Acknowledging that dur-

ing the oral stage, the actions associated with bolus preparation and bolus transport are quite different, it has been suggested that the classical description of three stages of swallowing be retained but the oral stage be described as having two separate phases: the oral preparatory phase and the oral transport phase (Perlman, 1994).

Although the oral stage of swallowing has also been referred to as the *buccal* stage, the role of the lips and tongue in both oral preparation and bolus propulsion support the term *oral* as conceptually more accurate. Additionally, it can be argued that because both the pharynx and the larynx are active during the second stage, *pharyngolaryngeal* more accurately describes the event. However, the path that the bolus is intended to travel is only through the pharynx; consequently, it seems appropriate to retain the traditional term of pharyngeal stage.

PERIPHERAL CONTROLS OF SWALLOWING

The following section describes the peripheral controls associated with the first two

15

stages of deglutition. Application of this information will follow in those chapters addressing the interpretation of diagnostic techniques and the decision-making processes associated with intervention.

Four pairs of cranial nerves (CN V, VII, IX, and X) convey afferent information on taste and general sensation associated with deglutition, and five pairs of cranial nerves (CN V, VII, IX, X, and XII) are responsible for the efferent control of the first two stages of deglutition. This chapter contains graphs of the functional components of the oral and pharyngeal stages of deglutition, which some readers may find more meaningful if they also have an illustrated neuroanatomy text open while reading this chapter.

Oral Stage of Deglutition

The oral preparatory phase involves manipulation of the food bolus and can employ the lips, jaw, tongue, soft palate, muscles of mastication, and buccal muscles. When the food bolus requires mastication, the oral preparatory phase can be further subdivided into an initial transport phase during which the tongue moves the food posteriorly until it is placed between the molars, and a reduction phase during which the bolus is chewed until it is ground into small pieces and mixed with sufficient saliva to be swallowed (Hiiemae & Crompton, 1985; Hiiemae, Thexton, & Crompton, 1978; Schwartz, Enomoto, Valiquette, & Lund, 1989; Thexton, Hiiemae, & Crompton, 1980). Following bolus reduction, the material is again placed on the tongue and then transported to the oropharynx for passage through the pharynx and into the esophagus. The components to the oral stage of deglutition are represented in Figure 2–1.

In humans as well as other species, the reduction phase can be still further subdivided into a fast opening, fast closing, and slow closing phase of mandibular movement. The fast opening stage occurs when the mandible descends; the fast closing stage occurs as the mandible ascends; and the slow closing phase begins when the teeth make contact with the food in preparation for the grinding process (Ahlgren, 1967; Appenteng, Lund, & Seguin, 1982; Hylander & Crompton, 1986; Luschei & Goodwin, 1974).

During the oral preparatory phase, the soft palate is generally in contact with the pharyngeal aspect of the posterior tongue. One can hypothesize that this posiitoning of the velum permits an individual to continue with respiration and assists in keeping the bolus in the mouth during the oral preparatory phase of the swallow. Intersubject and intrasubject variability can occur during the oral preparatory stage depending on such factors as the taste, temperature, viscosity, and size of the bolus, as well as individual anatomy, level of oral sensitivity, and rate of salivary secretion and viscosity of saliva (Cleall, 1965; Dantas et al., 1990; Inoue et al., 1989; Kapila, Dodds, Helm, & Hogan, 1984; Luschei & Goodwin, 1974; Plesh, Bishop, & McCall, 1986; Proffit, Kydd, Wilskie, & Taylor, 1964; Sonies, Ship, & Baum, 1989; Takada, Miyawaki, & Tatsuta, 1994; Thexton et al., 1980).

Once the bolus has been adequately prepared and positioned on the tongue, the oral transport phase begins. During this phase, the velum elevates, the lips and buccal muscles contract, the posterior aspect of the tongue depresses, and the remainder of the tongue presses against the hard palate as it propels the bolus toward the oropharynx (Lowe, 1980). It has been shown that the perimeter of the tongue remains in contact with the alveolar ridge while the posterior portion of the tongue blade first performs a centripetal motion and then a centrifugal motion. The centrifugal action defines the period during which the tongue is propelling the bolus toward the pharynx. (Kahrilas et al., 1993).

The muscle primarily responsible for active depression of the mandible during mastication is the lateral pterygoid, with assistance from the geniohyoid and, possibly to some extent, the anterior belly of the digastric. Elevation of the mandible is the result of contraction of the temporalis, masseter, and medial pterygoid muscles. Except for the geniohyoid muscle, which is innervated by the cervical plexus, all

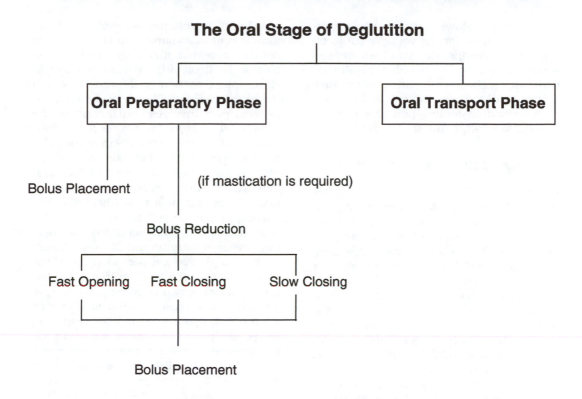

Figure 2–1. A schematic representation of the oral stage of deglutition.

other muscles of mandibular movement are innervated by CN V.

Two facial muscles, the buccinator and orbicularis oris, contribute to the oral stage of swallowing. The buccinator flattens the cheek and holds the bolus in contact with the teeth and the orbicularis oris opens, closes, protrudes, and inverts the lips. Although the lips are, at times, referred to as an oral sphincter, that is anatomically not correct. The orbicularis oris muscle is not a sphincter; it is a muscle that is composed of four quadrants originating from the modiolus (Lightoller, 1925).

Movement of the tongue is very important during the oral stage of the swallow. Movement patterns produced by the tongue are typical of the movements of a muscular hydrostat (Kier & Smith, 1985). The intrinsic muscles of the tongue have no bony attachment and are classified by the orientation the muscle fibers: longitudinal, vertical, and transverse. The extrinsic mus-

cles of the tongue—genioglossus, hyoglossus, and styloglossus muscles—have one stable attachment,and the free end decussates with muscle fibers in the body of the tongue. The genioglossus and styloglossus are antagonists and assist in positioning the tongue in the oral cavity. Additionally, it has been shown that the genioglossus inserts into the hyoid bone and sends fibers that blend with the middle constrictor (Doran & Baggelt, 1972). It is possible that the stylohyoid muscle plays a contributory role during oral preparation by elevating and retracting the base of the tongue; there have been no electromyographic (EMG) studies to confirm this statement.

There has been found to be an age-dependent change in the duration of the oral stage of the swallow. As an example, in an ultrasound examination of swallowing on 22 males and 25 females ranging from 18 to 74 years of age, Sonies et al. found that the oral stage of the swallow was generally slower for the elderly subjects than those for the younger subjects, and for all groups, dry swallows were of longer duration than bolus swallows. Older subjects were inclined to produce extra hyoid gestures, which are frequently described as tongue pumping (Sonies, Parent, Morrish, & Baum, 1988).

Pharyngeal Stage of Deglutition

During the oral transport phase, the bolus is propelled posteriorly and intraoral pressure is increased. The oral transport phase and pharyngeal stage of the swallow can be described as a single pressure-driven event during which the mouth and pharynx form a continuous tube with four valves: the lips, velopharyngeal port, larynx, and cricopharyngeal sphincter. Closure of the lips, tension in the buccal muscles, closure of the velopharyngeal port, and closure of the true and false vocal folds along with the pistonlike motion of the tongue and contraction of the pharyngeal muscles result in an increase in pressure within the tube. Meanwhile, the opening of the upper esophageal sphincter results in a pressure differential which likely assists in directing the bolus from the pharynx into the esophagus. Once the bolus enters the oropharynx, a sequence of rapid, coordinated motions occurs that assists in propelling the bolus into the upper esophagus. Animal studies have shown that if any aspect of the swallow is ablated, either by nerve sectioning, muscle excision, or desensitization, the sequence of muscle contraction for the remaining structures remains unaltered (Doty & Bosma, 1956; Miller, 1972).

Temporal measurements made from videofluoroscopic images of human swallows revealed that the time from the entrance of the bolus into the oropharynx to passage of the bolus into the esophagus was approximately 800 ms (McConnel, Cerenko, Jackson, & Guffin, 1988). This was in agreement with the average of 800 ms contraction time of the superior pharyngeal constrictor muscle during the normal swallow in adults (Perlman, Luschei, & Du Mond, 1989).

Although simultaneous measures of oral muscle contraction and velar elevation have not been reported, it is likely that the muscles of the floor of the mouth contract in close approximation to the time at which the velum elevates. Closure of the velopharyngeal port involves contraction of the levator veli palatini for elevation and contraction of the horizontal fibers of the palatopharyngeus for medial movement of the pharyngeal walls; contraction of the musculi uvulae, which can help to prevent eversion of the soft palate, is likely also occurring at that time. Closure of the velopharyngeal port prohibits entry of the bolus into the nasopharynx; additionally, closure of the velopharyngeal port along with the tight closure of the lips, contraction of the buccal muscles, and pressing of the tongue against the anterior portion of the hard palate and against the molars results in the production of increased oral and pharyngal pressures. Mean peak pressure just below the soft palate in the oropharynx was found to be independent of volume, viscosity, or gender and to average 10.9 (±3.9) kPa (Perlman, Schultz, & Van-Daele, 1993). When the sensor was placed at the level of the base of the tongue, the mean maximum pressure was reported at 16.3 kPa (Cerenko, McConnel, & Jackson, 1989). These two pressure studies were performed with the pressure sensors placed 180 degrees out of phase from one another; directional differences along with the differences in placement likely accounted for the differences in pressure magnitude.

The temporal relationship for pressure changes along the length of the pharynx has been reported from combined manometry and videofluoroscopy (Cerenko, et al., 1989; Kahrilas, Logemann, Lin, & Ergun, 1992; McConnel, Cerenko, & Mendelsohn, 1988; Robbins, Hamilton, Lof, & Kempster, 1992; Sokol, Heitmann, Wolf, & Cohen, 1966). Using videofluoroscopy and a solid state manometer with transducers at four sites in the pharynx, McConnel et al., (1988) measured pharyngeal pressures while observing the location of the bolus. He interpreted his results to suggest that the passage of a bolus through the pharynx was more dependent on tongue driving pressure and negative pressure developed in the pharyngeal esophageal segment than on the function of the pharyngeal constrictor muscles. Rather, he interpreted the pharyngeal constrictor pressure to function as a clearing force rather than as a driving force. When sectional measurements of pharyngeal shortening were made it was found that there is variation in the amount of shortening that occurs in different portions of the pharynx, with the greatest amount of shortening reported in the portion of the pharynx between the valleculae and the superior margin of the arytenoid. Halfway through the swallow, the average elevation of the arytenoid and upper esophageal sphincter was found to be 22 mm (Kahrilas et al., 1992); this is a considerable amount of shortening for a small area of the pharynx. Additionally, it has been observed that maximal pharyngeal shortening with a 10 ml swallow is maintained for 200 ms longer than it was held for a 5 ml swallow (Kahrilas et al., 1992).

As the bolus enters the oropharynx, the false vocal folds and true vocal folds contract. That closure helps to protect the airway from penetration. Additionally, the epiglottis covers the laryngeal aditus, providing further protection for the airway, reducing the irregularities of the pharyngeal conduit, and diverting the bolus into the pyriform sinuses. It is questionable whether the aryepiglottic folds contain muscle fibers that can contribute to laryngeal closure (VanDaele, Perlman, & Cassell, 1995). Swallows most often occur during the expiratory phase of respiration and include a period of apnea lasting from as short as 0.3 s to a maximum 2.5 s followed by additional expiration (Clark, 1920; Miller & Sherrington, 1915; Selley, Ellis, Flack, Bayliss, and Pearce, 1994; Selley, Flack, Ellis, & Brooks, 1989; Smith, Wolkove, Colacone, & Kreisman, 1989).

Using intramuscular needle electrodes, Hrycyshyn and Basmajian (1972) studied submental EMG activity in the mylohyoid, genioglossus, anterior belly of the digastric, and geniohyoid in normal swallowing adults. They found that individuals had different firing orders for these muscles and that the firing order even varied from swallow to swallow for the same individual; approximately 43% of their subjects had no activity from the anterior belly of the digastric. Nevertheless, the floor of mouth complex contracts as the oral transport phase begins; it is only the order of contraction of the muscles of the floor of mouth that varies. The duration of the contraction of the muscles of the floor of the mouth during swallow is approximately 1 s (Hrycyshyn & Basmajian, 1972). As the muscles of the floor of the mouth contract, the hyoid bone is pulled into an anterior-superior position. The motion of the hyoid along with the contraction of the thyrohyoid muscle elevates the larynx and causes the epiglottis to invert (VanDaele et al., 1995). From measures obtained with a modified electroglottograph and solid state manometer, it has been reported that the larynx begins to move approximately 330 ms before the onset of the oropharyngeal pressure wave (Schultz, Perlman, & VanDaele, 1994).

A direct relationship has been found between the anterior-superior movement of the hyoid bone and the amount of opening of the cricopharyngeus muscle during the swallow (Jacob, Kahrilas, Logemann, Shah, & Ha, 1989). Thus it appears that the opening of the cricopharyngeus muscle is related to both relaxation of the muscle and a passive mechanical operation.

A breakdown in the efficiency of the swallow can result from biomechanical or physiological changes in the anatomical structures involved in performing a swallow. Thus, conditions affecting the structure or function of any of the oral, pharyngeal, laryngeal, or esophageal musculature can influence the integrity of the swallow and result in dysphagia.

There is every reason to suspect that all muscles of the pharynx participate in deglutition. Likewise, except for the cricothyroid muscle, which has not been found to contribute to swallowing function, it is likely that all other laryngeal muscles are active during deglutition. Whereas the role of the suprahyoid muscles in swallowing can be assumed, the importance, if any, of the infrahyoids has not been addressed. The mylohyoid, geniohyoid, thyrohyoid, and at times, the anterior belly of the digastric are primarily responsible for the elevation of the hyoid bone and larynx, which contribute significantly to safe bolus passage.

Some data on physiological aspects of the anatomical structures involved in swallowing have been acquired. Doty and Bosma (1956) performed a study in which they recorded electromyographic activity from 11 pairs of muscles in anesthetized monkeys, cats, and dogs. The temporal relationships were highly constant regardless of the method of stimulation (superior laryngeal nerve stimulation, stimulation of the pharynx with a cotton swab or with a rapid injection of a stream of water). Method of stimulation did not alter the duration, amplitude, or temporal pattern of the swallow. When the duration of the pharyngeal contraction was compared across age groups, the average speed of contraction was not found to differ with age; however, there was considerable variability among the elderly dysphagic subjects that was not evident among young dysphagic patients or young normal subjects (Borgstrom & Ekberg, 1988). This is an area that needs further investigation.

It has been shown that the superior pharyngeal constrictor is a muscle of reflexive function; for example, the superior pharyngeal constrictor was found to be 60% as active during gagging as during swallowing, but only 6% as active during prolongation of the vowel /a/ and 23% as active during production of a heavily stressed /k/ in the final position of a word (Perlman et al., 1989). It is reasonable to assume that the middle and inferior pharyngeal constrictors are also more active during deglutition than during tasks related to phonation or respiration.

INNERVATION OF MUSCLES ASSOCIATED WITH THE ORAL AND PHARYNGEAL STAGES OF DEGLUTITION

Cranial Nerve V

Two divisions of the trigeminal nerve, the mandibular branch and the maxillary branch, contain fibers that transmit oral sensation (Figure 2–2). The mandibular division conveys impuses from the mucous membranes of the anterior two thirds of tongue (lingual n), cheek (buccal n), floor of mouth (lingual n), lower teeth and gums (lingual/internal alveolar), the skin of the lower lip and jaw (mental n), and the temporomandibular joint (auriculotemporal n). The maxillary division conveys information from the mucous membranes of the nasopharynx (pharyngeal br), the hard and soft palates (greater/lesser palatine nn, nasopalatine n) the upper teeth (superior alveolar n), and the tonsils (lesser palatine n).

Except for proprioceptive fibers from the neuromuscular spindles, the cell bodies of the afferent fibers of the fifth nerve are contained in the trigeminal ganglion. The sensory nucleus of CN V is often referred to as a series of three contiguous nuclei that extend from the upper midbrain to the upper cervical segments of the spinal cord (Pansky, Allen, & Budd, 1988). Afferent fibers enter the pons and divide into an ascending and descending limb. The ascending limb conveys impulses for touch and pressure and terminates in the principal sensory nucleus. Pain and temperature fibers comprise the descending limb and these fibers give off branches to the nucleus of the spinal trigeminal tract. Fibers from the principal sensory and spinal trigeminal nuclei ascend and eventually terminate in the ventral posteriormedial (VPM) nucleus of the thalamus.

Impulses from the stretch receptors in the muscles of mastication are conveyed to the mesencephalic nucleus of cranial nerve V. Proprioceptive fibers conveying pressure and kinesthetic information from the teeth, periodontium, hard palate, and joint capsules also terminate in this nucleus. Because much of the input to this nucleus comes from stretch receptors, and because impulses from stretch receptors in other parts of the body are relayed to the cerebellum, it has been hypothesized that fibers from the mesencephalic nucleus project to the cerebellum (Carpenter, 1978).

The motor nucleus of CN V is located in the tegmentum of the pons; it receives fi-

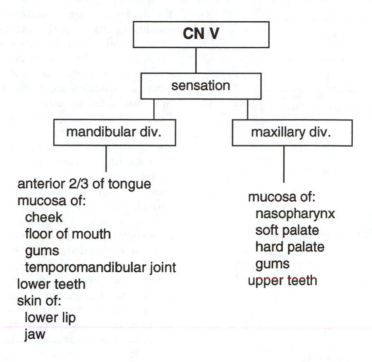

Figure 2–2. Afferent controls for deglutition from CN V.

bers from the trigeminal sensory nuclei and from the contralateral cerebral cortex. Of the muscles related to swallowing, the efferent root innervates the mylohyoid muscle, anterior belly of the digastric, and the four muscles of mastication: the temporalis, masseter, and medial and lateral pterygoid muscles (Figure 2–3).

The mylohyoid muscle elevates the hyoid bone and tongue and is active in chewing, swallowing, and sucking. If the jaw is fixed, the anterior belly of the digastric muscle elevates the hyoid bone; if the hyoid bone is fixed, the anterior belly of the digastric depresses the jaw. The temporalis muscle, masseter muscle, and medial pterygoid muscles each elevate the mandible. The lateral pterygoid muscle depresses and protrudes the mandible. Alternate contraction of the contralateral pterygoid muscle results in side-to-side movement of the mandible.

Cranial Nerve VII

Fibers for the facial nerve travel via the chorda tympani nerve and convey taste sensation from the anterior two thirds of the tongue (Figure 2–4). Cell bodies of the sensory neurons are in the geniculate ganglion. Some taste fibers may travel via the greater petrosal nerves. Afferent fibers enter the solitary fasciculus and terminate on cells in the rostral and lateral portion of the nucleus tractus solitarius (NTS). In the NTS, these fibers are joined by afferent fibers from the posterior third of the tongue (CN IX) and from the epiglottis (CN X). Most of the signals from the taste fibers ascend unilaterally to the VPM nucleus of the thalamus and pass through the internal capsule to terminate in the insula; other taste fibers travel to the hypothalamus and probaby influence autonomic function.

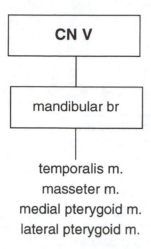

Figure 2–3. Muscles of mastication.

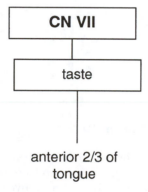

Figure 2–4. Afferent controls for deglutition from CN VII.

The facial motor nucleus is located in the ventrolateral part of the pontine tegmentum. After a rather convoluted course, the fibers emerge at the lateral border of the pons. Motor fibers innervate the muscles of facial expression and visceral efferent fibers supply parasympathetic preganglionic impulses to the pterygopalatine and submandibular ganglia. Fibers from these ganglia innervate the submandibu-

lar and sublingual salivary glands, the lacrimal glands, and mucous membranes of the nasal and oral cavities. A reduction of salivary secretions can have a dramatic effect on the efficiency of a swallow. The most extreme examples occur after radiation therapy, but difficulty due to disease, medication, and to advanced age can also occur.

After leaving the stylomastoid foramen, the motor root divides into four branches that supply, among others, the muscles of facial expression of the upper and lower face, the platysma muscle, the stylohyoid muscle, and the posterior belly of the digastric muscle. The muscles of facial expression have varying levels of participation in swallowing; only those known to participate in deglutition are listed (Figure 2–5); however, it is possible that others contribue to deglutition, allbeit subtly.

The buccal branch of the facial nerve divides into a superior and an inferior branch. The superior branch innervates muscles that are associated with facial expression; of those, the contraction of the orbicularis oris plays an important role in holding food in the mouth and the levator anguli oris muscle in elevating the angle of the mouth and compressing the lips; this compression may contribute somewhat to a good oral seal. Among other muscles, the inferior branch innervates the orbicularis oris and the buccinator. The orbicularis oris of the lower lip performs the same as the portion of the muscle innervated by the superior counterpart; that is, it opens, closes, protrudes, inverts, and twists the lips. The buccinator muscle flattens the cheeks and holds food in contact with the teeth.

Two suprahyoid muscles are innervated by the facial nerve. The digastric branch innervates the posterior belly of the digastric and the stylohyoid muscles. The posterior belly of the digastric and the stylohyoid elevate are recognized for their ability to retract the hyoid bone, a motion that is not desirable during swallowing; thus, it is likely that these muscles are inactive during the swallow. However, it is possible that the stylohyoid muscle plays a contributory role during oral preparation by elevating and retracting the base

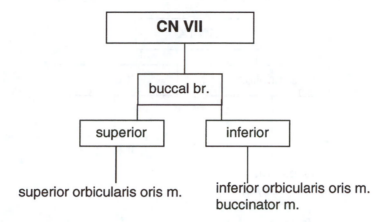

Figure 2–5. Muscles of the lower face that contribute to deglutition.

of the tongue; there have been no studies to confirm this statement.

Cranial Nerve IX

The glossopharyngeal nerve transmits visceral sensation from the pharynx as well as taste sensation from the posterior third of the tongue and touch, pain, and thermal sensation from the mucous membrane of the oropharynx, palatine tonsils, the faucial pillars, and the posterior third of the tongue (Figure 2–6). The cell bodies of these afferent fibers are in the petrosal ganglion. The afferent fibers all enter the NTS, and numerous projections are sent to the reticular formation. Little is known about secondary projections to the thalamus and cortex, but these pathways do apparently exist.

This nerve innervates only one muscle, the stylopharyngeus. On contraction, the stylopharyngeus muscle elevates and dilates the pharynx. This muscle may be very important for a safe swallow, but it has not been studied as yet. The neurons that supply the efferent fibers to the stylopharyngeus muscle are located in the rostral portion of the nucleus ambiguus. Also, CN IX supplies secretomotor impulses to the parotid gland; the visceral efferent fibers that innervate the parotid gland arise from the inferior salivatory nucleus. All other portions of the nerve are sensory.

Cranial Nerve X

This cranial nerve is heavily associated with deglutition. Of the two medullary sensory nuclei of the vagus, the nucleus associated with deglutition is the NTS. The inferior ganglion of the vagus is the site of origin of fibers for both general sensation and taste (Figure 2–7). General sensation from the mucosa of the pharynx is conveyed via the the pharyngeal plexus, which includes fibers from the internal laryngeal nerve and likely from the recurrent laryngeal nerve, as well as from the glossopharyngeal nerve.

The internal branch of the superior laryngeal nerve conveys general sensation from the mucosa of the laryngopharynx, the epiglottis, laryngeal mucosa above the vocal folds, joint receptors in the larynx, and a small area on the posterior portion of the tongue. The recurrent laryngeal nerve conveys general sensation from the mucosa below the vocal folds and the mucosa of the esophagus; it also conveys secretomotor fibers to the mucous glands in the lar-

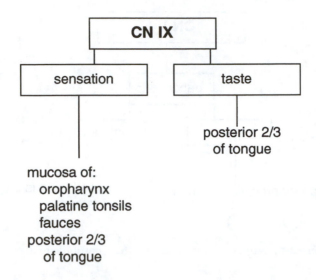

Figure 2–6. Afferent controls for deglutition from CN IX.

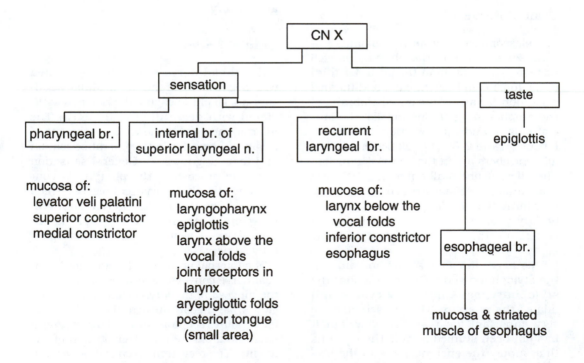

Figure 2–7. Afferent controls for deglutition from CN X.

ynx and laryngopharynx. The esophageal branch of the vagus conveys general sensation from the mucosa and striated muscle of the esophagus. Fibers transmitting taste sensation originate in the epiglottis. Taste fibers of CN X travel with those from CN IX.

Of the two medullary nuclei of the vagus nerve, the nucleus ambiguus, also known as the ventral motor nucleus, is the site of origin of axons that convey motor impulses via special visceral efferent fibers to all muscles of the soft palate (except the tensor veli palatini muscle) (Figure 2–8), the pharynx, and the larynx. The nucleus ambiguus is a column of cells that is located in the reticular formation. Caudal portions of this column form the cranial portion of the spinal accessory nerve (CN XI), and rostral portions give rise to the efferent fibers of CN IX.

Three efferent branches of the vagus are important to the motor aspects of swallowing. These are the pharyngeal, recurrent laryngeal, and external branch of the superior laryngeal nerve. The pharyngeal branch, which helps to form the pharyngeal plexus, is composed of afferent fibers from CN IX and efferent fibers from CN X.

The recurrent laryngeal branch contains fibers from the cranial portion of CN XI.

Fibers from the pharyngeal plexus innervate several oral-pharyngeal muscles (Figure 2–9). The palatoglossus muscle forms the anterior faucial pillar. On contraction the palatoglossus can either lower the soft palate or raise the posterior portion of the tongue. The palatoglossus is primarily antagonistic to the levator muscles; the muscle has a high elastic fiber content, which would assist in recoil of the elevated soft palate. The palatopharyngeus muscle forms the posterior faucial pillar; on contraction this muscle narrows the oropharynx and elevates the pharynx. The salpingopharyngeus muscle probably just fills in the gap at the lateral edge of the velum during velar approximation to the pharynx but may contribute somewhat to elevation of the nasopharynx. The levator veli palatini muscle elevates the soft palate, and the uvular muscle shortens and elevates the uvula. The superior and middle pharyngeal constrictor muscles perform a circular contraction of the pharynx and assist in bolus transport.

The recurrent laryngeal nerve innervates all intrinsic laryngeal muscles except for the

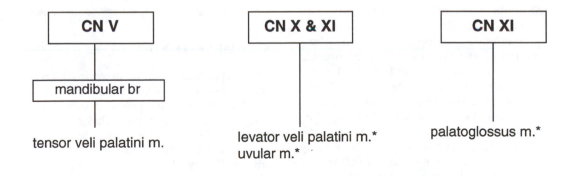

Figure 2–8. Muscles of the soft palate that contribute to deglutition.

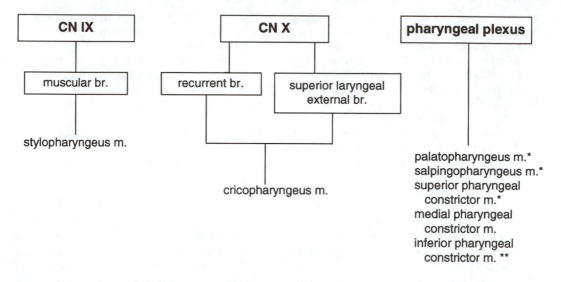

Figure 2–9. Muscles of the pharynx that contribute to deglutition.

cricothyroid, which has not been found to be involved in swallowing (Figure 2–10). Contraction of the thyroarytenoid muscles results in a shortening and thickening of the vocal folds as well as an adduction of the folds. Contraction of the transverse arytenoid muscles adduct the posterior, cartilaginous portion of the folds. Contraction of the oblique arytenoid muscle adducts the aryepiglottic folds and cartilaginous portion of the vocal folds. There is some disagreement as to the contribution of any muscle fibers in the aryepiglottic folds; this is due to the observation that many individuals do not have any muscle fiber in those folds (VanDaele et al., 1995). If there were any such contribution, the aryepiglottic muscle contraction would help to approximate the arytenoid cartilages to the epiglottic tubercle. Contraction of the lateral cricoarytenoid muscle adducts and lowers the vocal folds; to date, there have been no studies on the role, if any, of this muscle during swallowing. Only the posterior cricoarytenoid muscle abducts the vocal folds; this mus-

cle becomes activated at the completion of the swallow. The external branch of the superior laryngeal nerve of the vagus shares with the recurrent nerve in the innervation of the inferior pharyngeal constrictor muscle and the cricopharyngeus muscle.

Cranial Nerve XII

The hypoglossal nerve provides efferent stimulation to all of the intrinsic and most of the extrinsic muscles of the tongue (Figure 2–11). Fibers from this nerve originate in the hypoglossal nucleus in the medulla. Voluntary tongue movement is innervated by fibers derived from the corticobulbar tract. Fibers from the primary sensory nucleus of CN V and from the NTS enter the hypoglossal nucleus to activate reflexive actions such as sucking, chewing, and swallowing (Pansky et al., 1988). The four pairs of intrinsic muscles are innervated by this nerve. The superior longitudinal muscle shortens the tongue and turns the tip and lateral margins upward. The inferior longitudinal shortens the

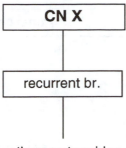

thyroarytenoid m.
transverse arytenoid m.
oblique arytenoid m.
lateral cricoarytenoid m.
posterior cricoarytenoid m.
thyroepiglottic m.

Figure 2–10. Muscles of the larynx that contribute to deglutition.

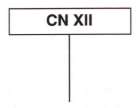

superior longitudinal m.
inferior longitudinal m.
transverse m.
verticalis m.
hyoglossus m.
genioglossus m.
styloglossus. m.

Figure 2–11. Muscles of the tongue that contribute to deglutition.

tongue and pulls the tip downward. The transverse muscle narrows and elongates the tongue, and the verticalis flattens and widens the tongue.

Of the extrinsic tongue muscles innervated by CN XII, the hyoglossus retracts and depresses the tongue when the hyoid is fixed; if the tongue is fixed as occurs during the swallow, the muscle elevates the hyoid. The posterior fibers of the genioglossus muscle bring the tongue tip forward, and the anterior fibers help to retrude the tongue; its fibers also help to make the tongue concave, which assists in forming a channel for transport of a bolus.

The styloglossus muscle draws the tongue upward and backward. The geniohyoid and thyrohyoid muscles are also innervated by CN XII. The geniohyoid muscle participates in the swallow by drawing the hyoid bone up and forward, and the thyrohyoid muscle participates by elevating the thyroid cartilage to the hyoid bone.

Cervical Plexus

The cervical plexus is formed from the anterior division of spinal nerves C1 to C4. Three infrahyoid muscles—the sternohyoid, omohyoid, and sternothyroid—serve to depress the hyoid bone (Figure 2–12). The omohyoid muscle also provides a dorsal and a lateral pull on the hyoid. Little is known about the action of these muscles at the end of a swallow.

Along with the downward traction on the hyoid by those muscles innervated by the ansi cervicalis, there are suprahyoid muscles that play an important role in the elevation of the hyoid bone and the larynx; the suprahyoid muscles receive innervation from cranial nerves V, VII, and XII. Whereas the thyrohyoid is the most important muscle for laryngeal elevation, the muscles most likely to be of major importance for hyoid elevation are the mylohyoid (CN V) and geniohyoid (CN XII). It is likely, however, that the digastric muscles and the stylohyoid also contribute to varying degrees to this elevation.

THE ESOPHAGUS AND THE ESOPHAGEAL STAGE OF DEGLUTITION

Segments and Topography

The esophagus, a long and flaccid muscular tube marked at both ends by short segments of tonically contracted muscle,

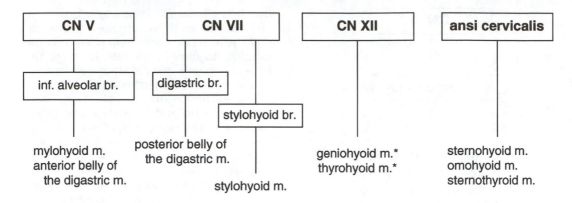

Figure 2–12. Suprahyoid and infrahyoid muscles associated with deglutition.

extends as a caudal continuation of the funnel-shaped pharynx and broadens into the baglike stomach in the abdomen (Fransen & Valembois, 1978). The two short contracted segments, called the upper and lower esophageal sphincters, demarcate the much longer esophageal body and separate it from the pharynx and stomach, respectively. The upper esophageal sphincter (UES) is also called the cricopharyngeal sphincter or cricopharyngeal segment. The lower esophageal sphincter (LES) is also called the gastroesophageal sphincter. A short segment of the esophagus, the cervical esophagus, lies in the neck rostral to the thorax, and another short part, the abdominal esophagus, lies in the abdomen below the diaphragm. The thoracic esophagus forms most of the length of the organ that lies within the thorax. The thoracic esophagus extends through the dorsal mediastinum, passing dorsal to the trachea and the aortic arch, then to the right side of the thoracic aorta, and finally ventral to the aorta. The esophagus then passes through the esophageal hiatus of the diaphragm to end at the cardiac orifice of the stomach.

The upper edge of the muscle that constitutes the upper esophageal sphincter lies about 16 cm from the upper incisors in humans, and the lower edge of the muscle that constitutes the lower esophageal sphincter is found at about 38 to 42 cm. Thus the full length of the esophagus, including both sphincters, is 22 to 26 cm, and the two sphincters are each about 2 cm long. These dimensions, of course, vary with body size.

Cervical Esophagus

The position of the esophagus can be reliably described in reference to the vertebral column. The cervical esophagus begins at the level of the transition between the second and third thoracic vertebral bodies (about the level of the suprasternal notch) and ends at the thoracic inlet. Elastic tissue containing a few fibromuscular bands joins it to the trachea ventrally. Loose connective tissue connects it to the spinal column dorsally. The recurrent laryngeal nerves that branch from the vagus nerves lie on both sides in a groove between the trachea and the esophagus. The carotid arteries lie a little farther away on both sides. The lateral lobes of the thyroid and the parathyroid glands they contain touch the cervical esophagus.

Thoracic Esophagus

As the esophagus enters the thoracic inlet, its general relationship to adjacent structures remains unchanged. As it deviates to the right to pass the aortic arch, that arch indents the esophagus to form a radiographic landmark, the aortic notch (also called the aortic groove or indentation). Just below the aortic notch, the esophagus passes dorsal to the tracheal bifurcation and then dorsal to the pericardium covering the left atrium. To the right, the parietal pleura covers the esophagus except where the azygos vein turns at the level of the fourth thoracic vertebra. To the left, above the aortic arch, the left subclavian artery and parietal pleura cover the esophagus; beyond the aortic arch, the aorta lies along the left side of the esophagus. At the level of the eighth thoracic vertebra, the esophagus curves away from the spinal column, passes ventral to the aorta, and enters the diaphragmatic hiatus.

The vagus nerves (also called the tenth cranial nerves), the esophageal plexus formed by the vagus nerves, and the vagal trunks all lie on the outer surface of the thoracic esophagus. The first five intercostal arteries and the hemiazygos vein pass behind it. The thoracic duct runs dorsal to the esophagus in the caudal part of the thorax, but it lies to the left, above the level of the fifth thoracic vertebra, between the esophagus and the parietal pleura posterolaterally, dorsal to the aortic arch and subclavian artery.

Abdominal Esophagus

A small hollow in the left lobe of the liver holds a part of the abdominal esophagus, touching its anterior and right sides. The musculotendinous loop formed by the right diaphragmatic crus surrounds the abdominal esophagus, and the spleen touches its left side in the abdomen. The length of the abdominal segment varies a little but it never exceeds about 3 cm. The lower esophageal sphincter occupies much of that length.

Diaphragmatic Hiatus and Phrenoesophageal Ligament

The musculotendinous tendinous sheets called the diaphragmatic crura arise from the anterior surfaces of the first four lumbar vertebrae. The right crus, passing

rostrally and ventrally to the right of the root of the celiac axis, splits into two bundles, which converge to form a loop about the esophagus. The left crus, passing to the left of the root of the celiac axis, does not form any part of the hiatus margin. Anatomic variations exist, however, so that the left crus may, in some people, enter to some degree into the ring of diaphragmatic muscle and tendon that surrounds the esophageal hiatus. The right crus is also the point of the attachment of the ligament of Treitz, the band of mesentery and connective tissue that suspends the end of the duodenum and the splenic flexure of the colon.

The esophagus is held within the esophageal hiatus by a fibroelastic ligament that arises from the subdiaphragmatic fascia and forms a seal about the organ. This fascial grommet, the phrenoesophageal membrane or ligament, constitutes two leaves or layers. The more rostral leaf forms a tentlike enclosure extending from the margins of the hiatus to insert in the circumference of the esophagus about 2 cm above the diaphragm. The more caudal layer, shorter and thicker, extends from the edge of the hiatus to merge with the peritoneal covering of the stomach. Fat lies between the two layers of the phrenoesophageal ligament in the enclosed space around the esophagus (Bombeck, Dillard, Nylus, 1966; Eliska, 1973; Mittal & Fischer, 1990). The vagal trunks and accompanying blood vessels pierce the phrenoesophageal ligament as they pass from the esophagus to the stomach.

Layers of the Esophageal Wall

Mucosa

The mucosa of the esophagus constitutes three layers of tissue: the epithelium, the lamina propria, and the muscularis mucosae. The mucosa is thrown into longitudinal folds when the esophagus is relaxed but these folds disappear on distensions of the organ (Desmet & Tytgat, 1974). The epithelium is a stratified squamous epithelium like that of the skin except for the lack of a stratum corneum (Orlando, Lacy & Toby, 1992). The striatum basalis extends between the epithelial basement membrane and the level where the nuclei of the squamous cells lie about one cell-diameter apart. The stratum spinosum extends between that level and the luminal surface to make up the zone in which the cells become flattened or squamous. As in the skin, the esophageal squamous epithelium is invaded by fingers of the underlying lamina propria called rete pegs or papillae. These normally extend less than two thirds of the distance to the surface but they reach farther in inflammation of the epithelium, because of epithelial thinning through surface desquamation (Schulze-Delrieu, Mitros, & Shirazi, 1982). The lamina propria is an areolar coat of connective tissue that lies just below the epithelium. It contains blood vessels and nerves. The muscularis mucosae, lying below the lamina propria, is described in the next section.

Submucosa

The submucosa is a thick layer of areolar connective tissue containing blood vessels, nerves, and mucous glands (Desmet & Tytgat, 1974). The submucosal blood vessels, small arteries and small veins, provide the blood supply to the overlying mucosa. The submucosal nerves constitute the ganglia and interganglionic bundles of the sparse submucosal plexus, described below. The submucosal glands are small racemose glands composed of mucous cells. They lie almost entirely in the submucosa, each gland draining to the luminal surface through a long excretory duct.

Muscularis Propria

The remainder of the esophageal wall, about half of its total thickness, constitutes the main muscle coat or the muscularis propria. This muscular layer also contains the major network of nerves in the esophagus, the myenteric plexus.

Sphincters and Muscular Layers of the Esophagus

The pharyngoesophageal junction and the UES: The upper esophageal (or pharyngoesophageal) sphincter reflects the operation of an anatomically distinct muscle, the cricopharyngeus, generally held to be a differentiated band of the inferior constrictor muscle of the pharynx. The cricopharyngeus muscle originates on both sides from the ends of the C-shaped cricoid cartilage and passes dorsal to the esophagus so that its contraction compresses the esophagus against the trachea. Some of its muscle bundles merge into those of the esophagus caudally, but the rostral margin of the cricopharyngeus is quite distinct. It has no median raphe dorsally to correspond to that of the musculature of the pharynx.

Esophageal Body

The musculature of the esophagus below the cricopharyngeus constitutes three layers: the outer longitudinal layer and the inner circular layer of the main muscle coat (the muscularis propria) and the muscle layer of the mucosa, the muscularis mucosae.

Muscularis Propria of the Esophageal Body

The muscularis propria constitutes striated muscle in the most rostral part of the esophageal body. A transition to smooth muscle occurs at 4 to 8 cm caudal to the cricopharyngeus. Smooth muscle alone or smooth muscle with occasional scattered fibers of striated muscle makes up the muscularis propria in the caudal two thirds of the organ. The transition from striated to smooth muscle usually lies a little more rostral in the inner circular layer of the muscularis propria than in the outer longitudinal layer.

The outer longitudinal muscle layer originates rostrally from the cricoid cartilage. One bundle emanates from each side of the cricoid cartilage and the two bundles then fan dorsally to fuse at the dorsal midline about 3 cm below the cricopharyngeus (Lerche, 1950). The V-shaped dorsal hiatus in the outer longitudinal muscle layer, formed by the edges of the two fanning longitudinal muscle bundles and the caudal border of the cricopharyngeus, the V-shaped area of Laimer, has no known functional significance. A coat of longitudinally oriented muscle fibers invests all the rest of the esophagus with a uniform thickness all the way to the stomach where it fuses with the corresponding outer longitudinal muscle layer of the stomach. This outer longitudinal muscle layer actually spirals slightly, turning about 90° between the pharyngoesophageal junction and the stomach. This spiral seems to have no functional significance. Rare muscle bundles diverge from the longitudinal muscle layer to fuse with the circular muscle layer all along the esophagus. Also rare bundles extend from the longitudinal layer to the trachea, the left mainstem bronchus and the left pleura (Lerche, 1950).

The inner circular muscle layer, thicker than the outer longitudinal layer, also spirals to form a tightly wound helix rather than a series of true rings. Its bundles deviate slightly from the true horizontal, the highest point of the loop being dorsal in the cervical esophagus, to the right in the upper thorax, ventral in the lower thorax, and to the left in the abdominal segment. This spiral arrangement has no demonstrated functional significance (Lerche, 1950).

Muscularis Mucosae of the Esophageal Body

The muscularis mucosae of the esophagus, composed of smooth muscle throughout the whole organ, begins as an extension of the elastic layer of the pharynx just below the level of the UES and extends to the esophagogastric junction where it fuses with the muscularis mucosae of the stomach. The muscularis mucosae is much thicker in the esophagus than it is in the other gastrointestinal viscera. Its thickness approaches the thickness of the longitudinal coat of the muscularis propria. The muscularis mucosae of the esophagus also differs from that of other viscera in that its muscle bundles run entirely in the rostrocaudal direction, whereas in the other viscera the bundles run in many directions within the plane of the mucosa (Christensen & Percey, 1984).

The functional significance of these special features of the esophageal mucosal muscle is not clear, just as the function of mucosal muscle in general throughout the gut is unclear. The various functions postulated for mucosal muscle in general include the compression of mucosal glands, the stirring of fluids at the epithelial surface, and the enhancement of lymph and blood flow through mucosal vessels. Since the esophagus contains few glands and is not an absorbing mucosa, such functions seem unnecessary there. The unusual strength of the esophageal mucosal muscle, however, and the unique longitudinal orientation of its muscle glands can be assumed to have some place in the unique function of the esophagus, the rapid and efficient peristaltic transport of a bolus. Exactly what that place is cannot yet be stated. Undoubtedly, the muscularis mucosae contributes to the considerable shortening of the organ that occurs as it contracts after a swallow, sharing that effect with the outer longitudinal muscle layer.

Musculature of the Gastroesophageal Junction and the LES

The outer longitudinal coat of the muscularis propria extends across the esophagogastric junction to fuse with the corresponding layer of muscle in the stomach. The circular muscle layer thickens slightly at the level of the esophagogastric junction, a thickening that is conspicuous in living tissue but not in dead tissue (Friedland, Kohatsu, & Lewin, 1971; Lieberman-Meffert, Allgower, Schmid, & Blum, 1979).

A complex structure was proposed long ago for the esophagogastric junction to account for various features seen radiographically (Figure 2–13). Thus, the term *gastroesophageal vestibule* is used to refer to the last 2 cm of the esophageal body. A muscular contraction ring called the *lower esophageal sphincter* or the *A-ring* marks its rostral end. Another contraction ring, the *constrictor cardiae*, marks the caudal end of the vestibule. A dilated segment of the esophagus just above the vestibule has been called the *esophageal ampulla* or *phrenic ampulla*. None of these radiographic features is evident in the neural and muscular anatomy of the region, nor does the physiology of the organ define these features. The whole gastroesophageal vestibule seems to be the lower esophageal sphincter. These structures, named and referred to only by radiologists (see also Chapter 6), seem to reflect the radiographic configuration of the organ as it is affected by various external influences in situ, most of the diaphragmatic crura and the phrenoesophageall ligament (Lin, Brasseur, Pouderoux, & Kahrilas, 1995).

The circular muscle layer, however, does exhibit a structural detail that may help to explain the sphincteric function of the LES (Figure 2–14). The muscle to the left side of the esophagogastric junction constitutes the most rostral bundles of the sling fibers of the stomach, part of the innermost oblique layer of gastric muscle. The circular muscle to the right side of the junction, called the clasp fiber, forms a continuous layer with the middle circular layer of gastric muscle (Lieberman-Meffert et al., 1979). Thus, the circular layer of the esophageal muscularis propria in the LES is continuous with both the circular and oblique layers of the muscularis propria of the stomach. The latter two layers are themselves not wholly separate throughout the stomach for they become continuous at about the level of the junction between the gastric body and antrum. The differences in function between these two layers of muscle in the stomach are not clear. And differences in function between the clasp fibers and sling fibers in the LES are also not clear. Presumably both muscular structures function in the tonic contraction and the transient relaxation that define the LES in physiological terms (Conklin & Christensen, 1994).

Extrinsic Nerve Supply to the Esophagus

The principal purpose of the esophagus, the transfer of food from the mouth to the stomach, results from the coordinated relaxation of its two sphincters (the UES and LES at its rostral and caudal ends) and the peristaltic contraction that sweeps the length of the conduit after a swallow (Conklin & Christensen, 1994). All three of these functions result from nervous impulses carried from the swallowing center in the brain stem to the esophagus by way of two major nerve pathways (Doty, 1968). Most of what we know of the neuroanatomy comes from the study of the opossum, but humans and other animals probably do not differ from the opossum in this respect.

Anatomic terminology distinguishes these two major extrinsic pathways as the *craniosacral* (or parasympathetic) and *thoracolumbar* (or sympathetic) neural pathways. The specific craniosacral and thoracolumbar nerve tracts leading to the esophagus from the central nervous system are called the *extrinsic nerves* of the esophagus. Within the esophageal wall, these extrinsic nerves make contact with another system of nerves not grossly apparent, the *enteric nerves*. These enteric nerves lie in two networks, one occurring as a sheet between the two main muscle layers and the other lying within the substance of the submucosa. The former, called the *myenteric plexus*, (or *Auerbach's plexus*), is much more complex and more dense than the latter (the submucosal or *Meissner's plexus*). The submucosal plexus is nearly devoid of nerve cells, containing mainly nerve fibers. The myenteric plexus probably provides essentially all of the nervous control of esophageal motor and secretory functions.

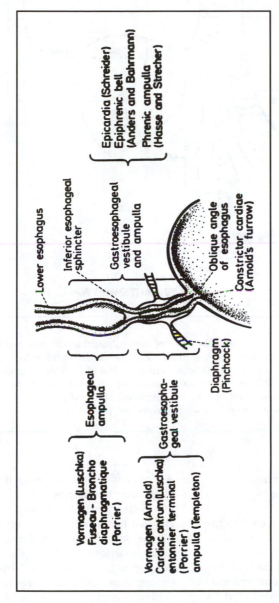

Figure 2–13. A diagram of the gastroesophageal junction to show structures commonly referred to by radiologists. The multitude of proper names in this figure indicates the intense interest given the subject at a time when its function could be studied only indirectly, by radiography (From "Basic data. Anatomy and Embryology by G. Fransen, & P. Valembois, 1994. In G. Vantrappen and J. Hellemans (Eds.), *Diseases of the Esophagus* (pp. 1–15). New York: Springer Verlag. Reprinted with permisssion)

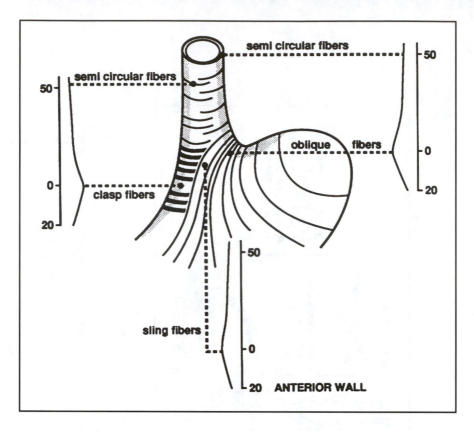

Figure 2–14. A diagram of the circular layer of musculature at the jiman esophagogastric junction. The thickest points in the wall lie in an oblique line at the junction. This indicates that sphincteric function probably resides in both sling fibers and clasp fibers (From Muscular Equivalent of the Lower Esophageal Sphincter by D. Lieberman-Meffert, D., M. Allgower, P. Schmid, & A. L. Blum, 1979, pp. 31–38. *Gastroenterology, 76,* with permission.)

Parasympathetic Innervation Through the Vagus Nerves

The vagus nerves provide the parasympathetic innervation to the whole esophagus. The vagal motor nerve fibers to the striated muscle of the rostral part of the esophagus arise from the nucleus ambiguus in the brain stem. Those directed to the smooth muscle of the caudal part of the organ originate in the dorsal motor nucleus, next to the nucleus ambiguus. The vagus nerves also receive fibers from the paravertebral sympathetic ganglia in the neck so that from that point on they are nerves of mixed parasympathetic and sympathetic composition.

A pharyngeal plexus, formed by the pharyngeal branches of the vagus nerves, lies on the outer surface of the middle pharyngeal constrictor and supplies the pharyngoesophageal junction. This plexus receives some contributions from the glossopharyngeal and spinal accessory nerves.

The recurrent laryngeal nerves, branches of the vagus nerves, innervate the cervical part of the esophagus. These two nerves pass dorsally, looping around the subclavian artery (on the right) and the aortic arch (on the left) to ascend to the neck in the lateral grooves between the contiguous esophagus and trachea, supplying both organs.

The upper thoracic esophagus receives branches both from the recurrent laryngeal nerves and from the vagus nerves themselves. Just below the hila of the lungs, the two vagus nerves break up into many branches, which mingle with branches from the sympathetic chain to form the esophageal plexus surrounding the esophagus in the lower thorax. Numerous branches from this plexus pierce the longitudinal muscle layer and enter into the substance of the esophageal myenteric plexus (MacGilchrist, Christensen, & Rick, 1991). The distribution density of these direct branches from the esophageal plexus to the esophageal myenteric plexus declines toward the stomach, generally corresponding with a decline in the density of nerve cells in the esophageal myenteric plexus.

About 6 cm above the diaphragm, the elements of the vagal esophageal plexus coalesce to form the vagal trunks, one to a few large nerves lying mainly anterior and posterior to the viscus. These pass through the diaphragmatic hiatus to enter the abdomen where they give off branches to the gastrointestinal viscera.

Sympathetic Innervation

The central connections of the sympathetic nerves to the esophagus occur over many segments, from the sixth cervical vertebra to the first lumbar vertebra, but most of them lie at the levels of the fourth to sixth thoracic vertebrae. The sympathetic fibers pass through the ventral spinal roots and the sympathetic chain. Some paravascular branches pass from the chain directly to the esophagus and others enter through the vagus nerves and the esophageal plexus. The proximal esophagus also receives branches from the stellate ganglion and the superior cervical ganglion. The distal esophagus also receives fibers from the celiac ganglion, mainly by way of the periarterial plexus of the left gastric artery.

Intrinsic Nerve Plexuses of the Esophagus

The most rostral ganglia of the esophageal myenteric plexus occur 1 to 2 cm caudal to the cricopharyngeus muscle. In its structure, consisting of ganglia (clusters or nodes or nerve cells and enteroglial cells) connected by interganglionic fascicles of nerve fibers (Christensen, Rick, Robison, Stiles, & Wix, 1983; Christensen & Robison, 1982), the myenteric plexus in the esophagus resembles that of the rest of the gut. The plexus differs from that of the rest of the gut, however, in the irregularity of its structure. The ganglia show a nonuniform or irregular pattern of distribution in the plane of the intermuscular space (the space between the two layers of the muscularis propria). Also, the ganglia vary enormously in size but they are comparatively small. Furthermore, many branching points of the interganglionic fascicles occur remote from a ganglion, and many small ganglia occur outside the main plexus of intersecting interganglionic fascicles, being connected to them by short stemlike fascicles. This virtually patternless structure of the esophageal myenteric plexus contrasts strongly with the quite regular polygons formed by the ganglia and interganglionic fascicles of the myenteric plexus in the gastric antrum, intestine, and colon.

The myenteric plexus of the esophagus also differs from that of the rest of the gut in its relative sparsity. The distribution density of nerve cells in the esophageal myenteric plexus is highest at the top of the smooth muscle segment, at the junction of the first and second one-thirds of the length of the organ. It falls progressively in both directions, rostrally and caudally, reaching a level at the esophagogastric junction which is about half that at the level of the striated-smooth muscle transition. Even at the striated-smooth muscle junction where the density is highest, it is considerably below that of the stomach and intestine.

The nerve cells of the myenteric plexus in the esophagus have very few dendrites and several axons (Christensen, 1988). That is, they are parvodendritic multiaxonal cells. The nerve cells that make up the myenteric plexus are not all alike. They differ from one another in relation to the neurotransmitters that they release in order to carry a stimulus from one nerve to another or from a nerve to muscle. In general, there must be three kinds of nerve cells in the myenteric plexus: sensory nerves, motor nerves, and interneurons (nerve cells that connect sensory nerve cells to motor nerve cells). Some of the motor nerves that regulate the contraction and relaxation of the smooth muscle release acetylcholine, and these nerves are called cholinergic nerves. The other class of motor nerves that regulate smooth muscle function release nitric oxide and these are called nitrergic nerves (Fang & Christensen, 1994a, 1994b; Fang, Christensen, & Rick, 1995;). Some other neurotransmitters present in the esophageal myenteric plexus, such as CGRP and substance P, probably characterize sensory nerves, and still others, like VIP, galanin, NP-Y, and bombesin, seem to identify nerves with more than one function (Christensen, Williams, Jew, & O'Dorisio, 1987a, 1987b, 1989; Fang & Christensen, 1994a).

Nitric oxide synthase-positive nerve fibers emanating from the myenteric plexus end abundantly in the circular layer of smooth muscle of the muscularis propria, but they are nearly absent from the longitudinal smooth muscle layer and muscularis mucosae except for a short segment just above the stomach. They are not to be found in either layer in the striated muscle of the proximal esophagus. In these striated muscle layers, the cells possess typical motor end plates, the endings of the somatic nerves to these striated muscles.

The ganglia of the esophageal myenteric plexus contain other structures that are absent from other parts of the gut, the intraganglionic laminar endings. These sensory structures, connected to the bipolar cells of the vagal sensory ganglia (the jugular and nodose ganglia), probably mediate parasympathetic reflexes and perhaps some sensations.

The submucosal plexus of the esophagus is exceedingly sparse, there being very few ganglia and only a tenuous plexus of nerve fiber bundles (Christensen & Rick, 1985). A subsidiary plexus of fine nerve fibers from the submucosal plexus extends into the lamina propria from which single nerve fibers depart to penetrate the squamous epithelium, ending near the luminal surface. These intraepithelial fibers presumably mediate mucosal sensation.

Muscle Cells and Interstitial Cells

The striated muscle of the rostral esophagus shows cells of both fast and slow muscle types. This muscle also contains muscle spindles, the specialized neuromuscular structures that mediate reflex responses to stretch.

The smooth muscle layers of the more caudal parts of the esophagus are made up of smooth muscle cells of typical form and size. No features distinguish one layer of smooth muscle from another throughout the esophageal body except for the specialized mesenchymal cells called the *interstitial cells of Cajal* (Christensen, Rick & Lowe, 1992; Christensen, Rick & Soll, 1987), which occur only in the circular muscle layer (Figure 2–15). These interstitial cells of Cajal resemble smooth muscle cells in size and in nuclear appearance, differing most notably in that they possess long branching processes. They are, however, not stained in conventional histology so the interstitial cells cannot be distinguished from smooth muscle at light microscopy unless some special differentiating stain, such as the zinc iodide-osmic acid stain, is applied. Such a stain shows that interstitial cells form 10% of more of the mass of the circular muscle layer. The interstitial cells lie in chains oriented along the bundles of muscle cells. Nerve fibers run along the chains, climbing over one interstitial cell after another. This arrangement implies that interstitial cells are involved in communication between the motor nerves and the circular muscle layer. Electron microscopy rein-

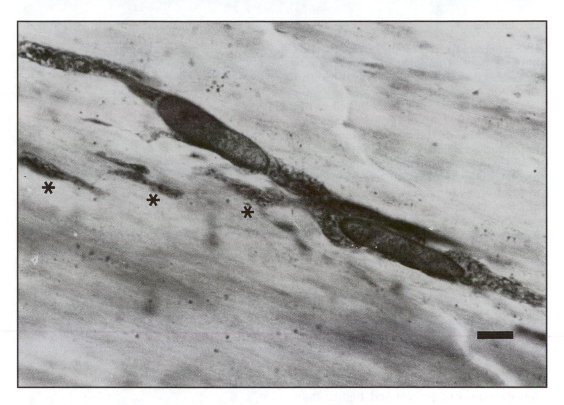

Figure 2-15. A photograph of two interstitial cells lying in the substance of the circular muscle layer of the opossum esophagus. Their oval nuclei are clear. The sinous processes, cut across in this thin section, are marked by asterisks. Zinc iodide-osmic acid stain. The bar indicates 5 mm.

forces this idea in showing a close apposition of nerve fibers to the interstitial cells and revealing the existence of specialized junctions between interstitial cells and smooth muscle cells.

The smooth muscle of the LES differs significantly from that of the circular layer of smooth muscle of the esophageal body (Christensen & Roberts, 1983; Seelig & Goyal, 1978). It possesses a larger of extracellular space, with prominent collagen fibrils and connective tissue. Also, the muscle cells themselves contain a greater mitochondrial mass and the mitochondria are somewhat differently located in the muscle cells. These findings support the conclusion from physiological studies that specialization in the smooth muscle itself defines the sphincter.

Connective Tissue and Extracellular Matrix of the Esophagus

Extracellular matrix is an important element in the cellular layers and the connective tissue layers of the esophageal wall. In the mucosa, matrix components maintain the structural integrity and the barrier functions of the epithelium (Toby & Orlando, 1991). In the lamina propria, and particularly the submucosa and the septa of the muscularis propria, the connective tissue matrix attaches muscle cells to each other, transmits their forces through the tissue and prevents deformity and tears of the organ (Gregersen et al., 1993; Tung et al., 1991).

Epithelium

Like all epithelia, the esophageal squamous mucosa limits the passage of compounds from the lumen to the interstitium and vascular spaces of the esophageal wall. Barrier functions are closely linked to the transport properties of epithelial cells and the properties of the matrix, which binds individual cells. Glycoconjugates, which bind the cells of the stratum spinosum of the esophageal mucosa together, are vital to the barrier functions of the esophageal mucosa. Upon their disruption, corrosives penetrate readily into the lamina propria, leading to edema, vascular congestion, and cellular infiltrates there and necrosis of epithelial cells (Orlando, Lacy, Toby, et al., 1992).

Lamina Propria and Submucosa

Collagen (specifically types I and III) is the most important component of the extracellular matrix in visceral smooth muscle. Collagen occurs in smooth muscle at a concentration of several-fold higher than that of skeletal or cardiac muscle and accounts for the comparatively great force and strain generation of smooth muscle. The distribution of so much collagen between smooth muscle cells has been likened to a "floating tendon." It is suspected that the muscle cells assemble and degrade much of the collagen between them. Collagen degradation is extremely slow. Collagen fibers pass from cell to cell in a three-dimensional network that enmeshes groups of cells into contractile units. In the submucosa, collagen fibers are arranged in a cross-ply arrangement; the orientation of fibers to the organ axis and to each other changes in opposite ways with distension and with shortening of the segment (Gabella, 1987). This fiber arrangement, therefore, allows for changes in gut size before any substantial loading of fibers occurs. Collagen fibers do not directly link up to the basal lamina of cells. Thin filaments intervene between collagen and basal lamina. These filaments consist primarily of fibronectin. Fibronectin is a glycoprotein that pro-

motes the migration, attachment, and differentiation of cells (Hukins, 1990). In visceral smooth muscle, fibronectin is thought to provide the link between smooth muscle cells and individual collagen fibers that provide the connective tissue network of septa and submucosa. Fibronectin exists both as a soluble form in plasma and lymph and an insoluble form in the extracellular matrix. Soluble fibronectin is taken up by specific cells that incorporate its insoluble form into the extracellular matrix.

Elastic fibers differ in their composition and loading properties from collagen fibers (Bonavina, Venturi, Columbo, et al., 1995; Gabella, 1983; Nagel, 1938). The distal esophageal wall contains more elastin and less collagen compared to the proximal wall. This arrangement could be responsible for the distensibility of the esophageal wall at the LES, which receives large contributions from the muscularis mucosae and especially the phrenoesophageal ligament, which is rich in elastic fibers.

SUMMARY

Accurate diagnosis and appropriate treatment of disordered swallowing first require understanding of the neuromuscular controls of the normal swallow. This chapter discusses the anatomic and neuromuscular controls of the three stages of swallowing: oral, pharyngeal, and esophageal. Whereas the role of the esophagus is to pass the food bolus into the stomach, the roles of the oral cavity and pharynx are broader. The mouth and pharynx are responsible for the transport of air for respiration, and they form the supralaryngeal portion of the vocal tract. Sensory and motor innervation to the muscles involved in the first two stages of deglutition are from cranial nerves V, VII, IX, X, and XII.

The esophagus constitutes three functional structures arranged in series, the upper esophageal sphincter, the esophageal body, and the lower esophageal sphincter. The upper esophageal sphincter is evident in the whole animal as a distinct muscle, the cricopharyngeus; the lower esophageal sphincter, evident grossly only in living tissues as a band of tonically contracted muscle, consists in part of the gastric sling fibers. The esophageal body, extending between these two sphincters, contains striated muscle in the rostral one-third. Special features characterize the morphology of the neural and muscular structures of the esophagus; these are reviewed in detail in this chapter.

MULTIPLE CHOICE QUESTIONS

1. Taste and sensation to the mouth and pharynx during deglutition is provided by
   a. CN V and VII
   b. CN V, VII, IX, and X
   c. CN IX and X
   d. V, VII and X

2. Which branch of CN X is important to the motor aspects of swallowing?
   a. pharyngeal branch
   b. recurrent laryngeal
   c. external branch of the superior laryngeal
   d. all of the above

3. The motor innervation of the upper esophagal sphincter is provided by
   a. CN IX
   b. CN X
   c. the splanchnic nerves
   d. all of the above

4. The circular layer of smooth muscle of the lower esophageal sphincter differs from that of the esophageal body in that
   a. it has a larger extracellular space
   b. its muscle contains a larger mitochondrial mass
   c. its mitochondria are located differently in the muscle cells
   d. all of the above

5. The principal neurotransmitter involved in esophageal motor function in humans is

a. nitric oxide
b. acetylcholine
c. norepinephrine
d. substance P

REFERENCES

Ahlgren, J. (1967). Kinesiology of the mandible. *Acta Odontologica Scandinavica, 25,* 593–611.

Appenteng, K., Lund, J., & Seguin, J. (1982). Intraoral mechanoreceptor activity during jaw movement in the anesthetized rabbit. *Journal of Neurophysiology, 48*(1), 27–37.

Bombeck, C. T., Dillard, D. H., & Nylus, L. M. (1966). Muscular anatomy of the gastroesophageal junction and role of phrenoesophageal ligament: Autopsy study of sphincter mechanism, *Annals of Surgery, 164*(4), 643–654.

Bonavina, L., Venturi, M., Colombo, L., Segalin, A., Mussini, E., & Peracchia, A. (1995). Elastic properties of the normal human esophagus: A biochemical study. *Gastroenterology, 108,* A-188.

Borgstrom, P. S., & Ekberg, O. (1988). Speed of peristalsis in pharyngeal constrictor musculature: Correlation to age. *Dysphagia, 2,* 140–144.

Carpenter, M. B. (1978). *Core text of neuroanatomy* (2nd ed.). Baltimore: Williams and Wilkins.

Cerenko, D., McConnel, F., & Jackson, R. T. (1989). Quantitative assessment of pharyngeal bolus driving forces. *Otolaryngology—Head and Neck Surgery, 100*(1), 57–64.

Christensen, J. (1988). The forms of argyrophilic ganglion cells in the myenteric plexus throughout the gastrointestinal tract of the opossum. *Journal of the Autonomic Nervous System, 24,* 251–260.

Christensen, J., & Percy, W. H. (1984). A pharmacological study of oesophageal muscularis mucosae from the cat, dog and American opossum. *British Journal of Pharmacology, 83,* 329–336.

Christensen, J., & Rick, G. A. (1985). Nerve cell density in submucous plexus throughout the gut of cat and opossum. *Gastroenterology, 89,* 1064–1069.

Christensen, J., Rick, G. A., & Lowe, L. S. (1992). Distributions of interstitial cells of cajal in stomach and colon of cat, dog, ferret, opossum, rat, guinea pig and rabbit. *Journal of the Autonomic Nervous System, 37,* 47–56.

Christensen, J., Rick, G. A., Robison, B. A., Stiles, M. J., & Wix, M. A. (1983). The arrangement of the myenteric plexus throughout the gastrointestinal tract of the opossum. *Gastroenterology, 85,* 890–899.

Christensen, J., Rick, G. A., & Soll, D. J. (1987). Intramural nerves and interstitial cells revealed by the Champy-Maillet stain in the opossum esophagus. *Journal of the Autonomic Nervous System, 14,* 137–151.

Christensen, J., & Roberts, R. L. (1983). Differences between esophageal body and lower esophageal sphincter in mitochondria of smooth muscle in opossum. *Gastroenterology, 85*, 650–656.

Christensen, J., & Robison, B. A. (1982). Anatomy of the myenteric plexus of the opossum esophagus. *Gastroenterology, 83*, 1033–1042.

Christensen, J., Williams, T. H., Jew, J., & O'Dorisio, T. M. (1987a). The distribution of VIP (vasoactive intestinal polypeptide) immunoreactive structures in the opossum esophagus. *Gastroenterology, 92*, 1007–1018.

Christensen, J., Williams, T. H., Jew, J., & O'Dorisio, T. M. (1987b). The distribution of vasoactive intestinal polypeptide (VIP) in the opossum esophagus in relation to function. *Experimental Brain Research, 16*, 102–106.

Christensen, J., Williams, T. H., Jew, J., & O'Dorisio, T.M. (1989). The distribution of substance P immunoreactive structures in the opossum esophagus. *Digestive Diseases and Sciences, 34*, 513–520.

Clark, G. A. (1920). Deglutition apnea. *Proceedings of the Physiological Society.*

Cleall, J. F. (1965). Deglutition: A study of form and function. *American Journal of Orthodontics, 51*(8), 566–594.

Conklin, J. L., & Christensen, J. (1994). Motor functions of the esophagus. In L. R. Johnson, J. Christensen, D. Alpers, E. D. Jacobsen, & J. Walsh (Eds.), *Physiology of the gastrointestinal tract* (3rd ed., chap. 4, pp. 33–40). New York: Raven Press.

Dantas, R. O., Kern, M. K., Massey, B. T., Dodds, W. J., Kahrilas, P. J., Brasseur, J. G., Cook, I. J., & Lang, I. M. (1990). Effect of swallowed bolus variables on oral and pharyngeal phases of swallowing. *The American Physiological Society, 258*, G675–G681.

Desmet, V. J., & Tytgat, G. N. (1974). Basic data. Histology and electron microscopy. In G. Vantrappen & J. Hellemans (Eds.), *Diseases of the esophagus* (pp. 1–15). New York, Springer-Verlag.

Doran, G. A., & Baggett, H. (1972). The genioglossus muscle: A reassessment of its anatomy in some mammals, including man. *Acta Anatomica, 83*, 403–410.

Doty, R. W. (1968). Neural organization of deglutition. In C. F. Code (Ed.), *Handbook of physiology. Section 6: Alimentary Canal* (Vol. 4, pp. 1861–1902). Washington DC: Motility Physiological Society

Doty, R. W., & Bosma, J. F. (1956). An electromyographic analysis of reflex deglutition. *Journal of Neurophysiology, 19*, 44–60.

Eliska, O. (1973). Phreno-oesophageal membrane and its role in the development of hiatal hernia. *Acta Anatomica* (Basel), *86*, 137–150.

Fang, S., & Christensen, J. (1994a). Colocalization of NADPH-Diaphorase activity and certain neuropeptides in the esophagus of the opossum (D. virginiana). *Cell and Tissue Research, 278*, 557–562.

Fang, S., & Christensen, J. (1994b). Distribution of NADPH-Diaphorase in the intramural plexuses of opossum and cat esophagus. *Journal of the Autonomic Nervous System, 46*, 123–133.

Fang, S., Christensen, J., & Rick, G. A. (1995). NADPH-diaphorase positive nerve fibers in smooth muscle layers of opossum esophagus: Gradients in density. *Journal of the Autonomic Nervous System, 52*, 99–105.

Fransen, G., & Valembois, P. (1978). Basic data. Anatomy and embryology. In G. Vantrappen & J. Hellemans (Eds.), *Diseases of the esophagus* (pp. 1–15). New York: Springer-Verlag.

Friedland, G. W., Kohatsu, S., & Lewin, K. (1971). Comparative anatomy of feline and canine gastric sling fibers (analogy to human anatomy). *Digestive Diseases and Sciences, 16*, 495–507.

Gabella, G. (1983). The taenia of the rabbit colon, an elastic vesceral muscle. *Anatomy and Embryology 167*, 39–51.

Gabella G. (1987). The cross-ply arrangement of collagen fibers in the submucosa of the mammalian small intestine. *Cell and Tissue Research, 248*, 491–497.

Gregersen, H., Gibersen, I. M., Rasmussen, L. M., & Tottrup, A. (1992). Biomechanical wall properties and collagen content in the partially obstructed opossum esophagus. *Gastroenterology, 103*, 1547–1551.

Hiiemae, K. M., & Crompton, A. W. (1985). Mastication, food transport and swallowing. In M. Hildebrand, D. Bramble, K. Liem, & D. B. Wale (Eds.), *Functional vertebrate morphology* (p. 262). Keknap.

Hiiemae, J., Thexton, A. J., & Crompton, A. W. (1978). Intra-oral food transport: The fundamental mechanism of feeding. In D. S. Carlson & J. A. McNamara (Eds.), *Muscle adaption in the craniofacial region* (p. 181). Ann Arbor: University of Michigan Press.

Hrycyshyn, A. W., & Basmajian, J. V. (1972). Electromyography of the oral stage of swallowing in man. *American Journal of Anatomy, 133*, 333–340.

Hukins, D. W. L. (1990). Dynamic aspects of connective tissue structure and function. In D. W. L. Hukins (Ed.), *Connective tissue matrix*. Boca Raton, LA: CRC Press.

Hylander, W. L., & Crompton, A. W. (1986). Jaw movements and patterns of mandibular bone strain during mastication in the monkey macaca fascicularis. *Archives of Oral Biology, 31*, 841–848.

Inoue, T., Kato, T., Masuda, Y., Nakamura, T., Kawamura, Y., & Morimoto, T. (1989). Modifications of masticatory behavior after trigeminal deafferentation in the rabbit. *Experimental Brain Research, 74*, 579–591.

Jacob, P., Kahrilas, P. J., Logemann, J. A., Shah, V., & Ha, T. (1989). Upper esophageal sphincter opening and modulation during swallowing. *Gastroenterology, 97*, 1469–1478.

Kahrilas, P., Logemann, J., Lin, S., & Ergun, G. (1992). Pharyngeal clearance during swallow: a combined manometric and videofluoroscopic study. *Gastroenterology, 103*, 128–136.

Kahrilas, P. J., Lin, S., Logemann, J.A., Ergun, G. A., & Facchini, F. (1993). Deglutitive tongue action: Volume accommodation and bolus propulsion, *Gastroenterology, 104*, 152–162.

Kapila, Y. V., Dodds, W. J., Helm, J. F., & Hogan, W. J. (1984). Relationship between swallow rate and salivary flow. *Digestive Diseases and Sciences, 29*(6), 528–533.

Kier, W. M., & Smith, K. K. (1985). Tongues, tentacles and trunks: The biomechanics of movement in muscular-hydrostats. *Zoological Journal of the Linnean Society, 83*, 307–324.

Lieberman-Meffert, D., Allgower, M., Schmid, P., & Blum, A. L. (1979). Muscular equivalent of the lower esophageal sphincter. *Gastroenterology, 76*, 31–38.

Lin, S., Brasseur, J.G., Pouderoux, P. and Kahrilas, P.J. (1995). The phrenic ampulla: Distal esophagus or potential hiatal hernia? *American Journal of Physiology*, G320–G327.

Lightoller, G. H. S. (1925). The modiolus and muscles surrounding the rima oris with some remarks about the panniculus adiposus. *Journal of Anatomy, 60*, 1–85.

Logemann, J. A. (1983). *Evaluation and treatment of swallowing disorders*. San Diego, CA, College-Hill Press.

Lowe, A. (1980). The neural regulation of tongue movements. In *Progress in Neurobiology* (pp. 295–344). New York: Pergamon Press.

Luschei, E. S., & Goodwin, G. M. (1974). Patterns of mandibular movement and jaw muscle activity during mastication in the monkey. *Journal of Neurophysiology, 37*, 954–966.

Magendie, F. (1836). Precis elementaire de physiologie. Paris.

MacGilchrist, A. J., Christensen, J., & Rick, G. A. (1991). The distribution of myelinated nerve fibers in the myenteric plexus of the opossum esophagus. *Journal of the Autonomic Nervous System, 35*, 227–236.

McConnel, F. M. S., Cerenko, D., & Mendelsohn, M. S. (1988). Manofluorographic analysis of swallowing. *Otolaryngologic Clinics of North America, 21*(4), 625–635.

McConnel, F. M.S., Cerenko, D., Jackson, R.T., & Guffin, T.N. (1988). Timing of major events of pharyngeal swallowing, *Archives of Otolaryngology—Head and Neck Surgery, 114*, 1413–1418.

Miller, A. J. (1972). Significance of sensory inflow to the swallowing reflex. *Brain Research, 43*, 147–159.

Miller, F. R., & Sherrington, C. S. (1915). Some observations on the bucco-pharyngeal stage of reflex deglutition in the cat. *Experimental Physiology and Cognate Medical Sciences, 9*, 147–186.

Mittal R.K., & Fisher, M.J. (1990). Electrical and mechanical inhibition of the crural diaphragm during transient relaxationof thelower esophageal sphincter, *Gastroenterology, 99*(5), 1265–1268.

Nagel, A. (1938). Das Bindegewebsgerust des menschlichen Oesophagus in seinen funktionellen Beziehungen zur glatten Muskulature und den Blutgesfassen. *Morphol Jahrbuch, 81*, 449–493.

Orlando, T. V., Lacy, E. R., Toby, N. A., et al. (1992). Barriers to paracellular permeability in rabbit esophageal epithelium. *Gastroenterology, 102*, 910–923.

Pansky, B., Allen, D. J., & Budd, G. C. (1988). *Review of neuroscience*. New York: Macmillan.

Perlman, A. (1994). Disordered Swallowing. In J. B. Tomblin, H. L. Morris, & D. C. Spriestersbach (Eds.). *Diagnosis in speech-language pathology* (pp. 361–382). San Diego, CA: Singular Publishing Group.

Perlman, A. L., Luschei, E. S., & Du Mond, C. E. (1989). Electrical activity from the superior pharyngeal constrictor during reflexive and nonreflexive tasks. *Journal of Speech and Hearing Research, 32*, 749–754.

Perlman, A. L., Schultz, J. G., & VanDaele, D. J. (1993). Effects of age, gender, bolus volume, and bolus viscosity on oropharyngeal pressure during swallowing. *Journal of Applied Physiology, 75*(1), 33–37.

Plesh, O., Bishop, B., & McCall, W. (1986). Effect of gum hardness on chewing pattern. *Experiemental Neurology, 92*, 502–512.

Proffit, W. R., Kydd, W. L., Wilskie, G. H., & Taylor, D. T. (1964). Intraoral pressures in a young adult group. *Journal of Dental Research, 43*(4), 555–562.

Robbins, J., Hamilton, J. W., Lof, G. L., & Kempster, G. B. (1992). Oropharyngeal swallowing in normal adults of different ages. *Gastroenterology, 103*, 823–829.

Schultz, J., Perlman, A. L., & VanDaele, D. J. (1994). Laryngeal movement, oropharyngeal pressure, and submental muscle contraction during swallowing. *Archives of Physical Medicine and Rehabilitation, 75*(2), 183–189.

Schulze-Delrieu, K., Mitros, F.A., & Shirazi, S. (1982). Inflammatory and structural changes in the opossum esophagus after resection of the cardia. *Gastroenterology, 82*(2), 276–283.

Schwartz, G., Enomoto, S., Valiquette, C., & Lund, J. P. (1989). Mastication in the rabbit: A description of movement and muscle activity. *Journal of Neurophysiology, 62*(1), 273–287.

Seelig, L. L., & Goyal, R. K. (1978). Morphological evaluation of opossum lower esophageal sphincter. *Gastroenterology, 75*, 51–58.

Selley, W. G., Ellis, R. E., Flack, F. C., Bayliss, C. R., & Pearce, V. R. (1994). The synchronization of respiration and swallow sounds with videofluoroscopy during swallowing. *Dysphagia, 9*(3), 162–167.

Selley, W. G., Flack, F. C., Ellis, R. E., & Brooks, W. A. (1989). Respiratory patterns associated with swallowing: Part 2. Neurologically impaired dysphagic patients. *Age and Ageing, 18*, 173–176.

Smith, J., Wolkove, N., Colacone, A., & Kreisman, H. (1989). Coordination of eating, drinking, and breathing in adults. *Chest, 96*(3), 578–582.

Sokol, E. M., Heitmann, P., Wolf, B. S., & Cohen, B. R. (1966). Simultaneous cineradiographic and manometric study of the pharynx, hypopharynx, and cervical esophagus. *Gastroenterology, 51*(6), 960–974.

Sonies, B. C., Parent, L. J., Morrish, K., & Baum, B. J. (1988). Durational aspects of the oral-pharyngeal phase of swallow in normal adults. *Dysphagia, 3*, 1–10.

Sonies, B., Ship, J., & Baum, B. (1989). Relationship between saliva production and oropharyngeal swallow in healthy, different-aged adults. *Dysphagia, 4*, 85–89.

Takada, K., Miyawaki, S., & Tatsuta, M. (1994). The effects of food consistency on jaw movement and posterior temporalis and inferior orbicularis oris muscle activities during chewing in children. *Archives of Oral Biology, 39*(9), 793–805.

Thexton, A. J., Hiiemae, K. M., & Crompton, A. W. (1980). Food consistency and bite size as regulators of jaw movement during feeding in the cat. *Journal of Neurophysiology, 44*(3), 456–474.

Toby, N. A. & Orlando, R. C. (1991). Mechanisms of acid injury to rabbit esophageal epithelium: Role of basolateral cell membrane acidification. *Gastroenterology, 101*, 1220–1228.

Tung, H. N., Schulze-Delrieu, K., Shirazi, S., et al. (1991). Hypertrophic smooth muscle in the partially obstructed opossum esophagus—The model: histological and ultrastructural observations. *Gastroenterology, 100*, 853–864.

VanDaele, D. J., Perlman, A. L., & Cassell, M. (1995). Contributions of the lateral hyoepiglottic ligaments to the mechanism of epiglottic downfolding. *Journal of Anatomy, 186*, 1–15.

3

Functional Controls
of Deglutition

A. Miller, D. Bieger, and J. L. Conklin

NEUROMUSCULAR CONTROL
OF SWALLOWING

The control of deglutition is a complex process that depends on a bewildering number of coordinated neuromuscular interactions between the central nervous system, the enteric nervous system, and the muscular components of the swallowing apparatus. This chapter will present a general overview of all the neural control mechanisms involved in the process of swallowing, followed by detailed descriptions of the neural and muscular processes that control each phase of swallowing.

Central Organization of Swallowing

The swallowing center is a complex organization of neural elements in the cortex and brain stem of the central nervous system. It is required to initiate and to coordinate the many muscles that are involved in the oral, pharyngeal and esophageal phases of swallowing. The patterns of discharge of the central neural swallowing pathway are fixed for the pharyngeal and esophageal phases of the swallow: multiple inhibitions and excitations of participating muscles occur in a constant order. The locations of all the constituent parts of the central swallowing pathway are not known fully. They include specific regions of the cortex and two primary sites the lower brain stem (Figure 3–1). The neurons in the brain stem that are involved in swallowing lie mainly in the dorsal region within and subjacent to the nucleus of the tractus solitarius, and in the ventral region around the nucleus ambiguus. In both regions, the neurons surrounding the reticular formation also are involved. The two regions are represented on both sides of the brain stem and are interconnected extensively, so that either side alone can coordinate the pharyngeal and esophageal phases of swallowing (Doty, 1968; Doty, Richmond, & Storey, 1967).

Although several cortical or subcortical regions modify the activity of the brain stem swallowing pathway, specific cortical regions may integrate with the lower brain stem to activate and control the oral, pharyngeal, and esophageal phases of swallowing (Car, 1970, 1973; Sumi, 1969, 1972a, 1972b). Swallowing is facilitated by mandibular movement and elevation of the tongue and can be initiated by tactile, pressure or liquid stimulation of the pharynx. This means that afferent inputs from these regions are critical to the control of normal swallowing. The efferent outflow from the central swallowing pathway (i.e., motor innervation) arises from many brainstem motor

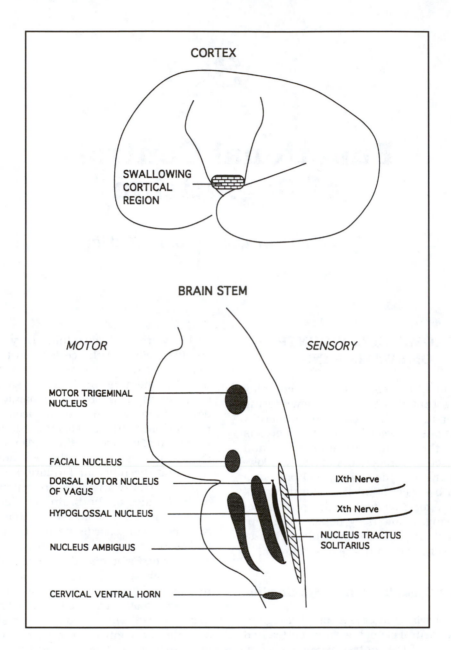

Figure 3–1. Schematic diagram of two primary regions of the central nervous system which compose the swallowing pathway involved with the pharyngeal phase. The brain stem and cervical spinal cord contain both the sensory and motor nuclei involved with the oral, pharyngeal, and esophageal phases. A region of the frontal cortex, anterior to the sensorimotor cortex, potentially has four subregions around a relatively discrete area that is suspected to integrate into the total control of swallowing. This diagram does not depict all of the central neural pathways that evoke swallowing when electrically stimulated and include regions of the hypothalamus, midbrain and pons.

nuclei and some cervical spinal motoneuron pools. Synaptic communication exists between the central swallowing pathway and the interneurons of the brain stem that control emesis and respiration (Bieger, Weerasuriya, & Hockman, 1978; Carpenter, 1989; Sumi, 1963). Most swallows in humans occur during a suspension of breathing in expiration; therefore, the functions of respiration and swallowing must be coordinated (Doty, 1968; Kawasaki, Ogura, & Takenouchi, 1965).

Cortex

Swallowing can be evoked by stimulating many different central neural pathways. Electrical stimulation of the primary motor cortex region does not elicit swallowing (Murray & Sessle, 1992), but stimulation of the anterolateral region immediately in front of the precentral cortex evokes swallowing that is often associated with mastication (Car, 1970, 1973, 1977; Miller & Bowman 1977; Sumi 1969, 1970). This region of the cortex elicits swallowing even if the primary motor cortex is destroyed, thus indicating its independence in the control of swallowing.

Pharyngeal and esophageal patterns of muscle contraction similar to those evoked by swallowing can be elicited after removing all of the cortical and subcortical regions above the brain stem, indicating that the neurons needed to program the pharyngeal and esophageal phases of swallowing reside in the brain stem. Still, specific cortical sites play a role in evoking and facilitating the initiation of swallowing. These cortical regions also modify the duration and intensity of the muscle activity that determines tongue movement, elevation of the hyoid bone, adduction of the vocal cords, and contraction of the upper esophagus during swallowing (Miller 1972a,b; Miller & Sherrington 1916). Stimulation of the prefrontal region elicits bilateral movements of the face and tongue, repetitive jaw movements, and, in selected regions, pharyngeal and esophageal swallowing (Kubota 1976). Detailed studies of the cortex using microelectrodes suggest that at least four cortical regions found bilaterally around the frontal cortex elicit swallowing when stimulated (Martin & Sessle, 1993).

Neural pathways from the anterolateral cortex descend through the internal capsule and subthalamic regions to the level of the substantia nigra and mesencephalic reticular formation region of the upper brainstem. Stimulation of this corticobulbar pathway, like stimulation of the cortical regions, evokes swallowing that is associated with mastication (Car 1970, 1973, 1977; Sumi, 1969, 1972b). The threshold for evoking swallowing depends on the frequency of the stimulus (Miller, 1972a, 1972b). Swallowing evoked reflexively by stimulating peripheral sensory nerves that innervate the major regions of the oropharynx is also frequency-dependent. This frequency-dependence suggests that descending, corticobulbar inputs and peripheral, sensory inputs synapse on a specific group of interneurons in the lower brain stem that are activated when the descending and/or peripheral inputs carry the correct excitatory code.

Reflex swallowing is facilitated from sites outside the corticobulbar pathway, in particular, the hypothalamus and midbrain ventral tegmental field. These are regions that control and integrate many visceral functions (Bieger, 1991; Bieger & Hockman, 1976; Bieger, Weerasuriya, & Hockman, 1978; Hockman, Bieger, & Weerasuriya, 1979). Exposing these neural structures to dopamine, a neurotransmitter that is intrinsic to this region, facilitates the evoking of swallowing. This suggests that the amygdalohypothalamic regions that integrate feeding with visceral and somatic responses modify the threshold for reflexively-evoked swallowing.

The studies described above indicate that several regions of the brain alter the threshold for reflexively evoked swallowing. These regions may be important pathways in the voluntary elicitation or facilitation of deglutition, and they may be critical in learning to integrate orofacial movements with swallowing. They may also integrate deglutition with other motor responses. The cortical and subcortical regions are not however, essential for the coordination of pharyngeal and esophageal muscle activity: sequential activation of the muscles involved in swallowing continues after cortical and subcortical inputs to brain stem are interrupted. The coordination of pharyngeal and esophageal muscle activity in swallowing continues normally in humans with extensive neurological damage to the cortex and in infants with severe central neural deficits involving the loss of tissue rostral to the midbrain. It also occurs in the normal human fetus before descending cortico-subcortical pathways that innervate the brain stem are developed (Doty 1968). All of this means that the brain stem contains the interneurons essential to the swallowing response (Miller 1972b; Miller & Sherrington 1916), but the cortex exercises significant control over the initiation of swallowing and the level of neuromuscular activity during swallowing.

Brain Stem

Two regions of the upper brain stem, at the level of the pons, evoke swallowing when stimulated (Amri, Car, & Jean, 1984; Car, Jean, & Roman, 1975; Sumi 1972b). These are the reticular formation immediately dorsal to the motor trigeminal nucleus and the region of the pons ventral to the motor trigeminal nucleus. The reticular formation, immediately dorsal to the motor trigeminal nucleus, receives input from peripheral fibers innervating receptive fields that evoke swallowing when stimulated. It also transmits information rostrally to the thalamus. Primary sensory fibers divide as they enter the brain stem. One subdivision synapses in the lower brainstem while the other proceeds rostrally to innervate interneurons within the upper brain stem, specifically the pons. (Car & Amri, 1982; Figure 3–2). Lesions in this region of the pons do not modify swallowing evoked by stimulating peripheral sensory nerves. This indicates that this part of the pons, while innervat-ed by sensory nerves that can initiate swallowing, is not essential to the reflex activation of deglutition.

The region of the pons ventral to the motor trigeminal nucleus is part of a cortical-subcortical loop that carries ascending and descending information between the cortex and subcortical regions (Sumi, 1972b). Stimulation of this region evokes both mastication and swallowing.

None of the pontine regions constitute the core of interneurons that controls the actual sequence of muscle activity during. Electrical stimulation of the cranial motor nuclei does not evoke swallowing, even though the muscles innervated by motoneurons located within pons, medulla, and the cervical spinal cord are involved in the sequential muscle activity of the pharyngeal and esophageal phases of swallowing. The program responsible for the sequential activation of specific pools of motoneurons that control swallowing resides within the lower brain stem swallowing pathway.

Activity of the Orofacial Musculature during the Oral Stage of Swallowing

The oral stage of swallowing consists of voluntary and reflexive components including mastication, bolus formation, and propulsion of the bolus by the tongue. The swallowing of water or materials associated with mastication recruits the elevator muscles of the mandible (the temporalis, masseter, medial pterygoid, and lateral pterygoid muscles) to stabilize the mandible, the suprahyoid, and infrahyoid muscles to position the hyoid, and the muscles of the tongue to move the bolus. (Cleall, 1965; Dubner, Sessle, & Storey, 1978; Hamlet, 1989; Hrychshyn & Basmajian, 1972; Laird, 1974; McNamara & Moyers, 1973; Thexton, 1973). The facial muscles are also activated during some swallows to develop an anterior seal of the lips. Sensory feedback from the oral cavity is needed so that the orofacial musculature is able to form a bolus that can be propelled into the pharynx by the

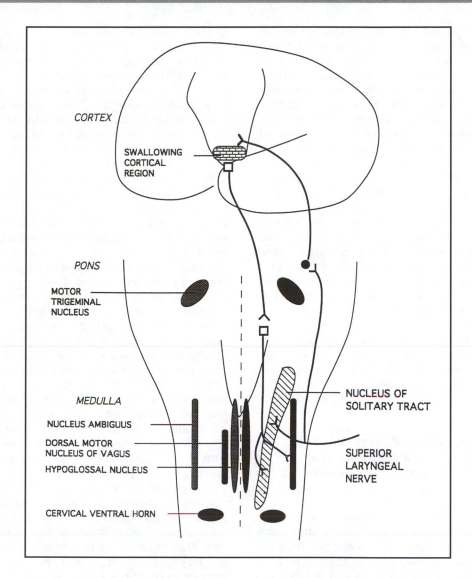

CORTEX

SWALLOWING
CORTICAL
REGION

PONS

MOTOR
TRIGEMINAL
NUCLEUS

MEDULLA

NUCLEUS AMBIGUUS

DORSAL MOTOR
NUCLEUS OF VAGUS

HYPOGLOSSAL NUCLEUS

CERVICAL VENTRAL HORN

NUCLEUS OF
SOLITARY TRACT

SUPERIOR
LARYNGEAL
NERVE

Figure 3–2. A schematic diagram of the lateral cortex and the dorsal view of the brain stem indicating that sensory input eliciting pharyngeal and esophageal swallowing is primarily carried by sensory fibers in the vagus (Xth) and glossopharyngeal (IXth) nerves. These fibers synapse in one of the sensory nuclei of the brain stem, the nucleus of the tractus solitarius, and simultaneously, send fibers more rostrally. The diagram suggests that a long brain stem-cortical reflex arc interacts with the brain stem to control pharyngeal and esophageal phases of swallowing. The oral stage appears to involve a different pathway in which the trigeminal sensory nuclei are involved.

tongue. The tongue, in particular, has touch and pressure receptors that provide complex sensory perception (Henkin & Banks, 1967). The type of bolus affects the recruitment of jaw-closing muscles (McNamara & Moyers, 1973), more activity occurs when greater stabilization of the mandible is needed. The primary motor nucleus involved in this process is the motor trigeminal nucleus of the pons.

Early in swallowing, the lips are sealed and the tongue, by activation of the genioglossus muscle, is positioned so that its anterior tip makes contact with the hard palate. This seals the oral cavity anteriorly. raising of the hyoid bone occurs during this time. Next, the intrinsic muscles of the tongue are recruited in a rostrocaudal sequence to propel the bolus into and through the pharynx. recruitment of the tongue muscles requires the activation of different motoneuron pools within the hypoglossal nucleus of the medulla.

Propulsive movements of the tongue can be elicited via a trigeminal-hypoglossal reflex (Thexton, 1973). Coordination of the jaw-closing muscles with the tongue and hyoid bone is dependent on sensory feedback which may involve receptors in the jaw-closing muscles and the supra- and infrahyoid structures. Sensory feedback concerning the size and consistency of the bolus modifies the activity of motoneurons in the motor trigeminal nucleus, hypoglossal nucleus and cervical spinal cord. Little information exists about this process.

Activity of the Pharyngeal and Parapharyngeal Musculature During the Pharyngeal Phase of Swallowing.

The pharyngeal and parapharyngeal muscles are striated muscles that exhibit tone at rest (i.e., the muscles are not flaccid). This tone represents the continuous activity of alpha motoneurons, somatic neurons that arise from cell bodies in the brain stem and upper cervical motor nuclei and innervate striated muscles of the gastrointestinal tract (Basmajian & Duttam, 1961; Christensen, 1987). Contraction of these muscles during swallowing is preceded by a brief decrease in their tone, which results from a decrease in efferent nerve activity (Bosma, 1957; Doty & Bosma, 1956).

The pharyngeal muscles contract in a fixed sequence during swallowing (Doty & Bosma 1956; Kawasaki et al., 1965). Lengthening the duration of this phase prolongs the activity of all the muscles, but the sequence of their activity remains the same. The genioglossus muscle, the major muscle protruding the tongue, is often active first. Additional muscles that are active in this first segment of the swallow, called the "leading complex," are those that raise the hyoid bone. The mylohyoid and hyoglossus muscles work in synchrony to raise the hyoid bone, while the geniohyoid and mylohyoid are simultaneously active to move it anteriorly (Matsumoto 1971). Muscles of the posterior tongue function as part of the ventral wall of the pharynx, and are activated with the superior pharyngeal constrictor to begin pharyngeal peristalsis.

The pharyngeal stage of swallowing begins as a bolus is driven into the posterior oral cavity by the propulsive activity of the tongue. The muscles that close off the nasopharynx (i.e., palatopharyngeus) and raise the soft palate (i.e., levator veli palatini) contract within the first segment of this sequence in coincidence with the inhibition of respiration. This seals the oropharynx from the nasopharynx so that nasopharyngeal reflux does not occur. At about the same time, the larynx elevates and the arytenoids move anteriorly to make contact with the epiglottis and close the laryngeal opening. Two types of pharyngeal contraction facilitate the movement of the bolus towards the esophagus. First, the pharynx shortens in its long axis, decreasing the distance a bolus must travel within the pharynx. Pharyngeal shortening also obliterates the laryngeal vestibule and the pyriform sinuses so that none of the bolus is caught in these recesses. The pharyngeal constrictor muscles are then activated in a fixed rostrocaudal sequence that generates a propulsive contractile wave which occludes the pharyngeal lumen behind the bolus as it sweeps caudally. This contraction clears all of the residue left behind the swallowed bolus towards the esophagus.

The muscles of the pharynx vary in their duration of contraction, contracting longer in the fully awake state than in the anesthetized state; the activity of each muscle varies from 400–700 milliseconds. The total duration of the pharyngeal stage is about 1 second. The timing and sequencing of these motor events takes place in the lower brain stem which sends signals to the motor nuclei from which the motorneurons that innervate the pharyngeal musculature arise. Lesions in the brain stem or peripheral cranial neuropathies can disrupt this sequence of events causing difficulty in the movement of boluses through the pharynx, the oral or nasopharyngeal reflux of the bolus, and/or the entry of the bolus into the larynx.

Although the pharyngeal stage of swallowing is a highly automated sequence of neuromuscular events, it can be modified by sensory feedback. Feedback mechanisms can modulate the threshold to evoke the pharyngeal stage of swallowing, modify the intensity of muscle activity during this stage, and alter the duration of the stage (Dodds et al., 1988; Ekberg, Olsson, & Sundgren-Borgstrom, 1988; Mansson & Sandberg, 1974, 1975a, 1975b). The genioglossus and the geniohyoid muscles discharge longer if the bolus is more dense (Hrychshyn & Basmajian 1972). The inferior pharyngeal constrictor and the cricopharyngeal muscles discharge longer during the later stages of the pharyngeal stage and demonstrate double discharges if they are detached at their laryngeal insertions and are sutured to their ipsilateral muscle (Shipp, Deatsch, & Robertson, 1970). The threshold to elicit repeated swallows is decreased by continuous feedback from the soft palate, pillars of fauces, tonsils, base of the tongue, and pharynx. Anesthetizing these mucosal regions with a topical anesthetic increases the time to evoke repeated swallows (Mansson & Sandberg 1974, 1975a, 1975b). Denervating the tongue and laryngeal muscles does not modify the sequence of swallowing in anesthetized animals (Miller 1972b) as deglutition depends on a strong central control.

The activation of certain motor neurons supplying the muscles participating in the pharyngeal stage of swallowing is both preceded and followed by inhibition of their activity. The central swallowing pathway coordinates inhibition at several levels. There is a general inhibition of respiration with each pharyngeal phase of swallowing. The two sphincters, rostral and caudal to the esophagus, are inhibited with each pharyngeal stage: Sustained inhibition of esophageal activation occurs with repeated pharyngeal contractions. Finally, a sequential inhibition brackets the activation of each muscle during its recruitment in the pharyngeal stage. These observations suggest that reciprocal interactions with overriding inhibitory inputs occur between the central respiratory pathway and the swallowing pathway, and between the deglutition central pathway and other synaptic inputs to cranial motor neurons. Once the central swallowing pathway is triggered for the pharyngeal stage, it dominates the motoneurons for the muscles to be recruited within the pharyngeal stage.

Activity of the Upper Esophageal Sphincter

Closure of the Esophageal Inlet

Closure of the lumen at the esophageal inlet arises from three sources: active contraction of the cricopharyngeus muscle, the major muscular component of the upper esophageal sphincter (Car & Roman 1970b; Levitt, Dedo, & Ogura, 1965; Murakami, Fukuda, & Kirchner, 1972; Shipp, Deatsch, & Robertson, 1970), passive forces resulting from the viscoelastic properties of the tissue (Jacob, Kahrilas, Herzon, & McLaughin, 1990) and compression by adjacent structures. Tonic contraction of the cricopharyngeus muscle, like the generation of tone in the pharyngeal and parapharyngeal musculature, arises from the tonic discharge of the somatic motor nerves that arise in the brain stem. Tonic contraction of the upper esophageal sphincter is depressed in deep sleep and by anesthesia (Kahrilas et al., 1987), fluctuates with respiration (Car & Roman, 1970b; Levitt, Dedo, & Ogura, 1965; Kawasaki, Ogura, & Takenouchi, 1964), and increases with esophageal distention (Creamer & Schlegel, 1957; Enzmann, Harell, & Zboralske, 1977).

Opening of the Esophageal Inlet

The esophageal inlet opens as the upper esophageal sphincter muscle relaxes and is pulled forward during laryngeal ascent. Relaxation of the sphincter results from the cessation of tonic discharges of the somatic motor innervation to the cricopharyngeus and inferior pharyngeal constrictor. This is seen as the cessation of electromyographically recorded spikes from these muscles during swallow-induced relaxation of the sphincter (Asoh & Goyal, 1978; Shipp, Deatsch, & Robertson, 1970). The passive components of upper sphincter closure are overpowered by two processes (Cook et al., 1989; Jacob, Kahrilas, Herzon, & McLaughlin, 1990; Lang, Dantas, Cook, & Dodds, 1991). contraction of the infrahyoid and suprahyoid musculature elevates the hyoid and laryngeal structures and displaces them anteriorly to produce traction on the anterior portion of the sphincter. In addition, pressures generated in the bolus by the tongue and the pharyngeal musculature distend the sphincter segment. The inhibition of upper esophageal sphincter tone, passive opening of the sphincter due to shifts in position of the relevant structures, and the intrabolus pressure, are important for the normal passage of a bolus through the esophageal inlet. Impairment of any one can produce oropharyngeal dysphagia.

The inhibition of upper esophageal sphincteric tone is one manifestation of the central neural inhibition of pharyngeal and certain parapharyngeal muscles prior to initiation of the pharyngeal peristalsis. The powerful, transient contraction of the sphincter following its relaxation results from the patterned discharge of the nerves that produces the pharyngeal phases of deglutition. The tight coordination of the contractile behaviors of the pharyngeal muscles participating in the opening of the upper esophageal sphincter is controlled centrally by outputs from the brainstem swallowing pathway to the different cranial motor nuclei.

Esophageal Motor Function

The Striated Muscle Esophagus

Contraction of the striated muscle portion of the esophagus is controlled entirely by somatic lower motor neurons, the alpha motoneurons arising in the brainstem cranial motor nuclei (Andrew, 1956b; Code & Schlegel, 1968; Figure 3–2). Because this innervation is excitatory only, the absence of contraction in the striated muscle esophagus at rest reflects inactivity of these motor neurons. Swallow-induced peristaltic contractions of the striated muscle esophagus result from the sequential firing of these somatic nerves so that the muscles are activated in a rostrocaudal sequence along the esophagus (Goyal & Gidda, 1981; Goyal & Paterson, 1989; Hellemans & Vantrappen, 1967; Hellemans, Vantrappen, & Janssens, 1974; Hellemans, Vantrappen, Valembois, Janssens, & Vandenbroucke, 1968; Roman, 1966, 1986; Roman & Gonella, 1981; Roman & Tieffenbach, 1972; Sarna, Daniel, & Waterfall, 1977; Snape & Cohen, 1978; Tieffenbach & Roman, 1972).

A proximal bilateral vagotomy abolishes peristalsis in the striated muscle segment, but unilateral vagotomy does not (Binder et al., 1968; Carveth, Schlegel, & Code, 1962; Higgs & Ellis, 1965; Price, El-Sharkawy, Mui, & Diamant, 1979; Roman, 1966; Ueda, Schlegel, & Code, 1972), indicating that there is overlap of the peripheral motor innervation of the esophagus. Stimulation of the peripheral ends of the severed vagi causes the simultaneous contraction of the circular muscle of the striated muscle esophagus, not esophageal peristalsis (Gidda, Cobb, & Goyal, 1981). More direct physiological evidence has been provided by studies in which one vagus nerve was left intact while the central end of the other vagus nerve, which was severed, was used to reinnervate the sternomastoid muscles. Swallowing resulted in a sequential activation of the reinnervated motor units of the sternocleidomastoid which occurred simultaneously with peristalsis of the striated muscle esophagus (Roman, 1966).

Esophageal sensory afferents influence peristalsis in the striated muscle esophagus (Burgess, Kelly, Schlegel, & Ellis, 1969; Burgess, Schlegel, & Ellis, 1972; Clerc & Mei, 1985; Hollis & Castell, 1975; Jordan & Longhi, 1971; Longhi & Jordan, 1971). Esophageal distention initiates peristaltic contractions in the striated muscle esophagus. Bilateral proximal vagotomy abolishes this response, indicating that the sensory input must proceed to the central nervous system as part of the peristaltic reflex. These data also support the hypothesis that the progressive nature of the peristalsis results from central programming (Roman, 1966). There are minor variations in the characteristics of peristalsis in the striated muscle as a function of changes in bolus volume and temperature, indicating that sensory afferent inputs are capable of modulating the central vagal output that controls peristalsis in the striated muscle esophagus (Dodds, Hogan, Reid, Steward, & Arndorfer, 1973; Janssens, Valembois, Hellemans, Vantrappen, & Pelemans, 1974; Janssens, Valembois, Vantrappen, Hellemans, & Pelemans, 1973; Jordan & Longhi, 1971; Longhi & Jordan, 1971; Roman & Tieffenbach, 1972).

The Smooth Muscle Esophagus

There is no tonic or phasic contractile activity in the smooth muscle esophagus at rest. Swallow-induced peristaltic contractions of the smooth muscle segment of the esophagus, as in the striated muscle segments, are initiated centrally because bilateral cervical vagotomy abolishes them. Peristaltic contractions of the smooth muscle esophagus, unlike the striated muscle segment, do not arise from a programmed sequence of activation in central cranial motor nuclei: Electrical stimulation of the peripheral end of a severed vagus nerve initiates a progressive, rather than a simultaneous, contraction of the smooth muscle segment (Dodds, Christensen, Dent, Wood, & Arndorfer, 1978, 1979; Dodds et al., 1978; Gidda & Goyal, 1983a; Mukhopadhyay & Weisbrodt, 1975). Thus, the central swallowing center appears to be responsible for triggering

peristalsis in the smooth muscle segment, but not for organizing the progressive nature of the contraction (Figures 3–3 and 3–4). The progressive nature of peristalsis in the smooth muscle segment depends on a programming mechanism within the esophagus.

The role of the swallowing center as the trigger for peristalsis in the smooth muscle esophageal muscle is supported by the finding that successive pharyngeal swallows can inhibit peristaltic contractions already initiated in the smooth muscle and striated muscle segments (Dodds, Stef, & Hogan, 1976). Several lines of evidence support the hypothesis that peristaltic contractions of the smooth muscle esophagus are programmed peripherally. Peristalsis induced by esophageal distention in the smooth muscle esophagus is not abolished by bilateral ligation of the vagi (Kravitz, Snape, & Cohen, 1966; Ryan, Snape, & Cohen, 1977). Moreover, the smooth muscle segment of the opossum

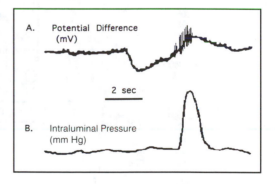

Figure 3–3. Schematic drawing demonstrating a simultaneous recording of myoelectrical activity (A) and intraesophageal pressure (B) at one location in the smooth muscle esophagus during swallow-induced peristalsis. Swallowing produces an immediate hyperpolarization of the circular smooth muscle membrane potential along the length of the smooth muscle esophagus. The hyperpolarization is followed by membrane depolarization and spike potentials. The increase in intraluminal pressure caused by circular muscle contraction correlates temporally with the spike potentials.

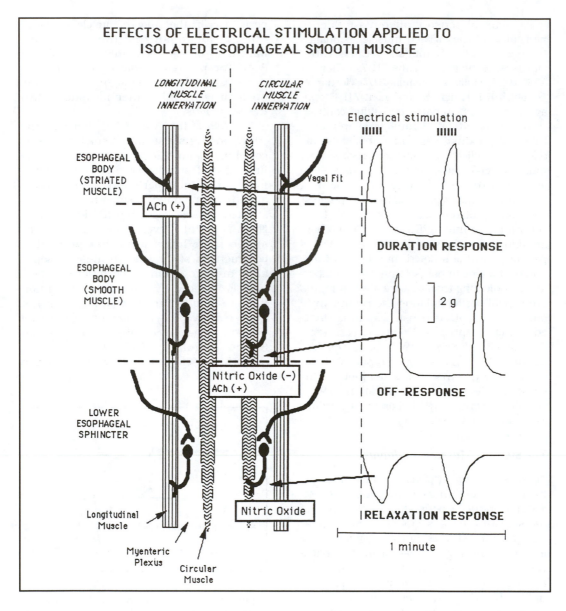

Figure 3–4. Schematic diagram indicating the effect of applying electrical field stimulation to different isolated strips of smooth muscle from the esophagus. Applying stimulation for several seconds to the longitudinal muscle induces contraction during stimulation labeled the "duration response." The duration response is due to activation of cholinergic excitatory nerve fibers. Applying stimulation to the circular esophageal muscle does not induce contraction until the stimulus turns off and is called the "off-response." There is a time delay between the end of the stimulus and the begining of the off-response that is called the latency. The duration of the latency increases along the length of the smooth muscle esophagus, such that the shortest latency is in muscle strips taken from near the junction of the smooth and striated muscle and the longest latency is in strips taken from adjacent to the lower esophageal sphincter. To some extent, the off-response depends upon both nitric oxide and cholinergic innervation. Applying electrical stimulation to circular muscle from the lower esophageal sphincter (LES), relaxes the muscle inducing a "relaxation response." The relaxation results from stimulation of intrinsic nerve fibers secreting nitric oxide.

esophagus can generate peristaltic contractions *in vitro* when isolated from the central nervous system: Simply pinching the esophageal muscle, distending a balloon in the lumen of the esophagus, or stimulation of the intrinsic nerves simultaneously throughout the length of the smooth muscle segment by an electrical field initiates a peristaltic sequence (Christensen, 1970a, 1978; Christensen & Lund, 1969).

Swallowing produces shortening of the esophagus that, like peristalsis, progresses in a rostrocaudal sequence, but occurs ahead of the peristaltic contraction (Sugarbaker, Rattan, & Goyal 1984b, Edmundowicz & Clouse 1991). The shortening is greater and lasts longer in the distal esophagus than in the proximal esophagus. It results from contraction of the longitudinal muscle layer, the distal half of which is composed of smooth muscle. Longitudinal muscle contraction occurs when nerves from the brainstem motor nuclei activate nerves that are intrinsic to the esophagus. These intrinsic esophageal neurons supply the longitudinal muscle layer and release acetylcholine when activated.

PERISTALSIS THROUGH THE TRANSITION ZONE. The striated muscle of the proximal esophagus begins to be infiltrated and replaced by smooth muscle about 4 cm caudal to the cricopharyngeus muscle in humans. Smooth muscle fibers progressively replace the striated muscle in the mid esophagus, and its caudal half is all smooth muscle. Peristaltic contractions sweep through this transition zone without a break. Computer simulations of esophageal peristalsis based on simultaneous radiographic and manometric measurements of esophageal peristalsis show that two contractile processes produce esophageal peristalsis (Brasseur & Dodds, 1991). One contractile sequence arises in the striated muscle esophagus and dies out over the transition zone. The other contractile sequence begins in the transition zone and strengthens in the smooth muscle segment. The uniformity of progression results from the overlap of these two contraction-generating systems. The swallowing center coordinates

the two contractile sequences by appropriately setting the timing of excitation of the somatic nerves to the striated muscles and the inhibitory nerves to the smooth muscle.

NEURAL INHIBITION OF THE LOWER ESOPHAGEAL SPHINCTER. When swallowing is not occurring, the stomach is partitioned from the esophagus by both a tonic contraction of the smooth muscle of the lower esophageal sphincter and contraction of the diaphragm (Altschuler, Boyle, Nixon, Pack, & Cohen, 1985; Mittal, Rochester & McCallum, 1988). Tonic contraction of the lower esophageal sphincter is due primarily to intrinsic properties of the muscle and is not the result of continuous neural activity since the muscle maintains tone when it is isolated from all central connections and is exposed to the neurotoxin tetrodotoxin. The lower esophageal sphincter begins to relax approximately 2 to 3 sec after initiation of the swallow, well after the peristaltic contraction begins in the proximal esophageal body. Its relaxation lasts 5 to 10 sec and may be followed by a transient contraction that represents the termination of the peristaltic contraction that sweeps the esophageal body. The muscle then returns to its resting level of tone. Relaxation of the lower esophageal sphincter results from the release of nitric oxide from myenteric nerves that supply its circular smooth muscle. These myenteric nerve cells are stimulated by neurons from the brainstem that are activated as part of the central swallowing program.

AFFERENT PATHWAYS

General Description

Afferent (sensory) pathways from the pharynx and larynx travel to the nucleus solitarius via the glossopharyngeal, trigeminal, and vagus nerves (Doty, 1968). Spinal afferents from the proximal esophagus, although sparse, arise from cervical and dorsal root ganglia (Hudson & Cunningham, 1985). The central projections of the spinal afferents are not known. Vagal afferents arising from within the wall of the esophagus terminate in a specific region on the medial aspect of the solitary tract called the central subnucleus (Altschuler, Bao, Bieger, Hopkins, & Miselis, 1989). Afferents from the rostral esophagus project to the rostral parts of the central subnucleus. The sensory endings of afferent fibers to the pharynx and proximal esophagus innervate muscle spindles that are found in this striated muscle. Tension receptors are thought to send their sensory fibers to the ganglia in the myenteric plexus (Asaad, Abd-El Rahman, Nawar, & Mikhail, 1983).

The sensory fibers innervating the smooth muscle segment of the esophagus are carried in both sympathetic and parasympathetic nerves (Christensen, 1984). The cell bodies of the vagal afferents reside in the nodose ganglia of the vagal nerves. Structures thought to be sensory, the intraganglionic laminar endings, are complex laminar arborizations within ganglia of the myenteric plexus and about the submucosal vessels (Rodrigo et al., 1982; Rodrigo, Hernandez, Vjdal, & Pedrosa, 1975a, 1975b). The esophageal mucosa contains terminal neural structures of various forms.

Sensory Properties of the Face and Oropharynx

Temperature Perception

The face and oral cavity are innervated by branches of the trigeminal nerve (Kerr, 1962). The facial skin is unique compared to the rest of the body skin because unmyelinated sensory fibers (i.e., C fibers) and the smallest myelinated fibers (i.e., A-delta) (Hensel & Huopaniemi, 1969; Iggo, 1969; Poulos, 1971) can supply the facial sensory.

The oral cavity has specific temperature-sensitive sites. When a cold stimulus is applied to that temperature-sensitive region, the subject recognizes the cold stimulus. These sites can be small (often 1 mm or less in diameter) so that the cold-sensitive sites, like those of the skin, presumably represent small regions innervated by a sensory fiber or fibers that respond to

the cold stimulus (Yamada, 1966, 1967). Warm spots also exist within the intraoral cavity. They are relatively discrete regions to which a fine probe of a certain temperature must be applied for the subject to perceive the stimulus. Most cold receptors innervating cold spots on the facial skin are beneath the surface (about 150–200 microns). Studies of cold spots on the tongue indicate that their receptive fields are 1 mm or less, are within 200 microns of the tongue surface, and are often innervated by the smallest myelinated fibers.

Temperature-sensitive spots appear to be in higher density in the anterior region of the mouth and are even more numerous on the facial skin than in the mouth. There is more representation and innervation of temperature-sensitive neurons in the regions of the tongue and palate that contact each other.

The sensory fibers that innervate the receptive fields for cold and warm spots discharge over a range of temperatures. A sensory fiber innervating a cold spot may respond to temperatures ranging from 17–37° C, whereas a fiber innervating a warm spot may respond to temperatures on the range of 30–43° C. A cold stimulus applied to a cold spot will increase the discharge of the sensory fiber innervating that region. In contrast, applying warmth to a cold spot will decrease the spontaneous discharge of the sensory fiber.

A few sensory fibers appear to respond to both temperature changes and mechanical stimuli (Burton, Terashima, & Clark, 1972). They are larger than the smallest myelinated fibers (i.e., A-delta) and are designated as medium-sized sensory fibers (i.e., A-beta). These fibers innervate the facial skin and the tongue and respond with increased discharges when the tongue is deformed or the temperature is shifted over the cooler temperatures (Poulos, 1971, Poulos & Lende, 1970).

Mechanoreceptors

The oral cavity is also innervated by sensory fibers that respond primarily to touch and pressure. Mechanical stimuli are perceived over many more regions of the oral cavity than are thermal stimuli. The tongue has a high density of mechanosensitive neurons. These mechanosensitive sites and their innervating sensory fibers are of two types: Those that respond only when the stimulus is applied and removed (i.e., fast adapting) and those that discharge as long as the stimulus remains (i.e., slow adapting). The most sensitive sites for the perception of light touch are the tip of the tongue and regions of the hard palate (Henken & Banks, 1967). These light touch-sensitive sites found are in higher numbers in the midline of the tongue and hard palate and become less dense laterally in each structure.

In terms of numerical representation, mechanosensitive sites are most numerous in the oral cavity, followed by chemosensitive sites, with the least representation devoted to thermosensitive sites. The most effective way to excite the mechanosensitive sensory fibers of the oral region is to apply the stimulus in a dynamic mode; that is, applying pressure with oscillating force will induce a more dynamic firing pattern from the sensory fiber.

Sensory Properties of the Pharynx and Larynx

The sensory innervation of the pharynx and larynx is distinctively different from that of the oral region, with the pharynx and larynx having more free nerve endings innervating the epithelium and fewer deep pressure-sensing mechanoreceptors (Andrew, 1956a; Sampson & Eyzaguirre, 1964; Sessle & Lucier, 1983; Storey, 1968a, 1968b). Among the mechanosensitive fibers of the oral, pharyngeal, and laryngeal regions, the fast-adapting fibers are most prominent within the oral cavity, and the slow adapting mechanoreceptors (which discharge throughout the duration of the stimulus) are most prominent on the epiglottis. Over the receptive fields of the glossopharyngeal nerve, vibration stimulates the mechanosensitive fibers to discharge at a higher rate than simple pressure, indicating again that dynamic stimulation is more effective in inducing a sensory fiber to respond.

Sensory Input Evoking Pharyngeal Swallowing

Each sensory fiber possesses specific membrane properties and receptors at its terminal that allow it to respond to a particular type of stimulus (Shinghai & Shimada, 1976). The sensory fiber transforms a stimulus into neuronal activity. However, the stimulus per se is not the key factor determining whether pharyngeal swallowing will be evoked or facilitated by a sensory input. We know this because not all receptive sites in the oral cavity, pharynx, and larynx are equally efficacious in evoking pharyngeal swallowing (Storey, 1968a, 1968b). Variations in the efficacy of a stimulus to provoke pharyngeal swallowing occurs because sensory afferent fibers that supply different receptive fields project central synaptic connections to different loci in the brain stem at the level of the medulla and/or pons. This means that a stimulus must activate sensory fibers that synapse at specific central neural sites to evoke or facilitate swallowing. Stimuli applied over the receptive field of the superior laryngeal (SLN) are the most effective in initiating pharyngeal swallowing (Doty, 1968; Miller & Dunmire, 1976; Miller & Loizzi, 1974; Storey, 1968a, 1968b). Activating fibers of the glossopharyngeal nerve (IX) can evoke swallowing, but their threshold to induce swallowing is higher (Snape, 1970, 1971). Stimulation of trigeminal fibers (V) innervating the oral region is unlikely to evoke swallowing (Lazara, Lazzara, & Logemann, 1986; Rosenbek, Robbins, Fishback, & Levine, 1991); and when the lingual nerve is stimulated, swallowing may even be inhibited after its initiation (Miller, 1982, 1986).

The type or modality of sensory input that evokes swallowing is also related directly to where the sensory fiber synapses within the CNS. Some sensory fibers bifurcate to synapse within the nucleus tractus solitarius (NTS) and more rostrally in the pons at the level of the supratrigeminal nucleus (Car, Jean, & Roman,

1975; Sumi, 1972a, 1972b). Mechanosensitive sensory fibers synapse mainly within the main trigeminal nucleus of the trigeminal nerve and some within the nucleus tractus solitarius. In terms of numbers alone, mechanical stimulation in the periphery excites more neurons of the trigeminal nucleus and nucleus of the tractus solitarius (NTS) than any other type of stimulus. Sensory fibers that are sensitive to chemical stimulation synapse both within the trigeminal sensory nuclei, particularly the spinal trigeminal nucleus, and the nucleus of the tractus solitarius (Sessle, 1973a, 1973b; Sessle & Henry, 1989; Sessle & Lucier, 1983). Chemical stimuli are the second-most effective activators of neural activity in these brainstem nuclei. The taste receptive sensory fibers synapse primarily within the nucleus tractus solitarius (Halpern & Nelson. 1965). Water receptors could be considered among these taste receptors (Shinghai & Shimada, 1976). A large number of central neurons throughout the trigeminal sensory nuclei (i.e., main sensory and spinal trigeminal nuclei) respond to both mechanical and cooling stimuli suggesting that some of these sensory inputs converge on the first central neurons (Torvik, 1956). Thermal stimuli are the least effective activators of central neurons within the brain stem.

Although sensory inputs synapse within both the trigeminal sensory nuclei and the nucleus of the tractus solitarius, only the sensory input to the nucleus of the tractus solitarius and its surrounding reticular formation initiates swallowing. Neurons within the nucleus of the tractus solitarius appear to be multimodal in their responses (Porter, 1963; Rudomin, 1968; Sessle, 1973a, 1973b): that is, several different types of stimuli can excite them (Miller & Sherrington, 1916). Sensory inputs from receptors for taste and some mechanosensation are carried from the anterior and posterior tongue by sensory fibers that synapse mainly in the nucleus of the tractus solitarius. The chorda tympani branch of the facial nerve, innervating the anterior tongue, and the glossopharyngeal branch, innervating the posterior one third of the tongue, send their sensory fibers carrying taste and some mechanosensation to the rostral nucleus tractus solitarius (Kerr, 1963, Rhoton, O'Leary, & Ferguson, 1966). The glossopharyngeal nerve innervates the dorsal and lateral surfaces of the posterior tongue, the posterior and lateral walls of the pharynx, the soft palate, the peritonsillar areas, and the posterior pillars. The fibers of the glossopharyngeal nerve supplying these regions carry mechanosensory input and taste including sensory input from water receptors (Shinghai & Shimada, 1976; Sinclair, 1970, 1971).

Some sensory fibers that synapse within the nucleus tractus solitarius bifurcate to send an ascending axon into the pons and rostrally to the cortex (Beckstead, Morse, & Norgren, 1980; Car, Jean, & Roman, 1975; Pritchard, Hamilton, Mors, & Norgren, 1986). Thus, some sensory inputs that initiate swallowing by activating the brainstem pathway are also transmitted to regions of the cortex that facilitate the initiation of swallowing. It is possible that during repeated swallowing a descending signal from cortical sites associated with swallowing decreases the threshold to evoke swallowing (Car, 1970, 1977). Experimental work in rabbits and monkeys demonstrates that simultaneous stimulation of specific cortical regions and a peripheral nerve, like the superior laryngeal nerve, will induce more swallows than stimulating either alone (Sumi, 1969).

The stimulation of several oral and pharyngeal regions with touch/pressure can elicit swallowing. The likelihood that a stimulus at given site will evoke a swallow is a function of the amount of pressure applied to the region. Light pressure applied to the anterior pillars evokes swallowing from approximately 50% of normal subjects (Pommerenke, 1928). This is the anatomical site that, when stimulated, elicits swallowing in the highest percentage of subjects. Heavy pressure is a more effective stimulus over the posterior pharyngeal wall, eliciting swallowing in approximately 50% of normal people. Fluids are most effective in eliciting swallowing when applied in the laryngeal region and, secondarily, around the portal region of the pharynx (Miller & Sherrington 1916; Storey, 1968a, 1968b). The most effective sites for thermal stimulation to induce swallowing are not known.

Criteria for a Sensory Input That Will Effectively Evoke Pharyngeal Swallowing or Facilitate Swallowing

If a sensory input is to be effective in evoking swallowing, several factors may be important. The stimulus must excite several receptive fields of a group of sensory fibers. The stimulus is most effective if it is applied in a dynamic, not a static, fashion; and vibration is more effective than constant pressure. The sensory fibers that are activated by a stimulus must provide a pattern of sensory input over a group of sensory fibers. The stimulus must activate sensory fibers that synapse within the nucleus of the tractus solitarius and its subjacent reticular formation. The cortical region associated with swallowing may be critical for eliciting swallowing or decreasing the threshold to the elicitation of swallowing by peripheral sensory inputs. It also may facilitate repeated swallowing. The cortical facilitation of swallowing may occur because repeated sensory stimuli recruit a cortical reflex arc that alters the brainstem threshold for eliciting swallowing. Fibers of the superior laryngeal nerve, many of which are responsive to liquids, carry the most effective sensory inputs to evoke swallowing.

With this information about the peripheral sensory system, we can evaluate the central neural pathway and review the evidence for its location and properties within the brain stem.

CENTRAL NEURAL STRUCTURES MODULATING SWALLOWING AND PERISTALSIS

Concepts About the Central Pattern Generator

Studies at the turn of the 20th century using electrical stimulation directly applied to the central nervous system provided the first demonstration that pharyngeal swallowing could be elicited from various regions of the CNS. Swallowing was elicited by stimulating selected areas of the cortex, certain deep subcortical sites like the amygdala and hypothalamus, and the brain stem (Miller & Sherrington, 1916). In many of these experiments, the brain stem and spinal cord were separated from the more rostral regions so that a completely unanesthetized and immobilized animal could be studied. Such studies indicated that swallowing was evoked when the lower part of the decerebrated preparation, the brain stem, was stimulated. In the 1960s, various investigators in France, Japan, the United States, and Canada began to study the brainstem region more thoroughly using electrical lesioning (selective ablation of neural structures), electrical recording, electrical stimulation, and microinjections of transmitters applied to local CNS regions to determine the sites most relevant and critical to pharyngeal and esophageal swallowing.

The logic used to determine the central neural pathway of swallowing arises from four ideas:

1. Electrical lesions in selected regions of the central nervous system should stop or interrupt the pharyngeal and/or esophageal stage of swallowing elicited by stimulating sensory and cortical inputs (Doty, Richmond, & Storey, 1967; Jean, 1972a, Weerasuriya, Bieger, & Hockman 1980). Ablating specific regions of the brain stem did interrupt swallowing, but studies of this type could not determine whether the lesion destroyed sensory fibers, cortical descending inputs, or the actual interneurons that control swallowing.

2. Microelectrode recordings made in or near single neurons of the brain stem must show that these neurons discharge in association with some external event related to swallowing, like the mylohyoid muscle contracting or esophageal muscle contraction (Jean, 1972b; Kessler & Jean, 1985b; Sumi,

1963–1964). Such recordings indicate that neurons in selected regions of the brain stem are activated at different times during swallowing. Some neurons discharge before or during the pharyngeal stage, other interneurons discharge at the start of the esophageal stage, and additional interneurons discharge very late in the esophageal stage (Figure 3–5). Data such as these are difficult to interpret because it is not possible to relate the pattern of activation of an interneuron to the role it plays in the initiation or patterning of swallowing. Are these interneurons initiating the sequential activation of pharyngeal and esophageal motoneurons, or are they among the interneurons that switch signals to the different motor nuclei (Tell et al., 1990)?

3. Electrical stimulation should directly excite neurons that are a part of the swallowing pathway (Car & Roman, 1970a; Jean & Car, 1979; Miller, 1972a; Roman & Car, 1967, 1970). Activation of the superior laryngeal nerve is the first step in a pathway that can induce swallowing, while stimulation of the glossopharyngeal (IXth) and trigeminal sensory nerves facilitate or inhibit the elicitation of swallowing. Electrical stimulation in various regions of the central nervous system (i.e., specific sites of the cortex, parts of the limbic pathway) and regions of the brain stem that include both the pons and medulla, evoke swallowing. Electrical stimulation of the motor nuclei sending motoneurons to muscles that are activated during the pharyngeal stage of swallowing produces contraction of those muscles, but it does not evoke pharyngeal swallowing. These findings suggest that, to initiate swallowing, an electrical stimulus must either excite the interneurons that drive or generate the sequential neuronal activation that produces swallowing or it must excite a pathway that synapses on the interneurons controlling swallowing. Swallowing is not elicited by an electrical stimulus that activates neurons downstream from these interneurons.

4. The local injection of potential synaptic transmitters in the swallowing pathway should evoke pharyngeal and esophageal swallowing (Bieger, 1984, 1991; Bieger, Weerasuriya, & Hockman, 1978; Kessler & Jean, 1991). Antagonists to these transmitters should prevent swallowing from being evoked by the stimulation of peripheral nerves or descending cortical pathways that normally elicit swallowing. These concepts are explored more fully later in this chapter.

Medullary Regions Involved in the Central Neural Pathway of Swallowing

Dorsal Region

Work done over the years in the laboratory of Andre Jean predominantly led to a working hypothesis that two regions of the brain stem are essential for the central control of the pharyngeal and esophageal phases of swallowing: One is in the dorsal region of the brain stem above the nucleus of the tractus solitarius and the other is in a more ventral site around the nucleus ambiguus (Jean, 1984, 1986, 1990; Kessler & Jean, 1985b, Jean, Kessler, & Tell, 1994) (Figure 3–6).

The following evidence suggests that the dorsal region of the medulla, around the nucleus tractus soliterius, is a vital part of the central neural control of the pharyngeal and esophageal stages of swallowing.

1. Sensory fibers innervating regions of the pharynx and larynx that evoke swallowing when stimulated, primarily fibers carried in the superior laryngeal nerve, synapse in the nucleus of the tractus solitarius and the adjacent reticular area of the dorsal region of the brain stem (Altschuler, Bao, Bieger, Hopkins, & Miselis, 1989; Jean & Puizillout, 1986). Lesions in the dorsal medullary region prevent electrical stimulation of the ipsilateral superior laryngeal nerve from evoking the pharyngeal and esophageal phases of swallowing. This means that sensory fibers of the

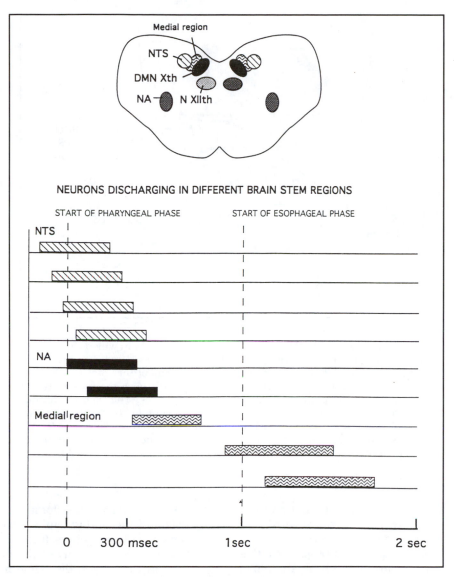

Figure 3–5. Schematic diagram depicting the cross-section of the medulla (*top*) in which specific sensory and motor nuclei are located. Extracellular recordings (*bottom*) from these regions by Jean (1972) indicate that neurons discharge both laterally and medially around the tractus solitarius and around the nucleus ambiguus. Neurons around the nucleus tractus solitarius can discharge (*length of hatched boxes on lower graph*) before the first muscle active in the pharyngeal stage and during various periods of the pharyngeal stage. Neurons around the nucleus ambiguus (*dark gray boxes*) discharge mainly during the pharyngeal phase. Neurons located in a "medial region" to the tractus solitarius discharge (*wavy line boxes*) during the late stages of the pharyngeal stage, or during different stages of the esophageal stage. The neurons are not sensory or motor neurons and will discharge even if the actual muscle contractions do not occur suggesting that they are an integral part of the central swallowing pathway. Abbreviations are: NTS = nucleus of the tractus solitarius; DMN Xth = dorsal motor nucleus of the vagus nerve (Xth); NA = nucleus ambiguus; N XIIth = hypoglossal nucleus of the XIIth cranial nerve; medial region = that area between the NTS and DMN Xth.

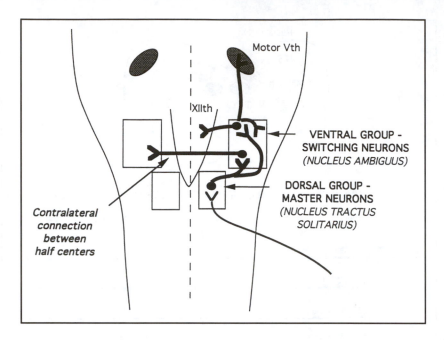

Figure 3–6. A schematic dorsal view of the brain stem in which the concept of the two primary sites composing the brainstem swallowing pathway are illustrated. The "dorsal region" around the nucleus of the tractus solitarius is hypothesized to contain the "master neurons," those neurons triggered into starting the pharyngeal and esophageal stages. The "ventral region" around the nucleus ambiguus is suggested to contain the "switching neurons," which send axons to other motor nuclei on the ipsilateral side and axons to the contralateral side to provide bilateral and overlapping control of the pharyngeal and esophageal muscles.

superior laryngeal nerve do not cross to the contalateral side before synapsing in the dorsal medullary region.

2. The sensory inputs that project into this dorsal medullary region have a minimal synaptic delay of 2–4 msec.

3. The specific cortical site that evokes swallowing when activated by electrical stimulation sends fibers to synapse in this same dorsal region of the brain stem, and lesions in the dorsal region prevent electrical stimulation of the cortex from evoking the pharyngeal and esophageal stages of swallowing. These data indicate that the dorsal region is at least a part of the central pathway controlling swallowing, most likely the initial neural entrance or afferent portal for inputs that modulate swallowing.

4. Interneurons in this dorsal medullary region of the brain stem are excited by sensory afferent fibers from the pharynx and larynx. Many of the interneurons in this region discharge in a patterned sequence at specific times during the pharyngeal and esophageal stages of swallowing. These data suggest that the dorsal region contains the first synaptic sites for the sensory inputs that evoking swallowing and that these interneurons, once excited, discharge at specific times during pharyngeal and esophageal swallowing. These bursts of sequential activity in the dorsal region occur even when sensory feedback from contraction of the pharyngeal and esophageal muscles is lost. This finding suggests that, when triggered into ac-

tion, the dorsal interneurons go through a preprogrammed pattern of activation. Jean's group refers to these dorsal interneurons as the "master" interneurons that set up a sequential pattern of activation which is transmitted to specific cranial motor nuclei.

5. The dorsal medullary region receives two types of sensory input. one type of sensory feedback is from mucosal receptors in the pharynx that respond to touch, pressure, chemicals, and water triggers. These sensory inputs facilitate the initiation and repeated activation of the pharyngeal stage of swallowing. The other type of sensory feedback is from mechanical receptors innervating the muscles that are activated during pharyngeal and esophageal swallowing. This sensory input affects the interneurons in the dorsal region that modify the motor output to muscles in the region from which the sensory information came. For example, an interneuron that discharges during the early esophageal stage of swallowing receives input when the upper esophagus is distended but not when the lower esophagus is distended.

6. A specific subarea of the dorsal region, an area between the tractus solitarius and the dorsal motor nucleus of the vagus, allows sensory inputs that initiate pharyngeal swallowing to elicit esophageal swallowing as well (Jean, 1972a, 1978). Electrical stimulation of the superior laryngeal nerve evokes both the pharyngeal and esophageal stages of swallowing. When this subarea is destroyed on one side of the brain stem, activation of the ipsilateral superior laryngeal nerve elicits the pharyngeal stage but not the esophageal stage of swallowing. Stimulation of the superior laryngeal nerve contralateral to the damaged subarea of the dorsal region still evokes both a pharyngeal and esophageal stage.

7. The microinjection of certain neurochemicals into the dorsal region evokes swallowing, whereas the microinjection of other chemicals inhibits the reflex elicitation of swallowing, as described later.

Medullary Regions Involved in the Central Neural Pathway of Swallowing

Ventral Region

The ventral region of the brain stem (i.e., the area around the nucleus ambiguus) also is involved in the swallowing pathway. This is not an accessory or supplemental area of control like certain subcortical areas or regions of the pons, but is a vital part of the central neural control of swallowing. Some of the evidence for this concept includes the following observations.

1. Sensory input from the superior laryngeal nerve reaches both the ventral and the dorsal regions of the brain stem; however, the synaptic pathways to the ventral region are longer than those to the dorsal region (7–12 msec). These data indicate that sensory inputs that elicit swallowing can affect the ventral region. Sensory inputs to this region may serve to modify the motor output during swallowing, and provide reflex control of laryngeal muscles. These observations do not mean that the pharyngeal stage of swallowing is triggered by sensory inputs at this ventral site.

2. Selected cortical regions that evoke swallowing when stimulated electrically send synaptic inputs to the ventral region. They project more synaptic inputs to the ventral region than to the dorsal region, and the latencies of these synaptic inputs are longer than those in the dorsal region. This information suggests that these cortical regions may modify the swallowing pathway or modulate the output of its motoneurons.

3. Excitation of interneurons in the ventral group by sensory inputs from the superior laryngeal nerve is prevented by selective lesions in the dorsal region of the medulla. This means that the dorsal group relays sensory inputs to the ventral region.

4. Neural elements of the ventral region around the nucleus ambiguus make extensive synaptic connections with

other neural structures associated with swallowing:

a. axons synapse in other motor nuclei involved in swallowing like the hypoglossal nucleus and the motor trigeminal nucleus (Jean, Amri, & Calas, 1983), and

b. axons connect with the contralateral brainstem region involved with swallowing.

5. Microelectrode recordings from the ventral region indicate that interneurons and motoneurons in the nucleus ambiguus discharge at specific times during the sequential activation of the pharyngeal and esophageal musculature during swallowing (Jean, 1978).

6. Removal of one cranial motor nucleus like the hypoglossal nucleus does not alter the sequential activation of motoneurons in other cranial motor nuclei, but the effects of lesions placed in the ventral region are not known.

Neuroanatomical Correlates— Medullary Circuitry

The anatomical identity of dorsal and ventral swallowing interneurons and their synaptic relationships with motoneurons innervating the upper alimentary tract musculature are only partially known at present. However, important clues have come from retro- and anterograde tracing experiments in which the inputs to various cranial nerve motor nuclei were examined (sheep: Amri & Car, 1988; Amri, Car & Jean, 1984; Amri, Car & Roman, 1990; Jean, Amri, & Calas, 1983; cat: Holstege et al., 1983; Loewy & Burton, 1978; monkey: Beckstead, Morse, & Norgren, 1980). In agreement with electrophysiological findings in sheep, dorsal group interneurons apparently lack direct connections with hypoglossal and trigeminal motoneurons (Amri & Car, 1988; Amri et al., 1984; Jean et al., 1983). Thus, in nonrodent species, projections from the NTS to trigeminal motoneurons have not been demonstrated (Beckstead et al., 1980; King, 1980; Loewy & Burton, 1978, Morest, 1967). The ventral interneurons would therefore appear to be obligatory links between dorsal interneurons and trigeminal motoneurons involved in swallowing. The postulated role of these cells as "switching" elements (Jean, 1984, 1990) or "command interneurons" (Amri & Car, 1988) accords with the observation that their efferent axons project collateral branches to the hypoglossal motor nucleus. The ventral interneurons are said to form part of the rhombencephalic reticular formation lying dorsomedially to the rostral portion of the nucleus ambiguus.

Tracing studies in the rat, however, show a direct linkage between dorsal (solitarial) interneurons and their motoneuronal targets (Norgren, 1978; Traverse & Norgren, 1983). More to the point, efferents from functionally identified deglutitive NTS loci can be traced to virtually all cranial nerve motor nuclei known to contain motoneurons active in swallowing (Hashim, 1989). As well, the premotoneuronal circuitry subserving the esophageal stage of swallowing is similarly organized, in that dorsal group interneurons are monosynaptically linked with esophagomotor neurons. Indeed, the pathway from the NTS subnucleus centralis to ambigual motoneurons is remarkable for its massiveness and the density of its terminal axons (Bieger, 1984, Cunningham & Sawchenko, 1989; Wang, Bieger, & Neuman, 1991). Ventral interneurons controlling esophagomotor output project to both the ambiguus and the solitarius complex (see later sections). Conceivably, reciprocal connections between ventral neurons and subnucleus centralis effect the coupling between the pharyngeal and esophageal stage of swallowing, as the subnucleus centralis reportedly does not receive afferents from other NTS regions (Cunningham & Sawchenko, 1989), including those containing buccopharyngeal stage interneurons.

The subnucleus centralis efferents are confined to the ipsilateral nucleus ambiguus, suggesting that esophageal motoneurons are controlled by ipsilateral interneurons. The converse arrangement has been inferred from split-brainstem experiments for pharyngeal motoneurons innervating the constrictor muscles (Doty et al., 1967).

Deglutitive activation of the inferior and middle constrictors in cats and dogs and of the inferior constrictor in monkeys arises from the contralateral hemimedulla, whereas all other motoneurons pools subserving the buccopharyngeal stage are under the control of the ipsilateral swallowing interneurons. The neuroanatomical correlates of the so-called "crossed constrictor phenomenon" (Doty et al., 1967) remain unknown to date.

Motoneuron pools active in the pharyngeal stage of deglutition also receive afferents from the caudal pontine reticular formation, specifically an area identified in the cat pontine tegmentum dorsomedial to the superior olivary complex (Holstege et al., 1983). The proposal that this area represents a pontine swallowing center does not appear to have much merit because: (a) its projections to brainstem motor nuclei are mainly crossed; (b) it does not overlap with the laterally adjacent deglutitive-masticatory region identified by Sumi (1972), (c) it fails to yield deglutitive responses when electrically stimulated, and (d) it does not contain cells that fire during the elicitation of reflex swallowing (Jean, 1990)

THE MOTOR NUCLEI AND THEIR PROJECTIONS

General Description of the Motor Output to the Striated Muscle Regions

The extrinsic motor nerves to the striated muscle regions of the pharynx and esophagus are somatic, not autonomic. Their nerve cell bodies reside in the brain stem, are defined as alpha motoneurons, and project axons that pass without synaptic interruption to innervate the striated muscle cells through motor end-plates. The neurotransmitter released at the end-plate is acetylcholine which activates nicotinic cholinergic receptors on the striated muscle. The cell bodies of neurons that innervate pharyngeal stage muscles reside in the trigeminal motor nucleus, the facial nerve nucleus, the nucleus ambiguus of

the vagus, the hypoglossal nucleus, and spinal segments Cl to C3. The motor efferents pass through cranial nerves (see Chapter 2). The trigeminal nerve (V) supplies the mylohyoid, tensor veli palatini, and digastric muscles. The facial nerve (VII) supplies the stylohyoid and posterior part of the digastricus. The glossopharyngeal nerve (IX) supplies the stylopharyngeus. The vagus nerve (X) innervates the levator veli palatini, the palatopharyngeus, salpingopharyngeus, thyroarytenoid, the pharyngeal constrictors and cricopharyngeus, as well as the laryngeal muscles and the striated muscle of the esophagus. The hypoglossal (XII) nerve supplies the thyrohyoid and geniohyoid muscles and the accessory nerve fibers (XI) are distributed through a branch to the vagus. The cricopharyngeus muscle is innervated by the vagus through a special branch in dog and cat (Kirchner, 1958; Lund 1965a, 1965b; Murakami, Fukuda, & Kirchner, 1972).

General Description of the Motor Output to the Smooth Muscle Regions

The terminal innervation of the smooth muscle of the esophagus arises outside the central nervous system within ganglia of the autonomic nervous system. The two divisions of the autonomic nervous system, the sympathetic, and parasympathetic. These divisions of the autonomic nervous system differ as to whether the ganglia are close to the central nervous system (sympathetic division) or the organ (parasympathetic division), and as to the origin of the central neurons (i.e., preganglionic) that synapse on the postganglionic neurons. The preganglionic fibers which synapse on these peripheral motoneurons of the autonomic, parasympathetic subdivision arise in the dorsal motor nucleus of the vagus and send their axons through the vagus nerves (Gidda & Goyal, 1983b). These preganglionic parasympathetic fibers synapse within ganglia of the myenteric plexus. They release acetylcholine that activates muscarinic and nicotinic receptors on myenteric neurons (Figure 3–7).

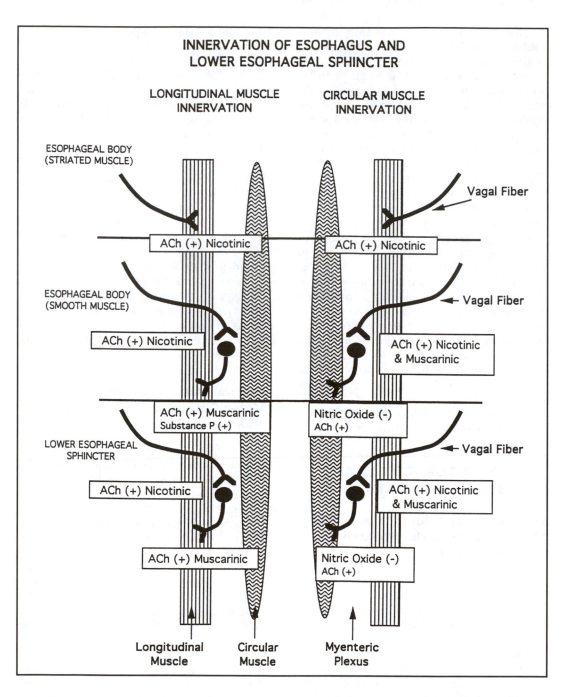

Figure 3–7. A schematic depicting the vagal innervation of the esophagus and lower esophageal sphincter and the intrinsic innervation (i.e., myenteric plexus) with its known or potential transmitters. Both longitudinal and circular muscle are depicted bilaterally but the innervation of the longitudinal muscle is illustrated on the left, and that for the circular muscle, on the right. ACh represents acetylcholine as a transmitter. The "+" symbol indicates that a transmitter excites the muscle to contract, while a "−" symbol indicates the transmitter prevents or stops a muscle from contraction due to its inhibitory influence.

As the vagi descend in the upper chest, they are joined by postganglionic sympathetic nerves passing from the superior cervical ganglion in some species, and from cervical and thoracic ganglia in other animals. Sympathetic fibers also reach the esophagus by way of perivascular nerves and from splanchnic nerves via the celiac ganglia. These sympathetic fibers to the esophageal body originate in preganglionic cells in spinal segments T5 and T6 (Andrew, 1956b; Weisbrodt, 1976). Those to the lower esophageal sphincter arise in spinal segments T6 to T10. Postganglionic sympathetic fibers terminate in the myenteric and submucosal plexuses and very few innervate the muscle directly (Baumgarten & Lange, 1964; Jacobowitz & Nemir, 1969; Cunningham & Sawchenko, 1990).

Functional Anatomy of Deglutitive Motoneurons.

Preparatory Stage

Although several studies have reported on the deglutitive firing patterns of hypoglossal nerve filaments or motoneurons (Car & Amri, 1988; Sumi, 1963, 1967, 1969, 1970; Travers & Jackson, 1992), little information is available on the deglutitive timing and recruitment of motoneurons innervating intrinsic and extrinsic tongue muscle groups during bolus transit through the oral cavity. Such information will have to be sought in unanesthetized, spontaneously feeding animals given the dependence of hypoglossal motor output on bolus variables. To complicate matters further, the tongue makes a critical contribution also to the pharyngeal stage. Extrapolations from anthropoid and nonanthropoid mammals also must take into account the divergent mechanism of bolus formation and preswallow transport. In the human, the preparatory stage may represent a specialized variation of "stage II transport" (Hiiema & Crompton, 1984; Palmer, Rudin, Lara, & Crompton, 1992) is absent. Fairly detailed accounts of the myotopical organization of trigeminal, facial, hypoglossal and hypobranchial motoneurons are available (see below).

Pharyngeal Stage

The relevant motoneuronal groups innervate muscles that (a) close the nasopharynx (levator and tensor veli palatini, palatopharyngeus) and the glottis (thyroarytenoid, lateral cricoarytenoid, aryepiglottic and oblique arytenoid); (b) shorten the pharynx and elevate the larynx (mylohyoid, geniohyoid, anterior digastric, stylohyoid, stylopharyngeus, salpingopharyngeus, thryohyoid), (c) propel the bolus (posterior tongue, hyoglossus, styloglossus); and (d) clear it from the pharyngeal lumen (superior, middle, and inferior pharyngeal constrictors). Opening of the esophageal inlet (pharyngoesophageal sphincter) occurs at the apex of laryngeal elevation (Cook et al., 1989; Kahrilas, Dodds, Dent, Logemann, & Shaker, 1988) and is preceded by a transient cessation of EMG activity and relaxation of active resting tonus in the inferior constrictor (cricopharyngeus and part of the thyropharyngeus) (Hellemans, Pelemans, & Vantrappen, 1981).

The relevant motoneuronal groups are described earlier. By virtue of their location in the motor nuclei of the Vth, VIIth, IXth, Xth, XIIth cranial nerves and the upper cervical (C_1–C_3) nerves, the pharyngeal stage motoneurons constitute an extensive array. However, their distribution is far from being random. A case in point are the motoneurons located in the nucleus ambiguus, which participates in the above substages (a, b, and d) of deglutition, and in all species examined displays a well-defined myotopic pattern, particularly with regard to the representation of the pharyngeal constrictors and laryngeal musculature (Bieger & Hopkins, 1987; Kitamura, Nagase, Chen & Shigenaga, 1993; Lawn, 1964; Molhant, 1911; Szabo & Dussardier, 1964; Yoshida et al., 1979). Pharyngomotor neurons form the bulk of the semicompact formation of the ambiguus complex, with inferior constrictor neurons lying rostrally to middle constrictor neurons and pharyngeal dilator neurons occupying the rostral pole of the complex. An orderly myotopic map of intrinsic tongue and associated substage b and c hypobranchial muscles is no less evident in the hypoglossal and supraspinal nuclei (Krammer, Rath, & Lischka, 19979; Uemura et al., 1979; Sokoloff & Deacon, 1992). Protrusor motoneurons make up ventral, ventromedial or intermediate, and retrusor motoneurons dorsal and dorsolateral columnar groupings, while motoneurons supplying transversely oriented muscle bundles lie medial to those supplying longitudinally oriented muscle groups (superior and inferior longitudinal, stylo-, palato- and hyoglossus). Motoneurons residing in the trigeminal (mylohyoid, anterior digastric, tensor veli palatini) and facial (stylohyoid, posterior digastric, labio-oral group) motor nuclei also show discrete myotopic groupings (Holstege, Graveland, Bijker-Biemond, & Schuddeboom, 1983; Landgren & Olsson, 1976; Matsuda, Uemura, Kume, Matsushima, & Mizuno, 1978; Mizuno et al., 1981; Welt & Abbs, 1990) and, as seen in the rat, occupy contiguous regions of the rhombencephalon.

Esophageal and Gastroesophageal Stage

Motor efferents to the striated tunica propria originate from a cell-dense subdivision of the ventral vagal complex, specifically that designated compact formation (commonly but inappropriately named "retrofacial nucleus") (i.e., the rostral portion of the principal column of the nucleus ambiguus; Bieger & Hopkins, 1987; Lawn, 1964; Molhant, 1912). Motor efferents to the two-layered smooth muscle tunica propria and the tunica muscularis mucosa consist of a two-neuron visceromotor pathway whose preganglionic neurons form part of the dorsal vagal complex (Niel, Gonella, & Roman, 1980) and whose terminal motor ganglia lie in the myenteric nerve plexus of the esophagus (plexus of Auerbach). The reported presence of some smooth muscle preganglionic efferent in the feline ventral vagal complex (Collman, Tremblay, & Diamant, 1993) requires confirmation by anterograde techniques; as well, it could reflect a more distal distribution of striated muscle fibers than presumed by the authors. The vagal pregan-

glionic motor elements are located at two separate levels of the dorsal vagal complex (Collman et al., 1993), suggesting the existence of two populations with dichotomous functional roles. This arrangement pertains to both the esophageal body and the gastroesophageal junction. Functional evidence implicates the caudal neurons as the long-sought origin of vagal fibers that mediate relaxation of the gastroesophageal junction (Rossiter et al., 1990). Caudal DMV neurons projecting to the esophageal body are logical candidates for vagal efferents responsible for *deglutitive inhibition*; those involved in *receptive relaxation* of the stomach would likewise be expected to have a nearby location.

Neurochemical Properties of Deglutitive Motoneurons

It is now well established that special visceral efferents to striated deglutitive muscles contain other putative mediators/ modulators beside acetylcholine. For instance, esophagomotor neurons of the ambigual compact formation (AMB_c) are immunoreactive for calcitonin gene-related peptide (CGRP), galanin, brain natriuretic peptide, and N-acetylaspartylglutamate (for review see Cunningham & Sawchenko, 1990). Furthermore, a subpopulation of rat AMB_c neurons expresses NADPH diaphorase activity, indicative of the presence of nitric oxide synthase. Levels of this nitritergic marker enzyme dramatically increase after injury of the cervical vagal trunk, and the same phenomenon is observed in the dorsal vagal complex (Hopkins, Bieger, de Vente, & Steinbusch, 1994).

Prima facie, the neurons of the dorsal vagal complex deviate even further from the general rule that deglutitive efferent pathways from medullary motor nuclei are essentially cholinergic. In the rat, the caudal neurons contain both choline acetyl transferase and tyrosine-hydroxylase (Armstrong, Manley, Haycock & Hersh, 1990; Manier et al. 1990; Ruggiero, Chau, Anwar, Mtui, & Golanow, 1993), that is, the respective marker enzymes for cholinergic and catecholaminergic cells. The absence of other catecholaminergic markers suggests the dopaminergic nature of these vagal efferents. Axotomy of the dorsal vagal neurons is followed by a rise in preprogalanin mRNA and a loss of tyrosine hydroxylase activity (Rutherfurd, Widdop, Louis, & Gundlach, 1992).

Apart from choline acetyltransferase and acetylcholine esterase, rat esophagomotor neurons possess butyrylcholine esterase activity (Nance, Hopkins, & Bieger, 1987; Tago, Maeda, McGeer, & Kimura, 1992). The latter enzyme also occurs in presumptive protrusor neurons in the hypoglossal nucleus.

Neurophysiology of Deglutitive Motoneurons

Probably all motoneurons active in deglutition participate to varying degrees in other physiological processes such as breathing, coughing, phonation, belching, gagging, retching, and vomiting. The same motoneurons of the Vth or XIIth cranial nerves may display both deglutitive, jaw opening reflex, and masticatory activity (Amri, Lamkadem, & Car, 1991; Car & Amri, 1982), indicative of the inherent multifunctionality of cranial nerve motoneurons. Furthermore, sensory afferent pathways relevant to swallowing also convey inputs utilized by these associated synergies and by the so-called "elementary reflexes." The latter can be thought of as representing segmental building blocks of motor programs organized at the rhombencephalic level (Doty, 1968).

These relationships need to be taken into account when motoneuronal responses are being recorded during reflex swallowing induced by electrical stimulation of the superior laryngeal nerve (SLN) (Sumi, 1969). Thus, at stimulus frequencies or patterns inappropriate for eliciting deglutition, graded excitatory responses occur in hypoglossal neurons at latencies consistent with mediation via an oligosynaptic relay. As the SLN stimulus frequency is increased, hypoglossal EPSPs show summation, leading to transient depolarization. With stimulus patterns in the optimal frequency range, a second, larger depolarizing response and spike discharge are seen that evidently represent deglutitive motor output as judged by its timing in relation to "leading complex" EMG activity. As explained earlier, the motoneuronal activity patterns observed under these conditions probably relate principally to the pharyngeal stage of deglutition (i.e., events normally occurring after stage II bolus transport is completed).

The deglutitive discharge is preceded and accompanied by a suppression of "elementary reflex activity" (Doty & Bosma, 1956), indicative of a collateral inhibition that may serve to disconnect the motoneurons from competing pattern generator circuits. In certain motor fibers or their muscles (viz. the mylohyoid, palatopharyngeus, genioglossus, geniohyoid, cricothyroid, thyrohyoid, middle and inferior pharyngeal constrictors), tonic or phasic (respiratory) activity ceases up to 200 msec before the onset of the pharyngeal stage "leading complex" EMG discharge (Cunningham & Basmajian, 1969; Doty & Bosma, 1956; Doty, Richmond, & Storey, 1967; Miller, 1972). However, no initial inhibition is seen in other muscles of the leading complex, including the posterior tongue, superior pharyngeal constrictor, and palatoglossus.

Extracellular microelectrode studies in sheep and rat by the Marseille group (Amri & Car, 1982; Car & Amri, 1982; Jean, 1972, 1978; Jean, Car, & Roman, 1975; Kessler & Jean, 1985) have provided detailed information about the activity of deglutitive neurons both in and outside the medullary areas known to contain motoneurons. As a general rule, it can be said that deglutitive motoneurons receive oligosynaptic sensory input from the regions of the upper elementary tract whose muscles they innervate. The characteristics of trigeminal motoneurons as identified by antidromic spike production or stimulation of the appropriate peripheral motor nerve branch, include: (a) absence of a resting discharge, (b) variable low frequency spike burst (≤50 Hz) during a SLN-induced swallow, (c) persistence of deglutitive activity during neuromuscular paralysis, (d) absence of a direct response to SLN stimulation; and (e) absence of a direct input from the cortical deglutitive pathway (Amri & Car, 1982; Car & Amri, 1982).

During a SLN-evoked reflex swallow, sheep hypoglossal motoneurons generate a deglutitive discharge that coincides with EMG activity in the geniohyoid muscle (Car & Amri, 1988). Average firing rates vary from 10–70 Hz, with peak instantaneous frequencies of 10–100 Hz. Compared with laterally adjacent swallowing interneurons ("perinuclear group II neurons"), the hypoglossal motoneurons do not show greatly differing latencies to ipsilateral SLN inputs (7–12 ms vs. 10–15 ms). However, as revealed in more recent work (Amri, Lamkadem & Car, 1991), only a minority of hypoglossal motoneurons with deglutitive activity appears to receive short-latency peripheral input via the SLN or lingual nerve. Not all hypoglossal cells discharge during swallowing, and some have spontaneous activity that is suppressed during deglutition. Intracellular recordings in cat hypoglossal neurons support the conclusion that deglutitive activation entails both simple EPSPs and complex EPSP-IPSP sequences (Tomume & Takata, 1099). Cat hypoglossal motoneurons are readily excited via oligosynaptic reflex loops with the SLN (Sumi, 1963, 1967).

Deglutitive motoneurons initially designated type 4 (Jean, 1972) are located in the nucleus ambiguus; they respond at a latency of 6–12 ms to ipsi- but not contralateral, SLN stimulation with a brief initial activity, exhibit an antidromic spike to stimulation of the cervical vagal trunk, and discharge at a mean rate 50 Hz during the buccopharyngeal stage. These attributes fit the description of laryngeal (possibly adductor) motoneurons. Putative ambiguus motoneurons, designated "early type 3" (Jean, 1972), have an initial response to SLN stimulation that resembles that of type 4 neurons; however, deglutitive discharges are characterized by a higher range of firing rates (50–250 Hz). These neurons are found in the caudal ambiguus complex, but their efferent axons do not project via the recurrent

laryngeal nerve. In the awake macaque (Macaca nemestrina), certain laryngeal motoneurons of the caudal nucleus ambiguus fire during a spontaneous swallow with a more vigorous discharge than during vocalization (Yajima & Larson, 1993), again illustrating the mul-tifunctionality of brainstem motor cells. Remarkably, few of these "deglutition-related" motoneurons display a respiratory cycle-related activity pattern.

Initial microelectrode recording studies (Jean, 1972) did not find evidence of esophageal motoneuronal discharges at levels of the sheep ambiguus where electrical microstimulation evokes short-latency esophagomotor responses (Jean, 1972b; Roman & Car 1967). The likely explanation is the failure of SLN-stimulated reflex swallows to propagate along the full length of the esophagus, particularly in the anesthetized animal. Subsequent studies (Jean, 1978, Jean & Car, 1979) have shown that the rostral portion of the nucleus ambiguus contains esophagomotor neurons projecting either via the pharyngoesophageal nerve to the proximal esophagus (type I neurons) or through the vagal trunk and recurrent laryngeal nerve to distal, thoracic and lower cervical segments of the esophagus (type II neurons). Type I but not type II neurons respond at short latency (7–12 msec) to ipsilateral SLN stimulation or cervical esophageal distention. Deglutitive burst activity with impulse rates of 15–40 Hz occurs 200–700 msec after the onset of mylohyoid EMG activity. Type II ambigual motoneurons lack oligosynaptic input from the SLN, discharge between 700 to 2,300 msec after the appearance of mylohyoid activity and produce impulse rates of 10–20 Hz. Their deglutitive discharge is markedly attenuated when the proximal esophagus is distended by a stationary balloon. Conversely, distention-induced tonic firing of type II neurons is interrupted for the duration of the pharyngeal stage of swallowing ("deglutitive inhibition"). The overall picture thus suggests (a) that the deglutitive motoneuron discharge rates progressively decline in the aboral direction; and (b) that distal levels receive inhibitory inputs form proximal levels.

In the rat, extracellular microelectrode mapping studies have revealed buccopharyngeal stage deglutitive discharges in presumptive motoneurons of the hypoglossal and ambiguus nuclei. When activated by ipsilateral SLN stimulation, these cells respond at latencies of 7–12 msec with an initial brief spike discharge and a subsequent 80–300 msec burst of firing that is synchronous with mylohyoid EMG activity or lags behind it for up to 140 msec. Firing rates range between 40 to 250 Hz, with extreme values of 400 Hz (Kessler & Jean, 1985).

The in vivo electrophysiological properties of rat esophagomotor neurons of the nucleus ambiguus compact formation (AMB$_c$) remain to be fully characterized. Based on preliminary work (Lu & Bieger, 1993; Lu, Neuman, & Bieger, 1993a), AMB$_c$ neurons fire rhythmically in a burst-pause pattern that is phase-locked with peristaltic pressure waves, recorded in the same segment from which local distention evokes a reflex discharge. Intracellular recordings from in vitro AMB$_c$ slice preparations demonstrate the absence of spontaneous discharges, the relatively low firing rates of these motoneurons during injection of depolarizing current, and a large spike after-hyperpolarization (Wang, Neuman, & Bieger, 1991a, 1991b; Wang, Bieger, & Neuman, 1991). Motoneuronal EPSPs are elicited from at least two different premotoneuronal afferent inputs. The major of these originates from subnucleus centralis of the solitarius complex, the more diffuse and smaller one from the intermediate reticular formation lying dorsomedial to the rostral pole of the nucleus ambiguus (Wang, Zhang, Neuman, & Bieger, 1993). Interestingly, microstimulation of the solitarioambigual pathway does not generate motoneuronal IPSPs. The solitarioambigual EPSP is complex. An initial high threshold component involves excitatory amino acid receptors (see below) and is though to make a critical contribution to action potential production (Wang, Bieger, & Neuman, 1991). Afferents from the rostral intermediate reticular formation generate EPSPs via nicotinic acetyl-

choline or excitatory amino acid receptors (Wang et al., 1993).

To date, virtually no information is available on the electrophysiological properties of vagal preganglionic neurons that innervate visceromotor ganglia of the smooth muscle esophagus.

PHARMACOLOGY OF SYNAPTIC TRANSMISSION IN CENTRAL DEGLUTITIVE PATHWAYS

General Considerations

The neuropharmacology of deglutition remained anecdotal until the mid-1970s. However, several past findings, not fully appreciated at the time, should be noted. Among these are the depressant effects of morphine (Meltzer, 1899; Wild 1847), myanesine, and nembutal (Doty, 1951) and the opposite action of strychnine (Doty, 1951), as well as Sumi's (1972) observation that GABA or lidocaine applied to the frontal cortex inhibits rhythmic deglutition when it is evoked by stimulation of the pons but not when it is evoked reflexively.

The study of chemical signals utilized by deglutitive neurons gained further impetus from pharmacological data obtained in the rat. In this species, diverse drugs administered by intravascular or other parenteral routes evoke rhythmic fictive swallowing under conditions of complete surgical anesthesia (Bieger, 1991). These observations first implicated specific transmitter receptor systems in CNS deglutitive pathways, principally those associated with brainstem monoamine neurons. As explained further below, receptors for monoamines such as dopamine, norepinephrine, and serotonin mediate quantifiable changes in centrally or reflexively generated, rhythmic swallowing activity. The presence of these receptor systems at different levels of the brain stem and forebrain provides the rationale for mapping their neural substrates by means of receptor-directed probes. The technique of choice for this purpose is pressure microphoresis of neuroactive chemicals from multibarrel glass micropipettes, as it enables patterned deglutitive motor output to be elicited on ejection of the appropriate test substance at doses small enough to provide meaningful topographical information. The advantages of this approach are threefold: (a) it permits identification of premotor substrates that generate deglutitive motor output, unlike microelectrode recordings which do not allow straightforward differentiation between premotor neurons and internuncial elements that generate inhibition of competing networks; (b) use of appropriate drug tools circumvents the problem of inadvertent activation of fibers of passage; and (c) the use of receptor antagonists can be helpful in determining if a particular receptor type is being activated within a specific pathway during a particular stage of swallowing.

Pharmacological investigations have been addressing the identity of neuromediators responsible for deglutitive control at several levels of the neuraxis. At present, interest is focusing on the pattern generator circuitry of the rhombencephalon and its intrinsic components, namely the nucleus of the solitary tract (NTS), the ventral vagal complex, and surrounding areas of the bulbar reticular formation. Relevant neuromediators involved in fast information transfer at this level include the excitatory amino acids, acetylcholine, GABA, and somatostatin.

Some information is also available on extrinsic components that generate central inputs for the modulation of the intrinsic circuitry. These utilize a wide range of neuromediators, including the catecholamines, serotonin, and various neuropeptides. The associated receptor systems operate at the level of segmental deglutitive reflex pathways and suprabulbar inputs from cortical, subcortical, diencephalic, and midbrain sources; most of which are not yet precisely defined (Hockman et al., 1979).

The next sections will briefly outline evidence implicating these putative transmitters and modulators in the neural control of deglutition.

Excitatory Amino Acids (EAA)

When microphoresed into discrete subnuclear regions of the rat NTS, S-glutamate and various EAA receptor agonists produce a diversity of deglutitive responses, encompassing the full-blown swallow sequence, its buccopharyngeal or esophageal components, or fractionation of the latter (Bieger, 1984; Hashim & Bieger, 1987, 1989; Hashim Bolger, & Bieger, 1989). Three general features of these responses are of particular significance: (a) their sharp anatomical localization, (b) their organized pattern, and (c) their potential rhythmicity.

EAA agonist-responsive deglutitive regions of the NTS can be delineated in enough detail to permit a reasonably accurate correlation between responsive loci and NTS subnuclear divisions. Loci that yield short latency complete swallows or the buccopharyngeal stage are coextensive with the intermediate and ventral subnuclei (i.e., the portion of the NTS adjacent to the medial aspect of the solitary tract (Bieger, 1984; Hashim 1989; Hashim & Bieger, 1989). According to a similar mapping study by Kessler and Jean (1991), in which several fold higher S-glutamate doses were employed in 100 to 500 times larger ejectate volumes, swallow response sites extend laterally into the subnuclei interstitialis and ventrolateralis. It thus remains to be determined if swallow-related extracellularly recorded unit activity in the latter two subnuclei (Kessler & Jean, 1985) indeed represents deglutitive premotor activation. Esophageal response loci are essentially confined to the subnucleus centralis (Bieger, 1984; Hashim 1989; Hashim et al., 1989; Hashim & Bieger, 1989) and conform to the rostro-caudal organotopical map of vagal viscerosensory afferents from the esophagus (Altschuler, Bao, Bieger, Hopkins & Miselis, 1989).

While buccopharyngeal and complete swallow responses become repetitive and rhythmic with increasing doses of different ionotropic EAA agonists, esophageal responses typically are nonrhythmic or monophasic events. Depending on the site stimulated, nonpropagating isolated cervical or distal, synchronous or peristaltic responses are seen. However, this distinction does not apply to metabotropic glutamate re-ceptor agonists such as 1-aminocyclopentane-1,3-dicarboxylic acid (ACPD) which not only produces rhythmic swallowing but also repetitive esophagomotor re-sponses (Lu et al., 1993b).

The rhythmic repetitive nature of EAA receptor agonist-induced buccopharyngeal swallowing invites comparison with other centrally programmed motor activities in which NMDA receptors contribute to the generation of oscillatory discharges in pattern generator neurons (Grillner et al., 1993; Sqalli-Houssaini, Cazalets, & Clarac, 1993). In vitro studies on slices of the solitary complex suggest that dorsal group swallowing interneurons may possess pacemakerlike properties (Tell & Jean, 1991a, 1991b, 1993; Tell, Fagni, and Jean, 1990). The rhythmogenic behavior of these neurons is thought to arise from a cyclical activation of voltage-operated inward calcium currents and outward potassium currents, the later being activated, in part, by an increase in intracellular calcium.

Based on the reported agonist efficacy or antagonist blocking potency of different EAA receptor subtype-selective ligands, it seems safe to conclude that all subtypes (AMPA, kainate, and NMDA) of ionotropic receptors are present on deglutitive neurons of the NTS (Hashim 1989; Hashim & Bieger, 1989; Jean, Kessler, & Tell, 1994; Kessler, Cherkaoui, Catalin, & Jean, 1990; Kessler & Jean, 1991) Furthermore, EAA receptors of these subtypes are probably activated during deglutitive reflex activity elicited by SLN stimulation (Hashim 1989; Jean, Kessler, & Tell, 1994), during secondary peristalsis evoked by esophageal distention (Bieger 1993, Lu et al., 1993a), or during fictive swallowing induced by the nonselective serotonin receptor agonist, ipazine (Hashim, 1989) and the GABA receptor blocker bicuculline (Wang & Bieger, 1991). These findings are consistent with an EAA-like transmitter being released from either deglutitive viscerosensory afferents (Schaffar, Pio, & Jean, 1990; Lu, Neuman, Reynolds, & Bieger, 1993) or

NTS interneurons generating deglutitive commands.

EAA receptor-mediated transmission plays an equally important role in information transfer from esophageal premotor neurons of the NTS subnucleus centralis (NTS$_c$) to motoneurons of the nucleus ambiguus (AMB). NMDA receptor blockade confined to the esophagomotor region of the AMB abolishes esophageal fictive peristalsis evoked by chemostimulation of the NTS$_c$ (Wang Bieger, & Neuman, 1991). Electrophysiological in vitro experiments show that these antagonists impair the ability of AMB motoneurons to generate the initial fast-rising phase of the excitatory postsynaptic potential (EPSP) evoked by stimulating afferents from the NTSC. Abolition of the fast NMDA receptor-mediated component of the EPSP leads to impaired spike production, thus providing a mechanistic explanation for the loss of esophagomotor output.

Injecting EAA agonists into the rat AMB and its immediate surround typically elicits a single contraction of the esophagus. Depending on the region of the AMB being stimulated, this response may (a) involve different segments or the full length of the organ, (b) be stationary or propulsive, and (c) be accompanied by a pharyngeal relaxation (Bieger 1984; Wang 1992; Wang, Bieger, & Neumann, 1991). The latter two response patterns suggest involvement of ventral group interneurons. Current-voltage relationships of AMB motoneurons determined in the presence of NMDA reveal a region of negative slope conductance at membrane potentials between -90 and -40 mV. The NMDA receptor-mediated inward current probably does not account for the full amplitude of the NTS$_c$-driven motoneuronal EPSP. This would be consistent with an involvement of additional EAA receptors such as those of the AMPA subtype.

Prolonged stimulation of EAA receptors either in vivo or in AMB slice preparations also fails to induce rhythmic activity of esophageal motoneurons or nearby reticular formation neurons (Bieger, 1984; Wang, 1992; Wang, Zhang, Neuman, & Bieger, 1993). However, other investigators (Dean,

Czyzk-Krzeska, & Millhorn, 1989) have suggested that neurons in the rostral AMB region (including the compact formation or "retrofacial" nucleus) are endowed with rhythmogenic properties. The strong possibility that these reflect nondeglutitive response patterns under control by the central pattern generator for respiration awaits further investigation.

Acetylcholine

Cholinergic mechanisms are integral to the transmission of deglutitive commands from the brain to peripheral effector organs and their intramural intrinsic nerve circuits. In at least two mammalian species, cholinergic mechanisms appear to participate also in generating the central motor pattern of esophageal peristalsis. In the rat, whose entire esophageal tunica propria consists of striated muscle, the central cholinergic link utilizes muscarinic cholinoceptors (Bieger, 1984, 1991, 1993); in the cat, whose tunica propria contains both striated and smooth muscle, central nicotinic cholinoceptors are mainly involved, but central muscarinic receptors may also contribute (Greenwood, Blank, & Dodds, 1992; Blank, Greenwood, & Dodds, 1989).

The principal site of muscarinic cholinergic control is the subnucleus centralis of the NTS (NTS_C) which forms the internuncial link between esophageal vagal afferents and esophagomotor efferents of the ambiguus (and presumably also the efferents of the dorsal vagal complex). NTS_C neurons require a muscarinic cholinoceptor-mediated input to be able to generate the premotor drive that engages esophageal motoneurons in the firing pattern appropriate for peristalsis. This input is most probably of central origin. The alternative hypothesis, that esophageal afferents themselves utilize Ach as their transmitter (Falempin, Teranax, Palouzier, & Chanoin, 1989), is not supported by pharmacological evidence demonstrating (a) the absence of atropine-sensitive EPSEs in these neurons (Lu, Neuman, Reynolds, & Bieger, 1993) and (b) the fail-

ure of muscarinic receptor blockade to suppress NTS_C neuronal activity that is evoked by esophageal distention (Lu et al., 1993a). Information about the source of central cholinergic afferents to the NTS_C is still incomplete. Retrograde tracer data point to the parvicellular reticular formation lying dorsomedial from the rostral portion of the ambiguus complex (Vyas, Wang, & Bieger, 1990; Wang, 1992).

As demonstrated in microstimulation studies (Bieger, 1984; Hashim & Bieger, 1987, 1989; Hashim et al., 1989; Wang & Bieger, 1991; Wang, Bieger, & Neuman, 1991), activation of muscarinic cholinoceptors gives rise to rhythmic patterned esophagomotor output that resembles secondary peristalsis and has been termed "fictive" (Bieger, 1991, 1993) because of its independence from relevant sensory stimulation and its quasi-purposiveness. Conversely, blockade of NTS_C muscarinic cholinoceptors abolishes swallow-induced esophageal peristalsis, whether deglutition is elicited by electrical stimulation of the solitarius complex or by pharmacological means (Bieger, 1984; Wang, 1992; Wang & Bieger, 1991). Evidence emerging from electrophysiological studies reveals that response properties of NTS_C neurons are profoundly affected by cholinergic input (Lu et al., 1993a; Lu, Neuman, Reynolds, & Bieger, 1993; Lu, Zhang, Neuman, & Bieger, submitted).

Distal esophageal distention triggers rhythmic secondary peristalsis that is phase-locked with a rhythmic burst-pause firing pattern in the NTS_C and ambigual esophagomotoneurons Local blockade of NTS muscarinic cholinoceptors causes the stimulus-response relationship to be shifted to higher pressures so that at normally effective pressure levels the burst-pause pattern of NTSC neurons is replaced by a sustained discharge and ambigual motoneurons fail to be activated.

In slice preparations, cells located in the NTS_C region respond to acetylcholine or muscarine with rhythmic burst discharges superimposed on pacemakerlike oscillations of the membrane potential.

Oblique slice preparations containing both the NTS_C and the esophagomotor portion of the nucleus ambiguus enable muscarinic agonist-evoked input from NTS_C cells to be recorded in their motoneuronal targets. The NTS_C-driven motoneuronal depolarizations exhibit a temporal pattern that replicates the rhythm of fictive peristalsis recorded in vivo. These observations justify the hypothesis that the central esophagomotor function generator is intrinsically capable of performing basic network operations in a sensory vacuum; in other words, the rhythm generator for esophageal peristalsis represents a neural network with hard-wired circuits for preprogramming of motoneuronal output.

Whether a central muscarinic cholinergic link also operates in other mammals is an unsettled issue. According to the prevailing view, antimuscarinic drug-induced esophagomotor deficits in humans are due mainly to peripheral parasympatholytic actions at the level of esophageal smooth muscle. It should also be noted that some studies reporting effects of atropine on esophageal peristalsis in the human suggest not only an unaltered responsiveness of the striated muscle portion (Dodds, Dent, Hogan, & Arndorfer, 1981; Paterson, Hynna-Liepert, & Selucky, 1991) but also the possible involvement of a noncholinergic mechanism that could trigger peristalsis in the smooth muscle portion via intramural inhibitory neurons (Dodds et al., 1981). Nevertheless, further investigation of atropine dosages equivalent to those employed in animal work would seem needed to (a) determine the potential effectiveness of antimuscarinic agents at disrupting pharyngoesophageal coupling and (b) rule out the possibility that these agents inhibit peristaltic progression not only in the smooth but also the striated muscle portion of the esophagus.

Since reflex-evoked propulsive activity proximal to an intraluminal distending balloon appears to be more readily blocked by antimuscarinic drugs than is primary peristalsis (Kendall, Thompson, Day, & Garvie, 1987), pharmacologic differences

between these two motility patterns may have to be reexamined as well.

Central cholinergic mechanisms also involve esophageal motoneurons of the ambiguus complex and the vagal preganglionic neurons projecting to myenteric motor ganglia of the esophagus. Ambigual neurons are endowed with nicotinic cholinoceptors that mediate a fast inward current, leading to burst discharges and contraction of the striated muscle tunic (Bieger, 1984; Wang, 1992; Wang, Neuman, & Bieger l991a). Focal stimulation with acetylcholine pulses applied to the rostral nucleus ambiguus produces various types of short-latency, nonrhythmic esophageal contractions that may involve the full length or different segments and may be propulsive or stationary. The motoneuronal cholinoceptors are believed to generate EPSPs elicited by focal microstimulation of the parvicellular intermediate reticular zone adjoining the dorsomedial aspect of the rostral nucleus ambiguus (Zhang, Wang, Vyas, Neuman, & Bieger, 1993). This region contains cholinergic neurons (Ruggiero, Giuliano, Anwar, Stornetta, & Reis, l9907 Tago, McGeer, McGeer, Akiyama, & Hersh, 1989) that may project not only to the ambiguus but also to the dorsal vagal complex (Lu et al., 1993a; Vyas, Wang, & Bieger 1990; Wang 1992).

As yet it is not clearly known how or if motoneuronal nicotinic cholinoceptor activation contributes to the regulation of esophagomotor output. Local blockade of these receptors with dihydro-β-erythroidine neither affects the production of solitario-ambigual EPSPs (Zhang et al., 1993) nor does it inhibit fictive peristalsis (Wang, 1992), although it disfacilitates responses to EAA-receptor stimulation (Wang et al., 1991a). As explained below, the nicotinic receptor-mediated excitation of esophagomotoneurons is subject to modulation by somatostatin, a putative transmitter in the solitario-ambigual pathway.

Since neurons of the dorsal vagal complex also possess functional nicotinic receptors (Ito, Fukuda, Nabekura & Oomura, 1989), nicotinic agonists should be able to activate preganglionic efferents to the smooth muscle esophagus. Whether this mechanism accounts for the ability of nicotine, given systemically, to elicit a single wave of esophageal peristalsis in the cat, is unclear, because the latter response involves the full length of the organ and is accompanied by relaxation of the pharyngoesophageal sphincter (Greenwood, Blank & Dodds, 1992). Furthermore, this nicotine effect exhibits an unusually long period of tachyphylaxis (1-2 days) suggesting the involvement of yet another mediator substance. In the rat, nicotine applied to the NTS surface elicits fictive rhythmic swallowing responses that show little tachyphylaxis (Lu & Bieger, unpublished data).

Gamma-aminobutyric Acid (GABA)

The involvement of medullary GABA neurons in deglutitive control is readily demonstrated in the rat. Localized activation of the $GABA_A$ receptor subtype within the NTS exerts a strong suppressant effect on both the buccopharyngeal and esophageal stage, whereas blockade of this receptor and its associated chloride channel by bicuculline and picrotoxin, respectively, gives rise to vigorous, repetitive swallowing activity (Wang 1992; Wang & Bieger, 1991). These actions not only can be shown to result from a unilateral interference with GABA-ergic transmission in the NTS, but also are localizable to the same subdivisions mentioned above, namely the intermediate, ventral and central subnuclei.

At pharyngeal premotor loci in the subnuclei intermedialis and ventralis, bicuculline ejection in subthreshold doses facilitates the excitant effect of S-glutamate or induces repetitive complete swallows at suprathreshold doses (0.5 pmol). Similarly at esophageal premotor loci in the subnucleus centralis, the GABA antagonist is effective at converting nonrhythmic responses to glutamate into rhythmic ones and, at sufficiently large doses (ca. 1 pmol), rhythmic esophageal contractions ensue.

Furthermore, subthreshold doses of bicuculline applied to the subnucleus centralis induce coupling between the pharyngeal and the esophageal stage, as evidenced by the conversion of incomplete (i.e., buccopharyngeal) into complete swallows.

It is therefore plausible to hypothesize that local GABA neurons provide tonic inhibitory input that maintains buccopharyngeal and esophageal NTS premotoneurons in a quiescent state. Removal of this inhibition releases a process of auto-excitation leading to rhythmic patterned motor output under the control of these premotoneurons. It is of interest that the autorhythmic activity involving the buccopharyngeal-esophageal pattern can be completely suppressed by the NMDA receptor antagonist, AP-7, whereas that involving the esophagus alone is suppressed by blockade of muscarinic cholinoceptors. Conceivably, therefore, the two pattern-generating subnetworks utilize different transmitter mechanisms for generating pacemakerlike oscillations of the constituent neurons. The electrophysiologic characteristics of rhythmogenesis under these conditions await further study.

Somatostatin

This peptide is present in NTS subnucleus centralis neurons projecting to esophago-motor neurons of the rat ambiguus complex (Cunningham & Sawchenko, 1989). Microphoretic application of somatostatin elicits variable and complex responses in the motoneurons when recorded intracellularly in slice preparations (Wang, Neuman, & Bieger, 1991b). Motoneuronal responsiveness to EAA receptor agonist stimulation is facilitated both in vivo and in vitro. Depletion in vivo of somatostatin from the intraambigual axon terminals is accompanied by a loss of fictive secondary peristalsis evoked by cholinergic stimulation of the ipsilateral solitarius complex (Neuman, Wang, Zhang, Vyas, & Bieger, 1993; Wang, 1992). In vitro depletion causes a loss of the NMDA receptor-dependent fast component of the motoneuronal EPSP, which can be transiently reversed by exogenous somatostatin (Wang, Zhang, Neuman, & Bieger, 1993).

As a putative co-transmitter in NTS subnucleus centralis efferents, somatostatin can thus be postulated to make a major contribution to information transfer between esophageal premotor and motor output stages. Because the peptide does not appear to be ubiquitously present throughout the subnucleus centralis, esophageal premotor neurons may constitute neurochemically distinct populations. What such heterogeneity implies functionally is yet to be determined. At the very least, it suggests additional levels of control by which fine tuning of esophagomotor output can be achieved. Since the somatostatinergic subpopulation should be in a strategic position to gate motoneuronal output, it would be of considerable interest to determine if cholinergic afferents impinge preferentially on this subpopulation. A corollary function of somatostatinergic input to ambigual motoneurons may be to down-modulate nicotinic cholinergic input from the parvicellular reticular formation.

Serotonin (5-hydroxytryptamine, 5-HT)

5-HT exemplifies a neuromediator substance that modulates rather than transmits signals between medullary function-generator neurons. Such a role comports with the preservation of deglutitive reflex responsiveness after 5-HT neurons or receptors are inactivated. Conversely, activation of 5-HT receptors can cause striking effects on deglutitive function. In view of the multitude of 5-HT receptor types in the brain and the multiplicity of response systems at different neuraxial levels, it is hardly surprising that 5-HT exerts multiple actions on deglutition (for review see Bieger, 1991). At the level of the basal forebrain and diencephalon, a facilitatory action predominates, as evidenced by the enhancement of reflex or fictive swallowing that results from intracerebral microinjection of the amine or injection of 5-HT precursor into the circle of Willis (Bieger, 1991; Hockman et al., 1979; Rupert, 1978) The topography of responsive forebrain loci largely overlaps with the distribution of basal forebrain thirst osmoreceptors (Blass, 1974). This would suggest an association with descending pathways that control motor aspects of drinking.

Since acutely decerebrated rats continue to respond to systemic 5-HT agonists with rhythmic fictive swallowing activity, the lower brain stem must contain major serotonin-sensitive target structures (Bieger, 1981). Among these, the NTS is probably most important. Activation of 5-HT receptors in this region of the medulla oblongata exerts both excitatory and inhibitory effects on the buccopharyngeal stage of swallowing. Excitation of $5\text{-}HT_2$ receptors leads to rhythmic swallowing with a concomitant increase or decrease in pharyngeal pressure, depending on the receptor subtype being stimulated (Bieger, 1981, 1991; Bieger & Neuman, 1991). Rapid desensitization of these receptors allows inhibitory effects to predominate.

The receptors responsible for inhibition probably belong to the $5\text{-}HT_{1A}$ subtype and have a higher threshold compared with that of the excitatory subtype. The preferential distribution of $5\text{-}HT_{1A}$ binding sites in the rat NTS subnucleus centralis (Thor, Blitz-Siebert, & Helke, 1992) agrees with the finding that fictive esophageal peristalsis evoked by muscarine or acetylcholine is inhibited by 5-HT microphoresed into the same subnucleus (Hashim & Bieger, 1987). The inhibitory response is also readily observed when a 5-HT precursor load is administered to animals pretreated with a monoamine oxidase inhibitor or an inhibitor of extracerebral aromatic amino acid decarboxylase (e.g., carbidopa). With nontryptamine 5-HT receptor agonists such as quipazine, chlorophenylpiperazine and 2,5-methoxyamphetamine or 5-HT releasing agents (e.g., fenfluramine), parenteral administration results in sustained deglutitive stimulation, as manifested by rhythmic fictive swallowing (Bieger, 1981; Clineschmidt & McGuffin, 1978; Tseng, 1978).

The source of serotoninergic projections to the deglutitive regions of the NTS is not exactly known, although a number of different 5-HT neuron groups of the brainstem have been shown by retrograde tracing methods to project to the NTS, including all the major raphe nuclei (pallidus, obscurus, magnus, pontis, dorsalis and medianus) and certain extra-raphe nuclei (medial lemniscal, pontine reticulotegmental, ventromedial paragigantocellular groups) (Schaffar, Kessler, Bosler, & Jean, 1988; Thor & Helke, 1987). However, in view of the technical shortcomings of this method, these observations cannot be regarded as definitive until corroborated by anterograde tracing techniques. Retrograde labeling studies of 5-HT afferent projections to functionally identified deglutitive loci in the NTS (Hashim, 1989) reveal a more restricted afferentation from only three raphe nuclei (viz. obscurus, magnus, and pontis).

The reported inhibition of reflex swallowing induced by electrical stimulation of 5-HT cell-rich brainstem regions (Kessler & Jean, 1986) must be viewed with caution, because the same areas also contain nonserotoninergic neurons with NTS projections and because excitation of fibers of passage would be unavoidable.

Overall, the emerging picture is compatible with the idea that 5-HT neurons of the brain stem are intermediary links by which projections descending from the forebrain diencephalon and upper brain stem may alter the excitability of the medullary motor pattern generator network controlling deglutition. The impulse traffic carried by these pathways may represent a penultimate step in the processing of sensory modalities relevant to feeding and drinking. In this functional domain, 5-HT neurons serve multiple and functionally dichotomous roles. Thus, the paradox that 5-HT receptor agonists with deglutitive excitant activity suppress intake of food or water, while those that induce hyperphagia may depress fictive swallowing, would seem to be more apparent than real. Clearly, however, this poses a big obstacle to the development of serotoninergic agents that would produce therapeutically useful "prodeglutitive" effects with systemic administration.

Catecholamines

The two major catecholamines of the CNS, dopamine and norepinephrine (noradrenaline), subserve deglutitive neuromodulator roles essentially analogous to that of serotonin (for reviews see Bieger, 1991; Hockman et al., 1979). A dopaminergic facilitatory system operates in a basal forebrain region that includes the lateral hypothalamo-preoptic continuum, the central amygdala, the sublenticular gray, and the nucleus accumbens. An inhibitory dopaminergic control mechanism exists in the brain stem The connectivity of these structures in relation to (a) cortical areas controlling deglutition and (b) subcortical descending projections to the tegmental areas of the brain stem is yet to be defined. It would be of particular interest to determine the relations between the basal forebrain areas mentioned and the dopamine neurons of the rostromedial substantia nigra, because cell loss in this part of the nucleus correlates with motor deficits in the head region (Bernheimer, Birkmayer, Hornykiewicz, Jellinger, & Seitelberger, 1973). A parallel pathogenic mechanism presumably underlies the well-documented occurrence of dysphagia, dysarthria, and drooling in patients medicated with classical neuroleptics (Ayd, 1961), as these agents are potent dopamine (D2) receptor antagonists. The "atypical" neuroleptic, clozapine, which is said to cause a preferential blockade of mesolimbic dopamine receptors, appears to carry an unprecedented risk of dysphagic manifestations (Bazemore, Ananth, & Tonkonogy, 1993).

Noradrenergic mechanisms prominently contribute to the deglutitive stimulant effects of drugs such as L DOPA, d-amphetamine, and certain CNS-permeant α_1-adrenoceptor agonists. The target structures are ill-defined neuroanatomically, but would again seem to include forebrain and brainstem regions, judged by the effectiveness of α_1 agonists at evoking fictive rhythmic swallowing on intracerebroventricular injection or application to the NTS surface (Bieger, 1991; Menon, Kodama, Kling, & Fitten, 1986). Noradrenergic inhibitory mechanisms (possibly α_2 adrenoceptor-mediated) may also play a role, the NTS having been implicated as a locus where microinjection of noradrenaline causes a depression of the swallowing reflex (Kessler & Jean, 1986). According to the latter authors, inhibition only ensues with NTS microinjection; however, excitation is obtained with NTS surface application at similar doses of noradrenaline (Bieger, 1991).

Opiopeptides

Although the classical studies by Meltzer (1899) and Wild (1847) demonstrated a depressant action of morphine on swallow-induced peristalsis of the esophagus, conclusive evidence for an involvement of opioid receptors in central deglutitive control has emerged only in recent years. To date, two types of opioid receptor-mediated deglutitive responses are known from experiments in the rat. The first is obtained with intracerebroventricular injection of the μ/δ agonist, D-ala2-met enkephalin-amide (DAMA) and consists of rhythmic fictive swallowing (Dzolcic, v.d. Lely, & v. Mourik, 1979). The second response type is commonly produced by nonpeptide opioid agonists with a relative preference for receptors (e.g., etorphine, levorphanol, methadone, morphine, meperidine) and involves inhibition of monoamine neuron-driven fictive swallowing with either systemic or intracerebroventricular administration of agonist. The nonselective opioid receptor antagonist, naloxone, not only nullifies the morphine inhibition, but also precipitates vigorous rhythmic swallowing in morphine-dependent rats (Bieger, Loomis, & Young, 1991; Menon, Tseng, Loh, & Clark, 1980).

As a general working hypothesis, it appears reasonable to consider these opioid actions on fictive swallowing to be the consequence of an interaction with inhibitory and excitatory monoaminergic system. At the level of the NTS, at least two other mechanisms would be expected to play a role, namely, (a) the well-known modulatory action of opioids on cholinergic transmission and (b) the release of opiopeptide modulator from NTS subnucleus

centralis neurons controlling esophageal peristalsis (Cunningham & Sawchenko, 1990; Cunningham, Simmons, Swanson, & Sawchenko, 1991). Experimental corroboration of either mechanism should shed new light on Meltzer's classical observations.

Other Putative Neuromediators in Deglutitive Pathways

Some neuropeptides are effective and potent stimulants of fictive swallowing activity when applied to the rat NTS (e.g., thyrotropin-releasing hormone [TRH], vasopressin, and oxytocin) (Bieger, 1991). All of these are present in afferents to the NTS, TRH probably as a co-transmitter in serotoninergic projections from the hindbrain raphe nuclei (Palkovitz, Mezey, Eskay, & Brownstein, 1986) while the other two peptides are likely mediators in hypothalamic projections from the paraventricular nucleus (Sofroniew & Schrell, 1981; Swanson & Sawohenko, 1983). The presence in rat subnucleus centralis cell bodies of nitric oxide (NO_2) synthase (Ohta et al., 1993) indicates the nitritergic nature of esophageal premotor neurons. Preliminary evidence (Lu et al., 1993b; in preparation) suggests that (a) NO_2 mediates inhibition of centralis neurons that may originate from the contralateral subnucleus and (b) NO_2 production is required for transmission of premotor input from subnucleus centralis to ambiguus motoneurons innervating esophageal striated muscle, and (c) NO_2 synthase histochemistry may provide a method for delineating the subnucleus centralis in mammals in which this NTS subdivision is yet to be identified (Bieger & Sharkey, 1993).

INTRINSIC MOTOR RESPONSES OF ESOPHAGEAL SMOOTH MUSCLE

The Smooth Muscle Esophagus

As discussed earlier, the progressive nature of the peristalsis in the smooth muscle esophagus, unlike the striated muscle segment, does not arise from a programmed sequence of activation in central cranial motor nuclei. Instead, the timing of peristalsis is set by neuromuscular interactions that are intrinsic to the esophagus. The electrophysiological events in the circular smooth muscle that underlie peristaltic contractions in vivo are well described (Rattan, Gidda, & Goyal, 1983; Sugarbaker, Rattan, & Goyal, 1984a). Swallowing and vagal nerve stimulation produce a prompt hyperpolarization of the circular muscle along the length of the smooth muscle esophagus. This hyperpolarization is followed by a transient depolarization of the plasma membrane and a burst of smooth muscle action or spike potentials (see Figure 3–3). The depolarization and spike potentials are associated with contraction of the circular muscle. The peristaltic nature of the contraction occurs because the duration of the hyperpolarization increases progressively along the length of the smooth muscle esophagus. The result is an incremental delay in the onset of circular muscle contraction that is seen as a peristaltic contraction. This hyperpolarization occurs when nerves from the brainstem motor nuclei activate neurons that are intrinsic to the esophagus. These intrinsic esophageal neurons supply the circular muscle layer of the esophagus and release nitric oxide when activated. The nitric oxide causes hyperpolarization of the muscle.

The cellular mechanisms that produce esophageal peristalsis are known because all of the mechanical and electrophysiological events described above are preserved in an isolated preparation of the smooth muscle esophagus from the opossum or cat. The preparation is a circumferentially oriented strip of the esophageal wall that is composed of the two muscular layers and the nerves of the myenteric plexus (see Figure 3–4). Stimulating the nerves intrinsic to the muscle strip with an electrical field activates a class of nerves called the *nonadrenergic, noncholinergic nerves*. We now know that this nonadrenergic, noncholinergic transmitter is nitric oxide or a substance that is able to release nitric

oxide in target tissues (Christink, Jury, Cayabyab, & Daniel, 1991; Du, Murray, Bates, & Conklin, 1991; Murray, Bates, & Conklin, 1994; Murray, Du, Ledlow, Bates, & Conklin, 1991; Tottrup, Svane, & Forman, 1991).

Selective stimulation of the NO_2 nerves produces a stereotyped contractile response of the circular muscle (Weisbrodt & Christensen, 1972). There is either no mechanical response or a small contraction that is attributable to direct muscle stimulation during the stimulus. Cessation of the stimulus is followed by a short period of mechanical quiescence prior to a transient circular muscle contraction. The time from the end of the stimulus to the beginning of the contraction is called the *latency period*, and the delayed contraction is called the *off-response* (Chan & Diamant, 1976). The latency period varies in muscle strips taken from along the length of the smooth muscle segment of the esophagus such that the latency is shortest in the proximal smooth muscle segment and lengthens progressively until it is longest just above the lower esophageal sphincter. The off-response also occurs when the vagal efferents supplying the smooth muscle esophagus are stimulated (Dodds, Christensen, Dent, Wood, & Arndorfer, 1978; Dodds et al., 1978), after a balloon distending the esophagus is deflated (Christensen, 1970a; Ryan, Snape, & Cohen, 1977) and when the whole esophagus is stimulated by localized electrical or mechanical stimuli (Christensen & Lund, 1969).

Electrical stimulation of intrinsic esophageal nerves produces a hyperpolarization of circular smooth muscle cells (Crist, Suprenant, & Goyal, 1987; Dektor & Ryan, 1982; Kannan, Jager, & Daniel, 1985; Serio & Daniel, 1988). A depolarization that may be associated with the generation of spike potentials follows the hyperpolarization. Smooth muscle spike potentials result from the opening of plasma membrane calcium channels and the inward movement of calcium ions. This increases the free cytosolic calcium ion concentration, activates the contractile machinery, and produces contraction of the circular muscle (Biancani, Hillemeier, Bitar, & Makhlouf, 1987; DeCarle, Christensen, Szabo, Templeman, & McKinley, 1983). Thus, the depolarization and spike potentials are the electrophysiological correlates of the mechanical off-response. The duration of the hyperpolarization and the timing of the depolarization increase in a monotonic fashion distally along the smooth muscle esophagus (Serio & Daniel, 1988). Thus, the timing of the off-response, and therefore the gradient in the latency period, depend on the timing of both the hyperpolarization and depolarization.

The cellular mechanisms that underlie nerve-induced hyperpolarization of the circular esophageal smooth muscle are debated. One body of evidence supports the hypothesis that both intrinsic nerve stimulation and exogenous nitric oxide hyperpolarize the plasma membrane by increasing potassium ion conductance (opening potassium channels) (Jury, Jager, & Daniel, 1985; Kannan, Jager, & Daniel, 1985; Murray et al., 1995; Sims, Vivaudo, Hillemeier, Biancani, Walsh, & Singer, 1990). Other evidence supports the hypothesis that intrinsic nerve stimulation results in a decrease in chloride ion conductance (closing chloride channels) (Crist, He, & Goyal 1991). Either mechanism should produce hyperpolarization.

Nitritergic and Cholinergic Control of Peristalsis

The genesis and timing of these nerve-induced electrophysiological events, the off-response and esophageal peristalsis, depend on the release of nitric oxide from intrinsic nerves supplying the circular muscle of the esophagus. Inhibitors of nitric oxide synthesis and scavengers of nitric oxide decrease the latency period in the distal esophagus to abolish the latency gradient along the length of the smooth muscle esophagus (Conklin, Murray et al., 1995; Murray, Du, Bates, & Conklin, 1991). The latency shortens because the duration of nerve-induced membrane hyperpolar-

ization of circular smooth in the distal esophagus shortens (Du, Murray, Bates, & Conklin, 1991). When given in high enough concentrations, inhibitors of nitric oxide synthase completely abolish the nerve-induced off-response, hyperpolarization, and depolarization of circular esophageal muscle. Thus, nitric oxide plays a key role in controlling the peripheral mechanisms responsible for generating peristaltic contractile sequences in the smooth muscle esophagus.

Inhibitors of nitric oxide synthesis or scavengers of nitric oxide also shorten the time between swallowing and the appearance of peristaltic contractions at all levels of the smooth muscle esophagus (Conklin, Murray, et al., 1995; Murray, Ledlow, Launspach, et al., 1995; Yamato, Spechler, & Goyal, 1992). The effect is most pronounced in the distal esophagus, making the contractions almost simultaneous along the smooth muscle segment. These studies support the hypotheses that nitric oxide and the nerve-induced membrane hyperpolarization it produces determine the timing of peristalsis.

Electrical stimuli of certain characteristics activate a population of cholinergic nerves supplying the circular smooth muscle of the esophagus (Crist, Gidda, & Goyal, 1984a, 1984b). These nerves produce circular muscle contraction shortly after the onset of stimulation. A similar response is seen with high frequency stimulation of vagal efferents (Dodds, Christensen, Dent, Wood, & Arndorfer, 1978). This cholinergic innervation plays a role in the generation of peristaltic contractions because atropine decreases the amplitude of peristaltic contractions produced by swallowing, vagal, or intrinsic nerve stimulation (Blank, Greenwood, & Dodds, 1989; Crist, Gidda, & Goyal, 1984, Dodds, Christensen, Dent, Wood, & Arndorfer, 1978, 1979; Dodds, Dent, Hogan, & Arndorfer, 1978). The importance of these nerves in setting the timing of esophageal peristalsis is debated. Earlier studies indicated that cholinergic nerve activity controls the timing of peristalsis in the proximal portion of the smooth muscle esophagus (Crist, Gidda, & Goyal, 1984a, 1984b). Those studies led to the hypothesis that the progressive nature of esophageal peristalsis results from gradients in the cholinergic and nonadrenergic, noncholinergic (nitric oxide) innervations of the smooth muscle esophagus. According to this hypothesis, the latencies of peristaltic contractions are short in the proximal esophagus because the cholinergic innervation is most dense there, and the latencies are long in the distal esophagus because the nitric oxide innervation is most dense there. This idea is consistent with anatomical evidence demonstrating a gradient in the density of nerve cells in the myenteric plexus along the esophagus (Christensen & Robison, 1982). It is not consistent with the observation that the number of choline acetyltransferase positive neurons does not differ along the esophagus (Seelig, Doody, Brainard, Gidda, & Goyal, 1984). Other observations do not support this hypothesis. Stimulating intrinsic esophageal nerves in vitro with electrical stimuli known to activate both nitric oxide and cholinergic nerves produces the stereotyped electrophysiological response described above, membrane hyperpolarization followed by depolarization and spike activity (Dektor & Ryan, 1982). The timing of these responses at any level of the smooth muscle esophagus is not changed after muscarinic receptor blockade by atropine (Serio & Daniel, 1988). In addition, atropine does not affect the timing of off-responses at any level of the esophagus. As pointed out above, inhibitors of nitric oxide synthesis preferentially shorten the time between swallowing and the appearance of peristaltic contractions in the distal smooth muscle esophagus to give a nearly simultaneous contraction. Adding atropine given after the inhibitor of nitric oxide synthesis changes the timing of these esophageal contractions smooth muscle little at all (Knudsen, Frobert, & Tottrup, 1994; Yamato Spechler, & Goyal, 1992). Finally, the velocity of peristalsis in the cat esophagus is increased by inhibitors of nitric oxide synthesis but is not altered by doses of atropine that decrease the amplitude of the contraction (Sifrim & Janssens, 1995). These data indicate that the nitritergic innervation determines the timing of peristalsis, and the cholinergic innervation determines the amplitude of peristaltic contractions.

Control of the Lower Esophageal Sphincter

Tonic Contraction of the Sphincter

The musculature of the lower esophageal sphincter is tonically contracted at rest (Hollaway et al., 1987). This tonic contraction appears to be a property intrinsic to the muscle and is not dependent on its innervation. The length-tension characteristics of the sphincter muscle differ from those of muscle from the esophagus or stomach. Stretching narrow strips of circular muscle cut from the sphincter generates much steeper length-tension curves (similar incremental increases in length generate greater force) than does stretching muscle strips from the adjacent esophageal body or the stomach (Christensen, Conklin, & Freeman, 1973). This increased force is not affected by drugs that antagonize neural function, so it is a myogenic property of the sphincter muscle. In addition, lower esophageal sphincter tone is not altered by close intra-arterial injection of tetrodotoxin in the opossum (Goyal & Rattan, 1976) and is reduced by only approximately 25% in the cat. The force is not passive (i.e., simply due to different viscoelastic properties of this muscle tissue), because the greater force generated by the sphincter muscle is abolished by agents that inhibit muscle contraction. Thus, the sphincter was defined as a muscular segment at the gastroesophageal junction that maintains a tone at rest.

The lower esophageal sphincter depends on both intracellular and extracellular pools of calcium for the maintenance of tone. Calcium channel antagonists do not abolish lower esophageal sphincter tone, but the removal of extracellular calcium results in a partial loss of sphincter tone (Biancani, Hillemeier, Bitar, & Makhlouf, 1987; DeCarle, Christensen, Szabo, Templeman, & McKinley, 1983). When intracellular stores of calcium are depleted in the absence of extracellular calcium, sphincter tone is lost (Murray, Du, & Conklin, 1992). Some studies suggest that the lower esophageal sphincter may be contracted tonically because its free cytoplasmic calcium is higher than that of adjacent esophageal body muscle (Schlippert, Schulze, & Forker, 1979).

There is evidence that special electrophysiologic properties of the smooth muscle plasma membrane may be responsible for the resting lower esophageal sphincter tone. Circular smooth muscle of the sphincter intermittently generates continuous spike activity that is not dependent on neuronal activity (Asoh & Goyal, 1978). Because these spike potentials result from the inward movement of calcium ions, the intermittent spike activity might, in part, explain maintained tone. However, abolition of spike activity results in only a minor attenuation of lower esophageal sphincter tone, indicating that mechanisms other than the influx of calcium ions during spike generation must be major contributors to the tonic contraction. Other studies indicate that the resting membrane potential of lower esophageal sphincter muscle is less negative than that of neighboring esophageal muscle cells. From this observation it is argued that the esophageal sphincter muscle tone partially depends on the smooth muscle membrane potential difference, with the tone increasing as the membrane potential becomes less negative (Zelcer & Weisbrodt, 1984). These findings led to the hypothesis that the more positive resting potential of sphincter muscle and its tonic contraction result from an increased calcium ion conductance. The validity of this hypothesis is yet to be determined, particularly as other investigators do not find a less negative resting membrane potential in smooth muscle cells from the lower esophageal sphincter (Conklin, Du, Murray, & Bates, 1993).

Muscle of the lower esophageal sphincter also differs biochemically from that of the adjacent stomach and esophagus. The myogenic tone of the sphincter is maintained entirely by aerobic mechanisms: As oxygen tension is reduced, tone is decreased in a 1:1 ratio (Christensen, 1982). Phasic contractions of the adjacent esophageal body continue little changed under anaerobic conditions. In addition, oxygen consumption by the sphincter muscle is low when it is unstretched, but increases sharply when stretched to generate a tonic contraction (Schulze-Delrieu & Crane, 1982). Stretching esophageal muscle produces neither the increase in tone nor the sharp increase in oxygen consumption seen in the sphincter muscle. The sphincter muscle is also able to utilize substrates not utilized by esophageal muscle and differs in other biochemical pathways (Robinson, Percy, & Christensen, 1984). Finally, studies of the contractile proteins from the sphincter muscle suggest that the maintenance of tone may result from higher levels of myosin phosphorylation in this muscle (Weisbrodt & Murphy, 1985).

The lower esophageal sphincter receives an excitatory cholinergic vagal innervation. A number of studies suggest that lower esophageal sphincter tone may, in part, be modulated by vagal activity and that this vagal influence is somewhat greater in the dog and cat than in the opossum (Dodds et al., 1978; Gonella, Neil, & Roman, 1979; Kravitz, Snape, & Cohen, 1966; Lind, Cotton, Blanchard, Crispin, & Dimopolos, 1969; Matarazzo, Snape, Ryan, & Cohen, 1976; Rattan & Goyal, 1974; Reynolds, El-Sharkawy, & Diamant, 1984). Activation of the cholinergic innervation increases the force of sphincter closure. Studies with cholinergic antagonists do not, however, support the idea that sphincter closure is to any major degree determined by tonic muscarinic activation in most animals. atropine, a muscarinic cholinergic antagonist, does not significantly reduce the force of sphincter closure in opossums or monkeys, but it does in dogs (Rattan, Coln, & Goyal, 1976; Zwick, Bowes, Daniel, & Sarna, 1976). In cats and humans, there are conflicting conclusions (Jensen, McCallum, & Walsh, 1978; Kelly and Friedland, 1967; Lind, Crispin, & McIver, 1968).

Sympathetic nerves that supply the lower esophageal sphincter are excitatory. They release norepinephrine that activates cholinergic parasympathetic motor neurons of the myenteric plexus (Christensen & Daniel, 1968; Fournet, Snape, & Cohen, 1979; Gonella, Neil, & Roman, 1979; Lund & Christensen, 1969). Adrenergic nerve destruction with 6-hydroxydopamine reduces the force of sphincter closure, but reserpine-induced depletion of norepinephrine does not. Alpha-adrenergic antagonists produce a small and transient reduction the force of sphincter closure in cats and opossums (Dimanno & Cohen, 1973). Thus, the sympathetic innervation influences the basal force of sphincter closure little.

There are many biologically active substances in the esophagus that could act as neurocrine, endocrine, or paracrine agents to modulate lower esophageal sphincter tone. No one hormone or nerve can be considered a major determinant of sphincter tone. Gastrin was once erroneously thought to control sphincter tone (Lipshutz, Hughes, & Cohen, 1972). Substance P participates in a local reflex pathway by which esophageal acidification raises sphincter pressure transiently in the cat (Reynolds, Ouyang, & Cohen, 1984). Motilin, a hormone thought to coordinate motor events throughout the gastrointestinal tract, contracts the sphincter (Gutierrez, Thanik, Chey, & Yajima, 1977; Meisner, Bowfes, Zwick, & Daniel, 1976). The prostaglandins (Daniel, Crankshaw, & Sarna, 1979a,b), dopamine (DeCarle & Christensen, 1976b; Mukhopadhyay & Weisbrodt, 1977; Rattan & Goyal, 1976), histamine (DeCarle & Christensen, 1976a; Kravitz, Snape, & Cohen, 1978; Rattan and Goyal, 1977a), serotonin (Rattan & Goyal, 1977b), met-enkephalin, and bombesin (Mukhopadhyay & Kunnemann, 1979) all affect the lower esophageal sphincter; however, none of these agents is a major contributor to the control of sphincter tone.

Relaxation of the Sphincter

Relaxation of the lower esophageal sphincter, whether by swallowing or by such things as esophageal distention, is neurogenic. The relaxation induced by swallowing is mediated vagally since it is abolished by bilateral vagotomy (Gonella, Neil, & Roman, 1977, 1979; Rattan & Goyal, 1974; Fournet, Snape, & Cohen, 1979; Goyal, & Rattan, 1973; Ryan, Snape, & Cohen, 1977; Tieffenbach & Roman, 1972). Distention of either the striated or smooth muscle esophagus results in lower esophageal sphincter relaxation. Sphincter relaxation caused by distention of the striated muscle esophagus is mediated via a central reflex that is eliminated by vagotomy (Cunningham, & Sawchenko, 1990; Hwang, 1954; Roman, 1966), but relaxation initiated by distention of the smooth muscle esophagus is mediated by an intrinsic reflex, and is not abolished by vagotomy (Paterson, Rattan, & Goyal, 1986; Price, El-Sharkawy, Mui, & Diamant, 1979; Roman, 1966; Kravitz, Snape, & Cohen, 1966; Ryan, Snape, & Cohen, 1977). The neural pathways that produce these reflexes are not fully defined (See also section 4c).

The electrophysiological correlate of lower esophageal sphincter relaxation, whether caused by swallowing, vagal nerve stimulation, or electrical stimulation of intrinsic nerves, is hyperpolarization of the smooth muscle membrane (Daniel, Taylor, & Holman, 1976; Rattan, Gidda, & Goyal 1983; Zelcer, & Weisbrodt, 1984). This hyperpolarization differs somewhat from that recorded from neighboring esophageal muscle in that it has a much longer time course and is not followed by membrane depolarization (Conklin, Du, Murray, & Bates, 1993). Thus, the mechanism by which off-contractions are generated in the esophageal body is not present in sphincter muscle.

The neural mediator of lower esophageal sphincter muscle hyperpolarization and relaxation is nitric oxide or a nitric oxide-releasing compound (Du, Murray, Bates, Conklin, 1991, Murray, Du, Ledlow, Bates, & Conklin, 1991, Yamato, Spechler, & Goyal 1992, Tottrup, Svane, & Forman, 1991). Inhibitors of nitric oxide synthesis competitively antagonize both the hyperpolarization and relaxation, and exogenously applied nitric oxide mimics both responses. Nitric oxide generation in the sphincter during intrinsic nerve stimulation has been measured (O'Meara, Conklin, & Murray, 1992). Histological techniques reveal nitric oxide synthase in myenteric plexus neurons of the esophagus, and nitric oxide synthase enzymatic activity can be measured in preparations of esophageal smooth muscle tissue (Tottrup et al., 1991, Torphy, Fine, Burman, Barnette, & Ormsbee, 1986). Finally, nitric oxide, like the activation of the intrinsic nerves, stimulates the guanylate cyclase of esophageal smooth muscle to increase the production of cGMP (Murray, Du, & Conklin, 1992, Torphy, Fine, Burman, Barnette, & Ormsbee, 1986; Gonella, Niel, & Roman, 1977).

At least two neuropeptides are proposed as neurotransmitters that may mediate lower esophageal sphincter relaxation in response to nerve stimulation. They are calcitonin gene-related peptide (CGRP) and vasoactive intestinal polypeptide (VIP). The only evidence for CGRP is that it relaxes lower esophageal sphincter muscle when applied exogenously and that CGRP-immunoreactivity can be found in neurons of the myenteric plexus (Rattan, Gonella, & Goyal, 1988). Vasoactive intestinal polypeptide relaxes lower esophageal sphincter muscle, anti-VIP antibodies partially antagonize nerve-induced relaxation of the muscle, and VIP-immunoreactivity is present in neurons of the myenteric plexus (Alumets et al., 1979; Biancani, Walsh, & Behar, 1984; Christensen, Williams, Jew, & O'Dorisio, 1987; Goyal, Rattan, & Said, 1980, Rattan, Grady, & Goyal, 1982; Rattan, Said, & Goyal, 1977; Siegel, Brown, Castell, Johnson, & Said, 1979). There is disagreement as to whether VIP

is released from the tissue during nerve stimulation (Biancani et al., 1984; Fox, Said, & Daniel, 1979). There is also evidence against VIP as the neurotransmitter mediating nerve-induced lower esophageal sphincter relaxation. Vasoactive intestinal polypeptide-induced relaxation is associated with an increase in cAMP levels in lower esophageal sphincter tissue, whereas nerve-induced relaxation is associated with a rise in cGMP levels (Barnette, Torphy, Grous, Fine, & Ormsbee, 1989). In addition, VIP does not mimic the hyperpolarization of the esophageal smooth muscle membrane potential that is characteristic of nerve stimulation (Daniel, Holmy-Elkholy, Jager, & Kannan, 1983). Thus, the role played by VIP in the relaxation process is not established. It is not likely to stimulate the generation or release of nitric oxide from nerves or other cellular elements of the lower esophageal sphincter since relaxations caused by VIP are not attenuated by inhibitors of nitric oxide synthesis (Tottrup, Svane, & Forman, 1991).

Many bioactive substances are capable of relaxing the lower esophageal sphincter. These include cholecystokinin (Fisher, Dimarino, & Cohen, 1975; Grossman, 1973; Resin, Stern, Sturdevant, & Isenberg, 1973), somatostatin (Bybee, Brown, Georges, Castell, & McGuigan, 1979), glucagon (Behar, Field, & Marin, 1979; Hogan, Dodds, Hoke, Reid, Kalkhoff, & Arndorfer, 1975; Jaffer, Makhlouf, Schorr, & Zfass, 1974; Siegel, Brown, Castell, Johnson, & Said, 1979), some prostaglandins (Brown, Beck, Feltcher, Castell, & Eastwood, 1977), especially prostaglandin E_1 (Goyal & Rattan, 1973), dopamine (De Carle & Christensen, 1976; Rattan & Goyal, 1976), the female sex hormones (Schulze & Christensen, 1977; Van Thiel, Gavaler, & Stremple, 1976), secretin (Behar, Field, & Marin, 1979; Siegel et al., 1979), neurotensin (Rosell et al., 1980; Thor & Rokaeus, 1983), and gastric inhibitory peptide (Sinar et al., 1978. None of these agents is cleary associated with nerve-induced relaxation of the sphincter.

REFERENCES

Altschuler, S. M., Bao, X., Bieger, D., Hopkins, D. A., & Miselis, R. R. (1989). Viscerotropic representation of the upper alimentary tract in the rat: Sensory ganglia and nuclei of the solitary tract and spinal trigeminal tracts. *Journal of Comparative Neurology, 283*, 248–268.

Altschuler, S. M., Boyle, J. T., Nixon, T. E., Pack, A. I., & Cohen. (1985). Simultaneous reflex inhibition of lower esophageal sphincter and crural diaphragm in cats. *American Journal of Physiology, 249*, G586–G591.

Amri, M., & Car, A. (1982). Étude des neurons déglutiteurs pontiques chez la brebis. II. Effets de la stimulation des adherences peripheriques et do cortex fronto-orbitaire. *Experimental Brain Research, 48*, 355–361.

Amri, M., & Car, A. (1988). Projections from the medullary swallowing center to the hypoglossal motor nucleus: A neuroanatomical and electrophysiological study in sheep. *Brain Research, 441*, 119–126.

Amri, M., Car, A., & Jean, A. (1984). Medullary control of the pontine swallowing neurones in sheep. *Experimental Brain Research, 55*, 105–110.

Amri, M., Car, A., & Roman, C. (1990). Axonal branching of medullary swallowing neurons projecting on the trigeminal and hypoglossal motor nuclei: Demonstration by electrophysiological and fluorescent double labeling techniques. *Experimental Brain Research, 81*, 384–390.

Amri, M., Lamkadem, M., & Car, A. (1991). Effects of lingual nerve and chewing cortex stimulation upon activity of the swallowing neurons located in the region of the hypoglossal motor nucleus. *Brain Research, 548*, 144–155.

Andrew, B. L. (1956a). A functional analysis of the myelinated fibers of the superior laryngeal nerve in the rat. *Journal of Physiology (London), 133*, 420–432.

Andrew, B. L. (1956b). The nervous control of the cervical esophagus of the rat during swallowing. *Journal of Physiology (London), 134*, 729–740.

Armstrong, D. M., Manley, L., Haycock, J. W., & Hersh, L. B. (1990). Co-localization of choline acetyltransferase and tyrosine hydroxylase within neurons of the dorsal motor nucleus of the vagus. *Journal of Chemical Neuroanatomy, 3*, 133–140.

Asaad, K., Abd-EI Rahman, S., Nawar, N. N. Y., & Mikhail, Y. (1983). Intrinsic innervation of the oesophagus in dogs with special reference to the presence of muscle spindles. *Acta Anatomica, 115*, 91–96.

Asoh, R., & Goyal, R. K. (1978). Electrical activity of the opossum lower esophageal sphincter in vivo. *Gastroenterology, 74*, 835–840.

Ayd, F. J. (1961). A survey of drug-induced extrapyramidal reactions. *Journal of the American Medical Association, 175*, 1054–1060.

Barnette, M., Torphy, T. J., Grous, M., Fine, C., & Ormsbee, H. S. (1989). Cyclic GMP: A potential mediator of neural and drug-induced relaxation of opossum lower esophageal sphincter. *Journal of Pharmacological Experimental Therapy, 249*, 524–528.

Basmajian, J. V., & Duttam, C. R. (1961). Electromyography of the pharyngeal constrictors and levator palati in man. *Anatomical Record, 139*, 561–563.

Bazemore, P.H., Ananth, R., & Tonkonogy, J.M. (1993). *Choking in psychiatric inpatients: Four year clinical review, 1989–1992.* Second Annual Scientific Meeting of the Dysphagia Research Society. Lake Geneva, WI.

Baumgarten, M. G., & Lange, W. (1964). Adrenergic innervation of the oesophagus in the cat (*Felis domestica*) and rhesus monkey (*Macaca rhesus*). *Zell Zellforschung, 95*, 529–545.

Beckstead, R. M., Morse, J. R., & Norgren, R. (1980). The nucleus of the solitary tract in the monkey: Projections to the thalamus and brain stem nuclei. *Journal of Comparative Neurology, 190*, 259–282.

Behar, J., Field, S., & Marin, C. (1979): Effect of glucagon, secretin and vasoactive intestinal polypeptide on the feline lower esophageal sphincter; Mechanisms of action. *Gastroenterology, 77*, 1001–1007.

Bernheimer, H., Birkmayer, W., Hornykiewicz, O., Jellinger, K., & Seitelberger, F. (1973). Brain dopamine and the syndromes of Parkinson and Huntington. *Journal of Neurological Sciences, 20*, 415–455.

Biancani, P., Hillemeier, C., Bitar, K. N., & Makhlouf, G. (1987). Contraction mediated by Ca^{2+} influx in esophageal muscle and Ca^{2+} release in the LES. *American Journal of Physiology, 253*, G760–G766.

Biancani, P., Walsh, J. H., & Behar, J. (1984). Vasoactive intestinal polypeptide: A neurotransmitter for lower esophageal sphincter. *Journal of Clinical Investigation, 73*, 963–967.

Bieger, D. (1981). Role of bulbar serotonergic neurotransmission in the initiation of swallowing in the rat. *Neuropharmacology, 20*, 1073–1083.

Bieger, D. (1984). Muscarinic activation of rhombencephalic neurons controlling esophageal peristalsis in the rat. *Neuropharmacology, 23*, 1451–1464.

Bieger, D. (1991). Neuropharmacologic correlates of deglutition: Lessons from fictive swallowing. *Dysphagia, 6*, 147–164.

Bieger, D. (1993). The brainstem esophagomotor network pattern generator: A rodent model. *Dysphagia 8*, 203–208.

Bieger, D., & Hockman, C. H. (1976). Suprabulbar modulation of reflex swallowing. *Experimental Neurology, 52*, 311–324.

Bieger, D., & Hopkins, D. A. (1987). Viscerotopic representation of the upper alimentary tract in the medulla oblongata in the rat: The nucleus ambiguus. *Journal of Comparative Neurology, 262*, 546–567.

Bieger, D., Loomis, C. W., & Young, I. (1991). Rhythmic fictive swallowing as an index of naloxone-precipitated morphine withdrawal in the rat. *Society of Neuroscience Abstracts, 17*, 330.

Bieger, D., & Neuman, R.S. (1991). *5-HT receptor subtypes mediating excitation and inhibition of fictive swallowing in the rat.* 5-Hydroxytryptamine-CNS Receptors and Brain Function. International Conference, Birmingham University, Birmingham, U.K.

Bieger, D., & Sharkey, K.A. (1993). Subnuclear organization of the solitarius complex: Can NADPH-diaphorase staining resolve any controversies? *Society of Neuroscience Abstracts, 19*, 320.

Bieger, D., Weerasuriya, A., & Hockman, C. H. (1978). The emetic action of L-Dopa and its effect on the swallowing reflex in the cat. *Journal of Neural Transmission, 42*, 87–98.

Binder, H. J., Bloom, D. L., Stern, H., Solitare, G. B., Thayer, W. R., & Spiro, H. M. (1968). The effect of cervical vagotomy on esophageal function in the monkey. *Surgery, 64*, 1075–1083.

Blank, E. L., Greenwood, B., & Dodds, W. J. (1989). Cholinergic control of smooth muscle peristalsis in the cat esophagus. *American Journal of Physiology, 257*, G517–G523.

Blass, E. M. (1974). Evidence for basal forebrain thirst osmoreceptors in rat. *Brain Research, 82*, 69–76.

Bloom, S. R. (1985). Calcitonin gene-related peptide immunoreactive sensory and motor nerves of the rat, cat, and monkey esophagus. *Gastroenterology, 88*, 151.

Bosma, J. F. (1957). Deglutition: Pharyngeal stage. *Physiological Review, 37*, 275–300.

Brasseur, J. G., & Dodds, W. J. (1991). Interpretation of intramural manometric measurements in terms of swallowing mechanics. *Dysphagia, 6*, 100–119.

Brown, F., Beck, B., Feltcher, J., Castell, D., & Eastwood, G. (1977): Evidence suggesting prostaglandins mediate lower esophageal sphincter (LES) incompetence associated with inflammation. *Gastroenterology, 72*, 1033.

Burgess, J. N., Kelly, K. A., Schlegel, J. F., & Ellis, F. I., Jr., (1969). Effect of esophageal mucosal denervation on the motility of the canine esophagus. *Journal of Surgical Research, 9*, 605–610.

Burgess, J. N., Schlegel, J. F. & Ellis, Jr., F. H. (1972). The effect of denervation of feline esophageal function and morphology. *Journal of Surgical Research, 12*, 24–33.

Burton, H., Terashima, S. I., & Clark, J. (1972). Response properties of slowly adapting mechanoreceptors to temperature stimulation in cats. *Brain Research, 45*, 401–416.

Bybee, E. E., Brown, F. C., Georges, L. P., Castell, D. O., and McGuigan, J. E. (1979): Somatostatin effects on lower esophageal sphincter function. *American Journal of Physiology, 237*, E77–E81.

Car, A. (1970). La commande corticale du centre deglutiteur bulbaire. *Journal of Physiology (Paris), 62*, 361–386.

Car, A. (1973). La commande corticale de la deglutition. II. Point d'impact bulbaire de la voie corticofuge deglutitrice. *Journal of Physiology (Paris), 66*, 553–575.

Car, A. (1977). Etude macrophysiologique et microphysiologique de la zone deglutitrice du cortex frontal. *Journal of Physiology (Paris), 73*, 945–961.

Car, A., & Amri, M. (1982). Etude des neurones deglutiteurs pontiques che la brebis. 1. Activite et localisation. *Experimental Brain Research, 64*, 345–354.

Car, A., & Amri, M. (1988). Activity of neurons located in the region of the hypoglossal motor nucleus during swallowing in sheep. *Experimental Brain Research, 69*, 175–182.

Car, A., Jean, A., & Roman, C. (1975). A pontine primary relay for ascending projections of the superior laryngeal nerve. *Experimental Brain Research, 22*, 197–210.

Car, A., & Roman, C. (1970a). Deglutitions et contractions oesophagiennes reflexes produites par la stimulation du bulbe rachidien. *Experimental Brain Research, 11*, 75–92.

Car, A., & Roman, C. (1970b). L'activité spontanee du sphincter oesophagien superieur chez la mouton. Ses variations au cours de deglutition et de la rumination. *Journal of Physiology (Paris), 62*, 505–511.

Carpenter, D. O. (1989). Central nervous system mechanisms in deglutition and emesis. In S. G. Schultz (Ed.), *Handbook of physiology: Gastrointestinal system* (Volume 1, Sec. 6, pp. 685–714). Washington, DC: American Physiological Society.

Carveth, S. W., Schlegel, J. F., & Code, C. F. (1962). Esophageal motility after vagotomy, phrenicotomy, myotomy, and myomectomy in dogs. *Surgery, Gynecology, and Obstetrics, 114*, 31–42.

Chan, W. W., & Diamant, N. E. (1976). Electrical off response of cat esophageal smooth muscle: an analog stimulation. *American Journal of Physiology, 23*, 233–238.

Christensen, J. (1970a). Patterns and origin of some esophageal responses to stretch and electrical stimulation. *Gastroenterology, 59*, 909–916.

Christensen, J. (1970b). Pharmacological identification of the lower esophageal sphincter. *Journal of Clinical Investigation, 49*, 681–691.

Christensen, J. (1975). Pharmacology of the esophageal motor function. *Annual Review of Pharmacology, 15*, 243–258.

Christensen, J. (1976). Effects of drugs on esophageal motility. *Archives of Internal Medicine, 136*, 532–537.

Christensen, J. (1978). The innervation and motility of the esophagus. *Frontiers of Gastrointestinal Research, 3*, 18–32.

Christensen, J. (1982). Oxygen dependence of contractions in esophageal and gastric pyloric and ileocecal muscle of opossum. *Proceedings of the Society of Experimental and Biological Medicine, 170*, 194–202.

Christensen, J. (1984). Origin of sensation in the esophagus. *American Journal of Physiology, 246*, G221–G225.

Christensen, J. (1987). Motor functions of the pharynx and esophagus. In L. R. Johnson (Ed.), *Physiology of the gastrointestinal tract* (pp. 595–612). New York: Raven Press.

Christensen, J., Conklin, J. L., & Freeman, B. W. (1973). Physiologic specialization at the esophagogastric junction in three species. *American Journal of Physiology, 225*, 1265–270.

Christensen, J., & Daniel, E. E. (1968). Effects of some autonomic drugs on circular esophageal smooth muscle. *Journal of Pharmacological and Experimental Therapy, 159*, 243–249.

Christensen, J., & Lund, G. F. (1969). Esophageal responses to distention and electrical stimulation. *Journal of Clinical Investigation, 48*, 408–419.

Christensen, J., Freeman, B. W., & Miller, W. (1973). Some physiological characteristics of the esophagogastric junction in the opossum. *Gastroenterology, 64*, 1119–1124.

Christink, F., Jury, J., Cayabyab, F., & Daniel, E. E. (1991). Nitric oxide may be the final mediator of non-adrenergic, non-cholinergic inhibitory junction potentials in the gut. *Canadian Journal of Physiology and Pharmacology, 69*, 1448–1458.

Cleall, J. F. (1965). Deglutition: A study of form and function. *American Journal of Orthodontics, 51*, 566–594.

Clerc, N., & Mei, N. (1985). Thoracic esophageal mechanoreceptors connected with fibers following sympathetic pathways. *Brain Research Bulletin, 10*, 1–7.

Clineschmidt, B.V., & McGuffin, J.C. (1978). Pharmacological differentiation of the central 5-hydroxytryptamine-like actions of MK212 (6-chloro-2) (1-piperazinyl)-pyrazine), para-methoxyamphetamine and fenfluramine in an in vivo model system. *European Journal of Pharmacology, 50*, 369–375.

Collman, P. I., Tremblay, L., & Diamant, N. E. (1993). The central vagal efferent supply to the esophagus and lower esophageal sphincter of the cat. *Gastroenterology, 104*, 1430–1438.

Conklin, J. L., & Du, C. (1992). Inhibitory junction potentials in opossum circular esophageal muscle: cGMP as an intracellular mediator. *American Journal of Physiology, 263*, G97–G101.

Conklin, J. L., Du., C., Murray, J. A., & Bates, J. N. (1993). Characterization and mediation of inhibitory junction potentials from opossum lower esophageal sphincter. *Gastroenterology, 104*, 1439–1444.

Conklin, J. L., Du, C., Schulze-Delrieu, K., & Shirazi, S. (1991). Abnormalities in the excitability of hypertrophic esophageal smooth muscle. *Gastroenterology, 101*, 657–663.

Conklin, J. L., Murray, J. A., Ledlow, A., Clark, E., Picken, H., & Rosenthal, G. (1995) Effects of recombinant human hemoglobin on opossum esophageal motor function. *Journal of Pharmacology and Experimental Therapeutics 273*, 762–767.

Cook, I. J., Dodds, W. J., Dantas, R. O., Massey, B. T., Kern, M. K., Lang, I. M., Brasseur, J. G., & Hogan, W. J. (1989). Opening mechanisms of the human upper esophageal sphincter. *American Journal of Physiology, 257*, G748–G759

Creamer, B., & Schlegel, J. (1957). Motor responses of the esophagus to distention. *Journal of Applied Physiology, 10*, 498–504.

Crist, J., Gidda, J. S., & Goyal, R. K. (1984a). Intramural mechanisms of esophageal peristalsis: roles of cholinergic and noncholinergic nerves. *Proceedings of the National Academy of Science, USA, 81*, 3595–3599.

Crist, J., Gidda, J. S., & Goyal, R. K. (1984b). Characteristics of "on" and "off" contractions in esophageal circular muscle in vitro. American *Journal of Physiology, 264*, G137–G144.

Crist, J., Gidda, J. S., & Goyal, R. K. (1986). Role of substance P nerves in longitudinal muscle contractions of the esophagus. *American Journal of Physiology, 250*, G336–G343.

Crist, J. R., He, X. D., & Goyal, R. K. (1991). Chloride-mediated inhibitory junction potentials in opossum esophageal circular muscle. *American Journal of Physiology, 261*, G752–G762.

Crist, J., Surprenant, A., & Goyal, R. K. (1987). Intracellular studies of electrical membrane properties of opossum esophageal circular smooth muscle. *Gastroenterology, 92*, 987–992.

Cunningham, D. P., & Basmajian, J. V. (1969). Electromyography of genioglossus and geniohyoid muscles during deglutition. *Anatomical Record, 165*, 401–409.

Cunningham, E. T., & Sawchenko, P. F. (1990). Central control of esophageal motility: Review. *Dysphagia, 5*, 35–51.

Cunningham, E.T., Jr., Simmons, D.M., Swanson, L.W., & Sawchenko, P.E. (1991). Enkephalin-immunoreactivity and messenger RNA in a discrete projection from the nucleus of the solitary tract to the nucleus ambiguus in the rat. *Journal of Comparative Neurology, 307*, 1–16.

Daniel, E. E., & Chapman, K. M. (1963). Electrical activity of the gastrointestinal tract as an indication of mechanical activity. *American Journal of Digestive Disorders, 8*, 54–60.

Daniel, E. E., Crankshaw, J., & Sarna, S. (1979a). Prostaglandins and tetrodotoxin-insensitive relaxation of opossum lower esophageal sphincter. *American Journal of Physiology, 235*, E153–E172.

Daniel, E. E., Crankshaw, J., & Sarna, S. (1979b). Prostaglandins and myogenic control of tension in lower esophageal sphincter *in vitro*. *Prostaglandins, 17*, 629–639.

Daniel, E. E., Holmy-Elkholy, A., Lager, L. P., & Kannan, M. S. (1983). Neither a purine nor VIP is the mediator of inhibitory nerves of opossum oesophageal smooth muscle. *Journal of Physiology (London), 336*, 243–260.

Daniel, E. E., & Posey-Daniel, V. (1984). Neuromuscular structures of the opossum esophagus: Role of interstitial cells of Cajal. *American Journal of Physiology, 246*, G305–G315.

Dean, J. B., Czyzyk-Krzeska, M., & Millhorn, D. E. (1989). Experimentally induced postinhibitoxy rebound in rat nucleus ambiguus is dependent on hyperpolarization parameters and membrane potential. *Neuroscience Research, 6*, 487–493.

DeCarle, D. J., & Christensen, J. (1976a). Histamine receptors in esophageal smooth muscle of the opossum. *Gastroenterology, 70*, 1071–1075.

DeCarle, D. J., & Christensen, J. (1976b). A dopamine receptor in esophageal smooth muscle of the opossum. *Gastroenterology, 70*, 216–219.

DeCarle, D. J., Christensen, J., Szabo, A. C., Templeman, D. C., & McKinley, D. R. (1983). Calcium dependence of neuromuscular events in esophageal smooth muscle of the opossum. *American Journal of Physiology, 232*, E547–E552.

Dektor, D. L., & Ryan, J. P. (1982). Transmembrane voltage of opossum esophageal smooth muscle and its response to electrical stimulation of intrinsic nerves. *Gastroenterology, 82*, 301–308.

Dodds, W. J, Christensen, J, Dent, J., Wood, J. D., & Arndorfer, R. C. (1978). Esophageal contractions induced by vagal stimulation in the opossum. *American Journal of Physiology, 235*, E392–E401.

Dodds, W. J., Christensen, J., Dent, J., Wood, J. D., & Arndorfer, R. C. (1979). Pharmacological investigation of primary peristalsis in smooth muscle portion of opossum esophagus. *American Journal of Physiology, 237*, E561–E566.

Dodds, W. J., Christensen, J., Dent, J., Wood, J. D., & Arndorfer, R. C. (1979). Pharmacological investigation of primary peristalsis in smooth muscle portion of opossum esophagus. *American Journal Physiology, 237*, E561–E566.

Dodds, W. J., Dent, J., Hogan, W. J., & Arndorfer, R. C. (1981). Effect of atropine on esophageal motor function in humans. *American Journal of Physiology, 240*, G290–G296.

Dodds, W. J., Hogan, W. J., Reid, D. P., Stewart, E. T., & Arndorfer, R. C. (1973). A comparison between primary esophageal peristalsis following wet and dry swallows. *Journal of Applied Physiology, 35*, 851–857.

Dodds, W. J., Stef, I. I., & Hogan, W. I. (1976). Factors determining pressure measurement accuracy by intraluminal esophageal manometry. *Gastroenterology, 70*, 117–123.

Dodds, W. J., Stef, J. J., Stewart, E. T., Hogan, N. T., Arndorfer, R .C., & Cohen, E. B. (1978). Responses of feline esophagus to cervical vagal stimulation. *American Journal of Physiology, 235*, E63–E73.

Doty, R. W. (1951). Influence of stimulus pattern on reflex deglutition. *American Journal of Physiology, 166*, 142–158.

Doty, R. W. (1968). Neural organization of deglutition. In C. F. Code (Ed.), *Handbook of physiology: Volume 4. Motility, Section 6. Alimentary Canal*, (pp. 1861–1902). Washington DC: American Physiological Society.

Doty, R. W., & Bosma, J. F. (1956). An electromyographic analysis of reflex deglutition. *Journal of Neurophysiology, 19*, 44–60.

Doty, R. W., Richmond, W. H., & Storey, A. T. (1967). Effect of medullary lesions on coordination of deglutition. *Experimental Neurology, 17*, 91–106.

Du, C., & Conklin, J. L. (1990). Inhibitory junction potentials in the opossum esophageal circular muscle: cGMP as an intracellular mediator. *Gastroenterology, 98*, A347.

Du, C., Murray, J., Bates, J., & Conklin, J. L. (1991). Nitric oxide: Mediator of nonadrenergic noncholinergic hyperpolarization of opossum esophageal muscle. *American Journal of Physiology, 261*, G1012–G1016.

Dubner, R. B., Sessle, B. J., & Storey, A. T. (1978). *The neural basis of oral and facial function*. New York: Plenum.

Edmundowicz, S. A., & Clouse, R. E. (1991). Shortening of the esophagus in response to swallowing. *American Journal of Physiology, 260*, G512–G516 .

Ekberg, O., Olsson, R., & Sundgren-Borgstrom, P. (1988). Relation of bolus size and pharyngeal swallow. *Dysphagia, 3*, 69–72.

Enzmann, E. R., Harell, G. S., & Zboralske, F. F. (1977). Upper esophageal responses to intraluminal distention in man. *Gastroenterology, 2,* 1292–1298.

Falempin, M., Ternaux, J. P. , Palouzier, B., & Chamoin, M. C. Presence of cholinergic neurons in the vagal afferent system: involvement in a heterogenous reinnervation. *Joumal of the Autonomic Nervous System, 28,* 243–250.

Fisher, R. S., Dimarino, A. J., & Cohen, S. (1975). Mechanism of cholecystokinin inhibition of lower esophageal sphincter pressure. *American Journal of Physiology, 228,* 1469–1473.

Fournet, J., Snape, W. J., & Cohen, S. (1979). Sympathetic control of lower esophageal sphincter function in the cat. Action of direct cervical and sphanchnic nerve stimulation. *Journal of Clinical Investigation, 63,* 562–570.

Fox, J. E. T., Said, S. l., & Daniel, E. E. (1979). Is vasoactive intestinal polypeptide (VIP) a neurotransmitter in the lower esophageal sphincter (LES) in the North American opossum? *Gastroenterology, 76,* 1134–1979

Gidda, J. S., Cobb, B. W. , & Goyal, R. K. (1981). Modulation of esophageal peristalsis by vagal efferent stimulation in opossum. *Clinical Investigation, 68,* 1411–1419.

Gidda, J. S., & Goyal, R. K. (1983a). Influence of successive vagal stimulation on contractions in esophageal smooth muscle of opossum. *Clinical Investigation, 71,* 1095–1103.

Gidda, J. S., & Goyal, R. K. (1983b). Swallow-evoked action potentials in vagal preganglionic efferents. *Journal of Neurophysiology, 52,* 1169–1180.

Gonella, J., Niel, J. P., & Roman C. (1977). Vagal control of lower oesophageal sphincter motility in the cat. *Journal of Physiology (London), 273,* 647–664.

Gonella, J., Neil, J. P., & Roman, C. (1979). Sympathetic control of lower oesophageal sphincter motility in the cat. *Journal of Physiology (London), 287,* 177–190.

Goyal, R. K., & Gidda, J. S. (1981). Relationship between electrical and mechanical activity in the opossum esophagus. *American Journal of Physiology, 240,* G305–G311.

Goyal, R. K., & Paterson, W. G. (1989). Esophageal motility. In S. G. Schultz, J. D. Wood, & B. B. Rauner (Eds.), *Handbook of physiology. Vol. 1. Motility and circulation, Section 6. The gastrointestinal system* (pp. 865–908). Bethesda, MD: American Physiological Society.

Goyal, R. K., & Rattan, S. (1973): Mechanism of the lower esophageal sphincter relaxation. Action of prostaglandin E_1 and theophylline. *Journal of Clinical Investigation, 52,* 337–341.

Goyal, R. K., & Rattan, S. (1976). Genesis of basal sphincter pressure: effect of tetrodotoxin on lower esophageal sphincter pressure in opossum in vivo. *Gastroenterology, 71,* 62–67.

Greenwood, B., Blank, E., & Dodds, W.J. (1992). Nicotine stimulates esophageal peristaltic contractions in cats by a central mechanism. *American Journal of Physiology, 262,* G567–571.

Grillner, S., Wallen, P., Dale, N., Brodin, L., Buchanan, J., & Hill, R. (1993). Transmitters, membrane properties and network circuitry in the control of locomotion in the lamprey. *Trends in Neuroscience, 10,* 34–41.

Grossman, M. I. (1973). What is physiological? *Gastroenterology, 65,* 994.

Gutierrez, J. G., Thanik, K. D., Chey, W. Y., & Yajima, H. (1977). The effect of motilin on the lower esophageal sphincter of the opossum. *American Journal of Digestive Diseases, 22,* 402–405.

Halpern, B. P., & Nelson, L. M. (1965). Bulbar gustatory responses to anterior and to posterior tongue stimulation in the rat. *American Journal of Physiology, 209,* 105–110.

Hamlet, S. L. (1989). Dynamic aspects of lingual propulsive activity in swallowing. *Dysphagia, 4,* 136–145.

Hashim M.A. (1989). *Premotoneuronal organization of swallowing in the rat.* Doctoral dissertation. Memorial University of Newfoundland, St. John's.

Hashim, M. A., & Bieger, D. (1987). Excitatory action of 5–HT on deglutitive substrates in the rat solitary complex. *Brain Research Bulletin, 18,* 355–363.

Hashim, M. A., & Bieger, D. (1989). Excitatory amino acid receptor-mediated activation of solitarial deglutitive loci. *Neuropharmacology, 28,* 913–921.

Hashim M. A., Bolger, G. T., & Bieger, D. (1989). Modulation of solitarial deglutitive N-methyl-D-aspartate receptors by dihydropyridines. *Neuropharmacology, 28,* 923–929.

Hellemans, J., Pelemans, W., & Vantrappen, G. (1981). Pharyngoesophageal swallowing disorders and the pharyngoesophageal sphincter. *Medical Clinics of North America, 65,* 1149–1171.

Hellemans, J., & Vantrappen, G. (1967). Electromyographic studies on canine esophageal motility. *American Journal of Digestive Diseases, 12,* 1240–1255.

Hellemans, J., Vantrappen, G., & Janssens, J. (1974). Electromyography of the esophagus. In *Diseases of the esophagus* (pp. 270–285). New York: Springer-Verlag.

Hellemans, J., Vantrappen, G., Valembois, P., Janssens, J., & Vandenbroucke, J. (1968). Electrical activity of striated and smooth muscle of the esophagus. *American Journal of Digestive Diseases, 13,* 320–334.

Henkin, R. I., & Banks, V. (1967). Tactile perception on the tongue, palate and the hand of normal man. In J. F. Bosma (Ed.), *Symposium on oral sensation and perception* (pp. 182–187). Springfield, IL: Charles C. Thomas.

Hensel, H., & Huopaniemi, T. (1969). Static and dynamic properties of warm fibers in the infraorbital nerve. *Pfluegers Archives, 309,* 1–10.

Higgs, B., & Ellis, F. H. H., Jr. (1965). The effect of bilateral supranodosal vagotomy on canine esophageal function. *Surgery, 58,* 828–834.

Hiiema, K. M., & Crompton, A. M. (1985). Mastication, food transport and swallowing. In M. Hildebrand, D. M. Bramble, K. F. Liem, & D. B. Wake (Eds.). *Functional vertebrate morphology* (pp 262–290) Cambridge, MA:, Harvard University Press.

Hockman, C. H, Bieger, D., & Weerasuriya, A. (1989). Supranuclear pathways of swallowing. *Progress in Neurobiology, 12,* 15–32.

Hogan, W. J., Dodds, W. J., Hoke, S. E., Reid, D. P., Kalkhoff, R. K., & Arndorfer, R. C. (1975). Effect of glucagon on esophageal motor function. *Gastroenterology, 69,* 160–165.

Hollaway, R. H., Blank, E. L., Takashashi, I., Dodds, W. J., Dent, J., & Sarna, S. K. (1987). Electrical control activity of the lower esophageal sphincter in unanesthetized opossums. *American Journal of Physiology, 252,* G511–G521.

Hollis, J. B., & Castell. D. O. (1975). Effect of dry swallows and wet swallows of different volumes on esophageal peristalsis. *Journal of Applied Physiology, 38,* 1161–1164.

Holstege, G., Graveland, G., Bijker-Biemond, C., & Schuddeboom, I. (1983). Location and motoneurons innervating soft palate, pharynx and upper esophagus. Anatomical evidence for a possible swallowing center in the pontine reticular formation. *Brain, Behavior and Evolution, 23,* 47–62.

Hopkins, D. A., Bieger, D., deVente, J., & Steinbusch, H. W. M. (1994). Nitric oxide synthase (NOS) and cGMP in the medulla oblongata after vagotomy. *Society for Neuroscience Abstract, 20.*

Hrychshyn, A. W., & Basmajian, J. V. (1972). Electromyography of the oral stage of swallowing in man. *American Journal of Anatomy, 33,* 335–340.

Hudson, L. C., & Cunningham, J. F. (1985). The origins of innervation of esophagus of the dog. *Brain Research, 326,* 125–136.

Iggo, A. (1969). Cutaneous thermoreceptors in primates and subprimates. *Journal of Physiology (London), 200,* 403–430.

Ito, C., Fukuda, A., Nabekura, J., & Oomura, Y. (1989). Acetylcholine causes nicotinic depolarization in rat dorsal motor nucleus of the vagus, in vitro. *Brain Research, 503,* 44–48.

Jacob, P., Kahrilas, P. J., Herzon, G., & McLaughlin, B. (1990). Determinants of upper esophageal

sphincter pressure in dogs. *American Journal of Physiology, 260,* G245–G251.

Jacobowitz, D., & Nemir, P. (1969). The autonomic innervation of the esophagus of the dog. *Journal of Thoracic Cardiovascular Surgery, 58,* 678–684.

Janssens I., Valembois P., Hellemans J., Vantrappen, G., & Pelemans, W. (1974). Studies on the necessity of a bolus for the progression of secondary peristalsis in the canine esophagus. *Gastroenterology, 67,* 245–251.

Janssens, J., Valembois, P., Vantrappen, G., Hellemans, J., & Pelemans, W. (1973). Is the primary peristaltic contraction of the canine esophagus bolus-dependent? *Gastroenterology, 65,* 750–756.

Jean, A. (1972a). Effet de lesions localisees du bulbe rachidien sur le stude oesophagien de la deglutition. *Journal of Physiology (Paris), 64,* 507–516.

Jean, A. (1972b). Localisation et activité des neurones deglutiteurs bulbaires. *Journal of Physiology (Paris), 64,* 227–268.

Jean, A. (1978). Localisation et activité des motoneurones oesophagiens chez le mouton. *Journal of Physiology (Paris), 74,* 737–742.

Jean, A. (1984). (1984). Brainstem organization of the swallowing network. *Brain, Behavior, and Evolution, 25,* 109–116.

Jean, A. (1986). Control of the central swallowing program by inputs from the peripheral receptors. A review. *Journal of Autonomic Nervous System, 10,* 225–233.

Jean, A. (1990). Brainstem control of swallowing: Localization and organization of the central pattern generator for swallowing. In A. Taylor (Ed.), *Neurophysiology of the jaws and teeth.* London: MacMillan Press.

Jean, A., Amri, M., & Calas, A. (1983). Connections between the ventral medullary swallowing area and the trigeminal motor nucleus of sheep studied by tracing techniques. *Journal of Autonomic Nervous System, 7,* 87–96.

Jean A., & Car, A. (1979). Inputs to the swallowing medullary neurons from the peripheral afferent fibers and the swallowing cortical area. *Brain Research, 78,* 567–572.

Jean, A, Car, A., & Roman, C. (1975). Comparison of activity in pontine versus medullary neurones during swallowing. *Experimental Brain Research, 22,* 211–220.

Jean, A., Kessler, J. P., & Tell, F. (1994). Nucleus tractus solitarii and deglutition: Monoamines, excitatory amino acids and cellular properties. In R. A. Baracco (Ed.) *Nucleus of the solitary tract* (pp. 355–369). New York: CRC Press.

Jean, A., & Puizillout, J. J. (1986, September). *Neurobiology of the nucleus of the solitary tract.* International Satellite Symposium of the 10th

Annual Meeting of the European Neuroscience Association. Marseilles, France.

Jensen, D. M., McCallum, R., & Walsh, J. H. (1978). Failure of atropine to inhibit gastrin-17 stimulation of the lower esophageal sphincter in man. *Gastroenterology, 75*, 825–827.

Jordan, P. H., & Longhi, J. E. (1971). Relationship between size of bolus and the act of swallowing on esophageal peristalsis in dogs. *Proceedings of the Society of Experimental Biology and Medicine, 137*, 868–871.

Jury, J., Jager, L. P., & Daniel, E. E. (1985). Unusual potassium channels mediate nonadrenergic noncholinergic nerve mediated inhibition of opossum esophagus. *Canadian Journal of Physiology and Pharmacology, 63*, 107–112.

Kahrilas, P. J., Dodds, W. J., Dent, J., Haeberle, B., Hogan, W. J., & Arndorfer, R. C. (1987). Effect of sleep, spontaneous gastroesophageal reflux, and a meal on upper esophageal sphincter pressure in normal human volunteers. *Gastroenterology, 92*, 466–471.

Kannan, M. S., Jager, L. P., & David, E. E. (1985). Electrical properties of smooth muscle cell membrane of opossum esophagus. *American Journal of Physiology, 248*, G342–G346.

Kawasaki, M., Ogura, J. H., & Takenouchi, S. (1964). Neurophysiologic observations of normal deglutition. I. Its relationship to the respiratory cycle. *Laryngoscope, 74*, 1747–1765

Kelly, M. L., & Friedland, H. L. (1967). Gastroesophageal sphinteric pressure before and after oral anticholinergic drug and placebo administration. *American Journal of Digestive Diseases, 12*, 823–833.

Kendall, G. P. N., Thompson, D. G., Day, S. J., & Garvie, N. (1987). Motor responses of the esophagus to intraluminal distension in normal subjects and patients with oesophageal clearance disorders. *Gut, 28*, 272–279.

Kerr, F. W. L. (1962). Facial, vagal and glossopharyngeal nerves in the cat. *Archives of Neurology, 6*, 264–281.

Kessler, J. P., Cherkaoui, N., Catalin, D., & Jean, A (1990). Swallowing responses induced by microinjection of glutamate and glutamate agonists into the nucleus tractus solitarius of ketamine-anesthetized rats. *Experimental Brain Research, 83*, 151–158.

Kessler, J. P., & Jean, A. (1985a). Inhibition of the swallowing reflex by local application of serotonergic agents into the nucleus of the solitary tract. *European Journal of Pharmacology, 118*, 77–85.

Kessler, J. P., & Jean, A. (1985b). Identification of the medullary swallowing regions in the rat. *Experimental Brain Research, 57*, 256–263.

Kessler, J. P., & Jean, A. (1986). Effect of catecholamines on the swallowing reflex after pressure microinjections into the lateral solitary complex of the medulla oblongata. *Brain Research, 386*, 69–77.

Kessler, J. P., & Jean, A. (1986). Inhibitory influence of monoamines and brainstem monoaminergic regions on the medullary swallowing reflex. *Neuroscience Letters, 65*, 41–46.

Kessler, J. P., & Jean, A. (1991). Evidence that activation of N-methyl-D-aspartate (NMDA) and non-NMDA receptors within the nucleus tractus solitarii triggers swallowing. *European Journal of Pharmacology, 201*, 59–67.

King, G. W. (1980). Topology of ascending brainstem projections to nucleus parabrachialis in the cat. *Journal of Comparative Neurology, 191*, 615–638.

Kirchner, J. A. (1958). The motor activity of the cricopharyngeus muscle. *Laryngoscope, 68*, 1119–1159.

Kitamura, S., Nagase, Y., Chen, K., & Shigenaga, Y. (1993). Nucleus ambiguus of the rabbit: Cytoarchitectural subdivision and myotopical and neurotopic representations. *Anatomical Record, 237*, 109–123.

Knudsen, A., Frobert, O., & Tottrup, A. (1994). The role of the L-arginine-nitric oxide pathway for peristalsis in the opossum oesophageal body. *Scandinavian Journal of Gastroenterology, 29*, 1083–1087.

Knudsen, M. A. Svane, D., & Tottrup, A. (1991). Importance of the L-arginine-nitric oxide pathway in NANC nerve function of the opossum esophageal body. *Digestive Diseases in Science, 9*, 365–370.

Krammer, E. B., Rath, T., & Lischka, M. A. (1979). Somatotopic organization of the hypoglossal nucleus: A HRP study in the rat. *Brain Research, 170*, 533–537.

Kravitz, J. J., Snape, W. J., & Cohen, S. (1966). Effect of thoracic vagotomy and vagal stimulation on esophageal function. *American Journal of Physiology, 238*, 233–238.

Kravitz, J. J., Snape, W. J., Jr., & Cohen, S. (1978). Effect of histamine and histamine antagonists on human lower esophageal sphincter function. *Gastroenterology 74*, 435–440.

Kubota, K. (1976). Motoneurone mechanisms: Suprasegmental controls. In B. J. Sessle & A. G. Hannam (Eds.), *Mastication and swallowing:. Biological and clinical correlates* (pp. 60–75). Toronto: University of Toronto Press.

Laird, W. R. (1974). Intermaxillary relationships during deglutition. *Journal of Dental Research, 53*, 127–131.

Landgren, S., & Olsson, K. Å. (1976). Localization of evoked potentials in the digastric, masseteric, supra- and intertrigeminal subnuclei of the cat. *Experimental Brain Research, 26*, 299–318.

Lang, I. M., Dantas, R. O., Cook, I. J., & Dodds, W. J. (1991). Videographic, manometric and electromyographic analysis of canine upper esophageal sphincter. *American Journal of Physiology, 260*, G911–G919.

Lawn A. M. (1964). The localization, by means of electrical stimulation, of the origin and path in the medulla oblongata of the motor nerve fibers of the rabbit esophagus. *Journal of Physiology (London), 174*, 232–244.

Lawn, A. M. (1966a). The nucleus ambiguus of the rabbit. *Journal of Comparative Neurology, 127*, 307–312.

Lawn, A. M. (1966b). The localization, in the nucleus ambiguus of the rabbit, of the cells of origin of motor nerve fibers in the glossopharyngeal nerve and various branches of the vagus nerve by means of retrograde degeneration. *Journal of Comparative Neurology, 127*, 293–306.

Lazara, G., Lazzarus, C., & Logemann, I. A. (1986). Impact of thermal stimulation on the triggering of the swallowing reflex. *Dysphagia, 1*, 73–77.

Leslie, R. A. (1985). Neuroactive substances in the dorsal vagal complex of the medulla oblongata, nucleus of the tractus solitarius, area postrema, and dorsal motor nucleus of the vagus. *Neurochemistry International, 7*, 191–211.

Levitt, M. N., Dedo, H. H., & Ogura, J. H. (1965). The cricopharyngeus muscle: an electromyographlc study in the dog. *Laryngoscope, 75*, 122–136.

Lind, J. F., Cotton, D. J., Blanchard, R., Crispin, J. J., & Dimopolos, G. E. (1969). Effect of thoracic displacement and vagotomy on the canine gastroesophageal junctional zone. *Gastroenterology, 56*, 1078–1085.

Lind, J. F., Crispin, J. S., & McIver, D. K. (1968). The effect of atropine on the gastroesophageal sphincter. *Canadian Journal of Pharmacology, 46*, 233–238.

Longhi, E. H., & Jordan, P. H., Jr. (1971). Necessity of a bolus for propagation of primary peristalsis in the canine esophagus. *American Journal of Physiology, 220*, 609–612.

Loewy, A. D., & Burton, H. (1978). Nuclei of the solitary tract: Efferent projections to the lower brainstem and spinal cord of the cat. *Journal of Comparative Neurology, 181*, 421–450.

Lu, W. Y., & Bieger, D. (1993). Secondary peristalsis in the rat. *Dysphagia, 9*, 77.

Lu, W. Y., Neuman, R. S., & Bieger, D. (1993a). Cholinergic innervation of esophageal premotoneurons—Central vs. peripheral source. *Dysphagia, 9*, 75.

Lu, W. Y., Neuman, R. S., & Bieger, D. (1993b). *Does nitric oxide contribute to the control of esophagomotor activity?* Dysphagia Research Society Second Annual Scientific Meeting, Lake Geneva. WI.

Lu, W. Y., Neuman, R. S., Reynolds, J., & Bieger, D. (1993). Muscarinic receptor activation modulates neuronal activity in the central subnucleus of the nucleus tractus solitarii (NTSC). *Society Neuroscience Abstract, 19*, 1524.

Lund, G. F., & Christensen, J. (1969). Electrical stimulation of esophageal smooth muscle and effects of antagonists. *American Journal of Physiology, 217*, 1369–1374.

Lund, W. S. (1965a). A study of the cricopharyngeal sphincter in man and in the dog. *Annals of the Royal College of Surgeons, England, 37*, 225–246.

Lund, W. S. (1965b). The function of the cricopharyngeal sphincter during swallowing. *Acta Otolaryngologica, 59*, 497–510.

Manier, M., Feuerstein, C., Passagia, J. G., Mouchet, P., Mons, N., & Geffard, M. (1990). Evidence for the existence of L-DOPA- and dopamine-immunoreactive nerve cell bodies in the caudal part of the dorsal motor nucleus of the vagus nerve. *Journal of Chemical Neuroanatomy, 3*, 193–205.

Mansson, I., & Sandberg, N. (1974). Effects of surface anesthesia on deglutition in man. *Laryngoscope, 84*, 427–437.

Mansson, I., & Sandberg, N. (1975a). Oro-pharyngeal sensitivity and elicitation of swallowing in man. *Acta Otolaryngologica, 79*, 140–145.

Mansson, I., & Sandberg, N. (1975b). Salivary stimulus and swallowing in man. *Acta Otolaryngologica, 79*, 445–450.

Martin, R. E., & Sessle, B. J. (1993). The role of the cerebral cortex in swallowing, *Dysphagia, 8*, 195–202.

Matarazzo, S., Snape, W. J., Jr., Ryan, J., & Cohen, S. (1976). The relationship of cervical and abdominal vagal activity in lower esophageal sphincter function. *Gastroenterology, 71*, 999–1003.

Matsuda, K., Uemura, M., Kume, M., Matsushima, R., & Mizuno, N. (1978). Topographical representation of masticatory muscles in the motor trigeminal nucleus in the rabbit: a HRP study. *Neuroscience Letters, 8*, 1–4.

Matsumoto, H. (1971). X-ray, T. V., cinematographical, and electromyographical studies on positional changes of the hyoid bone, especially in swallowing, maximum opening and closing of the mouth, and tongue movements. *Shika Gakuho, 77*, 533–544.

McNamara, J. A., Jr., & Moyers, R. E. (1973). Electromyography of the oral phase of deglutition in the rhesus monkey (Macaca mulatta). *Archives of Oral Biology, 18*, 995–1002.

Meisner, A. J., Bowfes, K. L., Zwick, R., & Daniel, E. E. (1976). Effect of motilin on lower esophageal sphincter. *Gut, 17*, 925–932.

Meltzer, S. J. (1899). On the causes of the orderly progress of the peristaltic movements in the esophagus. *American Journal of Physiology, 2,* 266–272.

Menon, M. K., Kodama, C. K., Kling, A. S., & Fitten, J. (1986). An in vivo pharmacological method for the quantitative evaluation of the central effects of alpha-l agonists and antagonists. *Neuropharmacology, 25,* 503–508.

Menon, M. K, Tseng, L. F., Loh, H. H., & Clark, W. G. (1980). An electromyographic method for the assessment of naloxone-induced abstinence in morphine-dependent rats. *Naunyn Schmiedeberg's Archive of Pharmacology, 312,* 43–49.

Miller, A. J. (1972a). Characteristics of the swallowing reflex induced by peripheral nerve and brain stem stimulation. *Experimental Neurology, 34,* 210–222.

Miller, A. J. (1972b). Significance of sensory inflow to the swallowing reflex. *Brain Research, 43,* 147–159.

Miller, A. J. (1982). Deglutition. *Physiological Review 62,* 129–184.

Miller A. J. (1986). Neurophysiological basis of swallowing. *Dysphagia, 1,* 91–100.

Miller, A. J., & Bowman, J. P. (1977). Precentral cortical modulation of mastication and swallowing. *Journal of Dental Research, 56,* 1154.

Miller, A. J., & Dunmire, C. (1976). Characterization of the postnatal development of the superior laryngeal nerve fibers in the postnatal kitten. *Journal of Neurobiology, 7,* 483–494.

Miller, A. J., & Loizzi, R. F. (1974). Anatomical and functional differentiation of superior laryngeal nerve fibers affecting swallowing and respiration. *Experimental Neurology, 42,* 369–387.

Miller, F. R., & Sherrington, C. S. (1916). Some observations on the buccopharyngeal stage of reflex deglutition in the cat. *Quarterly Journal of Experimental Physiology, 9,* 147–186.

Mittal, R. K., Rochester, D. F., & McCallum, R. W. (1988): Electrical and mechanical activity in the human esophageal sphincter during diaphragmatic contraction. *Journal of Clinical Investigation, 81,* 1182–1189.

Mizuno, N., Matsuda, K., Iwahori, N., Uemura-Sumi, M., Kume, N., & Matsushima, R. (1981). Representation of the masticatory muscles in the motor trigeminal nucleus of the macaque monkey. *Neuroscience Letters, 21,* 19–22.

Molhant, M. (1912). Le nerf vague. Étude anatomique et expérimentale. Deuxieme partie. Le noyau ambigu; les connexions anatomiques et la valeur fonctionelle du noyau central du vague et du noyaux ambigu. *Nevraxe, 13,* 309–316.

Morest, D. K (1967). Experimental study of the projections of the nucleus of the tractus solitarius and the area postrema in the cat. *Journal of Comparative Neurology, 130,* 277–300.

Mukhopadhyay, A. K., & Weisbrodt, N. W. (1975). Neural organization of esophageal peristalsis: Role of the vagus nerve. *Gastroenterology, 58,* 444–447.

Mukhopadhyay, A. K., & Weisbrodt, N. W. (1977). Effect of dopamine on esophageal motor function. *American Journal of Physiology, 232,* E19–E24.

Mukhopadhyay, A. K., & Kunnemann, M. (1979). Mechanism of lower esophageal sphincter stimulation by bombesin in the opossum. *Gastroenterology, 76,* 1409–1414.

Murakami, Y., Fukuda, H., & Kirchner, J. A. (1972). The cricopharyngeus muscle: an electrophysiological and neuropharmacological study. *Acta Otolaryngology, 311*(Suppl.), 1–19.

Murray, G. M., & Sessle, B. J. (1992). Functional properties of single neurons in the face primary motor cortex of the primate. 1. Input and output features of tongue motor cortex. *Journal of Neurophysiology, 7,* 747–758.

Murray, J., Bates, J. N., & Conklin, J. L. (1994). Nerve-mediated nitric oxide production by the opossum lower esophageal sphincter. *Digestive Diseases in Science.*

Murray, J., Du, C., & Conklin, J. L. (1992). Guanylate cyclase inhibitors: Effect on tone, relaxation and cGMP content of the lower esophageal sphincter. *American Journal of Physiology, 263,* G87–G90.

Murray, J., Du, C., Ledlow, A., Bates, J. N., & Conklin, J. L. (1991). Nitric oxide: Mediator of nonadrenergic noncholinergic responses of opossum esophageal muscle. *American Journal of Physiology, 261,* G40I–G406.

Murray, J., Ledlow, A., Launspach J., Evans, D., Loveday, M., & Conklin, J. L. (1995). The effects of recombinant human hemoglobin on esophageal motor function in humans. *Gastroenterology, 78.*

Murray, J, Shibata, E. F., Buresh, T. L., Picken, H., O'Meara, B. W. & Conklin J. L. (1995). Nitric oxide modulates a calcium-activated potassium current in muscle cells from opossum esophagus. *American Journal of Physiology.*

Nance, D. M., Hopkins, D. A., & Bieger, D. (1987). A reexamination of the innervation of the thymus gland in mice and rats. *Brain, Behaviour & Immunity, 1,* 134–147.

Neuman, R. S., Wang, Y. T., Zhang, M., Vyas, D., & Bieger, D. (1993). *Somatostatin (SST) is necessary for fast information transfer in vagal motoneurons.* Summer Neuropeptide Conference 1993, Martha's Vineyard, MA.

Niel, J. P., Gonella, J., & Roman, C. (1980). Localisation par la technique de marquage à la peroxydase des corps cellulaires des neurones ortho et parasympatiques innervant le sphincter inferieur du chat. *Journal de Physiologie (Paris), 76,* 591–599.

Norgren, R. (1978). Projections from the the nucleus of the solitary tract in the rat. *Neuroscience, 3,* 207–218.

Ohta, A., Takagi, H., Matsui, T., Hamai, Y., Iida, S., & Esumi, H. (1993). Localization of nitric oxide synthase-immunoreactive neurons in the solitary nucleus and ventrolateral medulla oblongata of the rat: their relation to catecholaminergic neurons. *Neuroscience Letters, 158*, 33–35.

O'Meara, B. W., Conklin, J. L., & Murray, J. (1992). Nitroblue tetrazolium inhibits NANC-mediated events in the opossum esophagus. *Gastroenterology, 103*, 1406.

Palkovitz, M., Mezey, E., Eskay, R. L., & Brownstein, M. J. (1986). Innervation of the nucleus of the solitary tract and the dorsal vagal nucleus by thyrotropin-releasing hormone-containing raphe neurons. *Brain Research, 373*, 246–251.

Palmer, J. B., Rudin, N. J,, Lara, G., & Crompton, A. W. (1992). Coordination of mastication and swallowing. *Dysphagia, 7*, 187–200.

Paterson, W. G., Hynna-Liepert, T. T., & Selucky, M. (1991). Comparison of primary and secondary esophageal peristalsis in humans: Effect of atropine. *American Journal of Physiology, 260*, G52–G57.

Pommerenke, W. T. (1928). A study of the sensory areas eliciting the swallowing reflex. *American Journal of Physiology, 84*, 36–41.

Porter, R. (1963) Unit responses evoked in the medulla oblongata by vagus nerve stimulation. *Journal of Physiology (London), 168*, 717–735.

Poulos, D. A. (1971). Trigeminal temperature mechanisms. In R. Dubner & Y. Kawamura (Eds.), *Oral-facial sensory and motor mechanisms* (pp. 47–72). New York: Appleton-Century-Crofts.

Poulos, D. A., & Lende, R. A. (1970). Response of trigeminal ganglion neurons to thermal stimulation of oral-facial regions. II. Temperature change response. *Journal of Neurophysiology, 57*, 518–526.

Price, L. M., El-Sharkawy, T. Y., Mui, H. Y., & Diamant, N E. (1979). Effect of bilateral cervical vagotomy on balloon-induced lower esophageal sphincter relation in the dog. *Gastroenterology, 77*, 324–329.

Pritchard, T. C,, Hamilton, R. B,, Mors, J. R., & Norgren, R. (1986). Projections of thalamic gustatory and lingual areas in the monkey, Macaca fascicularis. *Journal of Comparative Neurology, 244,* 213–228.

Rattan, S., Coln, D., & Goyal, R. K. (1976). The mechanism of action of gastrin on the lower esophageal sphincter. *Gastroenterology, 70*, 828–835.

Rattan, S., Gidda, J. S., & Goyal, R. K. (1983). Membrane potential and mechanical responses to vagal stimulation and swallowing. *Gastroenterology, 85*, 922–998.

Rattan, S., & Goyal, R. K. (1974). Neural control of the lower esophageal sphincter influence of the vagus nerves. *Journal of Clinical Investigation, 54*, 899–906.

Rattan, S., & Goyal, R. K. (1976). Effect of dopamine on the esophageal smooth muscle in vivo. *Gastroenterology, 70*, 377–381.

Rattan, S., & Goyal, R. K. (1977a). Effect of histamine on the lower esophageal sphincter in vivo: Evidence of action at three different sites. *Journal of Pharmacology and Experimental Therapy, 204*, 334–342.

Rattan, S., & Goyal, R. K. (1977b). Effect of 5-hydroxytryptamine on the lower esophageal sphincter in vivo. *Journal of Clinical Investigation, 59*, 125–133.

Reynolds, R. P. E., El-Sharkawy, T. Y., & Diamant, N. E. (1984). Lower esophageal sphincter function in the cat: Role of the central innervation assessed by transient vagal blockade. *American Journal of Physiology, 246*, G666–G674.

Resin, H., Stern, D. H., Sturdevant, R. A. L., & Isenberg, J. I. (1973): Effect of the C-terminal octapeptide of cholecystokinin on lower esophageal sphincter pressure in man. *Gastroenterology, 64*, 946–949.

Reynolds, J. C,. Ouyang, A., & Cohen, S. (1984). A lower esophageal sphincter reflex involving substance P. *American Journal of Physiology, 246*, G346–G354.

Rhoton, A. L., Jr., O'Leary, J. L., & Ferguson, J. P. (1966). The trigeminal, facial, vagal, and glossopharyngeal nerves in the monkey. *Archives of Neurology, 14*, 530–540.

Robinson, B. A., Percy, W. H., & Christensen, J. (1984). Differences in cytochrome C oxidase capacity in smooth muscle of opossum esophagus and lower esophageal sphincter. *Gastroenterology, 87*, 1009–1013.

Rodrigo, J., deFilipe, J., Robles-Chilida, E. M., Perez Anton, J. A., Mayo, I., & Gomez, A. (1982). Sensory vagal nature and anatomical access paths to esophagus laminar nerve endings in myenteric ganglia. Determination by surgical degeneration methods. *Acta Anatomica, 112*, 47–57.

Rodrigo, J., Hernandez, C. V., Vjdal, M. A., Pedrosa J. A. (1975a). Vegetative innervation of the esophagus. II. Intraganglionic laminar endings. *Acta Anatomica, 92*, 79–100.

Rodrigo, J., Hernandez, C. J., Vidal, M. A., & Pedrosa, J. A. (1975b). Vegetative innervation of the esophagus. III. Intraepithelial endings. *Acta Anatomica, 92*, 242–258.

Roman, C. (1966). Controle nerveux de peristaltisme oesophagus. *Journal of Physiology (Paris), 58*, 79–108.

Roman, C. (1986). Neural control of deglutition and esophageal motility in mammals. *Journal of Physiology (Paris), 81*, 118–133.

Roman, C., & Car, A. (1967). Contractions oesophagiennes produites par la stimulation de vague ou du bulbe rachidien. *Journal of Physiology (Paris), 59*, 377–398.

Roman, C., & Car, A. (1970). Deglutitions et contractions oesophagiennes renexes obtenues par la stimulation des nerfs vague et larynge superieur. *Experimental Brain Research, 11*, 48–74.

Roman, C., & Gonella, J. (1981). Extrinsic control of digestive tract motility. In L. R. Johnson (Ed.), *Physiology of the gastrointestinal tract* (pp. 289–333). New York: Raven Press.

Roman, C., & Tieffenbach L. (1971). Motricite de l'oesophage a musculeuse lisse apres vigatotomie: etude electromyographique (EMG). *Journal of Physiology (Paris), 63*, 733–762.

Roman, C., & Tieffenbach L. (1972). Enregistrement de l'activite unitaire des fibres motrices vagales destinees a l'oesophage du babouin. *Journal of Physiology (Paris), 64*, 479–506.

Rosell, S., Thor, K., Rokaeus, O., Nyquist, O., Lewenhaupt, A., Kager, L., & Folkers, K. (1980). Plasma concentration of neurotensin-like immunoreactivity (NTLI) and lower esophageal sphincter (LES) pressure in man following infusion of (Gln^4)-neurotensin. *Acta Physiologica Scandinavia, 109*, 369–375.

Rosenbek, J. C., Robbins, J. A., Fishback, B., & Levine, R. L. (1991). Effects of thermal application on dysphagia after stroke. *Speech and Hearing Research, 34*, 1257–1268.

Rossiter, C. D., Norman, W. P., Jain, M., Hornby, P. J., Benjamin, S., & Gillis, R. A. (1990). Control of lower esophageal sphincter pressure by two sites in dorsal motor nucleus of the vagus. *American Journal of Physiology, 256*, G899–G906.

Rudomin, P. (1968). Excitability changes of superior laryngeal, vagal and depressor afferent terminals produced by stimulation of the solitary tract nucleus. *Experimental Brain Research, 6*, 156–170.

Ruggiero, D. A., Chan, L., Anwar, M., Mtui, E. P., & Golanov, M. (1993). Effect of cervical vagotomy on catecholaminergic neurons in the cranieal divisions of the parasympathetidc nervous system. *Brain Research, 617*, 17–27.

Ruggiero, D. A., Giuliano, R., Anwar, M., Stornetta, R., & Reis, D. J. (1990). Anatomical substrates of cholinergic-autonomic regulation in the rat. *Journal of Comparative Neurology, 292*, 1–53.

Rupert, A. H. (1978). *Influences of serotonin on swallowing in the cat.* Doctoral thesis, University of Illinois, Urbana-Champaign.

Rutherfurd, S. D., Widdop, R. E., Louis, W. J., & Gundlach, A. L. (1992). Preprogalanin mRNA is increased in vagal motor neurons following axotomy. *Molecular Brain Research, 14*, 261–266.

Ryan, J. P., Snape, W. J., & Cohen, S. (1977). Influence of vagal cooling on esophageal function. *American Journal of Physiology, 232*, 159–161.

Sampson, S., & Eyzaguirre, C. (1964). Some functional characteristics of mechanoreceptors in the larynx of the cat. *Journal of Neurophysiology, 27*, 464–480.

Sarna, S. K., Daniel, E. E., & Waterfall, W. E. 1977. Myogenic and neural control systems for esophageal motility. *Gastroenterology, 73*, 1345–1352.

Schaffar, N., Kessler, J. P., Bosler, O., & Jean, A. (1988). Central serotonergic projections to the nucleus tractus solitarii: evidence from a double labeling study in the rat. *Neuroscience 26*, 951–958.

Schaffar, N., Pio, J., & Jean, A. (1990). Selective retrograde labeling of primary vagal afferent cellbodies after injection of [^{3}H] D-aspartate into the rat nucleus tractus solitarii. *Neuroscience Letters, 114*, 253–258.

Schlippert, W., Schulze, K., & Forker, E. L. (1979). Calcium in smooth muscle from the opossum esophagus. *Proceedings of the Society of Experimental Biology and Medicine, 162*, 354–358.

Schulze, K., & Christensen, J. (1977). Lower sphincter of the opossum in pseudopregnancy. *Gastroenterology, 73*, 1082–1085.

Schulze-Delrieu, K., & Crane, S. A. (1982). Oxygen uptake and mechanical tension in esophageal smooth muscle from opossums and cats. *American Journal of Physiology, 242*, G258–G262.

Seelig, L. L., Doody, P., Brainard, L., Gidda, J. S., & Goyal, R. K. (1984). Acetylcholinesterase and choline acetyltransferase staining neurons in the opossum esophagus. *Anatomical Record, 209*, 125–130.

Serio, R., & Daniel, E. E. (1988). Electrophysiological analysis of responses to intrinsic nerves in circular opossum esophageal muscle. *American Journal of Physiology, 254*, G107–G116.

Sessle, B. J. (1973a). Excitatory and inhibitory inputs to single neurons in the solitary tract nucleus and adjacent reticular formation. *Brain Research, 53*, 319–331.

Sessle, B. J. (1973b). Presynaptic excitability changes induced in single laryngeal primary afferent fibres. *Brain Research, 53*, 333–342.

Sessle, B. J., & Henry, J. L. (1989). Neural mechanisms of swallowing: neurophysiological and neurochemical studies on brain stem neurons in the solitary tract region. *Dysphagia, 4*, 61–75.

Sessle, B. J., & Lucier, G. E. (1983). Functional aspects of the upper respiratory tract and larynx: A review. In J. T. Tildon, L. M. Roeder, & A. Steinschneider (Eds.), *Sudden infant death syndrome* (pp. 501–529). New York: Academic Press.

Siegel, S. R., Brown, F. C., Castell, D. O., Johnson, L. R., & Said, S. I. (1979). Effects of vasoactive intestinal polypeptide (VIP) on the lower esophageal sphincter in awake baboons: Comparison with glucagon and secretin. *Digestive Diseases and Science, 24*, 345–349.

Shinghai, T., & Shimada, K. (1976). Reflex swallowing elicited by water and chemical substances. *Japanese Journal of Physiology, 26*, 455–469.

Shipp, T., Deatsch, W. W., & Robertson, K. (1970). Pharyngoesophageal muscle activity during swallowing in man. *Laryngoscope, 80*, 1–6.

Sifrim, D., & Janssens, J. (1995) Inhibitory and excitatory mechanisms in the control of esophageal peristalsis in cats. *Gastroenterology, 108*, A691.

Sims, S. M., Vivaudo, M. B., Hillemeier, C., Biancani, P., Walsh, J. V., & Singer, J. J. (1990). Membrane currents and cholinergic regulation of K+ current in esophageal smooth muscle cells. *American Journal of Physiology, 258*, G794–G802.

Sinar, D. R., O'Dorisio, T. M., Mazzaferri, E. L., Mekhjian, H., Cadwell, H. S. J. H., & Thomas, F. B. (1978): Effect of gastric inhibitory peptide on lower esophageal sphincter pressure in cats. *Gastroenterology, 75*, 263–267.

Sinclair, W. J. (1970). Initiation of reflex swallowing from the naso- and oropharynx. *American Journal of Physiology, 218*, 956–960.

Sinclair, W. J. (1971). Role of the pharyngeal plexus in initiation of swallowing. *American Journal of Physiology, 221*, 1260–1263.

Snape, W. J., Jr., & Cohen, S. (1978). Control of esophageal and lower esophageal sphincter function; neurohumoral and myogenic factors. *Frontiers of Gastrointestinal Research, 3*, 76–94.

Sofroniew, M. W., & Schrell, U. (1981). Evidence for direct projections from oxytocin and vasopressin neurons of the hypothalamic paraventricular nucleus to the medulla oblongata: Immunohistochemical visualization of both horseradish peroxidase transported and the peptide produced by the same neurons. *Neuroscience Letters, 22*, 211–217.

Sokoloff, A. J., & Deacon, T. W. (1992). Musculotopic organization of the hypoglossal nucleus in the cynomolgus monkey, Macaca fascicularis. *Journal of Comparative Neurology, 324*, 81–93.

Sqalli-Houssaini, Y., Cazalets, J. R., & Clarac, F. (1993). Oscillatory properties of thecentral pattern generator for locomotion in the neonatal rat. *Journal of Neurophysiology, 70*, 803–813.

Storey, A. T. (1968a). Laryngeal initiation of swallowing. *Experimental Neurology, 20*, 359–365.

Storey, A. T. (1968b). A functional analysis of sensory units innervating epiglottis and larynx. *Experimental Neurology, 20*, 366–383.

Sugarbaker, D. J., Rattan, S., & Goyal, R. K. (1984a). Mechanical and electrical activity of esophageal smooth muscle during peristalsis. *American Journal of Physiology, 246*, G145–G150.

Sugarbaker, D. J., Rattan, S., & Goyal, R. K. (1984b). Swallowing induces sequential activation of esophageal longitudinal smooth muscle during peristalsis. *American Journal of Physiology, 247*, G515–G519.

Sumi, T. (1963). The activity of brain-stem respiratory neurons and spinal respiratory motoneurons during swallowing. *Journal of Neurophysiology, 26*, 466–477.

Sumi, T. (1963–1964). Neuronal mechanisms in swallowing. *Pfluegers Archives Gesamte Physiologic Menschen Tiere, 278*, 467–477.

Sumi, T. (1967). The nature and postnatal development of reflex deglutition in the kitten. *Japanese Journal of Physiology, 17*, 200–210.

Sumi, T. (1969). Synaptic potentials of hypoglossal motoneurons and their relation to reflex deglutition. *Japanese Journal of Physiology, 19*, 68–79.

Sumi, T. (1969). Some properties of cortically evoked swallowing and chewing in rabbits. *Brain Research, 15*, 107–120.

Sumi, T. (1970). Activity in single hypoglossal fibers during cortically induced swallowing and chewing in rabbits. *Pfluegers Archives, 314*, 329–346.

Sumi, T. (1972a). Reticular ascending activation of frontal cortical neurons in rabbits, with special reference to the regulation of deglutition. *Brain Research, 46*, 43–54.

Sumi, T. (1972b). Role of the pontine reticular formation in the neural organization of deglutition. *Japanese Journal of Physiology, 22*, 295–314

Swanson, L. O. W., & Sawchenko, P. E. (1983). Hypothalamic integration: Organisation of the paraventricular and supraoptic nuclei. *Annual Review Neuroscience, 6*, 269–324.

Szabo, T., & Dussardier, M. (1964). Les noyaux d'origine du nerf vague chez le mouton. *Zeitschrift fur Zellforschung, 63*, 247–276.

Sweazey, R. D., & Bradley, R. M. (1987). Multimodal neurons in the lamb solitary nucleus: Responses to chemical, tactile and thermal stimulation of the caudal oral cavity and epiglottis. *Annals of the New York Academy of Science, 510*, 649–651.

Tago, H., McGeer, P. L., McGeer, E. G., Akiyama, H., & Hersh, L. B. (1989). Distribution of choline acetyltransferase immunopositive structures in the rat brainstem. *Brain Research, 495*, 271–297.

Tago, H., Maeda, T., McGeer, P. L., & Kimura, H. (1992). Butyrylcholinesterase-rich neurons in rat brain demonstrated by a sensitive histochemical method. *Journal of Comparative Neurology, 325*, 301–312.

Tell, F., Fagni, L., & Jean, A. (1990). Neurons of the nucleus tractus solitarius, *in vitro*, generate bursting activities by solitary tract stimulation. *Experimental Brain Research, 79*, 436–440.

Tell, F., & Jean. A. (1991a). Activation of N-methyl-D-aspartate receptors induces endogenous rhythmic bursting activities in nucleus tractus solitarii neurons: An intracellular study on adult rat brainstem slices. *European Journal of Neuroscience, 3*, 1353–1365.

Tell, F., & Jean, A (1991b). Bursting discharges evoked *in vitro*, by solitary tract stimulation or application of N-methyl-D-aspartate, in neurons of the rat nucleus tractus solitarii. *Neuroscience Letters, 124*, 221–224.

Tell, F., & Jean, A. (1993). Ionic basis for endogenous rhythmic patterns induced by activation of N-methyl-D-aspertate receptors in neurons of the rat nucleus tractus solitarii. *Journal of Neurophysiology, 70,* 2379–2390.

Thexton, A. J. (1973). Oral reflexes elicited by mechanical stimulation of palatal mucosa in the cat. *Archives of Oral Biology, 18,* 971–980.

Thor, K., and Rokaeus, O. (1983): Studies on the mechanism by which (Gln4)-neurotensin reduces lower esophageal sphincter (LES) pressure in man. *Acta Physiologica Scandinavia, 118,* 373–377.

Tieffenbach, L., & Roman, C. (1972). Role de l'innervation extrinsique vagale dans la motricité de l'oesophage a musculeuse lisse: Etude electromyographique chez le rat et le Babouin. *Journal of Physiology (Paris), 64,* 193–226.

Tomume, N., & Takata, M. (1988). Excitatory and inhibitory postsynaptic potentials in cat hypoglossal motoneurons during swallowing. *Experimental Brain Research, 71,* 262–272.

Torvik, A. (1956). Afferent connections to the sensory trigeminal nuclei, the nucleus of the solitary tract and adjacent structures—an experimental study in the rat. *Journal of Comparative Neurology, 106,* 51–141.

Tottrup, A., Svane, D., & Forman, A. (1991). Nitric oxide mediating NANC inhibition in opossum lower esophageal sphincter. *American Journal of Physiology, 260,* G385–G389.

Travers, J. B., & Jackson, L. M. (1992). Hypoglossal neural activity during licking and swallowing in the awake rat. *Journal of Neurophysiology, 67,* 1171–1184.

Travers, J. B., & Norgren, R. (1983). Afferent projections to the oral motor nuclei in the rat. *Journal of Comparative Neurology, 220,* 228–298.

Tseng, L. F. (1978). Effects of para-methoxyamphetamine and 2,5-dimethoxyamphetamine on serotonergic mechanism. *Naunyn Schmiedebergs Archive of Pharmacology, 304,* 101–105.

Ueda. 1., Schlegel, J. F., & Code, C. F. (1972). Electric and motor activity of innervated and vagally denervating feline esophagus. *American Journal of Digestive Diseases, 17,* 1075–1088.

Uemura, M., Matsuda, K, Kume, M., Takeuchi, Y., Matsushima, R., & Mizuno, N. (1979). Topographical arrangement of hypoglossal motoneurons: An HRP study in the cat. *Neuroscience Letters, 13,* 99–104.

Van Thiel, D.H., Gavaler, J.S., & Stremple, J. (1976). Lower esophageal sphincter pressure in women using sequential oral contraceptives. *Gastroenterology, 71,* 232–234.

Vyas, D., Wang, Y. T., & Bieger, D. (1990). Nucleus reticularis intermedialis—possible cholinergic source subserving esophageal peristalsis in the rat. *Society for Neuroscience Abstract, 16,* 730.

Wang, Y. T. (1992). *Brainstem mechanisms subserving oesophageal peristalsis in the rat.* Doctoral thesis, Memorial University of Newfoundland, St. John's.

Wang, Y. T., & Bieger, D. (1991). Role of solitarial GABA-ergic mechanisms in control of swallowing. *American Journal of Physiology, 261,* R639–R646.

Wang, Y. T., Bieger, D., & Neuman, R. S. (1991). Activation of NMDA receptors is necessary for fast information transfer at brainstem vagal motoneurons. *Brain Research, 576,* 260–266.

Wang, Y. T., Neuman, R. S., & Bieger, D. (1991a). Nicotinic cholinoceptor-mediated excitation in ambigual motoneurons of the rat. *Neuroscience, 40,* 759–767.

Wang, Y. T., Neuman, R. S., & Bieger, D. (1991b). Somatostatin inhibits nicotinic cholinoceptor-mediated excitation in rat ambigual motoneurons in vitro. *Neuroscience Letters, 123,* 236–239.

Wang, Y. T., Zhang, M., Neuman, R. S., & Bieger, D. (1993). Somatostatin regulates excitatory amino acid receptor-mediated fast excitatory postsynaptic potential components in vagal motoneurons. *Neuroscience 53,* 7–9.

Ward, S. M., Dalziel, H. H., Thornbury, K. D., Westfall, D., & Sanders, K. M. (1992). Nonadrenergic, noncholinergic inhibition and excitation in canine colon depend on nitric oxide. *American Journal of Physiology, 262,* G237–G243.

Weerasuriya, A., Bieger, D., & Hockman C. H. (1980). Interaction between primary afferent neurves in the elicitation of reflex swallowing. *American Journal of Physiology,. 239,* R407–R414.

Weisbrodt, N. W. (1976). Neuromuscular organization of esophageal and pharyngeal motility. *Archives of Internal Medicine, 136,* 524–531.

Weisbrodt, N. W., & Christensen, J. (1972). Gradients of contractions in the opossum esophagus. *Gastroenterology, 62,* 1159–1166.

Weisbrodt, N. W., & Murphy, R. A. (1985). Myosin phosphorylation and contraction of the feline esophageal smooth muscle. *American Journal of Physiology, 249,* C9–C14.

Welt, C., & Abbs, J. H. (1990). Musculotopic organization of the facial motor nucleus in Macaca fascicularis: A morphometric and retrograde tracing study with cholera toxin B-HRP. *Journal of Comparative Neurology, 291,* 621–636.

Yajima, Y., & Larson, C. R. (1993). Multifunctional properties of ambiguous neurons identified electrophysiologically during vocalization in the awake monkey. *Journal of Neurophysiology, 70,* 529–540.

Yamada, K. (1966). Gustatory and thermal responses in the glossopharyngeal nerve of the rat. *Japanese Journal of Physiology, 16,* 599–611.

Yamada, K. (1967). Gustatory and thermal responses in the glossopharyngeal nerve of the rabbit and cat. *Japanese Journal of Physiology, 17,* 94–110.

Yamato, S., Spechler, S. J., & Goyal, R. K. (1992). Role of nitric oxide in esophageal peristalsis in the opossum. *Gastroenterology, 103,* 197–204.

Yoshida, Y., Miyazaki, T., Hirano, M., Shin, T., Totoki, T., & Kanaseki, T. (1981). Location of motoneurons supplying the cricopharyngeal muscle in the cat studied by means of the horseradish peroxidase method. *Neuroscience Letters, 18,* 1–5.

Zelcer, E., & Weisbrodt, N. W. (1984). Electrical and mechanical activity of the lower esophageal sphincter in the cat. *American Journal of Physiology, 246,* G243–G247.

Zhang, M., Wang, Y. T., Vyas, D., Neuman, R. S., & Bieger, D. (1993). Nicotinic cholinoceptor-mediated EPSP in rat nucleus ambiguus. *Experimental Brain Research, 96,* 83–88.

Zwick, R. Bowes, K. L., Daniel, E. E., & Sarna, S. K. (1976). Mechanism of action of pentagastrin on the lower esophageal sphincter. *Journal of Clinical Investigation, 57,* 1644–1651.

4

Respiratory Function and Complications Related to Deglutition

Jeffrey L. Curtis and Susan E. Langmore

The respiratory and gastrointestinal passage share the oropharynx and hypopharynx as a result of their common origin in the embryonic foregut. With each deglutition, ingested liquids and solids pass anteriorly to posteriorly over the larynx and with each breath, air crosses in the opposite direction. Consequently, during each deglutition, the lungs are at risk for aspiration of swallowed materials. The lower airways and lung parenchyma are protected from aspiration by a series of defense mechanisms (Coleridge & Coleridge, 1994; Harada & Repine, 1985).

This chapter will describe these defenses and how they are adversely affected by instrumentation of the oropharynx, particularly by endotracheal intubation and tracheostomy. We will also consider the various clinical pulmonary syndromes that result from aspiration and the effect of reflux of gastrointestinal contents on bronchospasm.

INTERACTIONS BETWEEN DEGLUTITION AND RESPIRATION

Ventilation

Air flows passively into and out of the lungs with each breath because of differences between alveolar and ambient pressure. Inspiration occurs when alveolar pressure becomes subatmospheric owing to active contraction of the inspiratory muscles. If secretions, retained liquids, or food debris pool in the laryngeal vestibule, this subatmospheric pressure can suck them into the lungs. Normal expiration is a passive event driven by the elastic recoil of the chest wall when inspiratory muscle action ceases. In airflow obstruction (e.g., chronic bronchitis, emphysema) with expiratory airway collapse, expiration may actually be a forced active muscle contraction. Active muscle contraction during expiration may contribute to the high incidence of esophageal reflux in patients with chronic obstructive pulmonary disease (COPD) (Shapiro, Dobbins, & Matthay, 1989).

Respiratory muscles include the diaphragm; the muscles of the rib cage (parasternal, internal and external intercostals, and scalene); the abdominal muscles (internal and external obliques, transversus abdominis, and rectus abdominis), which are the primary muscles of expiration; and the muscles of the upper airways, which are essential to maintain airway patency. During quiet breathing, the diaphragm may be active. In contrast, in respiratory distress, many muscles of the shoulder girdle and neck are recruited. Respiratory muscle failure typically presents with hypercapnia (retention of CO_2) but may also be complicated by hypoxemia (low blood oxygen). All respiratory muscles including the diaphragm are entirely striated; hence, they may be involved in myopathies and myotonias, as well as in degenerative neurologic diseases (such as amyotrophic lateral sclerosis), disease of the neuromuscular junction (myasthenia gravis, botulism), and in inflammatory neuropathies (such as Guillain-Barré syndrome or porphyria) (Brin & Younger, 1988). Also see Chapter 11.

These types of neuromuscular diseases are thus associated with a restrictive ventilatory defect (i.e., decreased ability to inflate the lungs leading to weak cough, and potential hypercapnia and hypoxemia) as well as with increased propensity to aspirate owing to abnormalities in deglutition itself.

Normal and Pathologic Reflexes

The airways are protected from aspiration during deglutition by a variety of mechanisms including movement of the larynx superiorly and anteriorly, vocal fold apposition, repositioning of the aryepiglottic folds and epiglottis, and coordination of respiration and deglutition. Normal subjects always inhibit respiration during deglutition (swallow apnea) and normal

swallowing usually interrupts the expiratory phase of the respiratory cycle (approximately 80% of all swallows). After the swallow, normal subjects always resume breathing with an expiration (Coelho, 1987; Preiksaitis, Robins, & Diamant, 1992; Selley, Flack, Ellis, & Brooks, 1989). This pattern is seen with both bolus and nonbolus swallows (Preiksaitis et al., 1992).

Neurologic deficits cause incoordination between breathing and swallowing. In stroke patients, Selley noted that the respiratory pattern became variable as the spoon contacted the lips (Selley et al., 1989). He also noted inhalation immediately following the swallow in 43% of the trials, clearly an aberration from the normal pattern. Langmore and Murray (1991) corroborated that data in an unpublished study using seven patients with previous strokes. In addition to finding a number of swallows that were followed by inhalation, they also found that approximately 50% of the swallows were preceded by inhalation. While these data indicated that breathing swallowing coordination was sometimes abnormal, this clinical significance was highlighted by the finding that many of the swallows with documented aspiration were preceded by inhalation (8/9 swallows in which aspiration was documented by endoscopy or fluoroscopy). Thus, it appears that incoordination of breathing and swallowing can contribute to aspiration in patients with neurologic deficits.

Coordination of Breathing and Swallowing

(See also Chapter 3). Respiration and deglutition are thought to be controlled by brain stem nuclei in the medulla with interneurons connecting the two centers (Negus, 1949).

The ascending vagus nerves, with sensory receptors probably situated in the thorax, carry afferent impulses of this reflex to the medullary respiratory center, where a synapse with the recurrent laryngeal nerve causes the posterior cricoarytenoid muscle to abduct the vocal folds.

This activity in the intrinsic laryngeal musculature occurs several milliseconds prior to diaphragmatic descent, which is stimulated by activity in the phrenic nerve and causes inhalation to occur. Subsequently, just before actual expiration, the vocal folds adduct partially, valving the airflow through the glottis as expiration begins a few milliseconds later (Green & Neil, 1955).

For swallowing, a similar interplay occurs. The glottic closure reflex, carried by efferent fibers of the recurrent laryngeal nerve and manifest as complete vocal fold adduction, begins just prior to inhibition of diaphragmatic contraction. The nearly simultaneous signals to these two muscle groups are responsible for swallow apnea; it is virtually impossible to breathe and swallow at the same time. Miller and Loizzi (1974) also determined that the threshold for inhibiting respiration remains below that for evoking swallowing in the fully sensate animal, thus further protecting us from attempting to perform both activities simultaneously. Coordination between breathing and swallowing may also be altered in COPD, in part because of the rapid breathing rate and limited ability to alter their respiratory pattern. COPD patients more often swallow in the inspiratory phase and resume respiration with inspiration than normal controls (Shaker et al., 1992). These alterations may have consequences beyond aspiration: Nutrition is often suboptimal in patients with advanced COPD, in some cases leading to cachexia (Schols, Mostert, Soeters, Greve, & Wouters, 1989). Weight loss in advanced COPD may relate both to increased energy requirements (due to the high cost of breathing in these patients) and to decreased food intake. Arterial oxygen saturation declines during eating in some COPD patients; the inadequate dietary intake for energy expenditure is most pronounced in those with chronic hypoxemia (Coelho, 1987; Schols, Mostert, Cobben, Soeters, & Wouters, 1991). Even though there has not been rigorous proof that supplemental oxygen therapy is efficacious in this setting, quality of life is often improved by its institution in hypoxemic patients.

DEFENSE MECHANISMS OF THE LOWER RESPIRATORY TRACT

In the lung, oxygen is taken up by blood from air and carbon dioxide is released into the air from blood. The exchange of these two respiratory gases occurs across the interface of pulmonary capillaries and alveoli. Even small amounts of foreign material interfere with this gas exchange in multiple ways. Foreign solids may block small airways; liquids may reduce surfactant below the concentration necessary to maintain alveolar patency; and inflammation induced by aspirated material increases the distance between the inspired air and the blood within the alveolar capillaries. If the gas exchange areas of the lung become occluded, alveoli may collapse, and they may remain collapsed even after the obstruction is relieved. This collapse is termed atelectasis whether it is microscopic, involving only individual alveoli, or grossly evident, as in the collapse of entire lung lobes. On a chest radiograph, microscopic atelectasis can be inferred from a generalized decrease in lung volume, whereas atelectasis of larger segments is detected as focal infiltrates, which are usually wedge-shaped. Atelectasis is an important predisposing factor for development of pneumonia, both by impairing alveolar cellular defenses (see below) and by decreasing the efficiency with which secretions are cleared. Development of atelectasis is accelerated by a high inspired oxygen concentration, as occurs during mechanical ventilation and general anesthesia. In these settings, there is little or no nitrogen in the alveoli, so that if airflow is obstructed, alveoli rapidly collapse owing to absorption of oxygen. For all these reasons, it is imperative that the lower respiratory tract be protected against the introduction of foreign materials.

Mechanisms for Airway Clearance

The first line of defense against aspiration is the normal function of the larynx during deglutition, which includes laryngeal elevation, epiglottic depression, and glottic closure. These functions are described in Chapter 2. The upper esophageal sphincter, which is tonically contracted at rest, prevents material that refluxes from entering the pharynx and being aspirated (Winship, 1983). If aspirated material penetrates distal to the glottis, it is dealt with primarily by cough and mucociliary action within the conducting airways, which transmit respiratory gases (Figure 4–1). Aerody-namic size largely determines where within the respiratory tract particles will impinge. Once aspirated material reaches the gas exchange areas (terminal bronchi and alveoli), it must be dealt with by cellular mechanisms, because mucociliary clearance and cough do not function there. The vulnerable gas exchange regions of the lung are protected in part by the repeated branching of the airways. Particles tend to accumulate at the branch points, presumably owing to local turbulence (Clarke & Pavia, 1988; Schlesinger, Gurman, & Lipmann, 1982). Inhaled and aspirated particles may become trapped in the mucus that coats the airways.

Mucociliary Action

Mucus and the foreign particles entrapped in it are normally propelled toward the major airways and trachea by the beating action of cilia. This process has been termed the mucociliary escalator (Wanner, 1986). Cilia extend distally into the terminal bronchioles and proximally up to the larynx, where secretions are expectorated or swallowed. Cilia of adjacent airway cells beat in a coordinated fashion. Patients with defective ciliary function are at risk for repeated infections. Ciliary defects may be congenital, as in the immotile cilia syndromes or Kartagener's syndrome, or acquired, as occurs with general anesthesia or severe alcohol intoxication. Smoking acutely decreases ciliary beat frequency. Proper mucociliary clearance also depends on the physical properties of the mucus layer, which in health segregates into a viscous gel phase floating on a soluble phase in which the cilia beat. The physical properties of mucus are altered in cystic fibrosis (Barton & Lourenco, 1973), leading to secretions that are inspissated and difficult to clear. Patients with chronic bronchitis or bronchiectasis have deranged ciliary clearance due to excessive secretion of mucus and to patchy loss of ciliary coverage of epithelial cells.

Coughing is the forceful act of expelling air from the lungs through narrow air-

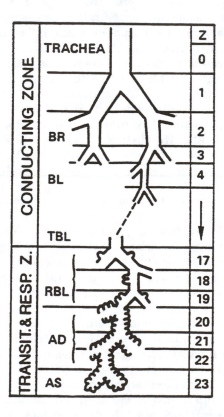

Figure 4–1. Normal human conducting airways and respiratory zone. BR, bronchus; BL, bronchiole; TBL, terminal bronchiole; RBL, respiratory bronchiole; AD, alveolar duct; AS, alveolar sac. (From *Morphometry of the Human Lung* by E. R. Weibel, 1963, p. 111. Berlin: Springer-Verlag, reprinted with permission)

ways (Leith, 1977). Cough is an involuntary reflex act, which can be triggered by stimulation of sensory receptors in the oropharynx, nasopharynx, larynx, and proximal segments of the lower respiratory tract (Coleridge & Coleridge, 1994). The afferent sensory paths for triggering cough are via the glossopharyngeal nerves in the oropharynx and via the superior laryngeal nerves for the rest of the larynx and pharynx (Sant'Ambrogio & Mathew, 1986). The reflex cough on penetration of the larynx by an oropharyngeal bolus may be decreased in the elderly, contributing to the severity of prandial aspiration (Feinberg, Knebl, Tully, & Segall, 1990). Supporting this observation, elderly subjects have been shown to have decreased sensation to inhaled ammonia (Pontoppidan & Beecher, 1960).

Cough generates extremely high linear sheer forces that sweep the tracheal surface. Coughing typically begins with a deep inspiration (Figure 4–2; Yanagihara, van Leden, & Werner-Kukuk, 1966). The glottis closes and pressures within both the thoracic and abdominal cavities increase to 50–100 mmHg as all the expiratory muscles contract simultaneously. Next the glottis opens abruptly, while subglottic pressure continues to rise. Because the posterior walls of the trachea and major conducting airways are not reinforced by cartilage, their lumens collapse, making the airway a narrow crescent. Expiratory airflow accelerates very rapidly, exceeding flows of 12 l/sec within 50 ms. This entire sequence may be repeated multiple times during a coughing episode without an additional inspiration, gradually taking the lung volumes down toward residual volume. Interestingly, glottic closure is not essential for effective cough; patients with permanent tracheostomies can be taught to cough effectively (Leith, 1977). Strength of expiratory muscles, especially of the diaphragm and abdominal muscles, is essential for cough to be effective. Cough is virtually ineffectual in paraparesis or quadriparesis.

Coughing is not necessarily due to aspiration. Persistent cough is a common symptom and has a broad differential diagnosis (Braman & Corrao, 1987; Irwin, Corrao, & Pratter, 1981). Frequent causes of cough are listed in Table 4–1 (for review, see Braman & Corrao, 1987; Irwin & Curley, 1991; Irwin, Curley, & French, 1990). Cough can have adverse effects, such as syncope, trauma to the lungs or thoracic structures (leading to pneumothorax, pneumomediastinum, or rib fractures), laryngeal edema, or bronchospasm. Cough may dangerously increase intracranial or intraocular pressure in patients with intracranial tumors, cerebral trauma, or glaucoma.

Strong mechanical or irritant stimulation of the laryngeal mucosa can induce bronchospasm (increased resistance to expiratory airflow), which can persist beyond the duration of coughing and apnea (Tomori & Widdicombe, 1969). Other potential adverse reflexes resulting from laryngeal irritation are bradycardia (at times asystole), hypertension, and increase in bronchial mucus production.

Irritant Properties of Aerosols

Water (often presumed innocuous for use in swallowing studies) may be considerably more likely to induce cough than isotonic saline, at least based on extrapolation from studies of inhaled aerosols in asthmatics. Eschenbacher and associates had nine subjects with mild asthma inhale various solutions while recording cough and measuring specific airway resistance (Eschenbacher, Boushey, & Sheppard, 1984). To evaluate the effects of altering osmolarity and ion concentration separately, the administered aerosols included hypo-osmolar distilled water (0 mOsm), iso-osmolar sodium chloride (308 mOsm), iso-osmolar dextrose in water (308 mOsm), hyperosmolar sodium chloride (1,232 mOsm), and a hyperosmolar solution of dextrose and sodium chloride (1,232 mOsm). Iso-osmolar solutions of sodium bromide, sodium gluconate, and lysine monoydrochloride were also used to determine whether the absence of a specific ion was important in causing cough or bronchoconstriction. Alteration in osmo-

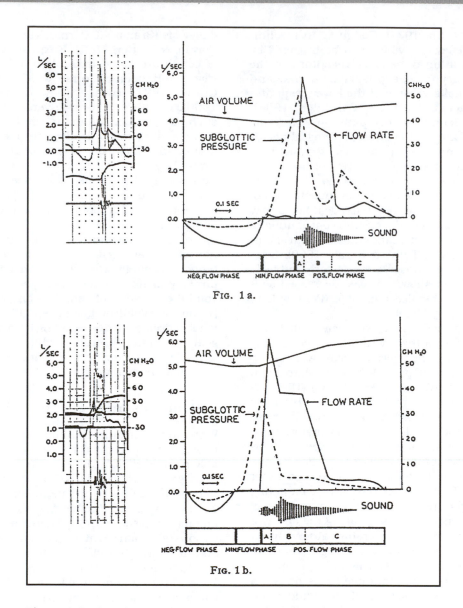

Figure 4–2. Simultaneous recordings of air flow, air volume, subglottic pressure, and acoustic signal in two single coughs. (From The Physical Parameters of Cough: The Larynx in a Normal Single Cough by N. Yanagihara, H. von Leden, & E. Werner-Kukuk, 1966. *Acta Oto-laryngologica (Stockholm)*, *61*, 495–510, reprinted with permission)

larity away from iso-osmolarity of inhaled aerosols was found to be a stimulus for bronchoconstriction in these subjects with mild asthma. Absence of ions in the presence of iso-osmolarity induced cough but not bronchoconstriction. Hence, the responses of cough and bronchoconstriction to inhaled aerosols can be separated.

TABLE 4–1. Differential diagnosis of persistent cough

Chronic bronchitis

Asthma

Bronchogenic carcinoma (or rarer benign tumors of the airways, mediastinum, or pleura)

Foreign body aspiration

Interstitial lung disease

Psychogenic

Gastroesophageal reflux

Lymphatic Clearance

The impermeability of the alveolar epithelium to solids means that foreign particles in the alveoli and respiratory bronchioles must be handled by cellular defenses (discussed below). In contrast, clearing the lung of liquids depends primarily on lymphatics. Lymphatics prevent edema by returning fluid from the interstitial compartment and carry foreign materials to the lymph nodes that are interspersed along their paths. Lymph nodes filter the lymphatic fluid, retaining particles and antigens (organisms and other material capable of triggering an immune response). Lung lymphatics begin as blind-ended vessels near the level of the respirator bronchioles (i.e., not within the alveolar walls or interalveolar septa); they join to form vessels of ever increasing size, which run adjacent to the bronchioles and arterioles. A separate lymphatic network drains the pleura (the membranous tissue covering the lungs and lining the inner chest wall). The liquid portion of lymph eventually is returned to the blood vessels via the thoracic duct, the major lymphatic vessel, which drains into the left subclavian vein.

The capacity of the lymphatics to clear liquids from the lungs is astounding: From 400–700 ml per day are removed in normal persons (Leckie & Tothill, 1965; Stewart, 1963). Lymphatics can clear the alveoli of macromolecules such as blood proteins resulting from alveolar hemorrhage (Meyer, Dominguez, & Bensch, 1969), but cannot remove particles such as aspirated food. A decreased net osmotic gradient into the lymphatics, from decreased serum albumin concentration (as seen in liver cirrhosis or nephrotic syndrome) or high hydrostatic pressure (as seen in congestive heart failure), markedly diminish the effectiveness of lymphatic clearance. Patients with these conditions are at increased risk of pneumonia. Decreased lymphatic clearance can also lead to collection of the fluid in the pleural space (a process known as a pleural effusion), in the interstitium (the supporting structures of the distal lung), or if severe, in the alveoli themselves where it impairs gas exchange and increases the susceptibility to infection.

CELLULAR IMMUNE DEFENSES OF THE LOWER RESPIRATORY TRACT

Alveolar Macrophages

The alveoli are protected primarily by the alveolar macrophages, which are capable of phagocytosis (the process of particle ingestion). Alveolar macrophages are common, occurring at an estimated frequency of one to two per alveolus. Alveolar macrophages originally derive from the bone marrow, but maintain their numbers within the lungs by in situ proliferation (Sawyer, 1986; Shellito, Esparza, & Armstrong,

1987). Alveolar macrophages can phago-cytose inhaled or aspirated pathogens and then carry ingested substances to region-al lymph nodes where immune responses are initiated by presentation to lympho-cytes (Harmsen, Muggenburg, Snipes, & Bice, 1985). Within the lung itself, alveolar macrophages have very limited ability to initiate immune responses (Kaltreider, Caldwell, & Byrd, 1986; Lipscomb et al., 1986; Mbawuike & Herscowitz, 1988). This is probably protective, because the lungs are potentially exposed to large numbers of antigens along with the 10,000–20,000 liters of air inspired daily. Were it easy for immune responses to be initiated in the lung parenchyma, the lung could become engorged with immune cells, interfering with gas exchange (Kaltreider, 1982).

For alveolar macrophages to kill patho-gens after their ingestion, they must be activated by factors or cytokines, like gamma interferon, secreted by lympho-cytes (Curtis & Schuyler, 1993). Lym-phocytes are white blood cells derived from bone marrow cells which regulate im-mune responses through their ability to recognize foreign substances. Lympho-cytes are divided into three major lin-eages: B cells, T cells, and natural killer (NK) cells.

Classes and Functions of Lymphocytes

All B cells directly recognize native (un-processed) antigens via surface immuno-globulin and produce antibody when acti-vated. Antibody secretion is crucial for opsonization of bacteria, which aids pha-gocytosis. Patients who are deficient in some or all antibody subclasses have an increased incidence of respiratory infec-tions. T cells respond only to antigens that have been processed and presented in conjunction with major histocompat-bility complex (MHC) molecules on the surface of antigen-presenting cells. Almost all T cells express either CD4 or CD8 sur-face receptors, which determine the class of MHC molecules to which the T cell re-

sponds. CD4[+] T cells respond to antigen presented by class II MHC molecules and primarily induce ("help") antibody pro-duction and maturation of cytotoxic T cells. A small group of CD4[+] function as class II-restricted cytotoxic cells, which can kill virally infected cells. CD8[+] T cells respond to antigen presented by class I MHC molecules; individual CD8[+] T cells either mediate cytotoxicity or suppress other immune effector cells. Class I MHC molecules are constitutively expressed by virtually all cell types. In contrast, class II molecules are expressed constitutively by only a few cell types, notably B cells; how-ever, class II MHC expression can be in-duced on many cells types by the cytokine gamma-interferon (Pober et al., 1983). Because of this requirement for antigen presentation in conjunction with MHC molecules, regulation by cytokines of the MHC expression of parenchymal cells such as fibroblasts and endothelial cells is central to the control of immune respons-es. Regardless of their MHC restriction (i.e, whether they express CD4 or CD8), mature T cells express a heterodimeric antigen receptor. In the vast majority, this antigen receptor is composed of ab chains; these cells mediate virtually all the function conventionally associated with T lymphocytes. The function of the small sub-set of T cells that express γδ T cells an-tigen receptors is far less well defined (Brenner, Strominger, & Krangel, 1988). Evidence suggests that γδ T cells, which are primarily distributed on mucosal sur-faces, may form an important link in host defense against a variety of pathogens (Janis, Kaufman, Schwartz, & Pardoll, 1989). NK cells are viewed as a separate lineage of lymphocytes although their re-lationship to lymphokine-activated killer (LAK) cells remains controversial (Lanier, Phillips, Hackett, Tutt, & Kumar, 1986). How NK cells recognize their targets, (tu-mors, dividing cells, or pathogens), is not understood. Within the lungs, NK cells are found primarily in the interstitium and are poorly represented in bronchoalveolar la-vages (Weissler, Nicod, Lipscomb, & Toews, 1987). Some investigators have detected very little functional activity of human pulmonary NK cells, possibly because of the suppressive effects of alveolar macrophages and surfactant (Bordignon et al., 1982; Robinson, Pinkston, & Crystal, 1984). To date, no specific lung diseases have been associated with abnormalities of NK function.

Lymphocytes are found within the lung in four distinct anatomic compartments: (a) in a marginated intravascular pool that differs in composition from peripheral blood (Pabst, Binns, Licence, & Peter, 1987), (b) in the interstitial spaces, (c) in the alveolar spaces, and (d) in organized lymphoid tissue. Organized lymphoid tissue includes lymphoid aggregates, both encapsulated and unencapsulated. The lung parenchyma of healthy humans contains relatively little organized lymphoid tissue and few parenchymal lymphocytes (Pabst, 1990). Hence, pulmonary immune responses are presumably initiated in regional lymph nodes and mediated largely by recruitment of lymphocytes and other leukocytes from extrapulmonary sources. The overwhelming majority of lymphocytes recovered from all lung compartments are T cells; B cells comprise fewer than 10% of recovered lymphocytes. These T cells are predominantly memory cells, that is, they are the progeny of cells that have been activated previously by encounter with an antigen. Deficiencies of lymphocyte function, as typified by infection with human immunodeficiency virus 1 (HIV-1), lead to pulmonary infection with a variety of opportunistic pathogens, notably *Pneumocystis carinii*, *Cryptococcus neoformans*, and mycobacteria including both *M. tuberculosis* and *M. avium-intracellulare* (Murray et al., 1984). The frequency and severity of these infections highlight the important role the immune system plays in preventing lung infection.

Neutrophils

Neutrophils or polymorphonuclear granulocytes are circulating white blood cells that defend against pathogenic bacteria and fungi. Deficiencies in neutrophil number or function markedly increase the risk for pneumonia. Normally, very few neutrophils are found in the alveoli or lung interstitium, whereas the normal pulmonary vasculature contains a large population of neutrophils, which are commonly termed marginated. This accumulation of neutrophils may have to do more with the size and rigidity of neutrophils relative to the alveoli capillary than to specific adhesion events (Doerschuk et al., 1990). Neutrophils and blood monocytes are recruited to the lung within hours of lung infection. Signals for recruitment include early response cytokines such as IL-1, tumor necrosis factor (TNF-α), which in turn induce expression of adhesion molecules and of longer acting chemotactic cytokines, known as chemokines, such as IL-8 and others (Springer, 1990). During this transmigration, activated neutrophils release products which kill pathogens but which are also potentially destructive to lung parenchyma, including reactive oxygen products, proteolytic enzymes, and products of lipid peroxidation (Jackson & Cochrane, 1988; Weiss, 1989).

In summary, minute amounts of inhaled or aspirated foreign substances can be handled by pulmonary lymphatics and resident alveolar macrophages. Recruitment of inflammatory cells from the bloodstream is essential to defend against larger amounts. The duration and magnitude of this inflammatory cell recruitment must be closely regulated, however, because of its potential for lung destruction. Experimentally, the lungs have markedly poorer ability to handle a given number of organisms when aspirated rather than inhaled, presumably because the higher focal inoculum in aspiration (Berendt, 1978).

Effect of Tracheal Intubation and Tracheostomy on Deglutition and Aspiration

Intubation of the trachea is needed for pressure mechanical ventilation, the currently preferred mode (Tobin, 1994). Tracheal intubation is not needed for negative pressure ventilation with iron lungs or cuirasses. However, it is much more difficult to provide high inspired oxygen contents with negative pressure ventilation, and the physical barriers these devices impose on the patient make delivery of nursing care difficult. For these reasons, negative pressure ventilation is rarely used at present except in patients with very chronic respiratory failure without the need for supplemental oxygen, as may occur in some patients with neuromuscular diseases.

The lower airways can be accessed either by translaryngeal endotracheal intubation (orally or nasally), or by tracheostomy, in which a tube is passed directly into the trachea through a surgical incision (Heffner, 1988). Endotracheal intubation can be readily performed and is easily reversible. Tracheostomy has advantages for chronic care: Tracheostomy tubes are more easily stabilized, permitting greater mobility; nasal and oropharyngeal hygiene is also much more easily maintained in the patient with a tracheostomy; patients with tracheostomies rarely suffer sinusitis or otitis media, a common complication of nasal or to a lesser degree oral endotracheal tubes.

The timing of the conversion from endotracheal intubation to tracheostomy is often controversial. Complication rates of endotracheal intubation and of tracheostomy, both acutely and chronically, are remarkably similar (McCulloch & Bishop, 1991; Stauffer, Olson, & Petty, 1981). However, the type of complications differ. Both are associated with mucosal damage to the trachea, potentially leading to tracheal strictures, with vocal fold granulomata, and with risk of aspiration (see below); serious bleeding and tracheoesophageal fistula formation is more common with tracheostomy. To complicate matters further, virtually all patients with tracheostomy and subsequent pathology have had preceding translaryngeal intubation. The current incidence of serious and persistent laryngeal pathology after prolonged intubation is estimated to be in

the 5–15% range (Weymuller & Bishop, 1990; Whited, 1983). The most important factor predisposing to injury of the respiratory tract mucosa is excessive pressure in the endotracheal tube cuff, especially in the critically ill with marginal perfusion of trachea and larynx. Therefore, it is imperative that cuff pressures be monitored daily. Laryngeal mucosal injury is usually evident within 7 days. Therefore, if prolonged mechanical ventilation becomes inevitable (e.g., when prolonged respiratory muscle weakness is anticipated), tracheostomy should not be delayed. Early and aggressive management of postintubation granulation tissue is warranted to prevent the development of laryngeal stenosis (Weymuller & Bishop, 1990). Aggressive use of both endoscopic debridement and local steroid injection has been advocated (Weymuller & Bishop, 1990)

Pathophysiology of Tracheal Intubation

Tracheal intubation can have profound effects on deglutition. Endotracheal tubes and, to a greater degree tracheostomies, tether the larynx inferiorly, preventing the normal protective elevation that occurs during deglutition. Tracheostomy also induces neurophysiologic changes in laryngeal function, such as desensitization of the larynx and increased threshold for protective reflexes such as the adductor response that accompanies swallowing. The adductor response, even when activated, may be weakened (Nash, 1988; Sasaki, Suzuki, Horiuchi, & Kirchner, 1977). All of these changes are thought to contribute to the high incidence of aspiration in patients with tracheostomies. The large balloon cuffs on contemporary high-compliance endotracheal and tracheostomy tubes can also impinge on the esophagus posteriorly and obstruct the passage of the swallowed bolus.

It is frequently assumed that a cuffed endotracheal tube protects against aspiration by occluding the path for entry. While it is true that massive aspiration is prevented as long as the balloon is inflated, endotracheal intubation does not prevent microaspiration (Nash, 1988). Moreover, prolonged placement of a cuffed endotracheal tube may lead to tracheomalacia and an ineffective seal. The tube also prevents the superior pathway of expired gas, which normally clears the larynx after swallowing. The incidence of aspiration is greater with tracheostomy than with simple endotracheal intubation (Cameron, Reynolds, & Zuidema, 1973). Even after extubation, prolonged and severe swallowing dysfunction may follow prolonged orotracheal intubation with or without tracheostomy (DeVita & Spierer-Rundback, 1990). Aspiration may also be seen in 27–35% of awake patients immediately after extubation from brief (<24 hour) endotracheal intubation (Burgess, Cooper, Marino, Peuler, & Warriner, 1979). Laryngeal incompetence, presumably due to transient laryngeal desensitization, can last up to 18 hours, long after recovery from inhalational anesthetics (although patients in these studies received analgesics). Tracheal intubation markedly diminishes the efficacy of cough. It prevents glottic closure, needed in the untrained patient for generating initial increased intrathoracic pressure. Tracheal intubation might also cause a decrease in lung volume (expressed as the volume at end expiration, the functional residual capacity or FRC that can predispose to atelectasis).

Intubation is associated with an extremely high rate of pneumonia (Levine & Niederman, 1991). The risk of nosocomial pneumonias has been estimated to be as high as 1% per day in patients receiving mechanical ventilation, based on use of culturing the lower respiratory tract with bronchoscopic protected specimen brushes (Fagon et al., 1988). Pneumonia associated with mechanical ventilation has a case fatality of roughly 50% in most series. Part of this high mortality doubtless reflects the severity of the underlying illness for which mechanical ventilation was instituted. Additionally, pneumonias in ventilated patients are frequently caused by organisms that are highly antibiotic resistant. Therapies to reduce other nosocomial complications in the critically ill patient may actually increase the risk of nosocomial pneumonia. Prophylaxis of the intubated patient against gastric stress ulceration with antacids or histamine receptor type-2 antagonists (e.g., cimetidine, ranitidine, famotidine) has generally been considered an important component of treatment of critically ill patients, especially those on mechanical ventilators. However, this therapy increases the risk of gastric colonization with gram-negative organisms (du Moulin, Hedley-White, Paterson, & Lison, 1982). Three randomized trials have indicated that prophylaxis with sucralfate (which does not alter gastric pH) is protective against gastrointestinal bleeding but is associated with fewer episodes of nosocomial pneumonia than therapies that alter gastric pH (Dachner et al., 1988; Driks et al., 1987; Tryba, 1987). One study has questioned the necessity for stress prophylaxis, based on the lack of difference in gastrointestinal bleeding between patients randomly assigned to sucralfate, cimetidine, or no prophylaxis (Ben-Menachem et al., 1994). Moreover, this study also found increased incidence of pneumonia in both treated groups compared to control. It has been suggested that the incidence of nosocomial gastrointestinal bleeding has decreased over the last decade, possibly owing to improved critical care nursing and supportive measures (Cook et al., 1994). Decontaminating the gut using nonabsorbable antibiotics in an attempt to reduce the incidence of nosocomial gram-negative pneumonias in patients with critical illness is popular in Europe, but is not commonly practiced in North America after the negative results of a randomized controlled clinical trial (Gastinne, Wolff, Delatour, Faurisson, & Chevret, 1992). Many clinicians feel that enteral feeding protects against gastric stress ulceration, although objective evidence of efficacy is lacking. Conversely, enteral feeding may be a risk factor for pneumonia in the patient on mechanical ventilation (Craven et al., 1986; Craven,

Steger, & Barber, 1991). At present the best safeguards against development of ventilator-associated pneumonia are meticulous attention to oral hygiene of the intubated patient to minimize bacterial colonization, frequent tracheal suctioning, and extubation as soon as feasible.

CLINICAL COMPLICATIONS OF ASPIRATION

Definition of Penetration and Aspiration

Some authors have distinguished penetration (the entry of oropharyngeal contents through the larynx distal to the true vocal folds, in some cases unassociated with respiration) from aspiration (passage of material into the lungs, often with the connotation of accompanying inspiration; Groher & Gonzalez, 1992; Kramer, 1989), whereas others have either equated the terms or used aspiration in both circumstances (Feinberg et al., 1990; Logemann, 1983). However, most pulmonary clinicians understand aspiration to denote delivery of material into the distal lung, although it is recognized that the process may be clinically silent. It is frequently stated that "the more liquid or fluid a substance, the more likely it will be aspirated and travel further into the respiratory system" (Feinberg et al., 1990). While reasonable, experimental or clinical data to verify this assertion are lacking.

The term aspiration pneumonia is applied to several distinct clinical entities. This often has led to considerable confu-

sion and even at times acrimonious dissent in the medical literature (Table 4–2). Four syndromes should be distinguished: (a) aspiration of large solids leading to acute upper airway obstruction or of large volume liquids leading to drowning and or near drowning; (b) aspiration of toxic fluids, including gastric or other acids and basic, mineral oils, or hydrocarbons; (c) aspiration of contaminated oral secretions or debris, which leads to infectious pneumonias, frequently from anaerobic organisms (Bartlett & Gorbach, 1975; Russin & Adler, 1989); and (d) chronic aspiration of small amounts of food or organic medications, leading to pulmonary fibrosis due to a granulomatous response (Table 4–3).

Acute Airway Occlusion

Acute upper airway obstruction due to aspiration of solids is an emergency: Obstruction can lead to death within minutes owing to immediate asphyxiation. This has been called the café coronary syndrome because it is frequently induced by hurried ingestion of large pieces of food by intoxicated individuals; it is also a prominent cause of death in nursing home patients. In the United States, the recommended emergency treatment of witnessed airway obstruction is the abdominal thrust known as the Heimlich maneuver (JAMA, 1986; Heimlich, 1981). The Canadian Heart Foundation recommends a combination of abdominal thrusts and back blows (Montoya, 1986; Redding, 1979). No controlled trials have compared the efficacy of the two treatments. Even when properly performed, the Heimlich

TABLE 4–2. Aspiration syndromes (and their potential outcomes).

Massive aspiration
    solids (acute airway obstruction)
    liquids (drowning/near drowning)
Toxic aspiration (toxic pneumonitis)
Aspiration of oral secretions (anaerobic or gram-negative lung infections)
Chronic aspiration of organic substances (pulmonary fibrosis)

TABLE 4–3. Predisposing factors for aspiration.

Decreased level of consciousness

    acute intoxication (alcohol, sedative medications)

    general anesthesia

    seizure

    cerebrovascular accident or transient ischemic attacks

    head trauma

Disorders of pharyngeal or esophageal structure or function

    tracheoesophageal fistula

    Zenker's diverticulum

Oropharyngeal dysphagia secondary to surgical resection, radiation therapy, chemotherapy

Oropharyngeal dysphagia secondary to neurological, neuromuscular, or connective tissue disease

    reflux esophagitis, gastroesophageal reflux,

    polymyositis, multiple sclerosis

Miscellaneous conditions

    tracheostomy

    nasogastric tubes

maneuver can be complicated by fractured ribs or pneumomediastinum (Redding, 1979). Smaller aspirated solids may pass through the larynx and lodge in the bronchi, usually of the lower lobes. Radiographs frequently do not demonstrate lobar or segmental consolidation acutely, leading to errors in diagnosis. Expiratory radiographs may be helpful to confirm location, by showing air trapping distal to the lesion. Foreign bodies can usually be removed bronchoscopically. Rigid bronchoscopes are mandatory for this purpose in children; fiberoptic bronchoscopes have been used in adults, but with a lower success rate than rigid bronchoscopes (60% vs. 98%) (Limper & Prakash, 1990). Persistent pneumonias or granulomatous inflammation are the most common sequelae of unremoved aspirated solid objects. Removal of foreign bodies may be complicated by postbronchoscopy pulmonary edema, especially when they have been present for a long time.

In patients with impaired cough who cannot clear the trachea, such as fully anesthetized patients, a volume of liquid equal to that of the central airways, (about 125–150 ml in an adult) would certainly be lethal due to simple asphyxia. This volume is known in respiratory physiology as the anatomic dead space, since it is the volume of inspired air that does not contribute to respiration. The effect of liquid that drains from the central airways into the lung parenchyma is more difficult to state categorically. Most data come from the analogous situation of near-drowning injuries. By convention, the term drowning is reserved for episodes that are fatal out of hospital, and near drowning used for those in which patients survive to receive emergency treatment (even if they die later). Up to 15% of drowning victims have no water distal to the larynx and die of asphyxia apparently triggered by reflex laryngospasm (Cot, 1931; Modell, 1976). Thus, aspiration of liquids might also lead to reflex laryngospasm and asphyxia, although we are not aware of data on this point.

It is difficult to extrapolate from either experimental or clinical data to definitively answer the question, how much aspirated material is likely to lead to significant lung injury? The injury probably depends on the nature of the aspirated material, the level of consciousness, and the person's ability to clear the airways. Even small solids (e.g., pills, peanuts) can be fatal if they lodge in the glottis and cannot be expelled. In near drowning, aspiration of water or isotonic liquids in large amounts leads to transient abnormalities of gas exchange but is unlikely to be fatal.

Toxic Aspiration Syndromes

Aspiration of toxic fluids causes a chemical pneumonitis or lung burn. The classic form was described in 1946 by Mendelson as a syndrome that followed aspiration of gastric contents in obstetric patients. Surprisingly, in that series there were no fatalities due to acid aspiration alone, in contrast to the high mortality in a later series (Cameron, Mitchell, & Zuidema, 1973). The pH and the volume of the aspirated fluid determine the degree of lung injury (Exharos, Logan, & Abbott, 1965; Greenfield, Singleton, & McCaffree, 1969; James, Modell, Gibbs, Kuck, & Ruiz, 1984; Wynne, Ramphal, & Hood, 1981). In dogs 1–4 ml/kg is necessary to cause significant injury (Greenfield, 1969). The corresponding volume would be approximately 50–300 ml for adult humans. pHs of below 2.5 seem necessary to cause significant acid injury (Teabeaut, 1952). Mechanical ventilation with high flow supplemental oxygen is frequently needed. The degree of hypoxemia often seems out of proportion to the amount of lung parenchyma involved based on the chest radiograph appearance. With acids, lung injury begins within minutes, making it virtually impossible to forestall. Gas exchange abnormalities occurred with aspiration of gastric contents at pH 5.9 (Schwartz, Wynne, Gibbs, Hood, & Kuck, 1980), but in that case oxygenation normalized within 4 hours.

The pathophysiology of other toxic aspirations, including petrochemical hydrocarbons, is believed to parallel that of acid injury. The lung injury seen in all these cases is manifested clinically as the adult respiratory distress syndrome (Figure 4–3).

Treatment of toxic aspiration pneumonitis is supportive, with provision of adequate oxygenation. As in other focal, air space-filling lung injuries, oxygenation can often be improved by the addition of positive end expiratory pressure, which is believed to help maintain the patency of alveolar units that would otherwise collapse and lead to shunting of oxygenated blood across the lung. More aggressive therapeutic maneuvers including bronchoscopic lung lavage and corticosteroids (Bannister, Sattilaro. & Otis, 1961; Downs, Chapman, Modell, & Hood, 1974; Gates, Huang, & Cheney, 1983; Lowrey, Anderson, Calhoun, Edmonds, & Flint, 1982) are of unproven benefit and may be detrimental. Prophylactic use of antibiotics remains controversial (Murray, 1979). Cultures obtained shortly after aspiration are usually sterile; antibiotics may select out resistant organisms. Immediate antibiotic prophylaxis does not prevent pneumonia (Lewis, Burgess, & Hapson, 1971) or improve mortality (Bynum & Pierce, 1976; Cameron, Mitchell, & Zuidema, 1973). However, once toxic pneumonitis is complicated by bacterial superinfection, which it is in 26–50% of cases, mortality increases; therefore, prompt treatment of infections is essential (Arms, Dines, & Tinstman, 1974; Bynum & Pierce, 1976). Prevention of acid aspiration by prophylactic reduction of gastric pH is no solution because, as discussed above, it actually increases the risk of bacterial pneumonias (Dachner et al., 1988; Driks et al., 1987; Tryba, 1987).

Bacterial Infections Associated With Aspiration

The term aspiration pneumonitis generally refers to the spectrum of anaerobic bacterial infections of the lungs and pleural space that result from aspiration of anaerobic organisms. Three somewhat distinct syndromes are distinguishable

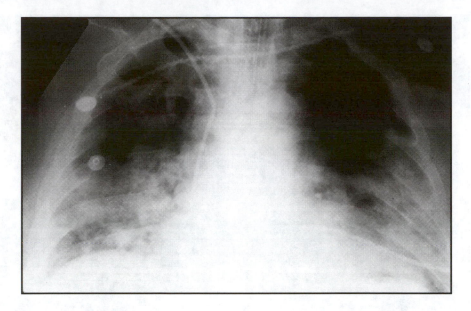

Figure 4–3. Anteroposterior (portable) chest radiograph showing diffuse lung injury (ARDS) following massive aspiration. 66-year-old man with a history of severe diabetes, hypertension, chronic renal insufficiency, and severe peripheral occlusion vascular disease, who was passed out and vomited while drinking orange juice for treatment of hypoglycemia.

within the spectrum of anaerobic pleuropulmonary infections: anaerobic pneumonitis, an indistinct lobar or segmental infiltrate; lung abscess, a usually spherical masslike lesion frequently with an air-fluid level; and empyema, an organized infection within the pleural space (i.e., between the lung and the chest wall; Figure 4–4). All anaerobic infections apparently begin as focal pneumonitis; if this pneumonitis is not adequately handled by immune cellular defenses, a focal abscess may develop. An empyema is believed to result from a pneumonitis that breaks into the adjacent pleural space. Development of these types of infectious complications presumably requires aspiration of a large inoculum of bacteria.

Anaerobic Pulmonary Infections

Anaerobic infections of all types present indolently. Patients frequently have only low grade fevers and night sweats, whereas constitutional symptoms such as weight loss, fatigue, and malaise are frequently profound; this constellation of symptoms may lead to a mistaken diagnosis of malignancy. Intermittent loss of consciousness (from epilepsy, alcoholism, substance abuse, or transient ischemic attacks), predisposes to anaerobic infections resulting from aspiration. These infections seem to relate to excessive colonization of the gingiva with anaerobic organisms, as classic anaerobic infections of the lower respiratory tract are distinctly uncommon in edentulous patients (Schachter, 1981). All aspiration syndromes most frequently involve the dependent segments of the lung. In the supine position, aspirations occur most commonly in the superior segments of the lower lobes, the posterior segments of the upper lobes, or somewhat less commonly in the posterior and medial basilar segments of the lower lobes. The most common of these locations, the superior segments, result in an infiltrate visi-

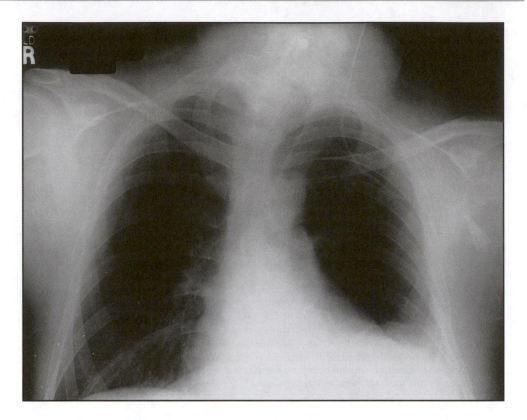

Figure 4–4. Posteroanterior chest radiograph showing aspiration pneumonia in patient with neuromuscular disease. 32-year-old man with C4 quadriparesis and recurrent aspiration pneumonias; note volume loss and left lower lobe collapse. Incidental note should be made of bullet fragments in cervical spine and (incorrect) cephalad placement of left subclavian catheter in jugular vein.

ble in the midlung fields on an upright chest radiograph (Figure 4–5).

Oral Secretions and Pneumonias

Most bacterial pneumonias of healthy outpatients are apparently acquired by aspiration of oral secretions. Only a few types of organisms (tuberculosis, histoplasmosis and other endemic fungi, *Legionella*, pneumonic plague, and anthrax) are acquired by inhalation. Hematogenous (bloodborne) spread accounts for a few types of pneumonias (tularemia, some cases of plague, some gram-negative pneumonias). In almost all other cases of outpatient bacterial pneumonias (including infec-

tions due to *Pneumococcus, Mycoplasma,* influenza, and *Chlamydia*) infection begins with the spread of organisms from the upper airways to the lung. Whether nosocomial pneumonias, especially those in mechanically ventilated patients, are also invariably acquired by aspiration of oropharyngeal secretion is controversial, although most appear to be (Scheld & Madell, 1991). A study of patients intubated for at least 72 hours demonstrated that continuous aspiration of subglottic secretions both decreased the incidence of ventilator-associated pneumonias (19.9 versus 39.6 episodes per 1000 ventilatory days; relative risk 1.98) and delayed the onset of those which occurred (12.0 ± 7.1 days versus 5.9 ± 2.1 days; Vallés, 1995).

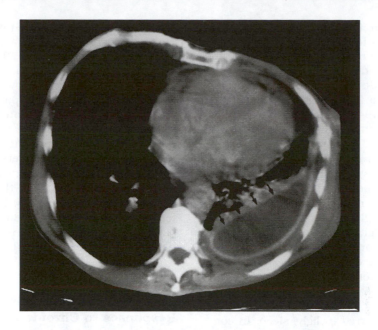

Figure 4–5. Computed chest tomography showing empyema in patient with recurrent aspiration. 65-year-old man with COPD and schizoaffective disorder. Note fluid collection within enhancing pleura (arrows); pleural fluid cultures grew hemolytic streptococcus and Bacteroides species.

An important finding was that in the study group the same pathogenic microorganisms that had been isolated from the subglottic secretions were later isolated bronchoscopically in 85% of cases. This finding further supports the significance of aspirated organisms from the oropharynx as a cause of nosocomial pneumonias.

However, an alternative cause of gram-negative and polymicrobial pneumonias in the critically ill patient is hematogenous spread of bacteria that translocate across the injured gut mucosa (Fiddian-Green & Baker, 1991). In hospitalized patients (including those in nursing homes), a wider spectrum of aspirated organisms is possible owing to colonization of the oropharynx by enteric gram-negative bacteria (Johanson, Pierce, & Sanford, 1969; Johanson, Pierce, Sanford, & Thomas, 1972). Thus, most pneumonias in all settings result from the spread of organisms from the mouth and upper airways to the

lungs, and aspiration of even small amounts of oral secretions would facilitate this spread.

The likelihood that pneumonia will result from a given episode in which oral secretions are aspirated reflects a balance between the size and virulence of the bacterial inoculum on one hand and the integrity of the patient's mechanical and immune defenses of the lungs on the other hand. Pharyngeal dysphagia predisposes to bacterial pneumonias because repeated or large-volume aspirations can overwhelm airway defenses. The term oral secretions is itself something of a misnomer, as the causative factor for pneumonia is the significant contamination of saliva with bacteria, and not the saliva itself, which is bacteriostatic (Gibbons & Houte, 1975). Although dysphagia is believed to cause aspiration of food and liquids and hence pneumonia, the evidence in the literature for linking these events is not uniformly strong. Some studies have found that patients who aspirated food or liquid were significantly more likely to develop pneumonia (Holas, 1994; Schmidt, 1994) but other studies have failed to find such an association (Croghan, 1994). Even normal persons may aspirate small amounts of oral secretions nightly. The best documented evidence of this comes from a study by Huxley and associates (1978) who performed lung scans after instilling Indium into the nasal pharynx of sleeping subjects through a 2-mm flexible catheter, the tip of which was placed 3 cm beyond the external nares. They instilled 10 ml of buffered saline containing the radiotracer in 1-mm aliquots every 30 minutes. They found that 9 of 29 normal subjects had positive scans, although all were minor and none occurred in light sleep. In contrast, 7 of 10 patients with stupor or coma aspirated, in many cases quite massively as documented by lung scanning. This single study has been widely quoted but never subsequently repeated, and its relevance to clinical practice can be questioned. For one thing, the rate of fluid instillation in that study was roughly twice that of normal resting salivary flow in the waking state (0.5 ml/hour; Helm et al., 1982), and was administered as a bolus, rather than continuously. Additionally, salivary flow virtually ceases during sleep in most subjects (Schneyer, Pigman, Hanahan, & Gilmore, 1956). Current standard practice is to advocate tube feeding rather than oral alimentation for the patient with recurrent aspiration, because tube feeding is believed to decrease the risk of aspiration. The controversies surrounding this issue and the indications for enteral feeding are discussed in detail in Chapter 16. However, owing in part to deficiencies in experimental design, existing data do not support unequivocally the hypothesis that aspiration is decreased by enteral alimentation compared to oral feeding or nasogastric tubes, nor that more distal placement of percutaneously introduced feeding tubes (jejunal versus gastric) is superior in preventing aspiration (Ciocon, Silverstone, Graver, & Foley, 1988; Cole, Smith, Molnar, & Shaffer, 1987; Feinberg et al., 1990; Lazarus, 1990; Olson, 1993; Sands, 1991). One small randomized trial showed decreased rate of pneumonia in 19 patients in the surgical intensive care unit randomized to endoscopic jejunal tube feedings compared to 19 similar patients randomized to gastric tube feedings (0 versus 2; Montecalvo et al., 1992). Larger randomized trials are needed to establish the cost–benefit ratio of enteral feedings. Percutaneous feeding tubes obviously do not prevent aspiration of oral secretions, with its inherent risk for development of pneumonia.

Granulomatous and Fibrotic Responses to Chronic Aspiration

Long-standing and repeated aspiration of small amounts of food has been identified traditionally as one cause of interstitial pulmonary fibrosis. Although there are some well-documented cases in which aspiration of food led to fibrosis (Coriat, Labrousse, Vilde, Tenaillon, & Lissac, 1984), most of these cases would today be classified either as late-fibrosis complicating diffuse alveolar damage triggered by the initial aspiration event, or as idiopathic pulmonary fibrosis. In other reports, aspiration was assumed because gastroesophageal reflux was demonstrated (Mays, Dubois, & Hamilton, 1976), or owing to esophageal dysmotility in diseases such as scleroderma, in which the underlying disease is now known to be associated with pulmonary fibrosis.

However, occult aspiration could plausibly induce pulmonary fibrosis in some cases. Experimentally, granulomatous pulmonary inflammation can be induced by intratracheal instillation of saline containing food particles (Moran, 1951; Wynne, 1982). Pathologic evidence of aspirated food particles may be difficult unless careful serial sections are performed (Knoblich, 1969).

Indications for Oropharyngeal Swallowing Examination

The following pulmonary problems merit an oropharyngeal swallowing examination: recurrent pneumonias compatible with aspiration, cough during or immediately after meals, or unexplained pulmonary fibrosis with a history compatible with aspiration. The workup for altered deglutition is discussed in detail in Chapter 5. Several points warrant discussion here. First, the ability to judge clinically which patients will aspirate is poor, especially using the traditional test of gag reflex in the posterior pharynx (DeVita & Spierer-Rundback, 1990; Horner & Massey, 1988; Linden, 1983; Splaingard, Hutchins, Sulton, & Chauduri, 1988). Systematic clinical evaluation for laryngeal dysfunction without videofluoroscopy may miss up to a third of cases (Linden, Kuhlemeier, & Patterson, 1993). A flexible endoscopic larnyngoendoscopy study is another exam that has been shown to be highly sensitive for detecting aspiration and other signs of pharyngeal dysphagia (Langmore, Schatz, & Olson, 1991). Second, although barium is preferred over iodinated ionic contrast media, which has well-known toxicity (Reich, 1969), barium swallow as the initial study for altered deglutition may also result in serious pulmonary injury if there is massive barium aspiration (Gray, Sivaloganathan, & Simpkins, 1989; Penington, 1993).

ROLE OF ALTERED DEGLUTITION AND ESOPHAGEAL REFLUX IN BRONCHOSPASM

The complex issues of the clinical features, pathophysiology, and management of gastroesophageal reflux have been reviewed by Jamieson and Duranceau (1988) and are discussed in Chapters 10 and 13 of this book. This section will be limited to a consideration of the influence of esophageal reflux on airway function.

An association between gastroesophageal reflux and bronchospasm has long been appreciated (Bray, 1934), and reflux is commonly considered a potential reason for refractory or difficult to manage asthma. It has been estimated variously that 30–60% of asthmatics have gastroesophageal reflux (Babb, Notaran-gelo, & Smith, 1970; Duclone, Van Devenne, & Jovin, 1987; Goodal, Earis, & Cooper, 1981); coincidence of the two disorders has been reported to be as high as 90% in one series, undoubtedly reflecting selection bias (Larrain, Carrasco, Galleguillos, Sepulveda, & Pope, 1991). Nevertheless, there is still controversy over the existence and relative importance of a causal link (Shapiro et al., 1989). In part, because both conditions are very common, and based on negative results of acid infusion testing on airway function, some authors have questioned whether the link is indeed etiologic (Ekstrom & Tibbling, 1987).

Two potential mechanisms have been suggested to account for this association: pulmonary aspiration of acidic gastric contents and vagally mediated reflex bronchospasm due to acid in the esophagus alone. Pulmonary aspiration has been demonstrated in patients with asthma and gastroesophageal reflux using scintigraphic imaging (Crausaz & Favez, 1988). It is also supported by the observation of dorsal laryngeal inflammation in many patients with chronic gastroesophageal reflux. It is likely that both mechanisms may contribute in different patients.

SUMMARY

Aspiration of foods, liquids or saliva is normally averted by coordination of respiration and deglutition. Swallow apnea usually interrupts expiration. After both bolus and nonbolus swallows, breathing is resumed during expiration in normal subjects. This coordination of breathing and swallowing is frequently lost in patients with strokes and in patients with advanced COPD. Patients with airways disease due to smoking or repeated pulmonary infection with bronchiectasis may simultaneously have deficient mucociliary clearance. Aspiration may lead to asphyxiation, atelectasis, bronchospasm, pneumonia, lung abscess with or without empyema, or rarely, pulmonary fibrosis. In the development of infectious complications of aspiration, poor oral hygiene and especially gingival disease with chronic anaerobic colonization appear to be of considerable importance. Whether an individual patient with depressed mental status or history of neurologic dysfunction will aspirate is difficult to predict based on clinical exam. Videofluoroscopy and flexible endoscopic laryngoscopy are complementary procedures in the systematic evaluation of deglutition.

MULTIPLE CHOICE QUESTIONS

1. The airways are normally protected from aspiration during deglutition by
   a. movement of the larynx superiorly and anteriorly
   b. vocal cord apposition
   c. repositioning of the aryepiglottic folds and epiglottis
   d. inhibition of respiration during deglutition (swallow apnea)
   e. all of the above

2. Afferent impulses for reflex suppression of respiration during swallowing are carried
   a. to the medullary respiratory center via the ascending vagus nerve
   b. to the medullary respiratory center via recurrent laryngeal nerve
   c. via the glossopharyngeal nerves from the oropharynx and via the superior laryngeal nerves from the rest of the larynx and pharynx

3. Aspirated solid material that reaches the gas-exchange areas (terminal bronchi and alveoli) is cleared by
   a. cough and mucociliary action
   b. by the "mucociliary escalator"
   c. by alveolar macrophages and lymphocytes
   d. by pulmonary lymphatics

4. In patients with tracheotomy tubes, the most important factor predisposing to injury of the respiratory tract mucosa is
   a. presence of a large bore diameter tube
   b. prolonged use of the tube (over 60 days)
   c. additional need for a respirator connected to the tracheostomy tube
   d. excessive pressure in the endotracheal tube cuff
   e. decreased airflow due to the diverted airway path

5. Nosocomial pneumonias, especially those in mechanically ventilated patients, are probably most often acquired by
   a. poor lung clearance mechanisms
   b. hematogenous spread of bacteria that translocate across the injured gut mucosa
   c. aspiration of oropharyngeal secretions
   d. migration of bacteria from endotracheal tubes, tracheostomy tubes, and ventilators into the lower airway.
   e. aspiration of refluxed gastric contents

REFERENCES

Arms, R., Dines, D., & Tinstman, T. (1974). Aspiration pneumonia. *Chest, 65,* 136–139.

Babb, R. R., Notarangelo, J., & Smith, V. M. (1970). Wheezing: A clue to gastroesophageal reflux. *American Journal of Gastroenterology, 53,* 230–233.

Bannister, W., Sattilaro, A., & Otis, R. (1961). Therapeutic aspects of aspiration pneumonitis in experimental animals. *Anesthesiology, 22,* 440–443.

Bartlett, J. G., & Gorbach, S. L. (1975). The triple threat of aspiration pneumonia. *Chest, 91,* 901–909.

Barton, A. D., & Lourenco, R. V. (1973). Bronchial secretions and mucociliary clearance. Biochemical characteristics. *Archives of Internal Medicine, 131,* 140–1444.

Ben-Menachem, T., Fogel, R., Patel, R. V., Touchette, M., Zarowitz, B. J., Hadzijahic, N., Divine, G., Verter, J., & Bresalier, R. S. (1994). Prophylaxis for stress-related gastric hemorrhage in the medical intensive care unit: A randomized, controlled, single-blind study. *Annals of Internal Medicine, 121,* 568–575.

Berendt, R. (1978). Relationship of method of administration to respiratory virulence of Klebsiella pneumoniae for mice and squirrel monkeys. *Infection and Immunity, 20,* 581–583.

Bordignon, C., Villa, F., Allavena, P., Introna, M., Biondi, A., Avallone, R., & Mantovani, A. (1982). Inhibition of natural killer activity by human bronchoalveolar macrophages. *Journal of Immunology, 129,* 587–591.

Braman, S. S., & Corrao, W. M. (1987). Cough: Differential diagnosis and treatment. *Clinics in Chest Medicine, 8,* 177–88.

Bray, G. (1934). Recent advances in the treatment of asthma and hay fever. *Practitioner, 133,* 368–379.

Brenner, M. B., Strominger, J. L., & Krangel, M. S. (1988). The γδ T cell receptor. *Advances in Immunology, 43,* 133–192.

Brin, M., & Younger, D. (1988). Neurologic disease and aspiration. *Otolaryngology Clinics in North America, 21,* 691–699.

Burgess, G. F., III, Cooper, J. R., Marino, R. J., Peuler, M. J., & Warriner, R. A., III (1979). Laryngeal competence after tracheal extubation. *Anesthesiology, 51,* 73–77.

Bynum, L., & Pierce, A. (1976). Pulmonary aspiration of gastric contents. *American Review of Respiratory Disease, 114,* 1129–1136.

Cameron, J., Reynolds, J., & Zuidema, G. (1973). Aspiration in patients with tracheostomies. *Surgery, Gynecology, and Obstetrics, 136,* 68–70.

Cameron, J. L., Mitchell, W. H. & Zuidema, G. D. (1973). Aspiration pneumonia. Clinical outcome following aspiration. *Archives of Surgery, 106,* 49–52.

Ciocon, J. O., Silverstone, F. A., Graver, L. M., & Foley, C. J. (1988). Tube feedings in elderly patients. Indications, benefits, and complications. *Archives of Internal Medicine, 148,* 429–433.

Clarke, S., & Pavia, D. (1988). Deposition and clearance. In J. Murray & J. Nadel (Eds.), *Textbook of respiratory medicine,* (Vol. 1, 313–331). Philadelphia: W. B. Saunders.

Coelho, C. A. (1987). Preliminary findings on the nature of dysphagia in patients with chronic obstructive pulmonary disease. *Dysphagia, 2,* 28–31.

Cole, M., Smith, J., Molnar, C., & Shaffer, E. A. (1987). Aspiration after percutaneous gastrostomy: Assessment by Tc-99m labeling of the enteral feed. *Journal of Clinical Gastroenterology, 9,* 90–95.

Coleridge, H. M., & Coleridge, J. C. (1994). Pulmonary reflexes: Neural mechanisms of pulmonary defense. *Annual Review of Physiology, 56,* 69–91.

Cook, D. J., Fuller, H. D., Guyatt, G. H., Marshall, J. C., Leasa, D., Hall, R., Winton, T. L., Rutledge, F., Todd, T. J., Roy, P. et al. (1994). Risk factors for gastrointestinal bleeding in critically ill patients. Canadian Critical Care Trials Group. *New England Journal of Medicine, 330,* 377–381.

Coriat, P., Labrousse, J., Vilde, F., Tenaillon, A., & Lissac, J. (1984). Diffuse interstitial pneumonitis due to aspiration of gastric contents. *Anaesthesia, 39,* 703–705.

Cot, C. (1931). *Les asphyxies accidentelles.* Paris: N. Maloine.

Crausaz, F. M., & Favez, G. (1988). Aspiration of solid food particles into lungs of patients with gastroesophageal reflux and chronic bronchial disease. *Chest, 93,* 376–377.

Craven, D., Kunches, L., Kilinsky, V., Lichtenberg, D., Make, B., & McCabe, W. (1986). Risk factors for pneumonia and fatality in patients receiving continuous mechanical ventilation. *American Review of Respiratory Disease, 133,* 792–796.

Craven, D., Steger, K., & Barber, T. (1991). Preventing nosocomial pneumonia: State of the art and perspectives for the 1990's. *American Journal of Medicine, 91,* S44–S53.

Croghan, J. E., Burke, E. M., Caplan, S., & Denman, S. (1994). Pilot study of 12-month outcomes of nursing home patients with aspiration on videofluoroscopy. *Dysphagia, 9,* 141–146.

Curtis, J. L., & Schuyler, M. R. (1993). Immunologically-mediated lung disease. In Baum, G. L. & Wolinsky, E. (Eds.), *Textbook of pulmonary diseases* (pp. 689–744). Boston: Little, Brown.

Dachner, F., Kappstein, I., Engels, I., Reuschenbach, K., Pfisterer, J., Krieg, N., & Vogel, W. (1988). Stress ulcer prophylaxis and ventilation pneumonia: Prevention by antibacterial cytoprotective agents? *Infection Control and Hospital Epidemiology, 9,* 59–65.

DeVita, M. A., & Spierer-Rundback, L. (1990). Swallowing disorders in patients with prolonged orotracheal intubation or tracheostomy tubes. *Critical Care Medicine, 18,* 1328–1330.

Doerschuk, C. M., Downey, G. P., Doherty, D. E., English, D., Gie, R. P., Ohgami, M., Worthen, G. S., Henson, P. M., & Hogg, J. C. (1990). Leukocyte and platelet margination within microvasculature of rabbit lungs. *Journal of Applied Physiology, 68,* 1956–1961.

Downs, J., Chapman, R., Jr., Modell, J. H., & Hood, C. I. (1974). An evaluation of steroid therapy in aspiration pneumonitis. *Anesthesiology, 40,* 129–135.

Driks, M., Craven, D., Celli, B., Manning, M., Burke, R., Garvin, G., Kunches, L., Farber, H., Wedel, S., & McCabe, W. (1987). Nosocomial pneumonia in intubated patients given sucralfate as compared with antacids or histamine type 2 blockers: The role of gastric colonization. *New England Journal of Medicine, 317,* 1376–1382.

du Moulin, G., Hedley-Whyte, J., Paterson, D., & Lison, A. (1982). Aspiration of gastric bacteria in antacid-treated patients: A frequent cause of postoperative colonisation of the airway. *Lancet, 1,* 242–245.

Duclone, A., Van Devenne, A., & Jovin, H. (1987). Gastroesophageal reflux in patients with asthma and chronic bronchitis. *American Review of Respiratory Disease, 135,* 327–332.

Ekstrom, T., & Tibbling, L. (1987). Gastroesophageal reflux and triggering of bronchial asthma. *European Journal of Respiratory Disease, 71,* 177–180.

Eschenbacher, W. L., Boushey, H. A., & Sheppard, D. (1984). Alteration in osmolarity of inhaled aerosols causes bronchoconstriction and cough, but absence of a permeant anion causes cough alone. *American Review of Respiratory Disease, 129,* 211–215.

Exharos, N., Logan, W., & Abbott, O. (1965). The importance of pH and volume in tracheal aspiration. *Journal of Thoracic and Cardiovascular Surgery, 79,* 275–282.

Fagon, J. Y., Chastre, J., Hance, A. J., Guiguet, M., Trouillet, J. L., Domart, Y., Pierre, J., & Gibert, C. (1988). Detection of nosocomial lung infection in ventilated patients. Use of a protected specimen brush and quantitative culture techniques in 147 patients. *American Review of Respiratory Disease, 138,* 110–116.

Feinberg, M. J., Knebl, J., Tully, J., & Segall, L. (1990). Aspiration and the elderly. *Dysphagia, 5,* 61–71.

Fiddian-Green, R. G., & Baker, S. (1991). Nosocomial pneumonia in the critically ill: Product of aspiration or translocation? *Critical Care Medicine, 19,* 763–769.

Gastinne, H., Wolff, M., Delatour, F., Faurisson, F., & Chevret, S. (1992). A controlled trial in intensive care units of selective decontamination of the digestive tract with nonabsorbable antibiotics. The French Study Group on Selective Decontamination of the Digestive Tract. *New England Journal of Medicine, 326,* 594–599.

Gates, S., Huang, T., & Cheney, F. (1983). Effects of methylprednisone on resolution of acid-aspiration pneumonitis. *Archives of Surgery, 118,* 1262–1265.

Gibbons, R. J., & Houte, J. V. (1975). Bacterial adherence in oral microbial ecology. *Annual Review of Microbiology, 29,* 19–44.

Goodal, R. J. R., Earis, J. E., & Cooper, D. N. (1981). Relationship between asthma and gastroesophageal reflux. *Thorax, 36,* 116–121.

Gray, C., Sivaloganathan, S., & Simpkins, K. C. (1989). Aspiration of high-density barium contrast medium causing acute pulmonary inflammation—report of two fatal cases in elderly women with disordered swallowing. *Clinics in Radiology, 40,* 397–400.

Green, J. H., & Neil, E. (1955). The respiratory function of the laryngeal muscles. *Journal of Physiology, 129,* 134–135.

Greenfield, L., Singelton, R., & McCaffree, D. (1969). Pulmonary effects of experimentally graded aspiration of hydrochloric acid. *Annals of Surgery, 170,* 74–86.

Groher, M., & Gonzalez, E. (1992). Mechanical disorders of swallowing. In M. Groher (Ed.), *Dysphagia: Diagnosis and management* (pp. 53–84). Boston: Butterworth-Heinemann.

Harada, R. N., & Repine, J. E. (1985). Pulmonary host defense mechanisms. *Chest, 87,* 247–252.

Harmsen, A. G., Muggenburg, B., Snipes, M.B. & Bice, D.E. (1985). The role of macrophages in particle translocation from lungs to lymph nodes. *Science, 230,* 1277–1280.

Heffner, J. E. (1988). Tracheal intubation in mechanically ventilated patients. *Clinics in Chest Medicine, 9,* 23–35.

Heimlich, H. (1981). Subdiaphragmatic pressure to expel water from the lungs of drowning persons. *Annals of Emergency Medicine, 10,* 476–480.

Helm, J., Dodds, W., Hogan, W., Soergel, K., Egide, M., & Wood, C. (1982). Acid neutralizing capacity of human saliva. *Gastroenterology, 83,* 69–74.

Holas, M. A., DePippo, K. L., & Reding, M. J. (1994). Aspiration and relative risk of medical complications following stroke. *Archives of Neurology, 51,* 1051-1053.

Horner, J., & Massey, W. (1988). Silent aspiration following stroke. *Neurology, 38,* 317–319.

Huxley, E. J., Viroslav, J., Gray, W. R., & Pierce, A. K. (1978). Pharyngeal aspiration in normal adults and patients with depressed consciousness. *American Journal of Medicine, 64,* 564–568.

Irwin, R. S., Corrao, W. M., & Pratter, M. R. (1981). Chronic persistent cough in the adult: The spectrum and frequency of causes and successful outcome of specific therapy. *American Review of Respiratory Disease, 123,* 413–417.

Irwin, R. S., & Curley, F. J. (1991). The treatment of cough. A comprehensive review. *Chest, 99,* 1477–1484.

Irwin, R. S., Curley, F. J., & French, C. L. (1990). Chronic cough. The spectrum and frequency of causes, key components of the diagnostic evaluation, and outcome of specific therapy. *American Review of Respiratory Disease, 141,* 640–647.

Issa, F. G., & Porostocky, S. (1994). Effect of continuous swallowing on respiration. *Respiratory Physiology, 95,* 181–193.

Jackson, J. H., & Cochrane, C. G. (1988). Leukocyte-induced tissue injury. *Hematology/Oncology Clinics of North America, 2,* 317–334.

JAMA (1986). Standards and guidelines for cardiopulmonary resuscitation and emergency cardiac care. *JAMA, 255,* 2905–2989.

James, C. F., Modell, J. H., Gibbs, C. P., Kuck, E. J., & Ruiz, B. C. (1984). Pulmonary aspiration—effects of pH and volume in the rat. *Anesthesia and Analgesia, 63,* 665–668.

Jamieson, G., & Duranceau, A. (Ed.) (1988). *Gastroesophageal reflux.* (pp. 281). Philadelphia: W. B. Saunders.

Janis, E. M., Kaufmann, S. H., Schwartz, R. H., & Pardoll, D. M. (1989). Activation of γδ T cells in the primary immune response to Mycobacterium tuberculosis. *Science, 244,* 713–716.

Johanson, W. G., Jr., Pierce, A. K., & Sanford, J. P. (1969). Changing pharyngeal bacterial flora in hospitalized patients: Emergence of gram-negative bacteria. *New England Journal of Medicine, 28,* 1137–1140.

Johanson, W. G., Jr., Pierce, A. K., Sanford, J. P., & Thomas, G. D. (1972). Nosocomial respiratory infections with gram-negative bacilli. The significance of colonization of the respiratory tract. *Annals of Internal Medicine, 77,* 701–706.

Kaltreider, H. B. (1982). Alveolar macrophages: Enhancers or suppressors of pulmonary immune reactivity? *Chest, 82,* 261–262.

Kaltreider, H. B., Caldwell, J. L., & Byrd, P. K. (1986). The capacity of normal murine alveolar macrophages to function as antigen-presenting cells for the initiation of primary antibody-forming cell responses to sheep erythrocytes in vitro. *American Review of Respiratory Disease, 133,* 1097–1104.

Knoblich, R. (1969). Pulmonary granulomatosis caused by vegetable particles: So called lentil pulse pneumonia. *American Review of Respiratory Disease, 99,* 380–389.

Kramer, S. (1989). Radiologic examination of the swallowing impaired child. *Dysphagia, 3,* 117–125.

Langmore, S. E., & Murray, J. T. (1991). *Coordination of respiration and swallowing in dysphagia.* Presented at Swallowing and Swallowing Disorders: From the Clinic to the Laboratory conference at Northwestern Universty, Evanston, IL.

Langmore, S. E., Schatz, K., & Olson, N. (1991). Endoscopic and videofluoroscopic evaluations of swallowing and aspiration. *Annals of Otolaryngology, Rhinology and Laryngology, 100,* 678–681.

Lanier, L. L., Phillips J.H., Hackett J. Jr., Tutt M., & Kumar V. (1986). Natural killer cells: Definition of a cell type rather than a function. *Journal of Immunology, 137,* 2735–2739.

Larrain, A., Carrasco, E., Galleguillos, F., Sepulveda, R., & Pope, C. E. D. (1991). Medical and surgical treatment of nonallergic asthma associated with gastroesophageal reflux. *Chest, 99,* 1330–1335.

Lazarus, B. A., Murphy, J. B., & Culpepper, L. (1990). Aspiration associated with long-term gastric versus jejunal feeding: A critical analysis of the literature. *Archives of Physical Medicine and Rehabilitation, 71,* 46–53.

Leckie, W. J. H., & Tothill, P. (1965). Albumin turnover in pleural effusions. *Clinical Sciences, 29,* 339–352.

Leith, D. E. (1977). Cough. In J. D. Brain, D. F. Proctor, & L. M. Reid (Eds.), *Respiratory defense mechanisms,* (Vol. 5, pp. 545–592). New York: Marcel Dekker.

Levine, S. A., & Niederman, M. S. (1991). The impact of tracheal intubation on host defenses and risk of nosocomial pneumonia. *Clinics in Chest Medicine, 12,* 523–543.

Lewis, R., Burgess, J., & Hapson, L. (1971). Cardiopulmonary studies in critical illness: Changes in aspiration pneumonia. *Archives of Surgery, 103,* 335–340.

Limper, A., & Prakash, U. (1990). Tracheobronchial foreign bodies in adults. *Annals of Internal Medicine, 112,* 604–609.

Linden, P., Kuhlemeier, K. V., & Patterson, C. (1993). The probability of correctly predicting subglottic penetration from clinical observations. *Dysphagia, 8,* 170–179.

Linden, P. S. A. (1983). Dysphagia: Predicting laryngeal penetration. *Archives of Physical Medicine and Rehabilitation, 64,* 281–284.

Lipscomb, M. F., Lyons, C. R., Nunez, G., Ball, E. J., Stanstny, P., Vial, W., Lem, V., Weissler, J. C., Miller, L. M., & Toews, G. B. (1986). Human alveolar macrophages: HLA-DR-positive cells that are poor stimulators of a primary mixed leukocyte reaction. *Journal of Immunology, 136,* 497–504.

Logemann, J. A. (1983). Evaluation and treatment of swallowing disorders (p. 249). San Diego, CA: College-Hill Press.

Lowrey, L., Anderson, M., Calhoun, J., Edmonds, H., & Flint, L. M. (1982). Failure of corticosteroid therapy for experimental acid aspiration. *Journal of Surgical Research, 32,* 168–172.

Martin, B. J. W., Logemann, J. A., Shaker, R., & Dodds, W. J. (1994). Coordination between respiration and swallowing: respiratory phase relationships and temporal integration. *Journal of Applied Physiology, 76,* 714–723.

Mays, E. E., Dubois, J. J., & Hamilton, G. B. (1976). Pulmonary fibrosis associated with tracheobronchial aspiration. A study of the frequency of hiatal hernia and gastroesophageal reflux in interstitial pulmonary fibrosis of obscure etiology. *Chest, 69,* 512–515.

Mbawuike, I. N., & Herscowitz, H. B. (1988). Role of activation in alveolar macrophage-mediated suppression of the plaque-forming cell response. *Infection and Immunity, 56,* 577–581.

McCulloch, T. M., & Bishop, M. J. (1991). Complications of translaryngeal intubation. *Clinics in Chest Medicine, 12,* 507–521.

Mendelson, C. (1946). The aspiration of stomach contents into the lung during obstetric anesthesia. *American Journal of Obstetrics and Gynecology, 52,* 191–205.

Meyer, E., Dominguez, E., & Bensch, K. (1969). Pulmonary lymphatic and blood absorption of albumin from alveoli. A quantitative comparison. *Laboratory Investigation, 20,* 1–8.

Miller, A. J., & Loizzi, R. F. (1974). Anatomical and functional differentiation of superior laryngeal nerve fibers affecting swallowing and respiration. *Experimental Neurology, 49,* 369–387.

Modell, J. H., Graves, S. A., & Ketover, A. (1976). Clinical source of 91 consecutive near-drowning victims. *Chest, 70,* 231–238.

Montecalvo, M. A., Steger, K. A., Farber, H. W., Smith, B. F., Dennis, R. C., Fitzpatrick, G. F., Pollack, S. D., Korsberg, T. Z., Birkett, D. H., Hirsch, E. F., et al. (1992). Nutritional outcome and pneumonia in critical care patients randomized to gastric versus jejunal tube feedings. The Critical Care Research Team. *Critical Care Medicine, 20,* 1377–1387.

Montoya, D. (1986). Management of the choking victims. *Canadian Medical Association Journal, 135,* 305–311.

Moran, T. J. (1951). Experimental food-aspiration pneumonia. *Archives in Pathology, 52,* 350–354.

Murray, H. W. (1979). Antimicrobial therapy in pulmonary aspiration. *American Journal of Medicine, 66,* 188–190.

Murray, J. F., Felton, C. P., Garay, S. M., Gottlieb, M. S., Hopewell, P. C., Stover, D. E., & Teirstein, A. S. (1984). Pulmonary complications of the acquired immunodeficiency syndrome. *New England Journal of Medicine, 310,* 1682–1688.

Nash, M. (1988). Swallowing problems in the tracheotomized patient. *Otolaryngology Clinics of North America, 21,* 701–709.

Negus, V. E. (1949). *The comparative anatomy and physiology of the larynx.* London: William Heinemann.

Olson, D. L., Krubsack, A. J., & Stewart, E. T. (1993). Percutaneous enteral alimentation: Gastrostomy versus gastrojejunostomy. *Radiology, 187,* 105–108.

Pabst, R. (1990). Compartmentalization and kinetics of lymphoid cells in the lung. *Regional Immunology, 3,* 62–71.

Pabst, R., Binns, R. M., Licence, S. T., & Peter, M. (1987). Evidence of a selective major vascular marginal pool of lymphocytes in the lung. *American Review of Respiratory Disease, 136,* 1213–1218.

Penington, G. R. (1993). Severe complications following a "barium swallow" investigation for dysphagia. *Medical Journal of Australia, 159,* 764–765.

Pober, J. S., Collins, T., Gimbrone, J. A., Cotran, R. S., Gitlin, J. D., Fiers, W., Clayberger, C., Krensky, A. M., Burakoff, J. S., & Reiss, C. S. (1983). Lymphocytes recognize human vascular endothelial and dermal fibroblast Ia antigens induced by recombinant immune interferon. *Nature, 305,* 726–729.

Pontoppidan, H., & Beecher, H. K. (1960). Progressive loss of protective reflexes in the airway with the advance of age. *JAMA, 174,* 2209–2213.

Preiksaitis, H. G., Mayrand, S., Robins, K., & Diamant, N. E. (1992). Coordination of respiration and swallowing: Effect of bolus volume in normal adults. *American Journal of Physiology, 263,* R624–R630.

Redding, J. (1979). The choking controversy: Critique of evidence on the Heimlich maneuver. *Critical Care Medicine, 7,* 475–479.

Reich, S. (1969). Production of pulmonary edema by aspiration of water soluble nonabsorbable contrast media. *Radiology, 92,* 367–370.

Robinson, B. W., Pinkston, P., & Crystal, R. G. (1984). Natural killer cells are present in the normal human lung but are functionally impotent. *Journal of Clinical Investigation, 74,* 942–950.

Russin, S. J., & Adler, A. G. (1989). Pulmonary aspiration. The three syndromes. *Postgraduate Medicine, 85,* 155–156, 159–161.

Sands, J. A. (1991). Incidence of pulmonary aspiration in intubated patients receiving enteral nutrition through wide- and narrow-bore nasogastric feeding tubes. *Heart Lung, 20,* 75–80.

Sant'Ambrogio, G., & Mathew, O. (1986). Laryngeal receptor and their reflex responses. *Clinics in Chest Medicine, 7,* 211–222.

Sasaki, C. T., Suzuki, M., Horiuchi, M., & Kirchner, J. A. (1977). The effect of tracheostomy on the laryngeal closure reflex. *Laryngoscope, 87,* 1428–1432.

Sawyer, R. T. (1986). The significance of local resident pulmonary alveolar macrophage proliferation to population renewal. *Journal of Leukocyte Biology, 39,* 77–87.

Schachter, E. (1981). Suppurative lung disease: Old problems revisited. *Clinics in Chest Medicine, 2,* 41–49.

Scheld, W., & Madell, G. (1991). Nosocomial pneumonia: Pathogenesis and recent advances in diagnosis and therapy. *Reviews of Infectious Diseases, 13* (suppl 9), S743–751.

Schlesinger, R., Gurman, J., & Lippmann, M. (1982). Particle deposition with bronchial airways. *Annals of Occupational Hygiene, 26,* 47–64.

Schmidt, J., Holas, M., Halvorson, K., & Reding, M. (1994). Videofluoroscopic evidence of aspiration predicts pneumonia and death but not dehydration following stroke. *Dysphagia, 9,* 9–17.

Schneyer, L., Pigman, W., Hanahan, L., & Gilmore, R. (1956). Rate of flow of human parotid, sublingual and submaxillary secretions during sleep. *Journal of Dental Research, 35,* 109–114.

Schols, A., Mostert, R., Cobben, N., Soeters, P., & Wouters, E. (1991). Transcutaneous oxygen saturation and carbon dioxide tension during meals in patients with chronic obstructive pulmonary disease. *Chest, 100,* 1287–1292.

Schols, A. M. W. J., Mostert, R., Soeters, P. B., Greve, L. H., & Wouters, E. F. M. (1989). Inventory of nutritional status in chronic obstructive pulmonary disease. *Chest, 96,* 247–250.

Schwartz, D. J., Wynne, J. W., Gibbs, C. P., Hood, C. I., & Kuck, E. J. (1980). The pulmonary consequences of aspiration of gastric contents at pH greater than 2.5. *American Review of Respiratory Disease, 121,* 119–126.

Selley, W. G., Flack, F. C., Ellis, R. E., & Brooks, W. A. (1989). Respiratory patterns associated with swallowing: Part 2. Neurologically impaired dysphagic patients. *Age Ageing, 18,* 173–176.

Shaker, R., Li, Q., Ren, J., Townsend, W. F., Dodds, W. J., Martin, B. J., Kern, M. K., & Rynders, A. (1992). Coordination of deglutition and phases of respiration: Effect of aging, tachypnea, bolus volume, and chronic obstructive pulmonary disease. *American Journal of Physiology, 263,* G750–G755.

Shapiro, M., Dobbins, J., & Matthay, R. (1989). Pulmonary manifestations of gastrointestinal disease. *Clinics in Chest Medicine, 10,* 617–643.

Shellito, J., Esparza, C., & Armstrong, C. (1987). Maintenance of the normal rat alveolar macrophage cell population: The roles of monocyte influx and alveolar macrophage proliferation in situ. *American Review of Respiratory Disease, 135,* 78–82.

Splaingard, M., Hutchins, B., Sulton, L., & Chauduri, G. (1988). Aspiration in rehabilitation patients: Videofluoroscopy vs. bedside clinical assessment. *Archives in Physical Medicine and Rehabilitation, 69,* 637–640.

Springer, T. A. (1990). Adhesion receptors of the immune system. *Nature, 346,* 425–434.

Stauffer, J. L., Olson, D. E., & Petty, T. L. (1981). Complications and consequences of endotracheal intubation and tracheostomy: A prospective study in 150 critically ill adult patients. *American Journal of Medicine, 70,* 65–76.

Stewart, P. B. (1963). The rate of formation and lymphatic removal of fluid in pleural effusions. *Journal of Clinical Investigation, 42,* 258–262.

Teabeaut, R. J. (1952). Aspiration of gastric contents. *American Journal of Pathology, 27,* 51–67.

Tobin, M. J. (1994). Mechanical ventilation. *New England Journal of Medicine, 330,* 1056–1061.

Tomori, Z., & Widdicombe, J. (1969). Muscular, bronchomotor and cardiovascular reflexes elicited by mechanical stimulation of the respiratory tract. *Journal of Physiology (London), 200,* 25–50.

Tryba, M. (1987). Risk of acute stress bleeding and nosocomial pneumonia in ventilated intensive care unit patients: Sucralfate vs antacids. *American Journal of Medicine, 83* (suppl. 3B), 117–124.

Vallés, J., Artigas, A., Rello, J., Bonsoms, N., Frontanals, D., Blanch, L., Fernández, R., Baigorri, F., & Mestre, J. (1995). Continuous aspiration of subglottic secretions in preventing ventilator-associated pneumonia. *Annals of Internal Medicine, 122,* 179–186.

Wanner, A. (1986). Mucociliary clearance in the trachea. *Clinics in Chest Medicine, 7,* 247–258.

Weibel, E. R. (1963). *Morphometry of the human lung* (p. 111). Berlin: Springer-Verlag.

Weiss, S. J. (1989). Tissue destruction by neutrophils. *New England Journal of Medicine, 320,* 365–376.

Weissler, J. C., Nicod, L. P., Lipscomb, M. F., & Toews, G. B. (1987). Natural killer function in human lung is compartmentalized. *American Review of Respiratory Disease, 135,* 941–949.

Weymuller, E. A., & Bishop, M. J. (1990). Problems associated with prolonged intubation in the geriatric patient. *Otolaryngology Clinics of North America, 23,* 1057–1074.

Whited, R. E. (1983). Posterior commissure stenosis post long-term intubation. *Laryngoscope, 93,* 1314–1318.

Winship, D. (1983). Upper esophageal sphincter: Does it care about reflux? *Gastroenterology, 85,* 470–472.

Wynne, J., Ramphal, R., & Hood, C. (1981). Tracheal mucosal damage after aspiration—a scanning electron microscope study. *American Review of Respiratory Disease, 124,* 728–732.

Wynne, J. W. (1982). Aspiration pneumonitis: Correlation of experimental models with clinical disease. *Clinics in Chest Medicine, 3,* 25–34.

Yanagihara, N., von Leden, H., & Werner-Kukuk, E. (1966). The physical parameters of cough: The larynx in a normal single cough. *Acta Oto-laryngologica* (Stockholm), *61,* 495–510.

5

Clinical Assessment of Dysphagia

Konrad S. Schulze-Delrieu
Robert M. Miller

ROLE OF THE CLINICAL EVALUATION

Dysphagia, or impaired swallowing, may severely affect one's quality of life. It may turn a pleasurable experience into torment. It can make patients dependent on feeding by others or on nonoral nutritional support. It can pose the constant threat of sudden airway obstruction or respiratory infections from aspiration. Along with a cranial nerve examination, the bedside evaluation of the patient should provide information on general health and social and cognitive ability. Is a generalized disease causing the dysphagia, or has the dysphagia led to a deterioration in general health? Has the patient been physically and emotionally able to compensate for any dysfunction? Is the swallowing dysfunction a source of isolation and depression? This knowledge affects the selection of the appropriate feeding modality and other aspects of diagnosis, prognosis, and management.

Swallowing may be impaired because of mechanical impingement on the bolus passage, lack of salivary secretions, weakness in the muscular structures propelling the bolus, or dysfunction of the neuronal

networks coordinating swallowing (Asher, 1984; Bonano, 1970; Buchholz, 1987b; Christensen, 1976; Hughes et al., 1987; Jones et al., 1985; Logemann, 1983; Pope, 1977; Weiden & Harrigan, 1986; Zerhouni, Bosma, & Donner, 1987). The bedside evaluation should identify the most likely sites and mechanisms for the disordered swallowing. The techniques used to do this are like those employed by all clinical disciplines: to define the nature of the problem by prompting the patient to describe the symptoms and clarify the symptoms through direct questioning. The clinician constantly compares the information provided by the history and examination to the manifestations of the various categories of swallowing disorders. The clinician may then define the patient's problem by category, syndrome, or, in some instances, a single disease entity (Batch, 1988 a, 1988 b; Bradley & Narula, 1987; Castell & Donner, 1987; Edwards, 1976).

Indications for Clinical Assessment of Swallowing

Table 5–1 lists symptoms and findings that are warning signs for the likely presence of impaired swallowing and the risk

TABLE 5–1. Warning Signs Associated with Dysphagia and Aspiration Risk.

Decreased alertness or cognitive dysfunction
• stupor, coma, heavy sedation, delirium, dementia, or profound mental retardation
• playing with food, inappropriate size of bites, talking or emotional lability during attempts to swallow

Changes in approach to food
• avoidance of eating in company
• special physical preparation of food or avoidance of foods of specific consistency
• prolonged meal time, intermittent cessation of intake, frequent "wash downs"
• compensatory measures (head and neck movements)
• laborious chewing, repetitive swallowing
• coughing and choking upon swallowing, increased need to clear throat

Manifestations of impaired oropharyngeal functions
• dysarthria
• wet, hoarse voice
• dysfunction of focal musculature (facial asymmetries, abnormal reflexes or dystonia, dyskinesias or fasciculations)
• drooling or oral spillage; pooling and pocketing of food
• frequent throat clearing

Patient complaints or observations of
• difficulty initiating a swallow
• sensation of obstruction of the bolus in throat or chest
• regurgitation of food or acid
• inability to handle secretions
• unexplained weight loss
• impaired breathing during meals or immediately after eating
• pain on swallowing
• leakage of food or saliva from tracheostomy site

of aspiration. The bedside evaluation should screen patients for the likelihood and seriousness of a swallowing impairment. Pain with swallowing, a sensation of sticking and obstruction during swallowing, or visible effort when swallowing are signs of discrete disease. This is so even when the sensation is intermittent, as it may be with organic strictures like Schatzki's rings (Schatzki, 1963), or made worse by emotional stress as has been observed in achalasia and esophageal spasm (Benjamin, Gerhardt, & Castell, 1979; Pope, 1989; Tucker, Snape, & Cohen, 1978; Vantrappen & Hellmans, 1974). Most patients seek help because they have recognized some malfunction of their swallowing (Ravich, Wilson, Jones, & Donner, 1989). Hospitalized or institutionalized patients may be unable to recognize or describe dysphagia, and accounts of swallowing problems must then be elicited

from attendants (Langmore, Schatz, & Olsen, 1988; Siebens, Trupe, Siebens, 1986).

Oral feeding problems are likely in patients whose neurologic disease has led to confusion or dementia (Buchholz, 1987a). Patients with poor judgment, sensory deficits, or poor motor coordination from brain damage may not possess the vigilance and physical ability to handle their food intake safely. Dysarthric speech with slow, labored, and slurred articulation, nasal air emission, and a hoarse or wet voice demonstrates impairment of muscle groups essential for effective oropharyngeal swallowing. Frequent coughing and choking on food or sputum signify impaired swallowing (Gerhardt & Winship, 1982; Kilman & Goyal, 1976). Strenuous chewing, labored swallowing, repetitive swallowing of a single bolus, and the prolongation of mealtime should be taken seriously, particularly if associated with disinterest in, or fear of, food and weight loss. Sialorrhea (excessive drooling) is of esthetic consequence and related to poor orolabial continence. Drooling is more ominous when due to poor pharyngeal clearance of secretions by periodic swallowing. Pooling of mucus or debris in the pharyngeal recesses (valleculae and pyriform sinuses) seen on laryngoscopy or videofluoroscopy implies poor bolus clearance and increased risk of aspiration (Jordan, 1977; Perlman, Booth, & Grayhack, 1994).

In addition to some neurologic disorders (Buchholz, 1987a; Gordon, Hewer, & Wade, 1987; Mayberry & Atkinson, 1986), impaired swallowing is a frequent complication, of some interventions to treat head and neck neoplasms (Linden & Siebens, 1983; McConnel et al., 1988) and of esophagitis and esophageal tumors (Moser et al., 1991). In many of these conditions the patient may be preoccupied with other symptoms, and the insight and foresight of the clinician is required to assess the potential for complications arising from a swallowing problem. The neurologic diseases commonly associated with abnormal swallowing include cerebrovascular accidents, traumatic brain injury, cerebral palsy, mental retardation and dementia, dyskinesias including Huntington's disease and Parkinson's disease, myasthenias, muscular dystrophies, degenerative disorders including multiple sclerosis, amyotrophic lateral sclerosis, and sleep apnea. Resection, dissection, or irradiation of the tongue, larynx, and pharynx are likely to cause mechanical and functional inadequacies. Enhanced swallowing and clearance of saliva are objectives in the treatment of cancers of the esophagus and of peptic esophageal strictures.

Components of Bedside Assessment

The swallowing history and physical examination determine the likely site and mechanism of the problem and guide in the selection of diagnostic tests and therapeutic measures. Does the process involve the oral cavity, the pharynx, the esophagus, or an interaction between all three (Jones et al., 1985)? Is the dysphagia caused by inflammation, dysfunction, or neoplasia localized specifically in the swallowing structures, or is it part of a systemic disease involving the deglutitory musculature or the central nervous system? Is the patient at risk for aspiration, or have respiratory complications already occurred (Cameron, Reynolds, & Zuindema, 1973; Elpern, Jacobs, & Bone, 1987; Greenbaum, 1976)? If so, are they likely to recur? The clinician uses history taking and the physical examination in an attempt to answer these questions, to formulate a preliminary diagnosis, and to select appropriate tests. The value of the clinical encounter is determined by the skill with which the clinician uses historical or physical clues to direct the search for additional evidence (Castell & Donner, 1987).

A history starts by prompting a patient to describe what is abnormal about swallowing and continues with questioning about associated symptoms and his or her general health status. The extent and intensity to which one probes for additional information follows from the likely nature of the swallowing disorder. If the history points to a mechanical obstruction, one ought to determine whether this has led to a preference for soft foods and to weight loss. If coordination and function appear affected, thorough questioning about problems with speech and other neuromuscular functions becomes essential. Thus, the examiner might find it expedient to expand immediately on items that seem relevant to the swallowing problem and may even complete a detailed neurologic history and examination.

If a swallowing problem occurs in an otherwise healthy individual, assigning it to a single category of clinical disorders and selecting definitive tests and treatments should be straightforward. If, however, dysphagia occurs against a background of multiple medical problems and complications, systematic inquiry into the contributing historical and physical factors is needed to arrive at a comprehensive assessment. Also, interactions between various diseases and problems need to be assessed, and follow-up questioning may be needed for many associated symptoms. If the problem seems to be multifactorial, it must be determined whether the intrinsic disease of the swallowing structures or the systemic disorder is primarily at fault. Which is more amenable to therapeutic intervention? Has management of other medical problems had a positive or negative effect on swallowing? Is suppression of one disorder paramount to patient survival, or is correction of the swallowing problem at the expense of the disorder of greater clinical benefit? Does the patient understand competing benefits and risks, and what is his or her preference? The clinical response of the patient may need periodic reassessment, and progress may be made only by trial and error with multiple diagnostic and therapeutic approaches.

SYMPTOMS AND SYNDROMES

Dysphagia, Odynophagia, Bolus Impaction, and Globus Sensation

Dysphagia may constitute difficulty in initiation of swallows or the feeling that, once swallowing starts, the passage of the bolus is impeded. Diagnostic probing strives to establish into which of the following categories an individual disturbance fits: oral, pharygneal, esophageal, or all three (Jones et al., 1985; Logemann, 1983). Is it a local mechanical and focal problem, or a functional and generalized problem? Characterization of the dysphagia by its type and timing may be all that is needed to identify the site and the mechanism responsible for the swallow disturbance. With *oropharyngeal* dysphagia, failure to completely clear the pharynx can result in airway penetration. *Esophageal* dysphagia may manifest itself as a substernal sticking sensation. If the patient points to the lower substernal area, the distal esophagus is very likely the site of obstruction. However, projection of

sensations into proximal fields is common, and patients with distal esophageal lesions may complain of symptoms in the neck. Timing is more accurate: a problem within 2 seconds is more likely to relate to an oropharyngeal process; after several seconds, an esophageal problem is indicated (Hamlet, Nelson, & Patterson, 1990). Table 5–2 provides a listing of historical data that are commonly useful in arriving at a clinical diagnosis. The table lists symptoms in a logical order for a history to progress. First, the subjective nature of the swallowing problem itself is defined. Associated symptoms are then explored as they relate directly to functions mediated by the swallowing musculature. Ancillary symptoms provide information on the sequelae of abnormal swallowing or the structure and function of organs that could secondarily impair swallowing. Table 5–3 lists historical data that are useful for diagnosing the site and the mechanisms responsible for the dysphagia.

Pain during swallowing, or odynophagia, indicates the disruption of mucosal integrity. Mucosal disruption occurs acutely with thermal, caustic, or radiation injuries. Subacutely or chronically, disruption is produced by infections (e.g., candidiasis, cytomegalovirus, or herpes infections of the oropharynx and esophagus). Caustic injury may be self-inflicted by infants or suicidal individuals by ingesting acidic or lye products or swallowing batteries. An often overlooked caustic injury of the oropharynx and esophagus results from the ingestion of corrosive drugs. Corrosive injury is particularly likely if high concentrations of drugs are taken with little fluid and the esophageal motility does not clear the material, particularly if the individual is supine and about to fall asleep. Common offending drugs are antibiotics (particularly tetracycline and derivatives), nonsteroidal antiinflammatory drugs (aspirin, indomethacin, ibuprofen, etc.), iron, anticholinergics, quinidine, and procainamide. Supine patients with pre-existing swallowing problems or a decreased sensorium are at particular risk for complications from such "pill esophagitis." If odynophagia

TABLE 5–2. Historical Data Used for Clinical Diagnosis of Dysphagia.

Site or timing of impairment
- oral (problems with chewing, bolus gathering, initiation of swallow)
- pharyngeal (problem immediately upon swallowing, choking after a long delay, suggestive of passage of residue from the pharynx into the larynx)
- esophageal (seconds after swallow, behind chest bone)

Onset, frequency and progression
- duration, sudden onset related to a specific event (stroke, pill impaction, etc.), or gradual
- frequency (constant, intermittent)
- progression and severity (including more and more foods and impairing nutrition and hydration?)

Aggravating factors and compensatory mechanisms
- food consistency (solids and/or liquids)
- temperature
- usefulness of sucking, turning, and tilting of head, etc.
- intermittent, constant, or fatiguing symptoms

Associated symptoms
- change of speech or voice
- weakness; lack of control of musculature, particularly of head and neck
- choking or coughing
- repetitive swallows or increased need to clear throat
- regurgitation (pharyngeal and nasal, or esophageal and gastric; immediately upon swallow, or long delay, undigested food, putrefied or secretions?)
- fullness/tightness in throat (globus sensation)
- pain, localized or radiating
- odynophagia (pain on passage of bolus)

Ancillary symptoms and evidence of complications
- loss of weight or loss of energy (including from dehydration)
- change in appetite; attitude toward food, toward eating in company; preparation of foods
- respiratory problems (cough, increased sputum production, shortness of breath, pneumonias and other respiratory infections)
- sleep disturbances (secondary to secretion management or regurgitation)
- changes in salivation (water brash or dry mouth)

occurs in gastroesophageal reflux disease, it signifies serious esophageal lesions, including erosions or the presence of a peptic ulcer in Barrett's esophageal metaplasia. Malignancies ulcerate as they advance and may also cause odynophagia. Any condition leading to odynophagia may also lead to continuous pain at rest, with sore throat and substernal chest pain. The symptoms of dysphagia and odynophagia indicate disease that directly involves the oropharynx or esophagus (Hurwitz, 1975). Both symptoms should be evaluated to the point of an adequate clinical explanation.

Rarely is dysphagia first detected during a physical examination, bedside observation, or diagnostic test. Patients themselves or their partners generally recognize that a problem with swallowing exists. Sometimes, the sensation of chronic fullness, tightness, or heaviness in the oropharynx or substernal area is assumed to relate to a problem in swallowing mechanisms and structures. If this sensation is centered in the lower neck and not affected by swallowing, it is called *globus sensation* or *pseudodysphagia* (Batch, 1988a, 1988 b; Bradley & Narula, 1987; Moloy & Charter, 1982; Wilson et al., 1987). If globus sensation is accompanied by pharyngeal dysphagia, it may relate to cricopharyngeal spasm. Otherwise, globus sensation occurs with a host of additional clinical conditions, including depression (Beck,

TABLE 5–3. Historical Data Used to Diagnose Sites and Mechanism Responsible for Dysphagia.

History Information	Site/Mechanism
Timing	
• Preswallow	Oral
• Immediately upon swallowing	Pharyngeal
• Several seconds after swallowing	Esophageal
Type	
• Chewing, bolus gathering, initiation	Oral
• Nasal regurgitation, coughing, choking	Pharyngeal
• Sensation of obstruction behind chest bone	Esophageal
Onset and progression	
• Lifelong problem (cerebral palsy, muscular dystrophy, etc.)	Oral-pharyngeal
• Sudden onset associated with a major event (cerebrovascular accident, head and neck surgery, etc.)	All stages
• Gradual progression associated with neurologic disease progression (Amyotrophic lateral sclerosis, Parkinson's, etc.)	
• Rarely lifelong (webs, congenital stenosis)	Esophageal
• Gradual onset and slow progression (peptic stricture, gastroesophageal reflux disease, achalasia, carcinoma, etc.)	
Frequency	
• Constant	Oral-pharyngeal
• Intermittent (lower esophageal ring, diffuse esophageal spasm)	Esophageal
• Constant and progressive (peptic stricture, carcinoma, scleroderma, achalasia)	
Bolus consistency	
• Liquids more than solids (CNS disease: cerebrovascular accident, amyotrophic lateral sclerosis, multiple sclerosis, etc.; CNS disease: poliomyelitis, neuropathies; myasthenia gravis; muscle disease: muscular dystrophy, polymyositis, lupus, etc.)	Oral-pharyngeal
• Solids more than liquids (local structural lesions: inflammation, head and neck surgeries, neoplasm, etc.; motility disorders of upper esophageal sphincter)	Esophageal
• Solid food only (lower esophageal ring, peptic stricture, carcinoma)	
• Solid or liquids (esophageal spasm, scleroderma, achalasia)	
Associated symptoms	
• Change in speech or voice, weakness or lack of motor control, coughing or choking, repetitive swallows, or need to clear throat, nasal regurgitation, drooling	Oral-pharyngeal
• Fullness or sensation of obstruction, chest pain, delayed regurgitation of gastric contents, chronic heartburn	Esophageal
Ancillary symptoms	
• Weight loss, dehydration, change in appetite or eating habits or attitude toward food, changes in salivation, pneumonia, hoarse voice, sleep disturbance (apnea, regurgitation)	Oral-pharyngeal
• Weight loss, respiratory problems (chronic cough, increased sputum production, chronic obstructive pulmonary disease, shortness of breath, asthma),	Esophageal

Ward, Mendelson, Mock, & Erbaugh, 1961; Cook, Dent, & Collins, 1989), and hence it does not have the same diagnostic relevance as dysphagia and odynophagia.

Oral dysphagia typically presents itself as difficulty in containing or manipulating a swallow. There is prolonged struggling with the bolus, but the involuntary pharyngeal and esophageal stages of swallowing may proceed normally once the swallow is triggered. Patients may compensate for failure to push the bolus backward with the tongue by using their fingers or lifting their chins. Oral stage dysphagia is part of the impairment of volitional functions and may be characteristic of post-surgery for oral cancer, dementia, pseudobulbar palsy, and cerebral palsy with oral motor incoordination (Hurwitz, 1975).

Pharyngeal dysphagia may present with patient complaints of coughing or choking on liquids more than on solids. Patients may report that water and other thin liquids like coffee or tea present the greatest problem. However, they may also complain of the sensation of food sticking because of an inability to propel a viscous bolus through the pharynx. When asymmetric impairments are present, patients may try to compensate by tilting or turning their heads, or by pressing against one side of their neck while swallowing. Saliva management is frequently a problem and may be experienced as an accumulation of phlegm in the throat due to pharyngeal stasis. In severe cases, tracheal aspiration will be evident. Concomitant problems of impaired phonation or speech may be reported (Bosma, 1967; Hurwitz, 1975).

Significant dysphagia may interrupt food intake. It may lead to repeated attempts to complete unsuccessful swallows or to dislodge the bolus through intake of additional fluids or retching. Patients may struggle to expel the bolus, or go through maneuvers such as hyperextension or even jumping up and down to advance it. Bolus impaction signifies the inability of the patient to dislodge a swallowed piece of food, usually a piece of meat. Patients with pharyngeal bolus impaction are at risk for impaired ventilation, respiratory arrest, or bolus aspiration. Patients with esophageal impaction are at risk for esophageal necrosis. Obstruction leads to hypersalivation, increasing the risk of aspiration.

In the case of neuromuscular disorders, the onset and the duration of dysphagia coincide with the paralysis resulting from cerebrovascular accidents or other manifestations of a disease. In esophageal malignancy, dysphagia begins with particulate foods and then progresses to difficulty with smaller bites or softer foods. Intermittent dysphagia only to solid foods is commonly seen in the "steak house syndrome" produced by a weblike protrusion of the squamocolumnar junction known as Schatzki's ring (Elpern et al., 1987). Peptic strictures resulting from gastroesophageal reflux disease (GERD) can lead to progressive dysphagia but lack the rapid progression and the decline in general health seen in cancers (Pope, 1989).

The consistency of the foods that produce dysphagia provide diagnostic clues. With neuromuscular dysfunction of the pharynx, liquids frequently cause greater problems with bolus gathering and clearance than more viscous materials. In the esophagus, mechanical obstruction is characterized by greater ease in swallowing liquids than solids, at least early in the disease. Esophageal motility disorders frequently cause almost as many problems with liquids.

Dysphagic patients may use multiple drugs for health maintenance but may experience enormous difficulties ingesting them. An inquiry into how such a patient handles specific preparations provides diagnostic clues and might prompt the selection of alternative medicine preparations or swallowing techniques.

Extensor posture and immobility of the neck and the oropharynx may compromise swallowing. Gravity and forward flexion of the head may facilitate swallowing. Patients with unilateral lesions of the oropharynx may find that bolus passage improves with rotation of their heads (Hurwitz, 1975; Olson, 1991). Patients with achalasia (Tucker et al., 1978) may enhance bolus passage by stretching the torso or distending the gastroesophageal junction with carbonated beverages.

Marked fatiguing is characteristic of myasthenia gravis. Individuals may function normally early in the day or into a meal, and later develop ptosis and dysphagia. Occasionally, the temperature of the bolus can exacerbate problems with swallowing. In muscular dystrophies, cooling can lead to myotonia and clonus of the oral-pharyngeal musculature. High pressure contractions of the esophagus may be elicited by very cold temperatures.

Associated Symptoms and Factors to take into Account

Even when the clinician has located the site of swallowing disturbance, the clinician ought to search for associated and ancillary symptoms. Symptoms that coexist with the dysphagia provide information on its origin; symptoms that are absent improve the prognostic outlook. Key issues involve the adequacy of secretions for lubrication and the clearance of secretions through periodic swallows without intermittent cough, excessive phlegm in the throat, or drooling; a tongue with strength, mobility, and coordination adequate to gather boluses and thrust them into the pharynx; a larynx with intrinsic musculature capable of closing the airway during swallowing and extrinsic musculature capable of securing it up and forward and under the tongue and simultaneously opening the esophageal inlet. Is the dysphagia but one manifestation of a systemic neurologic disease? Could the patient be a silent aspirator? Will the dysphagia cause devastating malnutrition or aspiration (Muz, Mathog, Rosen, Miller, & Borrero, 1987; Stein et al., 1990)? The following gives additional clinical information that may be important to characterize specific swallowing problems.

Eating Habits and Interest in Food

Patients may become indifferent to food or require a longer time to clear their trays. Some may handle a few bites and then tire. Disinterest in food may be a sign of depression. Abstinence may also be prompted by fear that eating will cause pain, aspiration, or social embarrassment through soiling. Mental or physical abilities may not be sufficient to recognize the components of a meal, or to perform the maneuvers necessary to cut, scoop, and introduce food into the mouth. Marginal respiratory reserve may produce fatigue during the course of a meal due to the requirement to cease breathing for each swallow.

Dehydration and Weight Loss

Dysphagic patients may maintain nutrition by adjusting their diet. Those with strictures may compensate with high caloric, semiliquid diets. Weight loss implies the swallowing problem is serious. Weight loss is common with esophageal cancers, but occurs when chronic infections or benign strictures limit nutrient intake. It is also a common problem in patients with progressive degenerative neurologic disease.

Patients with poor pharyngeal coordination may restrict the intake of liquids. Dehydration then leads to chronic fatigue, weakness, or faintness, particularly on assuming the upright position. Dysphagic patients may pass scanty, concentrated urine and become constipated.

Speech, Phonation, and Symptom Review of Neuromuscular System

In some instances neurologic problems affecting oropharyngeal swallowing also cause dysphonia and dysarthria. The speech may be slurred or the voice raspy (Shawker, Sonies, & Stone, 1984). Hoarseness and breathiness may point to primary laryngeal disease, if speech is otherwise articulate.

If speech or voice problems exist, did they occur at the same time as the swallowing problem? Are palsies, sensory and visual deficits, memory loss, or other neurologic deficits evident? Is the patient at risk from cerebrovascular accidents because of arterial hypertension, atrial fibrillation, or other significant cardiovascular disease? Is the patient suffering from a progressive dementia, Parkinson's disease, lower motor neuron disease, or muscular dystrophy?

A strong voice volume, clear phonation, and crisp articulation indicate normal muscle force and coordination of the articulatory, pharyngeal, and laryngeal musculature, at least for speech. This finding suggests that the investigator should focus concern on problems relating to the cricopharyngeus and the esophagus. However, one must be cautious because the muscle strength necessary for speech is much less than that required for swallowing. Poor pharyngeal clearance can lead to a wet quality of the voice or to a cough from overflow aspiration after multiple swallows. Dysphonia can be a sign of cricopharyngeal spasm (Gerhardt & Winship, 1982; Kilman & Goyal, 1976; Ossakow, Elta, & Colturi, 1987) accompanying esophageal disease, particularly gastroesophageal reflux (Jordan, 1977; Linden & Siebens, 1983; Olson, 1991).

Aspiration

One must determine to what extent the patient is at risk from aspiration (Muz et al., 1987). Have there been recurrent respiratory tract infections that cause one to suspect previous instances of aspiration? Are cough or dyspnea in the context of meals caused by current aspiration? What is the patient's capacity for airway clearance and ability to overcome respiratory complications?

The mechanism underlying aspiration can be deduced somewhat from its timing. For example, aspiration during swallowing can suggest poor pharyngeal control or inadequate airway closure. Aspiration as a consequence of reflux and regurgitation may be unrelated to swallowing and is particularly common after large meals, during recumbency, and sleep. Absence of a cough or other respiratory symptoms does not exclude the possibility of serious aspiration. Silent aspiration occurs with laryngeal anesthesia, chronic debilitation, and in dementia. Chronic expectoration of mucopurulent sputum, recurrent pulmonary infections, or a rapid decline in respiratory function should suggest silent aspiration.

Conditions that increase the risk for aspiration include depressed consciousness, a flat body position (particularly when combined with an inability to bend the neck), and intubation of the trachea or the esophagus (Sasaki et al., 1977).

Few patients will report such dramatic events as a previous need for Heimlich's maneuver because of choking spells and acute airway obstruction. However, patients may report an increased need to clear the throat, catch the breath, and cough during meals. Patients who do not trigger an efficient swallow (Bosma, 1967; Miller, 1986; Perlman & Liang, 1991; Perlman, Luschei, & Du Mond, 1989) may have a bolus enter the hypopharynx without adequate airway protection. The swallow normally diverts the bolus into the esophagus by mediating laryngeal ascent, inversion of the epiglottis, adduction of the vocal folds, and opening of the upper esophageal sphincter (UES). Patients with pharyngeal stasis and pooling of secretions and debris in the valleculae or pyriform sinuses may have overflow and spillage into the larynx only after repeated swallows. These patients often have chronically wet voices, may need to clear their throats periodically, and cough repeatedly even in the absence of recent intake. Patients with aspiration related to esophageal regurgitation may experience cough, wheezing, and respiratory distress primarily when recumbent. (See also Chapter 13, Esophageal Diseases.)

It is important to know whether cough occurs with all or only some swallows, and the effect of bolus consistency or of head position. Impaired swallowing of liquids is usually associated with neurologic disorders of the oropharynx, and aspiration-related phenomena may be less common but does still occur with somewhat viscous materials.

Oropharyngeal Competence

Closing the mouth with the lips and walling off the nasopharynx by elevation of the soft palate direct the bolus into the hypopharynx during swallowing. Absence of labial competence leads to drooling of saliva and food. Absence of palatal competence leads to a nasal voice quality on phonation and, if extreme, to nasal regurgitation. Healthy individuals may experience nasal regurgitation in unguarded moments associated with laughter or coughing.

Secretions, Dysgeusia, and Halitosis

A decrease in salivary secretions impairs the ability to masticate and to form a bolus. In extreme cases, patients may, upon chewing a dry cracker for 5 minutes, be found to have the crumbled pieces stuck to their tongue, palate, and gums. The mucous membranes can be dry even when patients are fully hydrated, and the tongue may become shriveled and fissured. Especially when combined with gingivitis and poor oral hygiene, bad breath *(halitosis)* may become pronounced and food may taste unpleasant *(dysgeusia)*. A decrease in salivary output occurs most commonly as an inflammatory destruction and atrophy of the salivary glands. This may be the result of radiation or of an autoimmune process as in Sjögrens or "sicca syndrome." Patients with sicca syndrome also have dry, itchy eyes and may develop keratoconjunctivitis, chronic arthritis, and other manifestations of autoimmune disease. They may have noticed a lack of tears, for instance, while cutting onions; and a strip of filter paper placed in the palpebral fissure will, after several minutes, be wet only over a few millimeters (Schirmer's test).

Increased salivation occurs in a variety of conditions. Hypersalivation is a consistent feature of acute esophageal bolus impaction, and the ability of patients to handle their own secretions is of concern in all conditions that obstruct the bolus passage. The acute intermittent occurrence of hypersalivation is known as *water brash*. Water brash is a reflex response to regurgitation of gastrointestinal secretions, which leads to prolonged esophageal exposure and heartburn. Salivary secretions are slightly salty tasting, but this is often compounded by the taste of bilious or acidic refluent in the mouth.

Gastroesophageal Reflux and Symptom Review of the Gastrointestinal System

Common complaints in gastroesophageal reflux disease include regurgitation of sour or bitter fluid, postprandial fullness and belching, food intolerance, and heartburn. Heartburn or *pyrosis* is an unpleasant sensation of a substernal burning, which can become painful. It is particularly common after acidic, spicy, sweet, or greasy meals. Antacids afford at least some relief from heartburn. If symptoms occur only after occasional large meals, the likelihood of significant sequelae is minimal. Massive regurgitation of gastrointestinal secretions upon stooping over or lying down; frequent heartburn, which over prolonged periods disrupts the sleep without any previous dietary excess; or heartburn associated with dysphagia or odynophagia imply that the patient is at high risk for esophageal, oropharyngeal, laryngeal, and bronchopulmonary reflux complications. Chest pain can accompany esophageal disease and frequently leads to concern about cardiac disease (Benjamin, et al., 1979; Pope, 1989; Tucker, et al., 1978). Patients who consume large amounts of antacids, including baking soda, may have a hiatus hernia, esophagitis or Barrett's esophagus (a replacement of squamous mucosa by columnar epithelium, primarily of an intestinal or gastric type associated with an increased risk of adenocarcinoma).

Gastroesophageal reflux and its complications can occur at any time in life, but significant symptoms and complications occur most commonly in middle-aged individuals who have had symptoms since childhood or early adulthood (and who may have family members with similar problems). Patients may have been told that they have peptic ulcer disease, gastritis, or a nervous stomach. Reflux may be acutely aggravated by delayed gastric emptying, gastric stasis, or gastric outlet obstruction. Particularly severe reflux occurs when competent closure of the gastroesophageal junction (Zamost et al., 1987) is ablated by operative resection, by scleroderma or its variant, the CREST syndrome (calcinois, Raynaud's vasospastic syndrome, esophagitis, sclerodactyly, and telangiectasis), or some other collagen-vascular disease.

Review of Structures Mediating Swallowing

It is of particular importance to know whether there is anything that could interfere with tongue function, laryngeal protection and closure, nasopharyngeal closure, UES opening, bolus propulsion, and pharyngeal clearance.

The tongue prepares for the swallow by collecting the bolus, the swallow is triggered as the bolus contacts anterior pharyngeal structures and the fauces, and the tongue drives the bolus into the pharynx in a pistonlike action. With loss of tongue function, the bolus may be misdirected, and there may be repetitive rolling movements and false starts. As the bolus escapes from the tongue, no swallow is triggered. Parts of the bolus may run over the base of the tongue and penetrate the fully exposed larynx. The delivery of the bolus from the pharynx into the esophagus will be less forceful.

Nasopharyngeal closure depends on the elevation of the soft palate. Without elevation, nasal regurgitation will occur and the voice assumes a nasal quality. Airway protection is accomplished by the anterior and superior movement of the larynx, tilting of the arytenoids, and inversion of the epiglottis. In addition, the vocal folds adduct. Impaired laryngeal elevation and protection is likely to result in aspiration during swallowing. Widening of the esophageal inlet depends on relaxation of the UES and the anterior traction exerted by the hyoid and laryngeal movement (Gerhardt & Winship, 1982; Kilman & Goyal, 1976). If sphincter compliance is impaired because of muscular fibrosis, there will be insufficient widening for rapid

bolus passage. Pharyngeal pressure will raise abnormally during swallowing. This *cricopharyngeal achalasia* may be associated with globus sensation, and may eventually be accompanied by formation of a hypopharyngeal or Zenker's diverticulum (Knuff, Benjamin, & Castell, 1982; Vantrappen & Hellmans, 1974). Large diverticula will give rise to regurgitation of putrid, undigested food between meals, or on manipulation of the neck. Pharyngeal peristalsis (a sequential contraction of the superior, middle, and inferior pharyngeal constrictors occurring against the background of longitudinal pharyngeal contraction and shortening) leads to eversion of the pharyngeal recesses and their clearance of any residue. Poor pharyngeal clearance leads to accumulation of residue in the valleculae and pyriform sinuses and leads to the risk of overflow airway penetration after multiple swallows (Logemann, 1987). Table 5–4 lists local processes that commonly cause dysphagia.

Review of General Health Status

The examiner must review the general status of the patient. Are there preexisting diseases and problems that will contribute to impaired deglutition or complicate the diagnosis and management? Does the patient suffer from chronic long-term problems such as diabetes or failure of the heart, lung (Stein et al., 1990), kidney, or liver, which require constant supervision and treatment? Does the patient suffer from a mood, behavioral, or personality disorder (Beck et al., 1961; Ravich et al., 1989)? Does an eating disorder exist? Is the patient competent to conduct his or her own affairs and to attend to his or her own physical needs, or is he or she dependent on the guidance or mechanical assistance of others? Is the patient on drugs that may interfere with alertness or impair swallowing by reducing salivary secretion or cause tardive dyskinesia? Are drugs causing dysgeusia or anorexia (Weiden & Harrigan, 1986)? Table 5–5 lists neurologic disorders commonly associated with swallowing problems.

TABLE 5–4. Local Processes Commonly Associated with Dysphagia.

Symptoms	Causes
Poor dentition	
Mucosal inflammation	Atrophy, radiation, corrosives (antibiotics, nonsteroidal antiinflammatories) or chemotherapy
	Infections (herpes/cytomegalovirus, streptococcus, candidiasis)
	reflux esophagitis
Impaired salivation	Atrophy (autoimmune–related or radiation)
	Drug–induced (dehydration, anticholinergics)
Webs, rings, strictures	(cricopharyngeal bar, postcricoid of Plummer-Vinson syndrome; lye strictures, Schatzki's ring)
Diverticula	(Zenker's diverticulum in hypopharynx, traction in epiphrenic)
Tumors	Cancers of lips, mouth, tongue
	Nasopharyngeal cancers or lymphomas
	Laryngeal cancers
	Squamous and adenocarcinomas of esophagus
	Pulmonary cancers invading or displacing esophagus
Structural defects	Congenital (cleft palate and others)
	Traumatic or operative (resection of tongue, mandible, pharynx, neck)
Defective support structures	Decreased mobility of local joints, spurs of cervical spine
	Operations on oropharynx, neck, and esophagus
	Arthritis, collagen-vascular diseases and skeletal deformities

Neuromuscular Diseases

Many inherited and acquired neuromuscular diseases may render individuals susceptible to problems with swallowing (Buchholz, 1987a) (see also Table 5–4 and Chapter 11). Oculopharyngeal dystrophy is particularly common among French-Canadians and leads to ptosis with its characteristic facial expression, followed by pharyngeal dysphagia. Myasthenia gravis may cause similar symptoms, with fatigue aggravated by muscle use and exercise. Patients with lower motor neuron disease, like amyotrophic lateral sclerosis, may experience early dysphagia as if they have atrophy of the tongue and pharyngeal muscles. The risk of aspiration and malnutrition is high. Patients with Parkinson's disease are prone to oral, pharyngeal, and esophageal dysfunction with swallowing. Rigidity of the tongue may interfere with bolus collec-

tion and propulsion. Pharyngeal musculature may be too weak to achieve bolus clearance. Esophageal contractions are often of excessive amplitude and duration, causing poor bolus transit and chest pain. A slowly progressive muscular atrophy, even of musculature not affected by the acute attack occurs in the wake of poliomyelitis. Palatal, pharyngeal, and laryngeal weakness may result in dysphagia and aspiration. Cerebrovascular accidents are a common cause of acute and chronic oropharyngeal dysphagia (Gordon et al., 1987). Dysphagia may be part of the syndromes of bulbar or pseudobulbar palsy (see Table 5–6). Stroke victims who experience dysphagia are more likely to succumb to pneumonia. Cortical strokes are less likely to cause significant and persistent dysphagia than brain stem strokes, but aspiration is a recognized complication of cortical strokes even when there is no alteration in consciousness (Perlman et al., 1994).

TABLE 5–5. Neurologic Disorders Commonly Associated with Dysphagia.

Diseases of cerebral cortex and brain stem
• cerebrovascular disease
  multiple lacunar infarcts involving corticobulbar tracts
  bilaterally; pseudobulbar palsy
  brain stem stroke with involvement of lower motor neurons
• altered state of consciousness (withdrawal, drugs, seizures, metabolic encephalopathies)
• multiple sclerosis, especially if complicated by bulbar or pseudobulbar palsy
• motor neuron disease (amyotrophic lateral sclerosis)
• poliomyelitis with bulbar involvement, residual dysfunction and progressive postpolio muscular atrophy
• Parkinson's disease, dystonias and dyskinesias
• Alzheimer's disease and other dementias
• head trauma
• cerebral palsy
• miscellaneous: neoplasms, encephalitis, meningitis, neurosyphilis

Diseases of cranial nerves
• chronic or neoplastic meningitis involving basilar meninges (lymphomatous, meningioma, retropharyngeal carcinoma)
• neuropathy (sarcoidosis, Guillain-Barré syndrome, facial nerve paralysis, diabetic vagal neuropathy)

Diseases of neuromuscular junction
• myasthenia gravis
• Eaton-Lambert syndrome (paraneoplastic impairment of acetylcholine release)
• botulism (food poisoning or intestinal colonization in infants)
• drugs (aminoglycosides, etc.)

Diseases of muscle
• dermatomyositis, polymyositis, sarcoidosis, and trichinosis
• metabolic myopathy (mitochondrial myopathy, Kearns–Sayre syndrome, thyroid myopathy)
• myotonic dystrophy
• oculopharyngeal and other dystrophies

TABLE 5–6. Differentiation of Dysphagia From Pseudobulbar and Bulbar (Paralytic) Palsy.

Paralytic (Bulbar)	*Pseudobulbar*
Lower motor neuron impairment	Bilateral upper motor neuron impairment
Mental status generally unaffected	Mental status affected; may include confusion, dementia, disorientation, spatial impairment or aphasia
Flaccid dysarthria (weak, breathy voice; marked hypernasality with nasal air emissions; loss of articulatory force)	Spastic dysarthria (strained voice, mild-moderate hypernasality; slow, imprecise articulation)
Rare emotional lability	Emotional lability common
Gag absent (unilateral or bilateral)	Generally hyperactive gag
Generally absent pathological reflexes	Pathologic reflexes present (suck, snout, rooting, jaw jerk)

Social and Physical Independence

Ambulatory individuals who hold jobs are more likely to respond to palliative and rehabilitative measures than institutionalized individuals or those unable to dress or feed themselves. To what degree is the patient able to learn compensations needed to overcome a handicap? To what degree is he or she recovering mental and physical abilities; or is the patient regressing? Is the disability caused by an acute trauma, infections, or operations? Is it related to a senile dementia or mental retardation? Is he or she able to remember instructions and comply with recommendations?

Drugs

The drug history should focus on agents that depress the level of consciousness and agents that may interfere with salivary secretions (Weiden & Harrigan, 1986), including diuretics and anticholinergic agents. Anticholinergic agents also can aggravate the gastroesophageal reflux. Additionally, attention should be paid to agents that may anesthetize the oral cavity and oropharynx, such as dental adhesives and throat lozenges. Table 5–7 lists classes of drugs, their medical indication and the mechanism by which they may interfere with swallowing.

THE PHYSICAL EXAMINATION

Clinical observations and the physical examination focus primarily on findings that relate to the cause of the dysphagia or are a consequence of it. In this, one proceeds largely in a sequence opposite to that used in the history. The examiner initially observes the general health and nutritional status of the patient, his or her alertness, degree of orientation and social independence, physical fitness and mobility, and the presence of intubation equipment or other prosthetic devices that might interfere with swallowing. From there, one proceeds to an assessment of the structural integrity of the head, neck, and oropharynx; testing of normal function of the nerves and muscles involved in mastication, swallowing, and bolus transport (see Chapter 2); and a systematic examination of other body parts. Observations made at any time during the physical examination will often lead to additional history taking. At the conclusion,

one may elect to test swallowing function at the bedside. The safety of such testing needs to be ensured. If there is evidence of recurrent or recent aspiration, or if the structures and function of the airway protective mechanisms are in question, it is best to omit this step. Otherwise, it is prudent to start the testing with small bits of something innocuous, like ice chips.

General Status

Is the patient in good general health and capable of functioning independently, or is the health and nutritional status precarious and the patient dependent on complex care and support? Is the patient robust enough to complete a comprehensive history, physical examination, and diagnostic testing? Is the examiner dealing with such severe illness and debility that interactions should be minimized?

Mental Status and Social Function

An individual's ability to recognize food and drink, to reach out for them, and introduce them into the mouth, chew, and finally swallow requires alertness, cognitive abilities, and spatial-temporal coordination of muscle movements. Is the patient fully alert and in possession of all cognitive abilities? If not, is the problem a depressed level of consciousness, a delirium or other state of temporary disorientation, or a permanent defect related to mental retardation or dementia? Patients with a depressed level of consciousness, from a disease process or from sedative drugs, might not initiate their own oral intake and are at increased risk for aspiration. Patients with severe muscle weakness or spatial incoordination may be unable to handle their intake, and patients with cognitive deficits because of delirium or dementia may not recognize food for what it is. Recovery might occur in conditions that were caused by trauma, acute illness, or drug treatment. In patients who have been chronically dependent on others to take care of all their personal needs, including feeding, assessments might need to be

TABLE 5-7. Medications Potentially Affecting Swallowing.

Product Category	Examples	Common Indications	Possible Effects
Neuroleptics (psychotropics) antidepressants	Elavil (tricyclic)	Relief of endogenous depression	Drying of mucosa Drowsiness
antipsychotics	Haldol	Management of patients with chronic psychosis	Tardive dyskinesia
	Thorazine	Tranquilizer; antiemetic	Extrapyramidal signs and symptoms (altered mental status; muscle rigidity)
Sedatives barbiturates	Phenobarbital Nembutal	Treatment of insomnia	CNS depressant (drowsiness causing decompensation of patients with cognitive deficits)
nonbarbiturates	Benadryl Phenergan	Antihistamine (allergic reactions); motion sickness	Drying of mucosa; thickening of bronchial secretions Drowsiness
Antihistamines	Cold and cough preparations	Relief of nasal congestion and cough	Drying mucosa Sedative effects
Diuretics	Lasix	Treatment of edema (e.g., associated with congestive heart failure)	Signs of chronic dehydration (dryness of mouth, thirst, weakness, drowsiness)
Mucosal anesthetics	Hurricaine (contains benzocaine)	Topical anesthetic used to aid passage of fiberoptic nasopharyngoscopes, control dental pain	Suppresses gag and cough reflex
Anticholinergics	Cogentin Cop	Adjunct in Parkinsonism therapy	Dry mouth and reduced appetite

restricted to identification of the cause of acute deterioration.

Physical Mobility

Swallowing proceeds optimally in the upright position with the head somewhat bent forward. Patients who are kept in the supine position with the neck extended do not have gravity in their favor and lose the protection of the airway that comes with an anterior tilt of the head. The indications for the supine position may need to be reviewed. If primarily for convenience of nursing care, an upright position during eating or drinking and for a period of time thereafter should be recommended. Some cervical spine diseases may prevent a patient from sitting upright, and can therefore cause a problem for safe swallowing (Zer-houni et al., 1987).

Tracheal or Esophageal Intubation

Indwelling cannulas may interfere with swallowing, increase the risk of aspiration, and interfere with effective clearance of aspirated material. By increasing oropharyngeal secretions, they increase the potential substrate for aspiration. Tracheal cannulas interfere with the ease of laryngeal ascent, thereby hampering the opening of the UES and the protection of the airway under the base of the tongue. By diverting the airstream, they also interfere with the protective closure of the glottis. Effective clearance of the airway during coughing depends on the buildup of subglottal pressure. The puncture of the airway at the tracheostomy site interferes with the patient's ability to increase subglottic pressure, and hence with protection and airway clearance. Even remote mechanical impedance from tracheostomies may leave local fistulas, scars, and deviations, and may cause functional impairments (Asher, 1984; Bonano, 1970; Greenbaum, 1976; Muz et al., 1987; Sasaki et al., 1977). It is generally agreed that, if a patient requires a cuffed tracheostomy tube to prevent aspiration, that patient should not be fed orally.

Nutritional and Hydration Status

Temporal wasting characterizes generalized malnutrition and muscular atrophy. Sunken eyeballs, dry mucous membranes, shriveling of the tongue, decreased skin turgor, hypotension, and elevated temperature may all result from dehydration.

Oropharyngeal Structures and Their Function

Examination of structures at rest is followed by palpation or inspection during performance of specific tasks. Are there any defects, such as a cleft palate or a resection of the mandible? Is the skin normal, or has scarring from operations, scleroderma, or radiation decreased its flexibility and interfered with opening of the mouth or laryngeal ascent? Table 5–8 provides an outline of the major aspects of a comprehensive clinical assessment of the functional integrity of the swallowing structures.

Speech and Phonation

Speech depends on the intact function of oral, laryngeal, and pharyngeal structures. Patients with pharyngeal weakness may have a wet quality to the voice because of pooling of secretions in the pharynx and spillage into the larynx. Patients with weakness of the palate may have hypernasal speech, and patients with processes interfering with tongue movement may have slurred speech. Breathiness of the voice and failure to phonate a clear (e–e–e) may indicate vocal fold paralysis indicating involvement of the recurrent laryngeal nerve (Logemann, 1983; Shawker et al., 1984).

In some instances, assessment of motor speech functions will require challenging the oral musculature by having the patient produce rapid alternating movements using the lips, tongue, and vocal mechanism (i.e., oral and phonatory diadochokinetics). Strength, range of motion, and the ability to vary muscular tension may

TABLE 5–8. Functional Integrity of Structures Involved in Swallowing

Speech and voice functions

adequacy of respiratory support including force of voluntary cough

voice (phonation and resonance)

speech (articulation and fluency)

Additional neuromuscular structures and their functions

facial expression (asymmetries including ptosis, frowning, lip closure)

mastication (strength of jaw closure, lateral movements)

tongue (bulk, strength, mobility, speed)

pharynx and soft palate (position and movement of uvula and epiglottis, symmetric and empty pharyngeal recesses)

internal laryngeal musculature (symmetry and movement of vocal folds)

external laryngeal musculature (position of larynx and its ascent upon swallowing)

reflexes (jaw jerk, suckling, gag, swallow)

sensations (stroke and pinprick, temperature, smell and taste)

Other supporting structures

adequacy of dentition or dentures

mucosa (moisture, tumor, inflammation, infection)

skull, spine, and articulations (fractures, resections, mobility, strength)

goiter, lymphadenopathy, or tracheal deviation

---

be evaluated in the labial and lingual muscles (Buchholz, 1987a, 1987b). The diagnosis of problems related to phonation may require laryngeal inspection using either a mirror exam, rigid pharyngolaryngoscope, with stroboscopy, or flexible nasolaryngoscope (Jordan, 1977).

Face, Cheeks, and Facial Nerves

Facial asymmetries occur both in lesions of the upper (UMN) and lower motor neurons (LMN). Generally, LMN disease tends to cause greater permanent difficulty with speech and lip seal than UMN disease. Patients with UMN weakness may have a unilaterally widened palpebral fissure and an inability to whistle, purse their lips, or inflate the cheeks. The nasolabial fold may be unilaterally absent, and in severe cases, patients may drool, loosing saliva from the angle of the mouth Figure 5–1 illustrates the muscles of facial ex-

pression in a patient with UMN impairment.

Tardive dyskinesias often lead to per-sistent involuntary movements of face, lips, and tongue, which could impair ingestion and preparation of a bolus for swallowing. These dyskinesias are often related to the use of drugs (anticholinergics, dopamines, and antihistamines). In patients suspected of having pseudobulbar palsy (patients with a history of arterial hypertension re-sulting in multiple strokes), one checks for pathological reflexes, including the snout reflex (lip-pursing response to touching the labial area), rooting (movement of the lips toward a brushing stimulus), or the palmomental reflex (contraction of muscles around the chin in response to stroking of the palm of the hand). These patients also exhibit extreme emotional lability. Induration of the skin around the mouth from scleroderma, operations, or irradiation may occasionally limit access to the oral cavity.

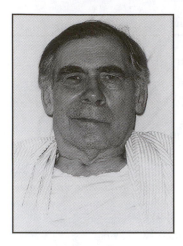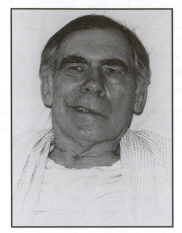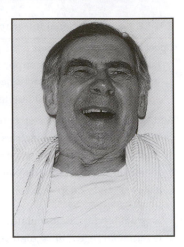

Figure 5–1. This series of photographs illustrates a patient with unilateral, left–sided, upper motor neuron facial weakness. (*Left*) With the muscles at rest, the widened palpebral fissure on the left side, flattened nasolabial fold, and droop at the corner of the mouth are evident. Notice the symmetrical wrinkles in the forehead. (*Middle*) When asked to grimace or bare his teeth, the patient contracts facial muscles on his right side, but has little movement on the left. (*Right*) However, when an emotional response is elicited, both sides of the face are activated, although the left–sided weakness remains noticeable.

The muscles of mastication can be palpated over the temples and above the angle of the mandible, and thus be assessed for bulk and force (Figure 5–2). The lateral movements of the mandible generated by the pterygoid muscles are important for food grinding, particularly in individuals with dentures (Figure 5–3).

Oral Cavity and Tongue

The condition of the teeth and the fit of dentures influence the patient's ability to masticate. The use of local anesthetics in denture adhesives may have a numbing effect and impair the initiation of swallowing. Normally, the mucous membranes of the oral cavity are covered by a film of mucus. Moisture is essential for bolus lubrication and initiation of the swallow. Absence of moisture can be a manifestation of dehydration or a drug-induced decrease in salivary secretion. Destruction of the salivary glands by inflammatory processes, such as the sicca syndrome or irradiation, also causes excessive dryness. Lack of moisture and lubrication can contribute to retention and decompostion of food residue in the oral cavity, with inflammatory fissuring and fungal overgrowth. Halitosis (bad mouth odor) may be pronounced.

The tongue is all-important in the collection of the bolus and in propelling it into the pharynx and esophagus, and one needs to assess its bulk and mobility. Atrophy and fasciculation of the tongue are often pronounced in LMN diseases and interfere with oral feeding in disease progression. UMN disease or cortical lesions may lead to spastic weakness of the tongue or its inability to perform its sequential functions (apraxia). Mobility and strength of the tongue are assessed by having patients protrude their tongue or push it into their cheek against the examiner's index finger. Deviation of the tongue from the midline is a feature of unilateral paralysis (Figure 5–4). Immobility of the tongue may also be caused by infiltrative processes, including tumors of the floor of the mouth and scarring.

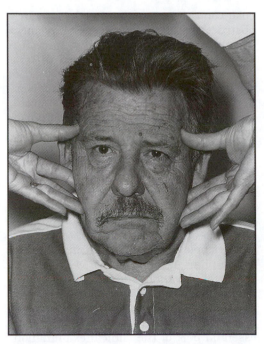

Figure 5–2. The major muscles of mastication can be palpated as the patient bites and opens the jaw. Placing the thumbs over the temporal muscles and the fingers over the masseters allows the examiner to feel for symmetrical contractions.

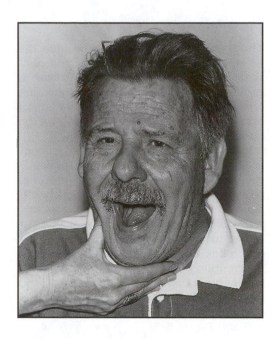

Figure 5–3. Grinding of food is accomplished by contraction of the pterygoid muscles to move the mandible in a lateral plane. Palpation of lateral jaw movement assesses strength and symmetry of movement.

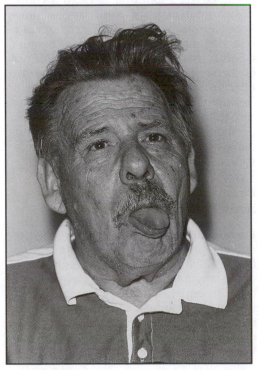

Figure 5–4. Deviation of the tongue on protrusion usually represents unilateral weakness. In this illustration, the tongue deviates to the patient's left side, consistent with his unilateral tongue weakness on the left side.

143

The Palate and the "Gag" Reflex

The normal palate moves to occlude the nasopharynx during swallowing and phonation, and failure to do so can lead to misdirection of the food bolus. Deviation of the uvula is suggestive of a unilateral paralysis. In general, deviation is to the stronger, contracting side.

Individuals vary greatly in their responsiveness to pharyngeal stroking. In some, the gag reflex is triggered with minimal provocation. In others, it is extremely difficult to trigger. Of greater diagnostic significance is a unilateral decrease or increase in the gag response. Testing of the gag reflex however provides little useful information on the intactness of the swallowing functions and on the safety of oral feedings. However, a lowered threshold is characteristic of pseudobulbar palsy (Table 5–6 and Figure 5–5).

Inspection of the Hypopharynx and Larynx

Some clinicians include an inspection of the hypopharynx and larynx as part of the clinical examination for swallowing. Visualization of the valleculae and pyriform sinuses may show signs of retained secretions and debris, which reflects the effectiveness of pharyngeal clearance. In some instances, spillage of secretions into the laryngeal aditus and their penetration through the glottis can be directly observed. Vocal fold mobility, for both abduction and adduction, can be assessed by direct visualization. Patients with suspected pathology of the larynx, either structural or functional, should be referred for more complete otolaryngologic examination (also see Chapters 7 and 12).

Examination of the Neck

One inspects and palpates for the presence of scars, tumors, and lymph nodes. Scars may indicate resection of structures involved in swallowing (larynx, strap muscles), or they may tether these structures and be associated with muscular contractures or atrophy. Goiters rarely obstruct the bolus passage. Enlargement of cervical lymph nodes may hint at a malignant lesion in the pharynx or be a manifestation of lymphoma. Deviation of the trachea from its normal midline position may be due to a mediastinal process, pleural scarring, or tumor. Stridor (a high-pitched sound during inspiration) may be audible only on auscultation over the trachea and indicates an obstruction in the upper airway, for instance, from laryngeal spasm or vocal fold paralysis. Head tilting and turning can be observed to assess normal mobility of the neck and appropriate support of the swallowing structures.

The single most important motor event in the pharyngeal phase of swallowing is laryngeal elevation and tilting. Laryngeal ascent protects the larynx and pulls the upper esophageal sphincter (UES) open. Palpation of the laryngeal elevation is an essential part of the clinical examination. To assess laryngeal ascent, the index finger is placed between the hyoid bone and notch of the thyroid cartilage with slight pressure (see Figure 5–6).

The larynx should be elevated a couple of centimeters on a voluntary swallow. Poor laryngeal ascent may be the result of resection, paresis, or paralysis of the musculature needed for elevation. Induration of the skin and subcutaneous structures after operations or irradiation may impair elevation. Particularly in elderly patients, the larynx may be in an abnormally low position (laryngoptosis) so that it cannot move into optimal position for airway protection during swallowing.

Examination of Other Body Parts and Systems

Examination of the chest may reveal significant problems with respiratory function related to aspiration or conditions in which any aspiration might have precarious consequences. An increased respiratory rate, a hyperinflated chest with reduced respiratory excursion, hypertrophy, and heavy dependence on neck muscles to move the rib cage all indicate problems with

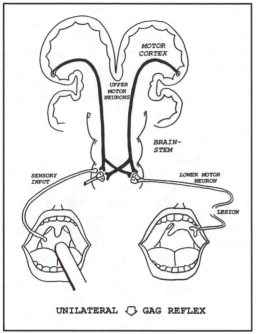

UNILATERAL ⬇ GAG REFLEX

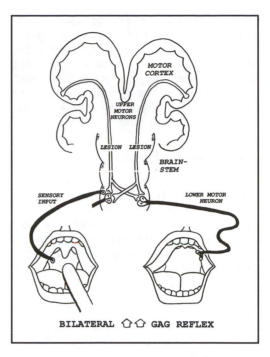

BILATERAL ⬆⬆ GAG REFLEX

Figure 5–5. Testing of gag reflex. In the gag reflex, stroking of the fauces or pharyngeal walls leads to an elevation of the palate. This is mediated by sensory and motor neurons of the IXth and Xth cranial nerves. With a unilateral lesion of a lower motor neuron, the gag reflex will be diminished or absent on the affected side (*Left*

photo). In the photo on the right, there is bilateral cortical representation for the muscles involved in the gag reflex. Bilateral lesions of the cortico-bulbar tracts result in a loss of upper motor neuron inhibition and bilateral hyperactive gag reflexes.

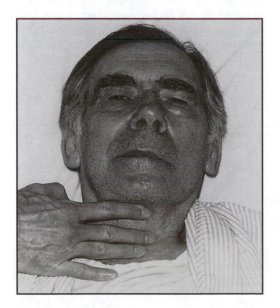

Figure 5–6. For evaluation laryngeal elevation and tilting, the examiner's finger is positioned between the hyoid bone and thyroid cartilage as the patient attempts to swallow. Note that the larynx is normally held in a position high up in the neck by its intrinsic musculature. Lack of muscle tone may lead to an abnormally low position (laryngoptosis).

ventilation and oxygen uptake. In this setting, the effort of eating, or even of minor aspiration, may precipitate respiratory decompensation. A reduced bulk and tone of abdominal and other respiratory muscles can reduce the forcefulness and effectiveness of bronchopulmonary clearance through coughing.

Cardiovascular System

Examination of the cardiovascular system can reveal the presence of arterial hypertension, arteriosclerotic disease (leading, for instance, to carotid stenosis from plaques), cardiac enlargement and arrhythmias, or valvular disease, which could be the source of emboli to the brain.

Muscoskeletal System

Examination of the musculoskeletal system may reveal deformities, particularly of the cervical spine, that interfere with normal mobility or indicate the presence of a muscular dystrophy, polymyositis, or scleroderma.

Bedside Testing of Swallowing

When the examiner has determined that it is safe to present test boluses, challenging the patient to take food, chew, and swallow can provide a great deal of diagnostic information. Clinicians may discover discrepancies between the patient's observations and their own, or may press the patient to clarify his or her complaints with regard to the timing, location, or nature of the problem. Table 5–9 outlines the major aspects of the bedside observation of swallowing functions.

Precautions and Contraindications

Clinical judgment regarding the relative safety of swallowing is critical. Obviously, the examiner would be more permissive with a generally healthy individual who is still eating than with a patient with preexisting respiratory compromise who had a sudden deterioration in swallowing.

The preceding history or physical examination might have indicated problems that will make bedside testing unnecessary or unsafe. These include cues for recent and continuous aspiration, the presence of severe dysarthria, impairment of mental status, respiratory compromise, or dysphonia, particularly if there is wet hoarseness. The findings of severely impaired cough, vocal fold paralysis, spillage into the larynx, or excessive retention of debris and saliva in the valleculae and pyriform sinuses are relative contraindications to the performance of bedside swallowing tests. Other signs that indicate an associated increased risk are lack of rapid and forceful elevation of the larynx, as observed by palpation of the neck during a dry swallow.

TABLE 5–9. Clinical Testing of Swallowing.

appropriate selection of food items, bolus size, coordination of orofacial movements with food delivery

effective mastication, complete and clearance

effective orolabial seal and arrest of speech

effortless swallow; no need to swallow again or perform additional maneuvers

no coughing, repeated clearing of throat, or respiratory difficulty or respiratory

characteristic swish and click heard on auscultation over side of the neck within 3 sec and splashing sound in epigastrium within 7 sec

ascent of larynx

no oropharyngeal residue or gurgling voice at end of swallow

Cough is the final protective mechanism against aspiration. Inadequacy of the cough reflex renders swallowing unsafe. The cough reflex consists of sensory and motor components. Cough is triggered in the larynx as the bolus interrupts the airstream. Loss of the reflex may result from laryngeal denervation or local anesthesia. The occurrence of cough is primarily a sign of laryngeal penetration and does not necessarily imply tracheal aspiration. The adequacy of the motor component of coughing should be judged by having the patient cough at will. If a voluntary cough is inadequate, one must be very cautious in determining the need for proceeding with test swallows. However, voluntary and reflex coughs may differ substantially in force and clearance function. Patients with cortical lesions of the brain may have an intact cough reflex but be unable to generate a good cough on command. Conversely, rare patients with selective cranial nerve damage can cough at will but have lost the reflex cough. If the sensory component of the cough is impaired, as it is with some neurologically compromised patients, aspiration may "silently" occur without eliciting this protective reflex.

The cough reflex may be influenced by the presence of a tracheostomy. Patients with a tracheostomy may not sense and thereby not protect the upper airway when laryngeal penetration occurs. The force of a cough is dependent on one's pulmonary capacity, ability to forcefully adduct the vocal folds, and ability to fix and contract the abdominal muscles. Patients with vocal fold paralysis or paresis may not be able to generate sufficient subglottal pressure to expel an aspirated bolus. Likewise, patients with insufficient pulmonary capacity, due to obstructive lung disease or cervical spinal cord injury, will not be able to initiate a strong cough. With denervation and resulting flaccidity of the auxiliary respiratory muscles, particularly the abdominals, many cervical spinal cord injury patients are unable to produce an adequately protective cough reflex.

Performance of Test Swallows

It is prudent to start this challenge with something as innocuous as ice chips, and if this is handled easily and without complication, to challenge the patient with more complex foods, eventually including those that historically give the most problems to the particular patient. Initially, one observes whether patients are able to recognize food components and to select, prepare, deliver, and hold a "mouthful" in their oral cavity. Does the patient initiate appropriate chewing movements, and are speech and respiration arrested on attempts to swallow? Is the swallow effortless, or does the patient try repeatedly and laboriously? Is one swallow enough to clear the mouth and the pharynx, and can the patient take swallows repeatedly in a rapid sequence without fatiguing, coughing, clearing the throat, increasing respiratory effort, or voice change? Does the patient need to make extraneous movements to initiate a swallow? If one auscultates the side of the neck, is there the characteristic swish and click produced by the epiglottis and the rush through the esophageal inlet? Is the phonation of an "e" as crisp as before the swallow? Also, on auscultation over the epigastrium, does a single major splash occur within 10 sec of the laryngeal ascent, or is this delayed with several minor arrivals barely enhancing the baseline gurgling of the stomach and intestines? This simple assessment of the effectiveness of primary esophageal peristalsis should be performed with the patient supine so as to eliminate gravity.

If one suspects that the patient has a problem with salivation, or with initiation of the swallow, with tongue function or pharyngeal clearance, reinspecting the oropharynx after mastication and swallowing attempts is revealing. Has food been squirreled away in the cheeks, or has it accumulated in the pharyngeal recesses? Have coarse dry particles been chewed up and impregnated with secretions to form a malleable bolus, or do they stick largely unchanged on the oral surfaces?

INTERPRETATION AND DECISION MAKING

Diagnostic Classification and Prognosis

The bedside encounter should lead to a formulation of the likely cause for the dysphagia, its prognosis, and management. The indications for specific tests, for the cessation of oral feeding or specific therapeutic measures should be elaborated. See Table 5–10 for main indications.

The diagnostic impressions formulated at this point have therapeutic and prognostic implications. Patients and caregivers require information about whether they are dealing with a remedial situation or one that will inexorably progress to the patient's demise. Remedial causes include virtually all benign diseases of the oropharynx and

the esophagus. Some neuromuscular disorders are remedial (myasthenia, polymyositis, and dyskinesias), others are expected to be followed by substantial recovery (recent cerebrovascular accident), and others to lead to ever greater problems with dysphagia and aspiration (motor neuron and other neurologic degenerative diseases). Successful treatment of malignant tumors of the oropharynx and larynx is often achieved at the expense of swallowing functions. Malignant tumors of the esophagus at the time of diagnosis are typically too advanced for curative treatment, but palliation of dysphagia resulting from the tumor can improve the patient's quality of life.

Diagnostic Studies and Referrals

Table 5–10 provides listings of tests according to the category of clinical disorder. If the bedside assessment points to a

TABLE 5–10. Diagnostic Studies or Therapeutic Measures Based on Clinical Evidence.

Structural lesion in larynx or pharynx
  laryngoscopy, pharyngoscopy
  (static) barium contrast study

Structural lesion in esophagus
  fiberoptic (thoracic) or rigid (cervical) esophagoscopy
  (static) esophagogram including full distention

Neuromuscular dysfunction of oral cavity, larynx, or pharynx
  (dynamic) laryngoscopy, fiberoptic endoscopic evaluation of swallowing or similar
  (dynamic) barium contrast, ultrasound, or similar
  neurologic evaluation
  electromyography

Neuromuscular dysfunction in esophagus
  dynamic barium contrast
  esophageal manometry, impedance planimetry
  gastroenterologic evaluation

Abnormalities of adjacent or support structures
  CAT scan or similar of head and neck or chest
  ENT, pulmonary evaluation

Serious aspiration, depression of sensorium, cognitive function, nutritional problems
  temporary: feeding tubes
    chronic: gastrostomies, jejunostomies, parenteral feeding

local mechanical process, diagnostic studies to assess the integrity of the swallowing structures are a primary choice. If one suspects lesions, pharyngoscopy and laryngoscopy are indicated. If it is unclear whether the pharynx or the esophagus is primarily involved, a barium contrast study is helpful. However, this will often need to be followed by esophagoscopic studies to document inflammatory changes, obtain biopsy material, or perform therapeutic dilatations. Endoscopy may be used as the primary diagnostic test if it is likely that a structural lesion will be encountered in the esophagus (see Chapter 13).

If the bedside assessment points to a problem in neuromuscular function of the pharynx or larynx, a dynamic endoscopic assessment of vocal fold and hypopharyngeal function and a videofluoroscopic examination can be helpful (see Chapters 6 and 7). If there is functional dysphagia of the esophagus (i.e., there is as much problem with the handling of liquids as with solids), considerable information may be gained by esophageal manometry (see Chapter 10). However, a dynamic contrast study can provide virtually the same information on the function of the esophagus as manometry, and at the same time demonstrate important information on oral and pharyngeal structure and function (see Chapter 6).

Normal swallowing involves many structures and functions, and many diseases that affect swallowing are dealt with by different disciplines. Referrals are typically indicated whenever multiple processes or multiple structures contribute to abnormal swallowing. Malignant tumors, for instance, may arise at multiple sites in the pharynx and esophagus, or a patient with pharyngeal paralysis might be at special risk if also suffering from GERD or chronic lung disease. Multidisciplinary approaches are particularly helpful with complex and severe abnormalities.

If the bedside assessment points to a primary neurologic cause of the dysphagia, its nature and treatment options need to be defined. This may include a diligent search of hitherto unknown cerebrovascular disease, Parkinson's disease, myasthenia, or other conditions for which the patient needs support or treatment. Imaging of the brain and brain stem with a CT scan or an MRI may confirm a suspected lesion. Doppler ultrasound in patients with carotid bruits, particularly if there is evidence for cerebrovascular ischemia, may be required.

If there is concern about aspiration, respiratory function tests and chest radiogram might be recommended. Oral feeding may be arrested until this issue is settled or when it has become clear that the patient is at high risk. For further details on these diagnostic issues see Chapters 6, 11, and 16.

SUMMARY

History taking and physical examination are important tools in the diagnostic classification of swallowing disorders. Often they allow, by themselves, the clinician to design appropiate strategies for care and to predict outcome. In other instances, the bedside assessment serves to aid the examiner in selecting appropriate tests and determining the need for referrals or management by multiple disciplines. The history proceeds from a definition of the swallowing problem appropriate to associated and ancillary (complicating) symptoms. The physical examination proceeds from a general assessment of the patient's physical and mental health to an assessment of swallowing structures and functions. Both history taking and physical examination seek to establish the adequacy and safety of oral food intake and to identify remediable causes of abnormal swallowing. Both provide indications for specific diagnostic tests, referrals, or therapeutic plans.

MULTIPLE CHOICE QUESTIONS

1. Relatives wheel into clinic their 78-year-old grandmother who has recuperated well from many little strokes over the last few years, but who will not eat properly anymore. As you approach her, the patient laughs at first, and then abruptly starts sobbing. As you try to examine her mouth, she gags. Which of the following findings are *not* part of her primary problem?

a. An exaggerated jaw jerk
b. Elevated blood pressure
c. Extreme forgetfulness
d. An enlarged thyroid gland (goiter)
e. Drooling

2. A 40–year–old man reports that, on several stressful occasions during the last 6 months, steak got stuck behind his lower chest bone. He admits to frequent heartburn and claims having had difficulties all his life with swallowing ice cream. He wears a wig and is scheduled to undergo cataract surgery. As he shakes hands with you, he admits that he can never easily release the grip. You should advise that he

a. be checked for an esophageal lesion
b. seek professional help for delusions or depression
c. avoid warm foods and beverages
d. be checked for a brain tumor
e. have a nerve biopsy

3. A 70–year–old retired teacher complains of constant fullness and phlegm in her throat and coughing spells with eating and drinking. Food passes best when she turns her neck and puts pressure on it. Important additional clues to the diagnosis would include the following:

a. a nasal voice
b. a remote history of poliomyelitis
c. residue in the pharyngeal recesses on a contrast study
d. painful "spasms" of throat
e. all of the above

REFERENCES

Asher, I. E. (1984). Management of neurologic disorders: The first feeding session. In M.E. Groher (Ed.), *Dysphagia: Diagnosis and management*, Boston: Butterworth.

Batch, A. J. G. (1988a). Globus pharyngeus. Part I. *Journal of Laryngology Otology, 102,*152–158.

Batch, A. J. G. (1988b). Globus pharyngeus. Part II. *Laryngology Otology, 102,* 227–230.

Beck, A.T. (1961). An inventory for measuring depression. *Archives of General Psychiatry, 4,* 561–571.

Benjamin, S. B., Gerhardt, D. C., & Castell, D. O. (1979). High amplitude peristaltic esophageal contractions associated with chest pain and/or dysphagia. *Gastroenterology, 77*(3), 478–483.

Bonano, P. C. (1970). Swallowing dysfunction after tracheostomy. *Annals of Surgery, 174,* 29–33.

Bosma, J. F. (1967). Deglutition; pharyngeal stage. *Physiological Review, 37,* 275

Bradley, P. J., & Narula, A. (1987). Clinical aspects of pseudodysphagia. *Journal of Laryngology and Otology, 101,* 689–694.

Buchholz, D. (1987a). Neurologic causes of dysphagia. *Dysphagia, 1,* 152–156.

Buchholz, D. (1987b). Neurologic evaluation of dysphagia. *Dysphagia, 1,* 187–192.

Cameron, J. L., Reynolds, J., & Zuindema, G. D. (1973). Aspiration in patients with tracheostomies. *Surgery, Gynecology, and Obstetrics, 136,* 68–70.

Castell, D. O., & Donner, M. D. (1987). Evaluation of dysphagia: A careful history is crucial. *Dysphagia, 2,* 65–71.

Castell, D. O., Knuff, T. H. E., Brown, F. C., Gerhardt, D. C., Brns, T. W., & Gaskins, R. D. (1979). Dysphagia. *Gastroenterology, 76,* 1015.

Christensen, J. (1976). Effects of drugs on esophageal motility. *Archives of Internal Medicine, 136,* 532–537.

Cohen, S., Laufer, I., & Snape, W.J.(1980). The gastrointestinal manifestations of scleroderma. *Gastroenterology, 79,* 155.

Cook, I. J., Dent, J., & Collins, S. M. (1989). Upper esophageal sphincter tone and reactivity to stress in patients with a history of globus sensation. *Digestive Disease Science, 34,* 672–676.

Edwards, D. A. (1976). Discriminatory value of symptoms in the differential diagnosis of dysphagia. *Clinical Gastroenterology, 5,* 49–57.

Ellis, F. H., & Corzier, R. E. (1981). Cervical esophageal dysphagia. *Annals of Surgery, 194,* 279.

Elpern, E. H., Jacobs, E. R., & Bone, R. C. (1987). Incidence of aspiration in tracheally intubated adults. *Heart and Lung, 16,* 527–531.

Gerhardt, D. C., & Winship, D. H. (1982). Cricopharyngeal disorders. In S. Cohen & R. D. Soloway (Eds.), *Diseases of the esophagus* (p. 121). New York: Churchill Livingstone.

Gordon, C., Hewer, R. L., & Wade, D. T. (1987). Dysphagia in acute stroke. *British Medical Journal, 295,* 411.

Greenbaum, D. M. (1976). Decannulation of the tracheostomized patient. *Heart Lung, 5,* 119–123.

Hamlet, S. L., Nelson, R.J., & Patterson, R. L. (1990). Interpreting the sounds of swallowing: fluid flow through the cricopharyngeus. *Annals of Otology, Rhinology Laryngology, 99,* 749–752.

Hughes, C. V., Baum, B. J., Fox, P. C., Marmary, Y., Yeh, C. K., & Sonies, B. C. (1987). Oral–pharyngeal dysphagia: A common sequela of salivary gland dysfunction. *Dysphagia, 1,* 173–177.

Hurwitz, A. L. (1975). Oropharyngeal dysphagia. *American Journal of Digestive Diseases, 20,* 313.

Jones, B., & Donner, M. W. (1989). How I do it: Examination of the patient with dysphagia. *Dysphagia, 4,* 162–172.

Jones, B., Ravich, W. J., & Donner M. W. (1985). Pharyngoesophageal interrelationships: Observations and working concepts. *Gastrointestinal Radiology, 10,* 225–233.

Jordan, P. H. (1977). Dysphagia and esophageal diverticula. *Postgraduate Medicine, 61,* 155–161.

Kilman, W. J., & Goyal, R. K. (1976). Disorders of pharyngeal and upper esophageal sphincter motor function. *Archives of Internal Medicine, 136,* 592.

Knuff, T. E., Benjamin, S. B., & Castell, D. O. (1982). Pharyngoesophageal (Zenker's) diverticulum: a reappraisal. *Gastroenterology, 82,* 734.

Langmore, S. E., Schatz, K., & Olsen, N. (1988). Fiberoptic endoscopic examination of swallowing safety; a new procedure. *Dysphagia, 2,* 216–229.

Larsen, G. L. (1981). Chewing and swallowing. In N. Martin, N. Holt, & D. J. Hicks (Eds.), *Comprehensive rehabilitation nursing* (pp. 174–185). New York: McGraw–Hill.

Linden, P., & Siebens, A. A. (1983). Dysphagia: Predicting laryngeal penetration. *Archives of Physical Medicine Rehabilitation, 64,* 281–284.

Logemann, J. A. (1983). *Evaluation and treatment of swallowing disorders.* San Diego: College-Hill Press.

Logemann, J. A. (1987). Criteria for studies of treatment for oral-pharyngeal dysphagia. *Dysphagia, 1,* 193.

Marguilies, S. I., Bruut, P. W., Donner, M. W., & Silbiger, M. L. (1968). Familial dysautonomia, a cineradiographic study of the swallowing mechanism. *Radiology, 90,* 107.

Mayberry, J. F., & Atkinson, M. (1986). Swallowing problems in patients with motor neuron disease. *Journal of Clinical Gastroenterology, 8,* 233.

McConnel, F. M. S., Cerenko, D., & Hersh, T.(1988). Evaluation of pharyngeal dysphagia with manofluorography. *Dysphagia, 2,* 187-195.

Miller, A. J. (1986). Neuropohysiological basis of swallowing. *Dysphagia, 1,* 91.

Moloy, P. J., & Charter, R. (1982). The globus symptom. Incidence, therapeutic response, and age

and sex relationships. *Archives of Otolaryngology, 108,* 740–744.

Moser, G., Vacariu–Granser, G., Schneider, C., Thalia–Anthi, A., Pokieser, P., Stacher–Jonotta, G., Gaupmann, G., Weber, U., Wenzel, T., Roden, M., & Stacher, G. (1991). High incidence of esophageal motor disorders in consecutive patients with globus sensation. *Gastroenterology, 101,* 1512–1521.

Muz, J., Mathog, R. H., Rosen, R., Miller, P. R., & Borrero C. (1987). Detection and quantification of laryngotracheopulmonary aspiration with scintigraphy. *Laryngoscope, 97,* 1180–1185.

Olson, N. R. (1991). Laryngopharyngeal manifestations of gastroesophageal reflux disease. *Voice Disorders, 24,* 1201–1213.

Ossakow, S. J., Elta, G., & Colturi, T. (1987). Esophageal reflux and dysmotility as the basis for persistent cervical symptoms. *Annals of Otology, Rhinology Laryngology, 96,* 387.

Perlman, A. L., Booth, B. M., & Grayhack, J. P. (1994). Videofluoroscopic predictors of operation in patients with oropharyngeal dysphagia. *Dysphagia, 9,* 90–95.

Perlman, A. L., & Grayhack, J. P. (1991). Use of the electroglottograph for measurement of temporal aspects of the swallow: Preliminary observations. *Dysphagia, 6.*

Perlman, A. L., & Liang, H. (1991). Frequency response of the Fourcin electroglottograph and measurement of temporal aspects of laryngeal movement during swallowing. *Journal of Speech and Hearing Research, 34,* 791–795.

Perlman, A. L., Luschei, E. L., & Du Mond, C. (1989). Electrical activity from the superior pharyngeal constrictor during reflexive and nonreflexive tasks. *Journal of Speech and Hearing Research, 32,* 749–754.

Pope, C. E. (1977). Motor disorders of the esophagus. *Postgraduate Medicine, 61,* 118–125.

Pope, C. E. (1989). Heartburn, dysphagia, and other esophageal symptoms. In M. H. Sleisenger & J. S. Gordtran, (Eds.), *Gastrointestinal disease,* (4th ed., p. 200). Philadelphia: W. B. Saunders.

Ravich, W. J., Wilson, R. S., Jones, B., & Donner, M. W. (1989). Psychogenic dysphagia and globus: Reevalaution of 23 patients. *Dysphagia, 4,* 35–38.

Sasaki, C. T., Suzuki, M., & Horiuchi, M (1977). The effect of tracheostomy on the laryngeal closure reflex. *Laryngoscope, 87,* 1428–1433.

Schatzki, R. (1963). The lower esophageal ring. *American Journal of Roentgenology, 90,* 805.

Shawker, T. H., Sonies, B. C., & Stone, M. (1984). Sonography of speech and swallowing. In R. Sanders, & M. Hill (Eds.), *Ultrasound annual* (pp. 237–260). New York, Raven Press.

Sieberns, H., Trupe, E., & Siebens, A.(1986). Correlates and consequences of eating dependency in institutionalized elderly. *Journal of American Geriatrics Society, 34,* 192.

Stein, M., William, A. J., & Grossman, F. (1990). Cricopharyngeal dysfunction in chronic obstructive pulmonary disease. *Chest, 97,* 347–352.

Straus, B. (1979). Disorders of the digestive system. In I. Rossman,(Ed.), *Clinical geriatrics* (2nd ed., pp. 266–289). Philadelphia: J.B. Lippincott.

Tucker, H. J., Snape, W. J., & Cohen, S. (1978). Achalasia secondary to carcinoma: Manometric and clinical features. *Annals of Internal Medicine, 89,* 315.

Vantrappen, G., & Hellmans, J. (1974). *Diseases of the esophagus* (p. 399). New York: Springer-Verlag.

Weiden, _., & Harrigan, M. (1986). A clinical guide for diagnosing and managing patients with drug–induced dysphagia. *Hospital Community Psychology, 37,* 396–398.

Wilson, J. A., Heading, R. C., Maran, A. G. D., Pryde, A., Piris, J., & Allan, P. L. R. (1987). Globus sensation is not due to gastroesophageal reflux. *Clinical Otolaryngology, 12,* 271–275.

Zamost, B. J., Hirschberg, J., & Ippoliti, A. F. (1987). Esophagitis in scleroderma. *Gastroenterology 92,* 421.

Zerhouni, E. A., Bosma, J. F., & Donner, M. W. (1987). Relationship of cervical spine disorders to dysphagia. *Dysphagia, 1,* 129–144.

6

Radiographic Contrast Examination of the Mouth, Pharynx, and Esophagus

Adrienne L. Perlman, Charles Lu, and Bronwyn Jones

A description of the use of a radiographic technique to study swallowing was first reported to the scientific community in 1898 (Cannon & Moser, 1898). Various food mixtures containing subnitrate of bismuth were presented to the goose, cat, dog, and horse, and the passage of the food bolus through the esophagus was observed during swallowing. Although the investigators stated that it was difficult to image the human swallow, they reported observations made on the swallow of a 7-year-old child. The investigators had the foresight to see promise for this new technique and were able to identify several problems that needed to be addressed before the human swallow could be satisfactorily imaged.

Observations on the oral and pharyngeal stages of human swallowing using x-ray were reported some years later. In a paper read before the Section of Otolaryngology at the Southern Medical Association, in 1926, Harris Mosher (Mosher, 1927) gave an in-depth description of the normal swallow of a roentgenologist colleague and swallowing as observed in patients with dysphagia. Series of still radiographs were organized in order to describe the sequential action.

With the advent of cinefluorography, the dynamics of swallowing could be observed more accurately. As the frequency of clinical research using dynamic studies of swallowing increased, cinefluorographic evaluation became recognized as a method for assessment (Ardran, Kemp, & Link, 1958; Cleall, 1965; Cohen & Wolf, 1968; Donner & Silbiger, 1966; Ekberg, 1982; Ekberg & Nylander, 1982; Ekberg & Sigurjonsson, 1982;). Since the development of the videotape recorder, the most frequently used method for assessing the functional components of the oral and pharyngeal stages of swallowing has become videofluorography (videotape recordings of the fluoroscopy).

During complete examination of the structures associated with swallowing, assessment includes both structure and function. Whereas the swallowing specialist will be more interested in the function of the mechanism, the radiologist will have the expertise to identify structural abnormalities. Consequently the combined effort of both specialists can contribute to the completeness of the examination.

There are three commonly used techniques for examining the pharynx with x-ray. Dynamic contrast pharyngography (videofluorography), rapid sequence with x-ray spot film, and double contrast pharyngography are the terms used to describe all three methods of pharyngeal examination. Rapid sequence with x-ray spot film is not advisable in the assessment of swallowing. That is because an intraluminal abnormality may be obscured by the dense barium and because the sequence cannot be repeated rapidly enough to capture the events associated with swallowing. Static images (double contrast pharyngography) are inappropriate for the assessment of the functional aspects of swallowing but may be important in the identification of structural abnormality. Thus, the use of dynamic contrast pharyngography, of which videofluorography is a form, is the technique of choice for assessing deglutition of the oral and pharyngeal stages of deglutition. However, a static double contrast pharyngogram provides additional information about the structure and mucosal surface of the epiglottis, valleculae, pyriform sinuses, the base of the tongue, and the lateral walls of the pharynx that can aid the radiologist in assessment of structural normality.

Videofluorography has been referred to by a variety of different names, including modified barium swallow; cookie swallow, rehabilitation swallow test, dysphagia diagnostic study, functional assessment of swallowing, videofluoroscopic swallow study, and videofluoroscopic evaluation of oropharyngeal swallowing function, to name a few. No matter what the name, the purpose and the basic protocol for this procedure are the same. However, the plenitude of names suggests that it is time to agree upon the nomenclature.

Videofluorography assesses the integrity of the oral and pharyngeal stages of deglutition; the cervical esophageal region is also observed. With this procedure, the examiner is able to determine the duration and completeness of bolus transit as well as the movement patterns of the mandible, tongue, velum, larynx, and to some extent, the pharyngeal wall and upper esophageal sphincter. Also, the symmetry of transport can be observed. Although a transverse view of the vocal folds cannot be obtained (this is best observed with endoscopy), penetration of material into the laryngeal vestibule and tracheobronchial aspiration can be observed.

This examination is performed in order to determine if patients can progress to or continue safe oral intake, if they are likely to meet their nutritional requirements with oral nourishment, or if it is advisable to find alternative methods of nutrition. Because of the psychological insult that can occur when patients are placed on tube feedings as well as the complications that can develop from nonoral methods of nourishment (Sitzmann, 1990), it is important to keep patients on oral intake whenever possible. A strength of the videofluoroscopic assessment is that the underlying cause(s) of aspiration can generally be determined. Also, the kinematics of the pharyngeal stage can be evaluated and various therapeutic measures can be tried as part of the evaluation procedure.

The clinical situations associated with the performance of the videofluoroscopic examination vary from institution to institution depending on the expertise and interest of the available specialists and on the type of caseload. Ideally the study should be performed collaboratively. The swallowing specialist should be especially trained in head and neck anatomy and physiology. Although in the majority of cases this is a speech-language pathologist, other health care professionals may have the required background and the appropriate interest. The examination is generally performed by the swallowing specialist and a radiologist. However, in some institutions, the swallowing specialist works with a specially trained radiology technologist. The diagnosticians should continuously consult during the study and should vary the procedure to tailor it to the individual patient. Common sense and continual reevaluation needs to be made of what compensations and decompensations are occurring during the examination.

The need to keep the procedure as brief as possible in order to limit the amount of radiation exposure to which the patient is subjected is its primary weakness. This is particularly apparent when attempting to evaluate the younger patient. Also, as mentioned above, there are more desirable methods for assessing the integrity of the larynx. Although cinefluorography allowed for a higher speed frame-by-frame analysis, videofluorography is limited to 30 frames per second. However, the radiation exposure is approximately half, the cost is less, and the turn-around time is immediate with videofluorography.

THE VIDEOFLUOROSCOPIC EVALUATION OF ORAL AND PHARYNGEAL SWALLOWING FUNCTION

Equipment and Supplies

If there is an attempt to limit the purchases to the least expensive equipment, only minimal information can be obtained and the examinations are not as useful as they would have been had proper equipment been purchased. For example, a time–date generator can add to the cost of the initial equipment, but without such a device, important temporal measurements cannot be made.

A commercial-quality 4-track SVHS recorder is probably the most durable and is strongly recommended. That instrument should have a jog and shuttle and frame lock capabilities; these are necessary for close examination and for the observations that must be made in slow motion. The advent of digital recording systems will further increase the image quality.

The videomonitor should have the resolution necessary for SVHS quality and have a picture reduction control. Also, an inexpensive microphone performs a valuable function. To name just a few advantages, on replay, the dialogue helps the examiner keep track of what the patient was swallowing, what type of instructions were being provided, and any problems experienced during the procedure.

Two other instruments, a time–date generator and a videoprinter, complete the instrumentation requirements. The time–date generator is needed to assess the duration of the oral preparatory phase, the extent of the delay in triggering the pharyngeal stage of the swallow, the duration of pharyngeal transit, and the duration of upper esophageal sphincter opening; it can, of course, also be used for assessing the duration of esophageal transit. Inadequate time resolution on the digital readout of the tape recorder precludes its use for performing these measurements. A time-date generator can provide information to the millisecond or centisecond depending on which instrument is purchased.

Because a "picture says a thousand words," including a print on the patient's report can be helpful in conveying information to the patient's physician. Black and white videoprinters are relatively inexpensive and extraordinarily useful.

Figure 6–1 shows a schematic representation of the recommended equipment as it is configured in a radiology suite. Most hospitals agree that it is efficient to have a duplicate recorder and monitor (most often in the speech pathology department) so that the time-consuming interpretation can be performed without interference with other radiologic procedures. When that is the case, the videoprinter is with the duplicate unit. Figure 6–2 is a schematic of the duplicate system. An instrument that is effective in quantifying the extent of displacement of important structures such as the hyoid bone or the thyroid cartilage is a measuring gauge (Perlman, VanDaele, & Otterbacher, 1995). That too becomes part of the duplicate system.

General Procedure

This protocol is described in detail in other sources (Logemann, 1993); therefore, only a short explanation will be provided here. Unlike esophageal motility studies, the

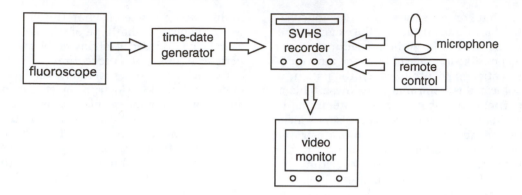

Figure 6–1. Recommended equipment as it is configured in a radiology suite.

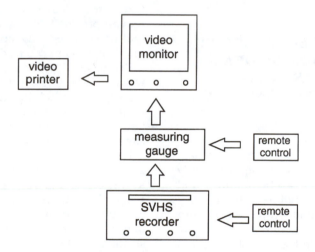

Figure 6–2. Recommended equipment for interpretation outside of the radiology suite.

patient is in a sitting or, on occasion, a standing position. Because a primary purpose of the study is to determine how safely a patient can manage oral intake, the situation is structured for success. Position is determined by the patient's physical and cognitive abilities as well as health status. For example, a patient who is ill or very weak should be positioned in a chair that provides adequate support and can be reclined if needed for rest during the procedure. There are now chairs that can be used to evaluate most adult patients. The

specialized chairs decrease the time it takes to position patients who are difficult to transfer and reduce the likelihood of technicians experiencing back injury while transferring patients.

Because the majority of information is obtained in the lateral plane, it is advisable to start with this view, but both lateral and P-A planes need to be evaluated. Signs that are observed better in the P-A plane can indicate a probable paralyzed larynx or pharynx as well as asymmetries related to mechanical dysfunction. Furthermore, because the area of concentration in the lateral plane is from the nasopharynx to C7 and from the lips to the vertebral column, a diverticulum may not be seen in the lateral view with some patients but it will be observable on the frontal or oblique view. If a patient is sitting on a hospital cart, it may be impossible to evaluate him or her in the A-P plane because of the metal back; obviously, sometimes there is no alternative. Figure 6–3 is a view of the lateral plane in which the structures of interest are identified.

Patients are given small boluses of varying viscosities in accordance with their level of tolerance. Bolus preparations range from 3 to 20 ml depending on the patient tolerance; most bolus presentations include 5 and 10 ml boluses and may proceed to 15 ml. These measurements should

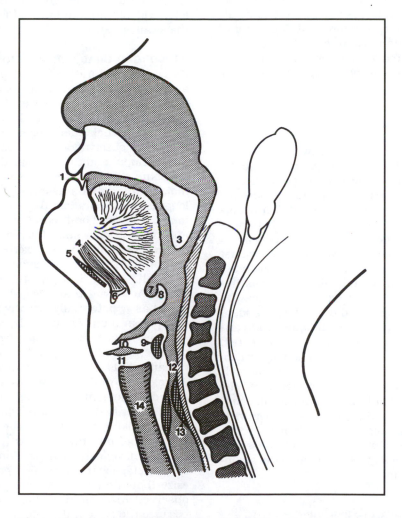

Figure 6–3. Lateral view showing normal adult anatomy. Structures are as follows: 1. lips; 2. tongue; 3. velum; 4. geniohyoid m; 5. mylohyoid m; 6. hyoid bone; 7. valleculae; 8. epiglottis; 9. arytenoid cartilage; 10. false vocal folds; 11. true vocal fold; 12. pyriform sinuses; 13. cricopharyngeus m; 14. trachea

be precisely made so that future examinations can be compared. Because of the variability among patients, no matter what the diagnosis, it is difficult to establish a firm protocol; the examiner must use good clinical judgment in selecting the bolus sizes and viscosities for presentation. Each examination is tailored to the individual patient depending on clinical evaluation and history. The examination is modified as it proceeds depending on the videofluorographic findings.

Because the swallow event can be exceedingly rapid, it is not possible to do an effective interpretation while performing the evaluation. Therefore, the videotape is interpreted at a later time, thus the recommendation of a duplicate recorder and monitor.

Interpretation

Assessment of the swallow includes observations of the oral and pharyngeal stages of the swallow. The following is a discussion of each observation and the possible underlying cause or causes of that observation; as research continues, other causes may become evident. It is important to remember that the swallowing specialist performs this examination in order to assess function. Within the limitations imposed by radiation exposure, once the underlying cause of the dysphagia is identified, compensatory techniques and variations in bolus presentation are tested. Interpretation of structural anomaly or neoplasm is performed by the radiologist. Although the swallowing specialist and the radiologist should be present at all studies, in case one is not available, it is vital that the radiologist be informed about swallowing function and that the swallowing specialist be familiar with structural problems.

The Oral Stage of Swallowing

DROOLING. Drooling is a common problem exhibited by children with cerebral palsy and by adults who have experienced neuro-

logic insult affecting oral sensation and weakness of the orbicularis oris (CN VII) muscle. Drooling is seen with decreased labial strength or decreased oral sensation.

Patients who have lost the ability to execute the pharyngeal stage of the swallow will drool because the mouth and pharynx can become filled with secretions; at times these individuals will find it necessary to carry around a small cup to expectorate their secretions. However, patients who are unable to execute the pharyngeal stage of the swallow are not candidates for a videofluorographic evaluation until the swallow returns.

PROLONGED ORAL PREPARATION TIME. If the combined duration for oral preparation and pharyngeal transit for a particular food consistency takes longer than 10 sec, patients are not likely to include that consistency in their diet (Logemann, 1983). Given this observation, the implications for malnutrition, and the associated complications, are obvious. There are presently four major explanations associated with prolonged oral preparation; they include xerostomia, decreased oral sensation, swallowing apraxia, and poor stimulus recognition.

When an individual has xerostomia, the oral preparation time increases (Liedberg & Owall, 1991; Sonies, Ship, & Baum, 1989). Any drug that dries the oral mucosa has a potentially negative effect on oral preparation. Additionally, xerostomia as a result of radiation therapy, systemic disease, or salivary gland hypofunction can affect this phase of the swallow.

Prolonged oral preparation is often observed in demented patients. In many of these patients the oral stage will be significantly prolonged, but after the bolus begins to spill into the pharynx (which puts the patient at risk for aspiration) the pharyngeal stage is triggered. One can hypothesize that the prolonged oral preparation observed in some demented patients is because the patient does not recognize the presence of food in the mouth, even though the afferent component of cranial nerves IX and X are intact. This may be a form of oral or gustatory agnosia, where *agnosia* is defined as the inability to recognize the import of sensory stimuli (Dorland, 1985). Prolonged oral preparation can occur when there is sensorimotor impairment such that the patient cannot sense the location of the bolus in the mouth or cannot produce the necessary movements of the tongue or jaw.

Apraxia of swallowing can also result in prolonged preparation. If this is suspected, it is advisable to provide no verbal instructions to the patient and to proceed with a very small bolus if a solid substance is presented. Patients with an apraxia of swallowing may have been able to do reasonably well during the clinical examination when test swallows were presented, but cannot execute a motor act on command. These patients may swallow an entire bolus of any volume or viscosity without oral preparation. These observations associated with deglutition are compatible with previous reports that the more severe the apraxia of speech demonstrated by a patient, the more profound the deficit in oral sensory perception (Rosenbek, Wertz, & Darley, 1973).

TONGUE PUMPING. From clinical observations, it appears that tongue pumping is likely to result from difficulty in triggering the pharyngeal stage of the swallow. *Tongue pumping* is different from *tongue thrusting* or from serial swallowing. Tongue thrusting, as referred to in this context, occurs with developmentally delayed children or with individuals who have experienced supranuclear injury; it is not the simple myofunctional problem that is sometimes reported in the speech or dental literature. Tongue pumping is a repeated rocking like motion preceding the swallow.

Some individuals may perform a long series of pumping motions during which the bolus spills into the pharynx, but no swallow is triggered. One reason for tongue pumping may be difficulty eliciting a swallow due to insufficient saliva (Mansson & Sandberg, 1975); it is likely that there are other explanations, such as decreased sensation, but further research is needed in this area. Tongue pumping

may also be seen in patients with "psychogenic dysphagia" (Barofsky, Buchholz, Edwin, Jones, & Ravich, 1994).

It is important to differentiate tongue pumping from myoclonus of the tongue and/or pharynx, which occurs in some neurologic conditions. Myoclonus is seen as rapid repetitive involuntary tremors of the involved structures.

SERIAL SWALLOWS. This behavior has also been termed *repeat swallowing* and *piecemeal swallowing*. When individuals who do not complain of dysphagia fill their mouth with too much of a good thing, there is a need to perform a series of swallows rather than one large bolus swallow; thus there are conditions where serial swallowing (three or more swallows per bolus) is normal.

Unlike tongue pumping, where the underlying cause is generally difficulty triggering a swallow, the primary cause of serial swallowing appears to be weakness of the oral or pharyngeal musculature. The individual may have difficulty forming a cohesive bolus that can be propelled into the pharynx during the oral transport phase of the swallow. Also, the inability to open the upper esophageal sphincter adequately or to clear the pharynx of residue can cause an individual to take several small swallows rather than one large swallow in order to safely clear the upper alimentary tract. Consequently, the examiner needs to differentiate between the piecemeal swallow where the patient executes a series of swallows and empties the mouth of a small portion of the bolus with each swallow and the repetitive swallows where the patient swallows repetitively to clear the pharynx of material either left behind or which they think is left behind. Serial swallowing has also been observed in patients who, for whatever reason, are afraid they will choke and therefore take small swallows as a protective technique, whether needed or not. There are others who swallow twice or more times as a learned behavior either consciously or unconsciously or, of course, as part of a treatment program.

POOR BOLUS FORMATION. The major underlying causes for poor bolus formation appear to be reduced tongue strength, reduced tongue range of motion, reduced lip strength, or discoordination. Lingual weakness as well as limitations in anterior-posterior motion or in the ability to dip or elevate the tongue tip, actions common to the oral stage (Dodds et al., 1989), can make it difficult to gather the bolus or to groove the tongue in the manner necessary for containment (Kahrilas, Lin, Logemann, Ergun, & Facchini, 1993). Furthermore, if the lips cannot seal sufficiently, the tongue must then take additional responsibility for increasing oral pressure during oral transport. In the absence of a tight labial seal, the tongue generally makes greater contact with the alveolar ridge, teeth, or palate; in doing so, the tongue configuration is altered. Thus, it becomes more difficult to contain a bolus, particularly a liquid consistency.

If the actions of the tongue are discoordinated, then logic suggests that the patient may have difficulty containing the bolus during the period of transport. This has been confirmed in studies of clinical populations (Kagel & Leopold, 1992; Stroudley & Walsh, 1991).

ORAL STASIS. As with poor bolus formation, residue in the mouth after the swallow can be due to tongue weakness, reduced tongue range of motion, or discoordination. Other causes include buccinator mucle weakness, oral structural alterations, and xerostomia. If the buccinator muscle is weak or paralyzed due to a CN VII injury, the patient is likely to exhibit a "squirreling" behavior in which bolus residue is contained in the lateral sulcus. This is often associated with decreased sensation and thus the patient is not aware of the food residue. After a total or partial glossectomy or lingual paresis or paralysis, it is difficult for the patient to clear the oral cavity.

The most common cause of xerostomia is medications; however, among the patients who complain of xerostomia and who are found to have moderate or severe dysphagia, postradiation atrophy of the salivary glands is often the cause of the lack of saliva. Xerostomia is also seen in patients with systemic disease such as connective tissue disorders, or of advanced age.

When barium residue is observed on the hard palate it indicates either tongue weakness or limited elevation due to surgical alteration. When the underlying cause is tongue weakness, the stasis generally increases as the viscosity of the bolus increases.

No matter what the cause of the oral stasis, it is advisable to clear the mouth with a swab or by oral suctioning after an examination so that the oral residue does not fall into the pharynx at a later time. This, of course, would put the patient at risk for aspiration.

POOR MASTICATION. The most likely causes for difficulty with mastication are weakness or absence of the muscles of mastication (temporalis, masseter, medial pterygoid for jaw closing, and lateral pterygoid for jaw opening). Jaw misalignment resulting from neurologic damage, surgical alteration, or as a characteristic of a congenital birth defect can also result in poor mastication. Discoordination can make it difficult to chew in the traditional rhythmical grinding fashion. Clinical observation of patients with Parkinson's disease or with Alzheimer's has suggested that these populations are likely to use a munching rather than grinding action. Poor dentition, malaligned teeth, or painful gums can also have an effect on the ability to grind food.

NASAL REGURGITATION. When velopharyngeal closure occurs during swallow, there is usually a notable "hump" where the levator veli palatini muscle has contracted and the palate is contacting against Passavant's cushion in the posterior pharyngeal wall (Figure 6–4), The presence of this visible sign of tight closure is not requisite for a successful swallow but its absence can indicate muscle weakness due to either velar or pharyngeal constrictor (superior)

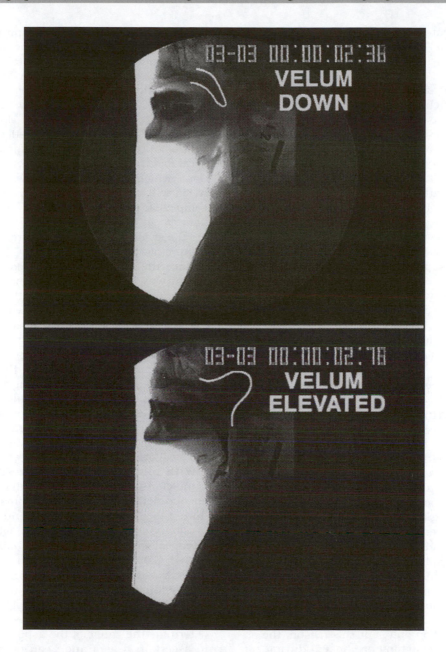

Figure 6–4. The velum is depressed during the oral preparatory phase, elevates during the oral transit phase, and remains elevated during the pharyngeal stage of the swallow.

weakness. Swallowing is a pressure-driven event and the closure of the velopharyngeal port does assist in development of this pressure, but the requisite minimal pressure and the extent of velopharyngeal closure have not been identified as yet.

When a food or liquid bolus is observed in the nasopharynx or flowing out the nose it indicates compromised velopharyngeal closure. This may be the result of incomplete closure associated with a congenital disorder, the result of palatal weakness or paralysis, or the effect of surgical alteration such as that associated with palatectomy. Discoordination causing a premature opening or delayed closure of the palate can also result in entry into the nasopharynx. Because the velar seal is of a short duration, it is possible for there to be retrograde flow as a result of some retained bolus in the pharynx even though the velar seal was adequate during swallow. In some instances, the onset of hypernasal speech and/or retrograde flow into the nasopharynx during a swallow can indicate velopharyngeal insufficiency associated with the early onset of neurologic disease such as amyotrophic lateral sclerosis (ALS). Also, an obstruction in the oropharynx or hypopharynx can send the bolus in the retrograde direction.

The Pharyngeal Stage of the Swallow

ASPIRATION. Although some patients will experience episodes of coughing or choking when food or liquid enters the larynx, many patients with dysphagia have decreased sensation in the larynx and exhibit no signs of discomfort when penetration occurs. These silent aspirators comprise a significant percentage of patients seen for videofluorographic evaluation (Linden, Kuhlemeier, & Patterson, 1993; Splaingard, Hutchins, Sulton, & Chaundhuri, 1988); errors in identification of aspiration range from 30% to 40% of patients in rehabilitation centers who were evaluated for dysphagia by clinical examination only. For this reason, the absence of coughing or choking during eating must not be interpreted as evidence of a safe swallow, and visual imaging of the swallow should be considered whenever there is a question as to the safety or efficiency of a swallow.

Aspiration can occur before, during, or after the swallow event. The time at which the aspiration occurs gives insight into the underlying cause of the patient's dysphagia. For example, if the aspiration is noted before the initiation of the swallow, the examiner should look for oral decompensation such as premature leakage or a delayed initiation of the swallow.

Aspiration during the swallow suggests inadequate vocal fold closure. Material may penetrate the laryngeal vestibule and be visible on the superior surface of the vocal folds as a result of a variety of situations, which are described below; this scenario will result in aspiration after the completion of the swallow. In order for the material to penetrate the vocal folds during the swallow, vocal fold closure must be compromised.

Once the swallow has been completed, the airway is opened for respiration or phonation and the larynx is in the resting position. Aspiration after the swallow can be observed as a result of residue from the valleculae, pharyngeal walls, or pyriform sinuses spilling into the open airway or from material that entered the vestibule during the swallow, falling through the now open glottis. Additionally, reflux from the esophagus can sometimes be observed spilling over the arytenoids and penetrating the larynx some time after the swallow.

With many procedures the study is completed when the patient exhibits tracheobronchial aspiration; with this procedure, the study should be continued with caution. Asking the patient to cough when laryngeal penetration or aspiration is observed may help to diminish the amount of aspirated material. Of course, if a patient exhibits gross aspiration the study is discontinued; but if the aspiration is less severe, small boluses are given to determine the cause of the aspiration and to ascertain if aspiration can be avoided by positioning the patient differently or presenting another bolus size or viscositiy. At this time there are no hard or fast rules because the extent of aspiration that individuals can experience without adverse effects is still an unknown. Common sense suggests that a patient who is acutely ill or who has a compromised respiratory system should be treated more conservatively than a patient who is past the acute stage, has good pulmonary function, and is ambulatory.

It is very important to have suctioning capabilities in the fluoroscopy suite and to have this equipment ready for action with all patients. Each day, before the procedure is performed, the suction equipment should be checked to ensure that it is ready for use if needed.

DELAYED INITIATION OF THE SWALLOW. The inability to trigger the pharyngeal stage of the swallow should have been identified during the clinical examination earlier performed. Obviously, if an individual has no swallow, it is not appropriate to perform a test of swallowing function. If by some error a patient is taken to radiology for a videofluoroscopic examination and it is evident there there is an absence of the pharyngeal swallow, the procedure should be discontinued.

From simultaneous videoendoscopy and ultrasound, we have learned that the hyoid complex usually begins to elevate before the bolus can be observed at the level of the base of tongue (Perlman & VanDaele, 1993). This elevation is considered the beginning of the pharyngeal stage of the swallow. A delayed initiation of the swallow begins when the bolus is observed spilling over the base of the tongue to the level of the ramus of the mandible and ends when the hyoid elevates as an indication that the swallow is triggered. If the bolus falls beneath the level of the valleculae, for example, into the pyriform sinuses or into the laryngeal aditus, the patient is likely to aspirate. When the swallow eventually triggers and the pharynx is shortened, the material in the pyriform sinuses is brought to the level of the laryngeal aditus and spillover into the laryngeal vestibule can easily occur. If the material has fallen into the laryngeal aditus, at the completion of the swallow the vocal folds will abduct and that material will likely fall into the open airway. Clinicians have reported observing filling of the valleculae and pyriform sinuses before the swallow by infants and adults who exhib-

it otherwise normal swallows. Given these clinical observations, one must be careful in determining that a swallow is abnormal on the basis of only this occurrence during examination. However, the event does put a person at greater risk for aspiration.

The severity of the delay can predict the likelihood of aspiration (Perlman et al., 1994); consequently, this temporal measurement is important. A delay of 1 sec or greater is, by rule of thumb, considered to be significant. The delay among healthy young adults is usually less than 200 ms, and in normal elderly it can be as long as 500 ms (Tracy et al., 1989).

The general consensus appears to be that decreased sensation in the posterior tongue and possibly into the pharynx is the most likely cause for a delay in triggering the swallow. Motor programming difficulty, possibly due to poor tongue control, is another likely cause.

The examiner must be careful to differentiate a delay in the initiation of the swallow from what has been called *premature bolus loss* or *premature leakage* (Logemann, 1993). A delayed initiation occurs when the tongue transfers the bolus into the pharynx but the swallow does not trigger in a timely manner. With premature bolus loss, a portion of the bolus breaks off from the main body of the bolus. That smaller bolus then flows over the base of the tongue and generally falls into the valleculae. In this case, the leakage is the result of the inability to maintain the bolus in the mouth owing to weakness or resection of oral structures. Once the body of the bolus is fully prepared a normal swallow event occurs.

REDUCED HYOID ELEVATION. The muscles of the floor of the mouth, specifically, the paired mylohyoid, geniohyoid, and anterior belly of the digastric muscles are primarily responsible for the anterior and superior movement of the hyoid bone during swallow. This motion plays a crucial part in moving the larynx forward, thus reducing the opportunity for aspiration. During a normal swallow, the hyoid bone has been reported to move an average of

9–12 mm anteriorly and 11–12 mm superiorly. (Jacob, Kahrilas, Logemann, Shah, & Ha, 1989; Perlman et al., 1995). Although the duration of hyoid movement is influenced by the size of a bolus, the extent of displacement is not significantly affected (Jacob et al., 1989).

When a patient with dysphagia exhibits reduced hyoid displacement, there is a 3.7 times greater likelihood of that patient experiencing aspiration than if the hyoid bone displaces properly (Perlman, Booth, & Grayhack, 1994). Although the critical distance that the hyoid must elevate has not yet been determined, there is notable value in measuring the displacement and assessing the improvement over time. This can be done with the method previously described (Perlman et al., 1995) or with more sophisticated computer programs (Caruso, Stanhope, & McGuire, 1989; Cordaro, 1993; Dengel, Robbins, & Rosenbek, 1991; Logemann, Kahrilas, Begelman, Dodds, & Pauloski, 1989).

When a supraglottic laryngectomy is performed, the hyoid bone generally is removed. This has a similar effect in that the larynx is not passively moved forward by the contraction of the muscles of the floor of the mouth and the anterior-superior motion of the hyoid.

REDUCED LARYNGEAL ELEVATION. Reduced laryngeal elevation is strongly associated with aspiration (Perlman, Grayhack, & Booth, 1992). Of 330 patients evaluated for complaints of dysphagia, Perlman et al. identified only 28 with reduced laryngeal elevation as opposed to 62 patients with reduced hyoid elevation. However, of the 28 patients with reduced laryngeal elevation, aspiration was noted in 23 (82%) patients. The superior movement of the larynx helps to bring the airway safely away from the path of the bolus. Along with the association to the hyoid motion, weakness of the paired thyrohyoid muscles would seriously affect this motion.

VALLECULAR STASIS. Because the valleculae are cuplike spaces on the lateral and anterior aspect of the epiglottis, clearance principally depends on epiglottic inversion. Seventy percent of patients with vallecular stasis have been found to have problems with epiglottic inversion (Perlman et al., 1992). Patients with mild vallecular stasis are almost twice as likely to aspirate as patients with dysphagia who do not demonstrate vallecular stasis; furthermore, the likelihood of aspiration increases as the severity of the stasis increases (Perlman et al.,1994).

Logemann (1993) comments on the importance of tongue-base movement to the clearance of the vallecular spaces. In support of Logemann, Perlman et al. (1992) also recognized the importance of intact oral function in relation to vallecular residue. Even though their study did not break down the various types of oral involvement (i.e., tongue-base retraction), the investigators found a significant relationship between vallecular stasis and oral stage dysphagia. Although this is likely to be important, there is probably more to the cause of vallecular stasis than tongue-base retraction.

It is difficult to determine the severity of the vallecular stasis from the lateral view. That is because the volumes retained in both valleculae are seen together. Consequently, it is best to determine the severity of retention from the P-A view.

Some patients who have an intact sensory system, and who experience vallecular stasis, will describe the sensation of food sticking in their throat. When asked to identify the location of this sticking, they will point to the level of the valleculae.

DEVIANT EPIGLOTTIC FUNCTION. The epiglottis, the lidlike, fibroelastic structure at the entrance to the larynx, inverts to cover the laryngeal aditus during swallowing. The epiglottis generally makes two distinct movements (Ardran & Kemp, 1951, 1952, 1967; Ekberg & Sigurjonsson, 1982). The first motion brings the epiglottis to the horizontal position and the second brings it to the completely downfolded position. The mechanism of epiglottic inversion during swallowing is the result of anterior movement of the hyoid bone, which brings the epiglottis to the horizontal position, and superior movement of the thyroid cartilage to approximation with the elevated hyoid. Thyrohyoid approximation then becomes the principal action for epiglottic downfolding below the horizontal plane (VanDaele, Perlman, & Cassell, 1995).

The geniohyoid and mylohyoid musculature appear to be the primary muscles responsible for anterior movement of the hyoid bone; the anterior belly of the digastric has been found to be less consistent in its contribution (Hrycyshyn & Basmajian, 1972). Because the epiglottis is a passive performer, when the structure does not move to the horizontal position or when it moves to the horizontal position but does not complete the second motion to complete inversion, the examiner should consider weakness of the muscles of the floor of the mouth as the likely cause for this phenomenon. The extent of laryngeal elevation should also be assessed. An absence of epiglottic downfolding can also occur because of calcification (Ardran, 1965) and has been seen in patients who have undergone radiation treatments.

Because patients are 4.4 times as likely to aspirate when they exhibit deviant epiglottic function (Perlman et al., 1994), it is important to assess the epiglottic motion during examination. If the valleculae are covered, as occurs with an excessively curled epiglottis, the bolus may cling to the inferior aspect of the epiglottis, slide along the base, and enter the larynx. Also, if the epiglottis does not complete the action of downfolding, the path of least resistance can be into the laryngeal vestibule rather than through the upper esophageal sphincter. In either instance, aspiration is likely.

A safe swallow can occur in the absence of the epiglottis. Some patients who have undergone supraglottic laryngectomy, including removal of the hyoid bone, epiglottis, and false vocal folds, have been observed using compensatory techniques, such as tight glottal closure during the swallow followed by throat clear-

ing after the swallow, that result in a safe swallow; others who have undergone this procedure are plagued with problems (Flores, Wood, Levine, Koegel, & Tucker, 1982; Rademaker et al., 1993). It is generally agreed that the supraglottic laryngectomy patient is less likely to have a safe swallow if there has been removal of an arytenoid cartilage; without the arytenoids, the glottis cannot close tightly.

PYRIFORM SINUS STASIS. If the pyriform sinuses are not cleared following the swallow, the underlying cause(s) may be related to reduced elevation of the hyolaryngeal complex, cricopharyngeal hypertonicity, poor pharyngeal constrictor function or discoordination. The cricopharyngeus muscle forms the floor of the pyriform sinuses and is the uppermost portion of the upper esophageal sphincter (UES). This C-shaped muscle inserts onto the lateral margins of the posterior aspect of the cricoid cartilage. Because of this attachment, the muscle is strongly affected by laryngeal movement.

For the pyriform sinuses to empty, it is necessary for the upper esophageal sphincter to open. The duration of UES opening during a normal swallow increases as bolus volume increases: 0.34 ms for a 1-ml volume; 0.45 ms for a 5-ml bolus; 0.50 for a 10-ml bolus; and 0.54 for a 20-ml volume (Jacob et al., 1989). The critical size and critical duration of this opening have not been documented.

Adequate opening of the UES appears to depend on two factors: relaxation of the cricopharyngeus muscle and an anterior pull resulting from the anterior–superior displacement of the larynx. If the UES opens adequately but closes prematurely, the pyriform sinuses will show retention after the swallow. Also, if the pharyngeal constrictor muscles are weak, the entire bolus may not be transported through the pharynx before the upper esophageal sphincter closes. In the case of weak pharyngeal muscle function there can be diffuse hypopharyngeal stasis including pyriform sinus and vallecular stasis. Diffuse wall stasis can also result from poor lubrication of the pharyngeal mucosa, such as that which occurs after radiation therapy; this too can result in pyriform sinus stasis.

It is difficult to determine the severity of the stasis from the lateral view. That is because the volumes retained in both pyriform sinuses are seen together. Consequently, it is best to determine the severity of retention from the AP view. This also allows for determination of symmetry of entrance through the cricopharyngeus and symmetry of pyriform sinus stasis.

If unilateral retention is visible in the AP view it is likely owing to unilateral weakness and it advisable to try techniques such as tilting the head to the functioning side or turning the head toward the nonfunctioning side. Turning helps the bolus travel the contralateral side, which may result in increased clearance. When unilateral retention is observed in the absence of weak pharyngeal constrictor function, a structural abnormality must be ruled out.

Some patients with an intact sensory system who experience pyriform sinus stasis will complain of the sensation of something sticking in their throat. When asked to identify the location, they will point to the level of the cricopharyngeus muscle. These patients may also complain of coughing or choking after eating. At times, the complaint of something sticking is not due to pyriform sinus stasis, and on examination the patient is found to have a cricopharyngeal bar or even gastroesophageal reflux. Thus careful follow-up must be made to this complaint.

REDUCED LARYNGEAL CLOSURE. Assessment of laryngeal competence is not done as easily with videofluorography as it is with laryngeal endoscopy; nevertheless, laryngeal closure can somewhat be assessed in the AP plane. By instructing the patient to extend the neck and say *eeee*, vocal fold motion can be observed. If the patient is instructed to say *ah*, sometimes the mandible will drop too far and the vocal folds will not be easily visualized. If there is a vocal fold paralysis, one fold will not move. Many times these patients

have aspirated and so the vocal folds have a barium coating that makes it easier to observe motion or lack of motion. After certain surgical procedures, the vocal folds and pyriform sinuses may no longer be at the same level in the horizontal plane; this can result in laryngeal penetration and aspiration.

The entrance to the larynx can be compromised by inadequate epiglottic inversion as explained above, by inadequate arytenoid adduction due to arytenoidectomy associated with supraglottic laryngectomy, or by the absence of vocalis muscle shortening associated with vocal fold paralysis. Additionally, bowing of the vocal folds, associated with senile changes in the viscoelastic properties of the vocal folds or with postendotracheal intubation can result in inadequate vocal fold closure during the swallow. Aspiration during the swallow is generally associated with inadequate laryngeal closure.

A safe swallow can occur in the absence of the vocal folds. That is to say, given adequate displacement of the hyolaryngeal complex and the preservation of sensation, the airway is still safeguarded; this has been demonstrated in patients who had undergone cricohyoid epiglottopexy (Laccourreye, Laccourreye, Menard, Weinstein, & Brasnu, 1990; Weinstein, Perlman, & Jones, 1990).

Patients who have a voice quality that can be described as breathy, weak, or hoarse should be considered as likely candidates for poor laryngeal closure. The weak, breathy quality may indicatie vocal fold paresis or paralysis. Dry hoarseness may also be indicative of a vocal fold pathology. A voice that appears to have a wet, hoarse quality suggests food, liquid, or secretions either on the vocal folds or in the laryngeal vestibule. These patients should be seen for a laryngeal examination.

CRICOPHARYNGEAL BAR. A cricopharyngeal prominence, sometimes referred to as a *cricopharyngeal bar, cricopharyngeal achalasia,* or *hypertrophy,* can be observed in both esophageal and pharyngeal abnormalities (Figure 6–5) (Jones, Ravich, Don-

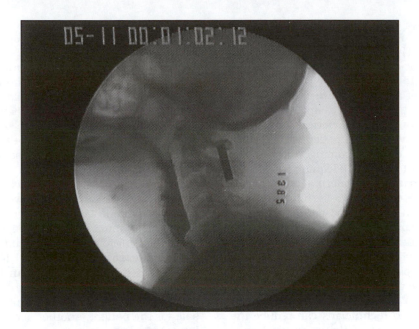

Figure 6–5. A cricopharyngeal prominence.

ner, & Kramer, 1985). Radiographic evaluation only provides information regarding the amount of cricopharyngeal opening or closing, and not information regarding the extent of relaxation or spasm, which manometry demonstrates. Therefore, the term cricopharyngeal achalasia should be reserved for manometric observations and not be a fluoroscopic term.

This prominence is sometimes seen in the following diseases: primary muscle disease (polymyositis), partial pharyngectomy, peripheral or central cranial nerve palsy, cerebrovascular disease affecting the brain stem, or other causes of pharyngeal paresis. Additionally, the bar is sometimes seen in patients who have reflux or other esophageal disorders, presumably as a secondary phenomenon, and in patients in which no known disease or disorder is present. If there is a question as to the presence of a bar, it becomes very visible on a prone, oblique swallow; that position can be used for confirmation if needed.

PURPOSE AND LIMITATIONS OF THE DYNAMIC VIDEOFLUOROSCOPIC ASSESSMENT OF SWALLOWING FUNCTION OF THE ORAL AND PHARYNGEAL STAGES

The videofluoroscopic examination of oropharyngeal swallowing function has become the gold standard for assessing the integrity of the oral and pharyngeal stages of the swallow. This procedure is not simply to detemine if a patient is aspirating or even why the patient is aspirating; rather, it helps the clinician determine if a patient can receive any nourishment by mouth, if the patient can receive sufficient nourishment by mouth for health and recovery, and if there are particular compensatory postures or particular volumes or viscosities that can help the patient return to oral intake.

There are four major limitations to this procedure. First, a patient is exposed to radiation. This limits the amount of information that can be obtained because it is necessary to keep exposure to a minimum. Second, not all patients are able to cooperate; albeit, this is only a small fraction of the patients who are referred for evaluation. Third, with some patients, the procedure can be time-consuming. And last, the dynamic study is not adequate for assessment of structural abnormality. With the appropriate equipment, the time required to position a patient and perform the procedure is considerably shorter than with less-than-ideal equipment, particularly the examining chair. Nevertheless, it does take time to prepare the barium presentations, position the patient (often an ongoing task), and present the material. The assistance of well-trained technicians can reduce the time commitment of the swallowing specialist considerably.

Contraindications

As stated earlier, this procedure is not appropriate for patients who lack a pharyngeal swallow. Patients who exhibit a decreased level of alertness, making it inadvisable for them to be on oral nourishment, should be evaluated after they become more alert. Patients who are extremely ill and are fed by tube, and for whom it is unlikely that sufficient nourishment can be obtained by mouth, may also be best served if the procedure is postponed until their condition improves. Furthermore, it is not appropriate to reevaluate a patient if no new or useful information will be obtained.

ASSESSMENT OF STRUCTURAL ABNORMALITIES OF THE PHARYNX

Structural abnormalities and mucosal lesions are best identified with the double contrast study of the pharynx rather than with single contrast combined with videofluoroscopy (Semenkovich, Balfe, Weyman,

Heiken, & Lee, 1985). The standard images for double contrast pharyngograms are anterior–posterior and lateral spot films (see Figure 6–6) while the patients blow against their pursed lips or phonate prolonged vowel sounds after swallowing high density barium sulfate, a 200% weight by volume or higher percentage of barium suspended in water. The aim of the examination is to obtain good mucosal coating and thus define surface structure. A bolus of as little as 15 ml can often be used to identify these abnormalities; however, in the case of a patient who is found to aspirate, the clinician must make a decision specific to that patient regarding the amount of barium to present. An individual for whom aspiration is not an issue can be given larger amounts depending on the patient's individual choice when cup drinking. When safe for the patient, another set of A-P and lateral view pharyngograms after an additional barium swallow will make interpretation and detection of the lesion better; also oblique projections sometimes add more valuable information, particularly when the examiner is looking for neoplasm or extent of the tumor.

Web

Most esophageal webs are in the cervical esophagus. The esophageal web is also known as the *cricopharyngeal web* because of its visibility in the upper esophagus, when the cricopharyngeus muscle is open widely. The web is easy to detect on barium swallow as it creates the "jet" phenomenon during the swallow when the barium passes through narrowed lumen. It can, however, be missed if the cervical esophagus is not fully distended. The web typically arises from the anterior wall of the cervical esophagus just above or below the cricopharyngeus, and is either semicircular (Figure 6–7) or circumferential in shape (Figure 6–8). The web is commonly seen in women with Plummer-Vinson syndrome but also has been reported in patients with ectopic gastric mucosa (Weaver, 1979; Williams, May, Krause, & Harned, 1987), benign mucosal pemphigoid, and

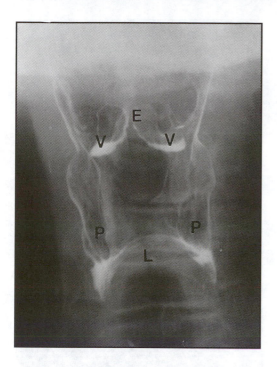 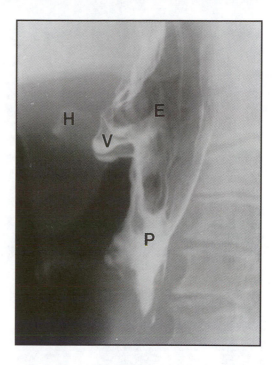

Figure 6–6. AP (*left*) and lateral (*right*) views show normal anatomical structure of the pharynx on double contrast pharyngogram. Larynx and trachea are outlined by air. E, epiglottis; L, larynx; P, pyriform sinuses; V, valleculae; H, hyoid bone.

epidermolysis bullosa dystrophica (Agha, Francis, & Ellis, 1983; Agha & Raji, 1982; Sharon, Greene, & Rachmilewitz, 1978).

Pharyngeal Diverticula

Various types of pharyngeal diverticula have been described. Most are symptom-free when small; however, once the diverticulum starts to cause regurgitation, the patient is more likely to complain of dysphagia.

A posterior hypopharyngeal (Zenker's) diverticulum is an outpouching through Killian's dehiscence just above the crico-pharyngeus circular muscle. It is general-ly accepted as an acquired diverticulum, pulsion in nature. When the outpouching is small, it may pool a small amount of barium briefly on the lateral view of the dynamic study. As it becomes larger, it tends to extend caudally and posteriorly to the esophagus. Very often it will flap to one side rather than being central in position (Figure 6–9).

During the dynamic videofluoroscopic examination of swallowing function, a Zenker's diverticulum is usually visible in the lateral view as the pharynx elevates. However, because the Zenker's is at the level of C_6–C_7, it can be missed during the dynamic study if the patient's shoulder is obscuring the view. Also, if the Zenker's is small, it can be missed on the AP view. Patients may have complaints of food "coming back up" hours after eating, continu-ous halitosis, or a bad taste in the mouth. Clinically it is important to differentiate the Zenker's diverticulum from gastro-esophageal reflux. However, most patients with Zenker's diverticulum have evidence of GERD (gastroesophageal reflux disease) and a prominent cricopharyngeus. Cook (Cook, Blumbergs et al., 1989; Cook, Gabb, et al., 1989) described patients with mano-metric studies and Zenker's showed raised

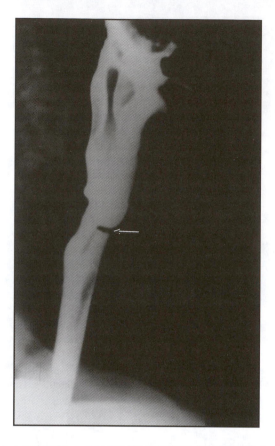

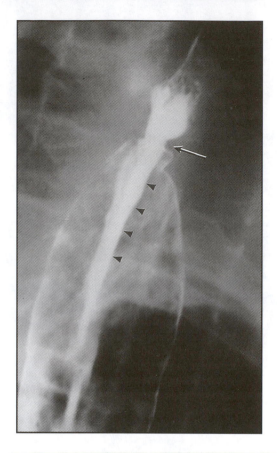

Figure 6–7. A smooth cervical web (*arrow*) at the anterior wall of the pharyngoesophageal junction on lateral view.

Figure 6–8. A 48-year-old lady with long-standing dysphagia. She complains of food hanging in the throat. A ring-form web is seen at the upper esophagus (*arrow*). There is a "jet" phenomenon (*arrow heads*).

intrabolus pressures prior to cricopharyngeus myotomy and diverticulectomy. Decreased intrabolus pressure after surgery was observed.

Oral-Pharyngeal-Laryngeal Cancers

Squamous cell carcinoma of the head and neck is generally visible by mirror examination or by endoscopy but there are some blind areas such as below the piriform sinus. Radiographic examination is not only able to detect the lesion but also gives infor-

mation regarding the extent of the lesion, especially when it is combined with CT or MRI. A dynamic contrast study or rapid sequence film may show an irregular, rigid segment of contrast-filled wall, or a filling defect. Usually these shadows represent only a small portion of the neoplastic lesions. On the other hand, a double contrast pharyngogram will outline the tumor against the air containing, barium-coated pharynx (Figures 6–10 and 6–11), thus giving a more accurate view of the tumor. Oblique views often add more information in determining the extent of tumor (Taylor, 1991)

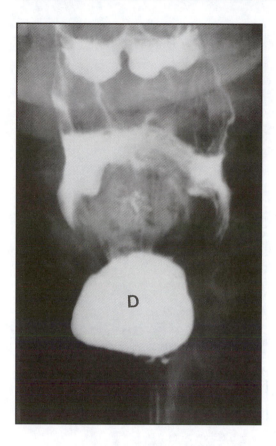
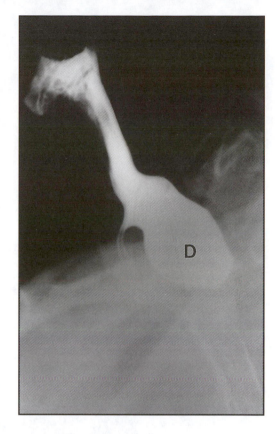

Figure 6–9. A large Zenker's diverticulum (D) full of barium is projecting posteriorly. AP (left) and lateral (right) views.

Postradiation or Postoperative Pharynx

Deformity of the pharynx is inevitable after surgical removal or radiation therapy. To interpret the radiographic examination, the radiologist needs to understand the surgical procedure, how long it is after surgery, and the patient's ability to swallow. Narrowing from scar versus tumor recurrence is difficult to differentiate on barium swallow. Fluoroscopic observation of restricted distensibility and good contraction seen at an area of narrowing may help in this distinction (Figure 6–12).

Radiation, on the other hand, does not disfigure the anatomical structures much. However, because of fibrotic change and inflammatory reaction from the radiation, muscular contraction will not function normally, and this increases the risk of aspiration (Figure 6–13).

Pseudoepiglottis

After total laryngectomy, the mucosa at the base of the tongue may be sutured in such a manner that a fold of tissue is formed that resembles an epiglottis. This cuplike structure can serve as a reservoir much the same as the epiglottis and valleculae. However, in the case of the total laryngectomy patient, aspiration is not an issue; thus, this retention can generally be eliminated by having the patient drink a thin liquid or water after a solid bolus

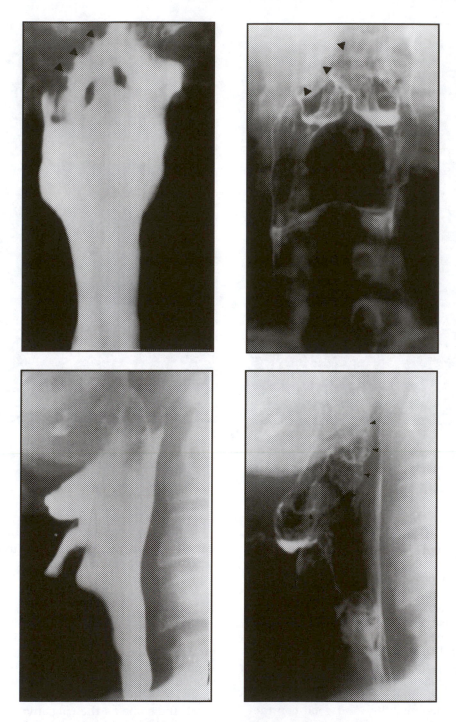

Figure 6–10. AP (*top*) view of a pharynx; single contrast (*left*) only shows some irregular contour (*arrow heads*) suggestive of a tumor. Double contrast (*right*) demonstrates the extent of the tumor (*arrow heads*) in the right tonsillar fossa. Lateral view (*bottom*) of the pharynx, single contrast (*left*) totally covers the mass but the tumor (*arrow heads*) is well outlined on double contrast (*right*).

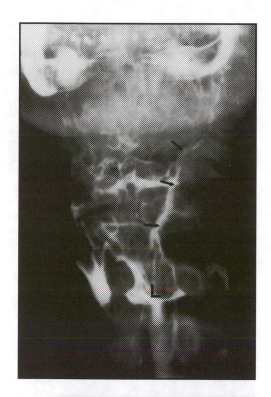

Figure 6–11. Double contrast, AP view shows a squamous cell carcinoma at the left lateral wall of hypopharynx (T). Aspirated barium outlines larynx (L).

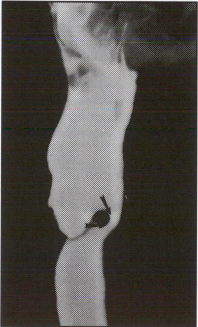
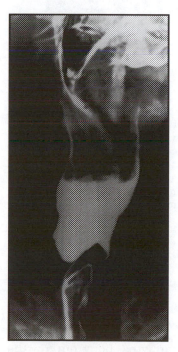

Figure 6–12. A patient with total laryngectomy. Gradual onset of dysphagia raised a question of recurrence. Barium swallow shows a severe narrowing (*arrow*) (*left*), but retains a good contraction (*right*). No recurrence was found on endoscopic examination and dilatation.

173

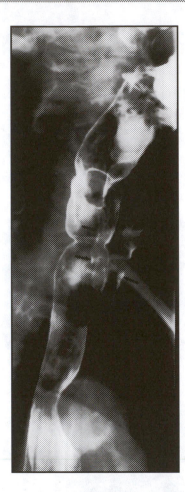

Figure 6–13. Oblique projection of a neck after barium swallow shows loss of normal contraction of the upper esophageal sphincter owing to previous radiation therapy at neck. Barium in the trachea from aspiration (*arrows*).

and by altering head position. The technique for clearance should be tested under fluoroscopy during the evaluation process.

Cervical Osteophytes

Cervical osteophytes, bony outgrowths from the cervical vertebrae, protrude into the pharynx and can cause dysphagia (Brandenberg & Leibrock, 1986; Zerhouni,

Bosma, & Donner, 1987; Lambert, Tepperman, Jimenez, & Newman, 1981). They have been observed, at times, to be large enough to block epiglottic downfolding and to cause pharyngeal stasis. Even when small, on rare occasion, they can be the underlying cause of the complaint of dysphagia; consequently, a swallowing evaluation should include assessment of the cervical spine. In a case report by Valadka, Kubal, and Smith (1995), a patient whose dysphagia was attributed to cervical osteophytes was later found to have a squamous cell carcinoma at the base of tongue and vallecula. Reports such as this reinforce the need for a complete diagnostic workup by various disciplines.

RADIOGRAPHIC EXAMINATION OF THE ESOPHAGUS

Technique

The techniques available for assessment include barium contrast examination with or without videorecording, CT especially cine-CT, and MR imaging. The latter two modalities are basically for organic lesions and are particularly useful for detecting any extrinsic lesion affecting the esophagus. These latter techniques are discussed elsewhere in this textbook. The routine procedure for barium examination of the esophagus should include a full column, mucosal relief, double contrast, and motility assessment.

The radiographic examination needs to be performed in different positions such as upright and recumbent and in anterior–posterior or both oblique projections. Preceding administration of the gas-producing granules, it is advisable to have the patient swallow in the AP and oblique projections with high density barium. At this time the examiner can check for aspiration, severe stricture, or obstruction. Obviously, if the patient is one who is at risk for aspiration the examiner should be sure to control the bolus size. If aspiration is evident, the study should proceed cautiously to determine with as few swallows as possible why the aspiration is occuring.

To obtain double contrast views of the mucosal structure, the upright position is easier to perform after having distended the stomach with gas-producing granules. Rapid gulping of a high-density barium in the upright, left posterior oblique projection to avoid operlapping with the spine usually will produce a well-distended double contrast view. A tube esophagogram may be necessary in a small percentage of patients.

If there is a low-grade or suspicious narrowing a barium tablet (EZ-EM Co.) should be used with plenty of water in order to evaluate the degree of the narrowing.

Unlike the examination of the oral and pharyngeal stages of swallowing, which are assessed in the upright position, the esophagus is also assessed in the recumbent position, which is imperative for assessment of esophageal peristalsis, as in the upright position the esophagus empties by gravity. At this time the full column and mucosal relief are also examined. Continuous drinking of low-density barium in the right anterior oblique recumbent position can achieve optimal distention of the entire esophagus and gastroesophageal junction. Placing a bolster under the ribs may improve distention. This is important for detecting not only intrinsic lesions in profile but also stenosis, rings and/or sliding hiatal hernia. Mucosal relief is attained by taking spot films of the collapsed esophagus after the patient has swallowed high density barium or barium paste to coat the mucosal surface.

In the recumbent position, normal peristalsis produces an inverted V configuration to the tail end of the barium bolus. A single swallow should be observed, as a second swallow obliterates the peristalsis. The wave should traverse the entire esophagus, and the esophagus should clear the bolus in approximately 8 sec (Castell, 1989). Injection of glucagon will lower the peristaltic contraction amplitude for as long as 25 minutes and will increase the proximal "escape" (see Functional Disorders of the Esophagus below), thus inter-

fering with the assessment of esophageal function (Mehran, Richards, Dent, Waterfall, & Stevenson, 1989). Glucagon also does not appear to improve the quality of double contrast images (Ott, Chen, & Gelfand, 1989)

When a patient is examined for a suspected esophageal disorder, it is important for the radiologic examination of the esophagus also to include the oral and pharyngeal stages of the swallow. This is because it has been reported that approximately 35% of symptomatic patients have simultaneous disorders of the pharynx and esophagus; furthermore, the level of a lesion does not necessarily correspond to the site of the patients' symptoms (Jones et al.,1985).

Functional Disorders of the Esophagus

Abnormal function in the esophagus is generally described as either a decrease in the frequency of peristaltic waves in response to a swallow, failure of the wave to progress along the esophagus to the gastroesophageal (GE) junction, or complete absence of peristalsis. Proximal escape is a common phenomenon that occurs at the thoracic inlet/aortic arch level where the peristaltic wave appears to stop and then start again a few centimeters lower in the esophagus, with a small volume of bolus being left behind in the esophagus. It is thought to represent poor "communication" between the striated and smooth muscle. These patients sometimes complain of the sensation of food sticking in the thoracic inlet or substernal level; often the sensation only occurs with solid foods. The sign of proximal escape is reproducible by barium swallow examination, and will be abolished by drinking water to clear the retained bolus in the upper esophagus. Distal escape on the other hand appears as a weakening of the stripping contraction as it approaches the lower esophagus and will result in regurgitation of the barium into the proximal esophagus instead of complete emptying of the bolus. This needs to be differentiated from spasm or a distal esophageal stricture with incomplete emptying. A stricture is usually detectable on fluoroscopic observation or on radiographic images. Esophageal distension is commonly associated with a stricture, whereas with aperistalsis the esophagus is uniform in caliber. Both proximal and distal escape are often seen in patients with gastroesophageal reflux (GER).

Achalasia and Pseudo-achalasia

Achalasia is characterized by absent or incomplete relaxation of the lower esophageal sphincter (LES), and eventually absent primary peristalsis in the esophageal body of the esophagus owing to degeneration of the ganglion cells in Auerbach's plexus. With severe dilatation, the esophagus becomes atonic and somewhat elongated in a "sigmoid" configuration. Barium esophagography usually reveals a "bird's beak" appearance at the level of the LES. Barium retention depends on the tightness of the LES. Intermittent opening of the beaked segment results in barium dribbling into the gasless stomach, and the sphincter then closes abruptly until the hydrostatic pressure in the esophageal lumen is again greater than the raised pressure in the LES. The narrowed segment usually has normal longitudinal mucosal folds that traverse the segment leading to the normal gastric cardia (Figure 6–14). Achalasia must be distinguished from pseudo- or secondary achalasia due to cancerous invasion of the LES segment such as from gastric or pancreatic cancer (Figure 6–15). In early achalasia, only the LES may be affected whereas in late achalasia there will also be absence of peristalsis. A variant has been described by Bondi, Goodwin, and Garett (1972), namely *vigorous achalasia*, which is characterized by mild to moderate dilatation with spontaneous esophageal body contractions after swallow. Some of these patients present with severe chest pain. Some experts consider diffuse esophageal spasm, vigorous achalasia, and achalasia as a spectrum of the same disease.

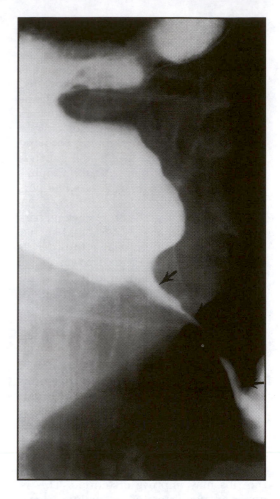

Figure 6–14. Achalasia. Bird's beaking with normal mucosal folds through the narrowed LES (*arrows*). Esophagus is enormously dilated and tortuous.

Scleroderma

In scleroderma, a connective tissue disorder that commonly affects the esophagus, progressive atrophy and fibrosis of the smooth muscle of the esophagus results in loss of peristaltic contraction. One swallow of the barium bolus in the prone position will show loss of the peristaltic wave in the smooth muscle portion of the esophagus, usually below the level of the aortic arch, with failure of esophageal emptying. As the LES pressure is low in scle-

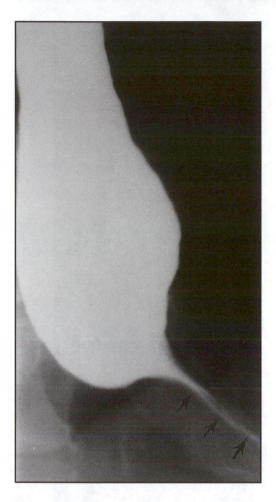 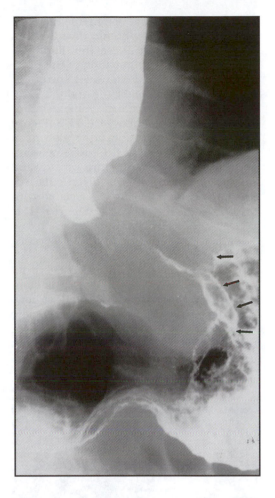

Figure 6–15. Pseudo-achalasia. (*Left*) smooth, tapered narrowing at distal esophagus (*arrows*), which is indistinguishable from acha- lasia. However, other spot film (*right*) demon- strates a cancer at the gastric cardia (*arrows*).

roderma and the GE junction is patulous, GER is common, resulting in peptic esophagitis, stricture, or shortening of the esophagus. There is also an increased incidence of Barrett's esophagus and adenocarcinoma of the esophagus.

Esophageal Diverticula

There are two types of diverticulum, *pulsion* and *traction*. A pulsion diverticulum results from localized high pressure pushing the mucosal and submucosal layers through a weakened muscle layer. A traction diverticulum results from a localized adhesion of the esophagus to a mediastinal structure (e.g., lymph node, trachea), and is composed of all layers of the esophageal wall. The pulsion diverticulum will neither contract nor completely empty, whereas the traction diverticulum may do both. Thus, the pulsion diverticulum will result in the complaint of dysphagia and the traction diverticulum may not.

The more common types of pulsion diverticula are Zenker's in the pharyngoesophageal segment, and epiphrenic near the diaphragm. The epiphrenic diverticulum is mostly seen just above the diaphragmatic hiatus. The summation of the pressure resulting from the muscles surrounding the diaphragmatic hiatus and the lower esophageal sphincter can cause a buildup of pressure just above the LES (Figure 6–16). These diverticula may also form above a stricture, and it is extremely important to exclude a stricture with careful evaluation. Some pulsion diverticula can be in an unusual location associated with trauma; some are idiopathic (Figure 6–17).

Corkscrew Esophagus

This motility disorder has also been described as *presbyesophagus* as it is commonly seen in the elderly population; however, the term *corkscrew esophagus* is more appropriate as the disorder is not limited to the elderly. The disorder results from tertiary contractions that are nonpropulsive,

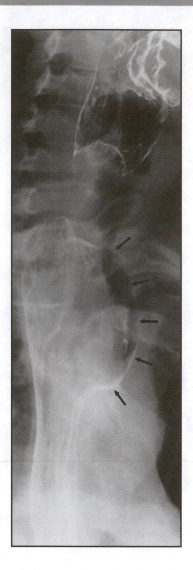

Figure 6–17. A 28-year-old man complains of dysphagia since childhood. At age 4 months, he had an operation for thymic cyst. Esophagogram shows a large, noncontractile diverticulum in the upper esophagus (*arrows*).

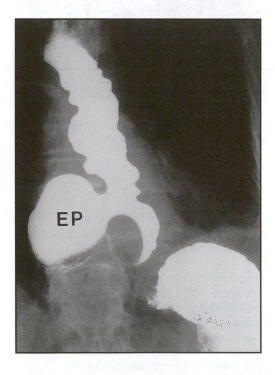

Figure 6–16. A large epiphrenic diverticulum (EP) with diffuse spasm of the lower esophagus.

simultaneous ring contractions of the esophagus at various levels. This is usually observed in the distal half of the esophagus and gives the radiographic appearance of a corkscrew. If the disorder is intermittent, the patient may complain of dysphagia, but a solid bolus may not hang in the esophagus and the radiologist may observe only mild, intermittent, tertiary contractions. In very severe cases, the bolus will hang up in the esophagus and the patient may develop one or multiple outpouches between the ring contractions (Figure 6–18). Manometry may be necessary to clarify this.

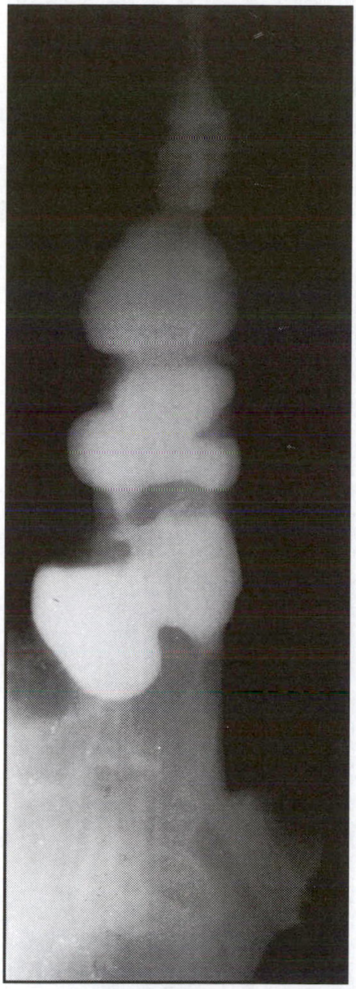

Figure 6–18. A 79-year-old man with the complaint of severe dysphagia. Esophagogram shows multiple simultaneous ringlike contractions in the lower two thirds of the esophagus, with multiple outpouchings.

Nutcracker esophagus is a manometrically diagnosed condition in which there are very high pressure contractions in the esophagus associated with normal peristalsis. The patient may complain of severe chest pain. In these patients the peristaltic wave appears normal during radiographic study.

Gastroesophageal Reflux (GER)

The primary diagnostic tool for the detection of reflux is not radiographic examination; rather, it is 24-hour pH probe monitoring. Unprovoked, spontaneous reflux on barium study was seen in only 26% of subjects proven to have GER by 24-hour pH probe monitoring (Thompson, Koehler, & Richter, 1994). However, the morphologic changes from the acid reflux can be recognized on radiographic study. Mucosal fold thickening around the gastroesophageal junction, fixed transverse ridges, ulceration or erosion, stricture or ring formation, intramural pseudodiverticulosis, Barrett's columnar-lined esophagus, and cancer are all associated with reflux. A sliding hiatal hernia may be found in patients with GE reflux, but there may be reflux throught a patulous GE junction without a hiatal hernia being present.

GE reflux may produce changes in esophageal motor function such as spasm, loss of the peristaltic wave, and segmental escapes. Secondary changes may be present such as prominence of the cricopharyngeus or even a cricopharyngeal bar.

GER RELATED ORGANIC LESIONS

Radiography is useful for detecting the morphologic changes produced by GER, ranging from superficial mucosal change such as edema or erosions to deep ulceration, stricture, intramural pseudodiverticulosis, and development of cancer. Radiographically superficial changes are hard to detect.

Reflux Esophagitis

Thickening of mucosal folds and inflammatory polyps (Figure 6–19) around the gastroesophageal junction shown on double contrast or mucosal relief x-ray picture may suggest reflux esophagitis, although the findings are nonspecific. Sometimes an inflammatory polyp is indistinguishable from a submucosal mass.

High quality double contrast examination is capable of demonstrating superficial erosions (Figures 6–20 and 6–21). Diffuse granular or nodular appearance of the esophagus, though nonspecific, may be seen in GER (Figure 6–22). This needs to be differentiated from infectious esophagitis or glycogic acanthosis.

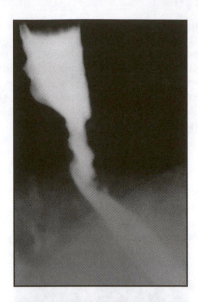

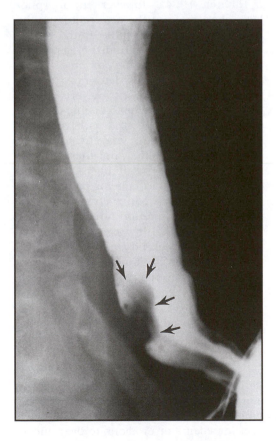

Figure 6–19. An esophagogastric polyp (*arrow*) is shown in a sliding hiatal hernia (note the gastric folds traversing the hiatus) near the GE junction in a patient with GERD.

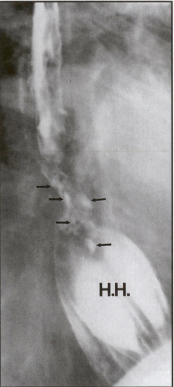

Figure 6–20. Irregular narrowing at distal esophagus on single contrast (*top*) simulating cancer. Actually, patient has multiple erosions (*arrows*) at the GE junction (*bottom*) on double contrast. HH, hiatal hernia.

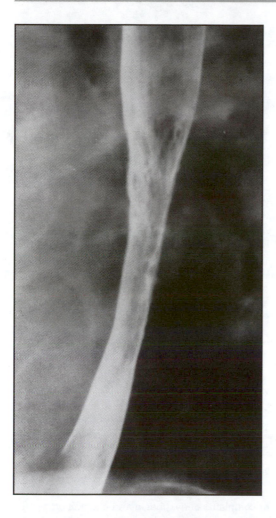

Figure 6–21. Multiple punctate barium collections associated with fine nodules and smooth narrowing approximately 5-cm long in the distal one third of the esophagus. Endoscopy and biopsy revealed erosive esophagitis without Barrett's esophagus.

Peptic ulcers are demonstrable with meticulous barium swallow examination (Figure 6–23). Ulcer shape may be round, ovoid, or linear, and single or multiple. A linear ulcer is usually oriented longitudinally and may be accompanied by radiating folds, resulting in mild segmental narrowing. Ulcers are located in the lower half of the esophagus, most commonly in the distal end, but can be as high as the aortic arch level.

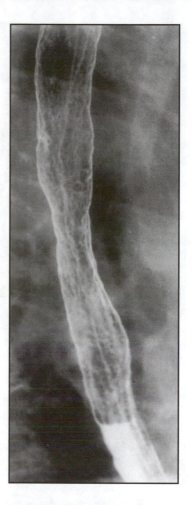

Figure 6–22. Diffuse granularity and nodularity are seen on double contrast esophagogram. The patient complains of severe heartburn.

Stricture

Long-standing or chronic recurrent ulcerations from GER may result in a benign stricture. Radiographically this is seen as a concentric smooth, tapered narrowing without an overhanging shelf (Figure 6–24). On barium swallow, an overhanging edge from proximal distention may mimick a shelf and this may be confused with a neoplastic lesion (Figure 6–25). Differential diagnosis of these two conditions is important. The neoplastic lesion is a rigid

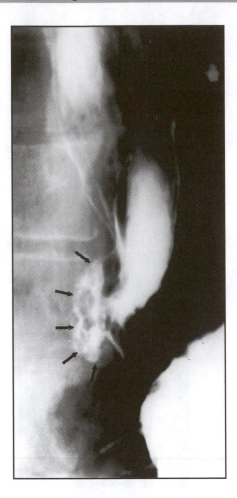 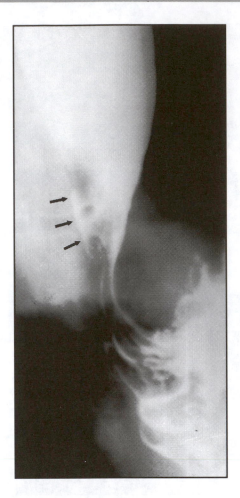

Figure 6–23. Benign peptic ulcer (*Left*) a patient complains of dysphagia and choking on eating. Esophagogram demonstrates a large, deep ulcer (*arrows*) in the right lateral wall of the distal esophagus and focal spasm. Barium contrast seen in the bronchi is from aspiration. (*Right*) ulcer becomes smaller (*arrows*) without focal spasm after medical treatment.

structure; therefore, a shelf usually is present on both ends of the narrowing if maximum distention of the esophagus is obtained (Figure 6–26). Endoscopic biopsy is important for any questionable lesions and to make the diagnosis of Barrett's esophagus.

Barrett's Esophagus

The squamous cell epithelium of the esophagus may be replaced by columnar epithelium as the result of chronic GER, a change known as the *columnar-lined* or *Barrett's esophagus*. Radiographic diagnosis of Barrett's esophagus is difficult and is poorly correlated with endoscopic findings. (Agha, 1986; Chen, Gelfand, Ott, & Wu, 1985; Levine, 1988; Levine, Dillon, Saul, & Laufer, 1986). A stricture remote from the GE junction in the mid-esophagus or proximal esophagus, or a large ulcer remote from the GE junction should raise the possibility of Barrett's esophagus (Chernin, Amberg, Kogan, Morgan, & Sampliner, 1986). Biopsy is important, as the

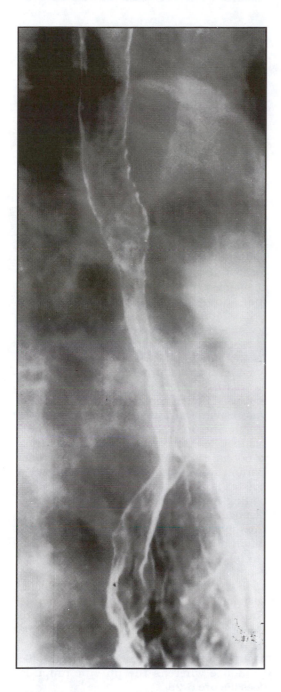

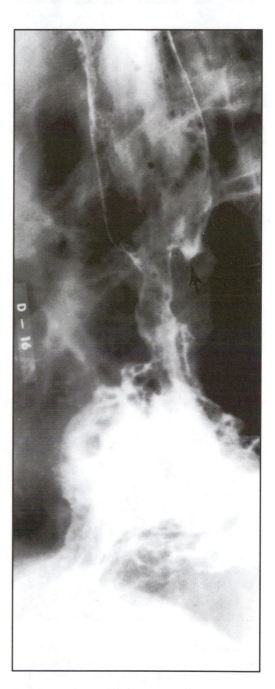

Figure 6–24. A smooth, tapered narrowing in the distal esophagus. A large hiatal hernia and some scarring are at the proximal end of the narrowing. Biopsy shows benign chronic esophagitis.

Figure 6–25. Prone swallow shows an irregular narrowing in the distal end of the esophagus and a large hiatal hernia. An overhanging edge at the proximal end of the narrowing (*arrow*) mimics a shelf often seen in a cancer. Surgery revealed benign peptic stricture.

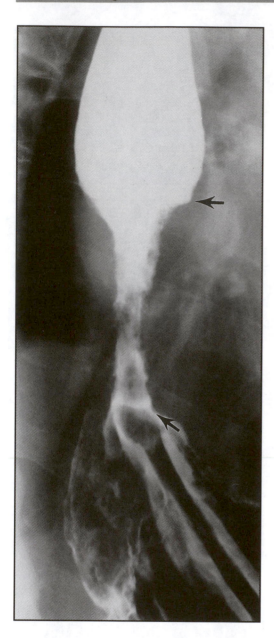

Figure 6–26. A 73-year-old man complains of progressive dysphagia in the past 6 months. He had a history of reflux esophagitis in the past 17 years. The esophagogram shows a long segment of irregular narrowing in the distal esophagus and a large hiatal hernia. Shelf is seen at both proximal and distal ends of the narrowing. Adenocarcinoma in association with Barrett's esophagus was found at endoscopy and biopsy.

condition is known to have the potential for dysplastic change and the development of adenocarcinoma. Interestingly, many patients found to have Barrett's esophagus on biopsy fail to give a history of reflux symptoms, possibly related to an insensitivity of the esophageal mucosa to chronic acid reflux. Others have a long history of severe reflux symptoms such as heart burn or chest pain.

Hiatal Hernia

There are two types of hiatal hernia: sliding or axial, and paraesophageal or rolling. In sliding hiatal hernia, the GE junction is located above the diaphragm, whereas in the paraesophageal hernia, it is in the normal subdiaphragmatic location (Figure 6–27). Mixed hernias combine the characteristics of both. Classically the sliding type is associated with reflux symptoms, whereas the paraesophageal is not. A transient, small sliding hiatal hernia may be seen in the normal person during the swallow. This is caused by the contraction of the esophagus resulting in transient shortening of its length. The presence of a sliding hiatal hernia may be associated with GER but a hernia is not an essential factor for GER disease. Barium swallow in the prone position over a bolster is the best way to demonstrate a sliding hiatal hernia, which needs to be distinguished from a phrenic ampulla (gastroesophageal vestibule), a segmental dilatation of the distal esophagus, about 2–3 cm in length, just proximal to the gastroesophageal junction. This segment corresponds to the lower esophageal sphincter segment, demarcated by a muscular ring contraction at the rostral end (refer to Chapter 13). In a sliding hiatal hernia, the herniated portion of the stomach does not contract as part of the esophageal peristaltic sequence whereas the phrenic ampulla does (Figure 6–28).

Lower Esophageal Ring

Ring-type narrowings in the lower esophagus and GE junction include the muco-

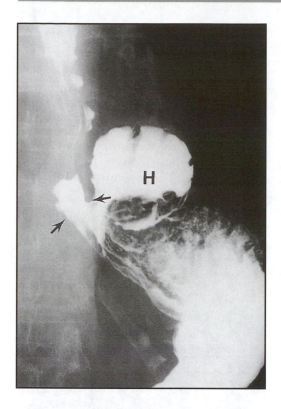

Figure 6–27. Paraesophageal hiatal hernia. The gastroesophageal junction (*arrow*) is below the diaphragm. Part of the gastric fundus has herniated (*H*) above the diaphragm beside the esophagus.

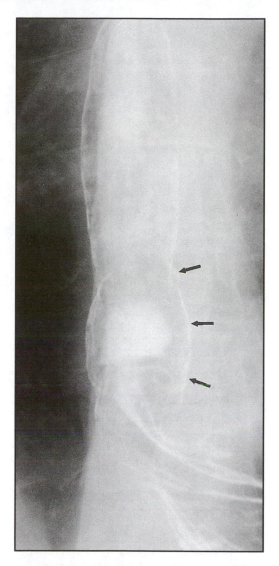

Figure 6–28. A small sliding hiatal hernia and a phrenic ampulla (*arrows*) in a 63-year-old man without GER symptoms.

sal ring, a muscular contraction and strictures due to peptic narrowing. The mucosal ring is known as *Schatzki's* or *B ring*, which is located at the gastroesophageal junction and consists of an epithelial mucosal layer. It appears as a thin, uniform ring type of narrowing. The length is usually less than 3 mm (Figure 6–29). Schatzki's description referred to a stenotic mucosal ring, becoming symptomatic always if smaller than 13–14 mm, often symptomatic if 14–18 mm, and rarely symptomatic if wider than 20 mm. These rings can easily be treated with dilatation.

A *muscular A* or *Wolf ring* is a thick smooth narrowing located 2–3 cm cephalad to the GE junction; this ring will change

in thickness and depth on contraction. The muscular ring is the upper margin of the lower esophageal sphincter and is the rostal demarcation of the phrenic ampulla.

Long-standing reflux esophagitis may result in peptic stricture and form a variable degree of concentric narrowing. This

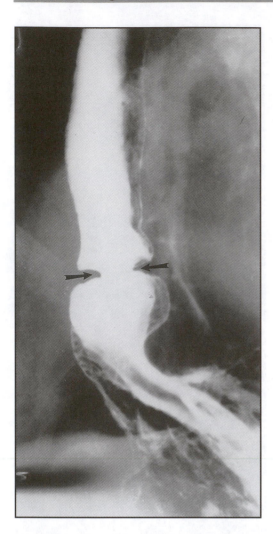

Figure 6–29. A small sliding hiatal hernia with a smooth, ringlike form narrowing (Schatzki's ring) at the GE junction (*arrow*).

condition has a higher incidence of Barrett's esophagus; therefore, it needs endoscopic biopsy.

The epithelial and peptic rings sometimes narrow so much that patients may complain of dysphagia for solid food. Fluoroscopic examination with a 13-mm barium tablet (E-Z EM Co.) with plenty of water in the upright position is valuable unless the lumen is obviously narrower than the size of the tablet.

Intramural Pseudodiverticulosis

This disease entity was first reported as an intramural diverticulosis (Mendl, McKay, & Tanner, 1960). Deep, small, multiple outpouchings in the wall of the esophagus are the radiographic manifestion of ectasia of intramural glands and therefore were termed intramural *pseudo*-diverticulosis in 1974 (Beauchamp, Nice, Belanger, & Neitzschman, 1974; Figure 6–30). The

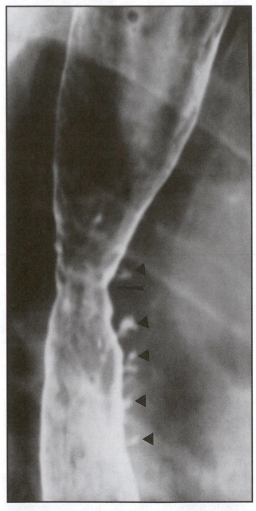

Figure 6–30. The patient has long history of GER with progressive dysphagia. The esophagogram shows a narrowing at the aortic arch level (*arrow*). Multiple deep, small outpouchings (*arrow heads*) represent intramural pseudodiverticulosis.

appearance is so characteristic that it rarely needs a differential diagnosis or biopsy.

The lesion is thought to be related to nonspecific inflammation from long-standing GER or prior infection such as candidiasis. It is often accompanied by some narrowing of the esophageal lumen. It may be an incidental finding during routine upper GI examination although most of the patients complain of dysphagia, probably due to the stricture rather than the pseudodiverticula themselves.

INFECTIOUS ESOPHAGITIS

Infectious esophagitis may be caused by bacteria, viruses, and fungi. Opportunistic esophagitis is seen in immunocompromised patients receiving steroids, chemotherapy, antibiotics, radiation, or in other causes of immune suppression such as with diabetes or AIDS patients.

Monilia

Candida albicans, a normal flora in the mouth, is the most common agent resulting in opportunistic esophagitis. When it involves the esophagus and becomes pathogenic, the patient will experience dysphagia, odynophagia, and chest pain. On double contrast examination, the esophagus shows multiple nodular lesions of various size, representing the yellowish plaques on the mucosal surface. Shagginess is another radiographic manifestation in most cases of candidiasis. The findings are similar to the condition known as *glycogen acanthosis* of the esophagus in which there are small nodules of intracellular glycogen deposits. This is seen in normal individuals, and the esophagus in this condition does not show the shagginess of moniliasis and is asymptomatic (Mitros, 1988). In candidiasis some patients cannot gulp the barium rapidly because of odynophagia. Then the radiograph may just show a shaggy contour and irregularity in a poorly distended esophagus. In some cases candidiasis will appear as a cobblestone pattern (Figure 6–31). Wall (1992) described a masslike lesion in

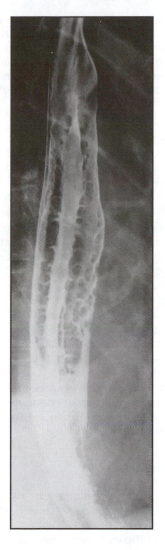

Figure 6–31. Patient on chemotherapy for malignant lymphoma developed dysphagia and odynophagia. Diffuse plaques and cobblestoning are shown on the esophagogram. Candida was found on brush biopsy.

localized candida infection, and deep ulcers superimposed with plaquelike lesions in severe esophagitis. The peristaltic contraction in some cases of candidiasis is decreased or atonic but spasm is more common. Rarely, moniliasis will result in stricture (Ott & Gelfand, 1978). Intramural pseudodiverticulosis may also follow moniliasis if healing of the infection results in scarring of the neck of the mucous glands.

Viruses

The most common type of viral infection is herpes simplex type I and cytomegalovirus. Viral infection starts with a vesicle but quickly becomes an ulcer after rupture of the vesicle. In practice, radiologic demonstration is at the ulcer stage, with single or multiple discrete ulcers surrounded by edema (Figure 6–32). Giant or confluent ulcers are occasionally seen in patient with AIDS (Balthazar, Megibow, Hunick, Cho, & Beranbarum, 1987). Other radiologic features include mucosal thickening, granular-nodular mucosal pattern, and plaquelike lesions (Teixidor et al., 1987; Meyers, Durkin, & Lover, 1975). Herpes esophagitis was recently described in a group of male patients with no sign of immunocompromise (Shortsleeve & Levine, 1992).

Tuberculosis

As AIDS patients increase in number so do the tuberculosis cases. Chest x-ray may be negative, and dysphagia may be the first clinical symptom (Schneider, 1976). Nonspecific ulceration and narrowing of the esophagus sometimes with sinus tracts to the mediastinum will be shown on esophagogram.

Idiopathic Esophageal Ulcer in Acquired Immunodeficiency Syndrome.

In AIDS, a large, sometimes penetrating ulcer in the middle to distal esophagus can occur early in the course of the disease after seroconversion. These patients usually complain of odynophagia without any clinical evidence of opportunistic in-

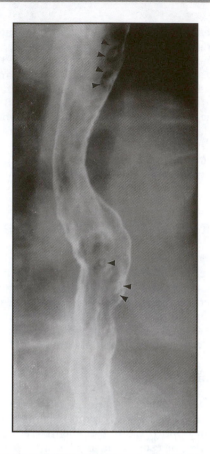

Figure 6–32. Patient is on steroids for sideroblastic anemia. Double contrast esophagogram reveals multiple ulcers with surrounding edema (*arrow heads*). Herpes simplex virus was found at the site of the lesions on endoscopy.

fection. Human immunodeficiency virus itself is suspected as the pathogenic agent. Radiographically the lesions are giant (bigger than 2.5 cm) and located in the mid or distal esophagus (Frager, Kotler, & Baer, 1994.). They respond well to corticosteroid therapy (Wilcox & Schwartz, 1992).

OTHER NONINFECTIOUS ESOPHAGITIS AND STENOSIS

Stenosis can be congenital stenosis or result from an unknown etiology (Figure 6–33),

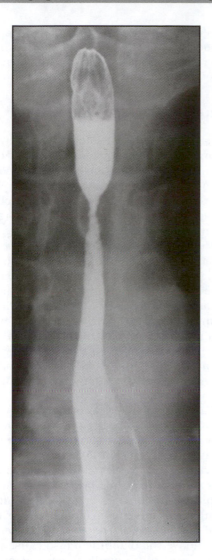

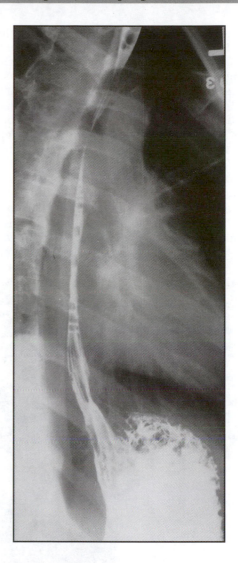

Figure 6–33. Unknown cause of benign upper esophageal narrowing in a 64-year-old man who has no trauma or inflammatory history. Dysphagia for several years is improved after balloon dilatation.

Figure 6–34. Six months after lye ingestion in suicide attempt. Diffuse narrowing of the entire esophagus is shown on barium esophagogram. The appearance is benign.

from postradiation, from post-chemical burn such as lye or acid swallow (Figure 6–34), or be post-traumatic or iatrogenic. Radiographically, these narrowings appear smoothly tapered on maximal distention but depending on the degree of damage to the esophageal wall can still show peristaltic contraction.

NEOPLASTIC LESIONS

A mass of intrinsic origin can be differentiated from extrinsic lesions based on the radiographic appearance. Intrinsic lesions include lesions in the mucosa, submucosa or muscle layer. Demonstration of the lesion tangentially and enface view on esophagogram is important for accurate evaluation. Abrupt cutoff of the mucosal folds is seen in masses arising from the mucosa, whereas submucosal or extrinsic lesions will show effacement or stretching of the esophageal mucosal folds. A shelflike sharp edge is present in in-trinsic lesions of either mucosal or submucosal origin (Figure 6–35). Ulceration is more often seen in mucosal or submucosal lesions but can also be seen if extrinsic malignancy directly invades the esophageal wall. The surface of the mass is usually smooth in both submucosal and extrinsic masses, and irregular, nodular, and/or

ulcerated in malignant mucosal tumors. Good quality double contrast eso-phagogram is essential for the diagnosis of superficial mucosal lesions.

External Masses

Enlarged goiter, particularly in an intrathoracic location, may be a cause of dysphagia. Esophagogram shows a smooth extrinsic compression at the thoracic inlet corresponding to a mass seen on chest x-ray, or increased uptake of radiotracer on nuclear imaging.

Mediastinal masses such as thymoma, teratoma, adenopathy, or mass from bronchogenic origin may narrow the esophageal lumen by simple compression or direct invasion (Figure 6–36). If the mass directly invades the esophagus, there will eventually be destruction of the mucosa and fistula formation (Figure 6–37). The radiographic appearance on barium esophagogram will be the same regardless of the type of the mass.

Vascular anomalies located in the mediastinum such as aberrant right subclavian artery or pulmonary sling may cause esophageal compression. Aberrant right subclavian artery passes behind the esophagus, pulmonary sling between the esophagus and trachea. An enlarged heart (particularly enlargement of the left atrium) and tortuosity of the descending aorta just above the diaphragm also cause posterior and anterior displacement of the lower esophagus, respectively.

Intrinsic Masses

Intrinsic lesions include mucosal lesions such as cancer and submucosal lesions such as leiomyomas. Dysphagia is late with intrinsic tumors because the remainder of the esophageal wall not involved by tumor can expand to accommodate the bolus until the lesion is concentric or almost concentric, when luminal narrowing results. Often the small or flat lesion is incidentally found on routine barium upper GI tract examination. Bleeding

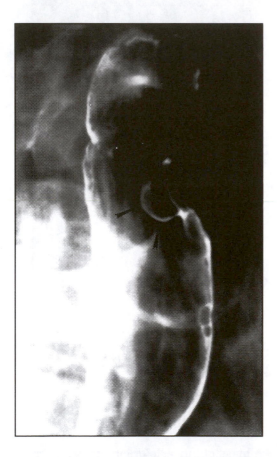

Figure 6–35. A 48-year-old man with 1-year history of dysphagia and choking. Esophagogram reveals a 1.5-cm sized, smooth polyp (*arrow*) on the anterior wall of the upper esophagus. The lesion is sharply demarcated. Biosy shows an inflammatory polyp.

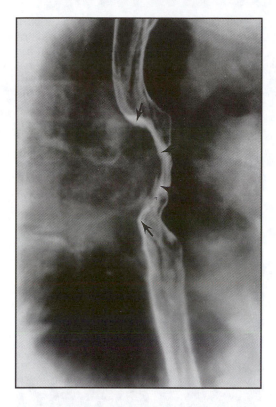

Figure 6–36. Left posterior oblique view of the mid esophagram reveals a smooth external mass, smooth owing to compression from bronchogenic carcinoma (*arrows*). There are smooth edges on both ends of the compression. No esophageal destruction is seen. The lumen is narrowed by compression from this mass.

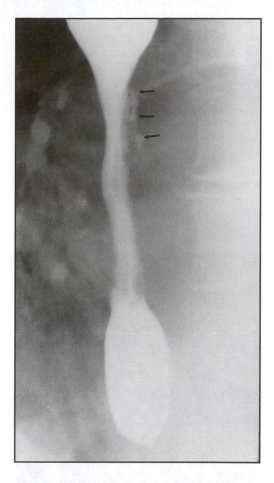

Figure 6–37. A narrowed segment, about 7 cm in length, in the mid to lower esophagus without shouldering mimics a benign lesion, yet there is an area of mucosal destruction with irregular barium collection (*arrows*) at the proximal site end, suggesting ulceration or excavation. This is suggestive of extrinsic malignancy invading the esophageal wall. Sqamous cell carcinoma of the lung was the histological diagnosis.

or hematemesis may be the first symptom.

Some benign mucosal lesions are the adenoma, the papilloma, and the inflammatory polyp. The shape of the mass can be discoid, sessile, or pedunculated. The lesion always shows abnormal mucosal pattern such as abrupt cutoff of mucosal folds, nodularity, or ulceration. The origin of the growth is demonstrable if the lesion is pedunculated.

Carcinoma

Carcinoma is the most common malignant tumor of the esophagus. As the car-cinoma progresses, it grows into a fungating mass, with or without ulceration, or spreads by both longitudinal and circumferential growth and infiltration. As the esophagus has no serosa and as it has an extensive lymphatic drainage, spread is fast and the overall prognosis of esophageal carcinoma is poor. However, if the cancer is detected and resected at an early stage when the cancer is confined to the mucosa and submucosa, the prognosis is very favorable (Baba, Kaku, Sakata et al., 1994; Yoshinaka, Shimazu, Fukumoto, Baba, 1991; Figure 6–38). When the tumor grows circumferentially it becomes an annular narrowing, the so-called "apple-core" lesion.

Early carcinoma in previously benign peptic structure and early adenocarcinoma in Barrett's esophagus may be very difficult to diagnosis radiographically. Therefore, biopsy should be performed in such cases for early detection (Levine et al., 1986).

There is a form of cancer known as *varicoid* carcinoma in which submucosal infiltration produces a nodular or tortuous mucosal pattern, resembling esophageal varices (Figure 6–39). Differential diagnosis is possible with fluoroscopy, for observing the changing size and pattern in varices compared to the rigid, noncontractile varicoid tumor (Figure 6–40).

Necrotic ulceration or excavation is another appearance which radiographically appears as an irregular ulcer in a well-demarcated tumorous mass (Figure 6–41).

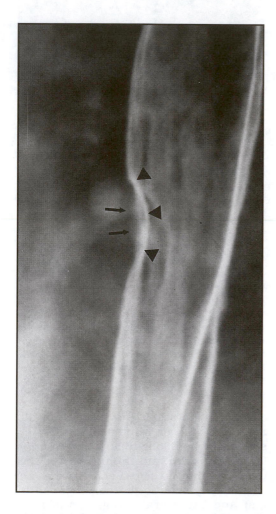 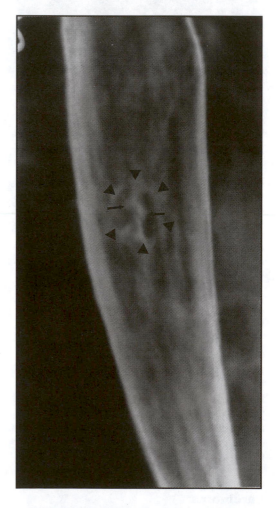

Figure 6–38. Early esophageal cancer; (*Left*) profile and (*right*) en face views of a squamous carcinoma (*arrow heads*) detected in an asymptomatic patient. The cancer invasion is limited to submucosa. Small ulcer (*arrow*) is present at the center of the lesion.

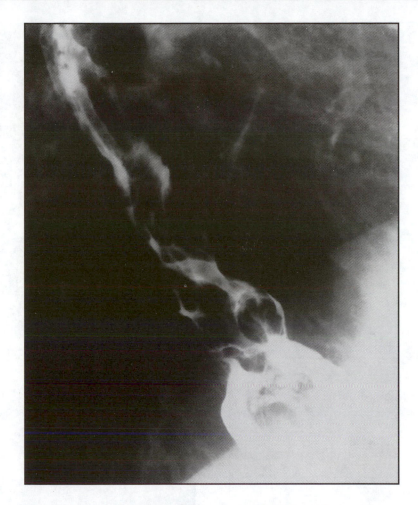

Figure 6–39. An advanced adenocarcinoma from Barrett's esophagus. The tumor is varicoid in appearance.

Submucosal and Intramural Tumors

Submucosal (intramural) tumors include leiomyoma, neurofibroma, fibroma, lipoma, hemangioma, and sarcomatous change of the above-mentioned lesions. It can be difficult to differentiate benign from malignant submucosal tumors but rapid growth and increase in size favors malignancy. Biopsy may be necessary for diagnosis of malignant change. Carcinoid, metastatic melanoma, certain types of metastatic carcinomas, or lymphoma (although rarely in the esophagus) will show the same radiographic appearance but more rapid growth, and formation of the central necrotic cavity may lead to the appearance of the so-called "target" or "bulls-eye" lesion.

Carcinosarcoma

Carcinosarcoma has mixed carcinomatous and sarcomatous elements and has a characteristic appearance. It is extremely bulky, resulting in expansion of the esophageal lumen and is often pendunculated, resulting in an intraluminal filling defect on esophagogram (Figure 6–42).

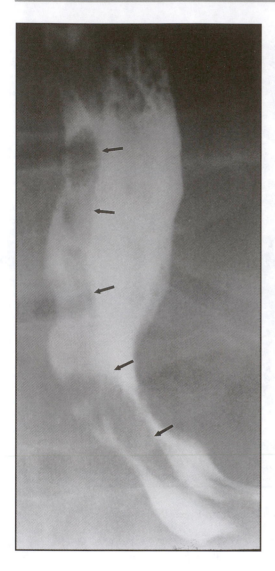

Figure 6–40. (*Left and right*) lower esophageal varices in a patient with portal hypertension. The engorged veins (*arrows*) are changing in size and shape during respiration.

SUMMARY

A barium contrast study is an effective tool for evaluating functional and morphological disorders of the pharynx and esophagus. It is less expensive than many other procedures and is noninvasive. In most instances this should be the initial examination for a patient complaining of dysphagia. Functional assessment of the pharynx must be performed with a dynamic imaging technique, preferably videofluorography, but a combination of videofluorography and spot films is necessary when assessing both the pharynx and esophagus. A full understanding of the physiological and anatomical bases of deglutition and of radiologic technique, and the

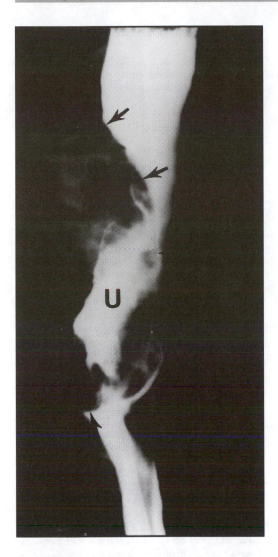

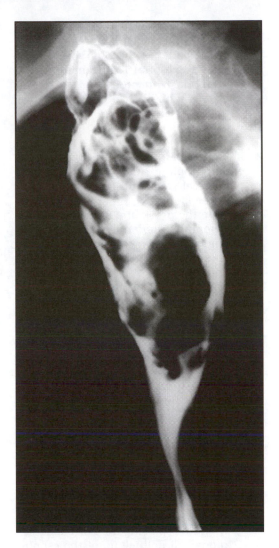

Figure 6–41. A large fungating mass with central ulceration (*U*) or excavation narrowing the esophageal lumen at the upper esophagus. There is a sharp shelf (*arrows*) at proximal and distal ends of the lesion. Advanced squamous carcinoma with mediastinal involvement was found at thoracotomy.

Figure 6–42. A large lobulated and pedunculated mass expanding the lumen in the upper esophagus. The finding is characteristic for carcinosarcoma.

proper selection of assessment technique based on the clinical history and tailored to each individual patient, are important for accurate diagnosis.

MULTIPLE CHOICE QUESTIONS

1. Purposes of a videofluoroscopic examination of oral and pharyngeal swallowing function include determining

a. if a patient can either progress to or continue safe oral intake.

b. if the patient is likely to meet his or her nutritional requirements with oral nourishment.

c. if it is advisable to find alternative methods of nutrition.

d. if there is a tumor.

2. If aspiration is observed during a videofluoroscopic examination of oral and pharyngeal swallowing function, the general rule is to

a. stop the procedure immediately

b. attempt to determine the underlying cause(s) for the aspiration while keeping risk to the patient at a minimum

c. continue with all bolus volumes and viscosities listed in the protocol

d. routinely recommend the patient become npo

3. Concerning gastroesophageal reflux (GER)

a. Clinical diagnosis of GER should rely on fluoroscopic observation of barium examination.

b. Abnormalities associated with GER include intramural pseudodiverticulosis, stricture, ulceration or erosion, squamous cell carcinoma, and absence of esophageal peristalsis.

c. Hiatal hernia is essential for GER.

d. Barrett's esophagus is columnar epithelium replacing the normal squamous cell epithelium of the esophagus as the result of chronic GER.

4. Which of the following statements are true concerning esophageal tumor?

a. Tumors causing dysphagia can be intrinsic or extrinsic.

b. Esophageal cancer has an overall poor prognosis because of late detection.

c. Carcinosarcoma is characterized by the presence of a bulky mass, often with pedicle, and appears as an intraluminal filling defect.

d. Radiographically, it is easy to differentiate a benign intramural tumor from a malignant intramural tumor.

REFERENCES

Agha, F. P., Francis, I. R., & Ellis, C. N. (1983). Esophageal involvement in epidermolysis bullosa dystrophica. *Gastrointestinal Radiology, 8,* 111–117.

Agha, F. P., & Raji, M. R. (1982). Esophageal involvement in pemphigoid, *Gastrointestinal Radiology, 7,* 109–112.

Agha, E. P. (1986). Radiologic diagnosis of Barrett's esophagus: Critical analysis of 65 cases. *Gastrointestinal Radiology 11,* 123–130

Ardran, G. (1965). Calcification of the epiglottis. *British Journal of Radiology, 38,* 592–595.

Ardran, G., & Kemp, F. (1951). The mechanism of swallowing. *Proceedings of the Royal Society of Medicine, 44,* 1038–1040.

Ardran, G., & Kemp, F. (1952). The protection of the laryngeal airway during swallowing. *British Journal of Radiology, 25,* 406–416.

Ardran, G., & Kemp, F. (1967). The mechanism of the larynx, Part II: The epiglottis and closure of the larynx. *British Journal of Radiology, 40,* 372–389.

Ardran, G. M., Kemp, F. H., & Lind, J. (1958). A cineradiographic study of bottle feeding. *British Journal of Radiology, 31,* 11–22.

Baba, Y., Kaku, Y., Sakata, H., Tomimatsu, H., Shimizu, H., Takemoto, N., Takegoshi, T., Karneo, S., Shirochi, T., Tateishi, H., Matsubara, T., Ueda, M., Kato, H., & Yanagisawa, A., (1994). Roentgenologic diagnosis of intramucosal carcinoma of the esophagus. *Stomach and Intestine, 29,* 301–317.

Balthazar, E.J., Megibow, A. J., Hulnick, D., Cho, K. C., & Beranbaum, E., (1987). Cytomegalovarius esophagitis in AIDS: Radiographic features in 16 patients. *American Journal of Roentgenology 149,* 919–923.

Barofsky, I., Buchholz, D., Edwin, D., Jones, B., & Ravich, W. (1994). Characteristics of patients who have difficulty initiating swallowing. *Dysphagia, 9*(4), 264.

Beauchamp, J. M., Nice, C. M., Belanger, M. A., & Neitzschman, H. R. (1974). Esophageal intramural pseudodiverticulosis. *Radiology, 113,* 273–276

Bondi, J. L., Godwin, D. H., and Garett, J. M. (1972). "Vigorous" achalasia, its clinical interpretation and significance, *American Journal of Gastroenterology, 58*(2), 145–55.

Brandenberg, S., & Leibrock, L. G. (1986). Dysphagia and dysphonia secondary to anterior cervical osteophytes. *Neurosurgery, 18*(1), 90–93.

Cannon, W. B., & Moser, A. (1898). The movements of the food in the oesophagus. *American Journal of Physiology, 1,* 435–444.

Caruso, A., Stanhope, S., & McGuire, D. (1989). A new technique for acquiring three-dimensional orofacial nonspeech movements. *Dysphagia, 4*(2), 127–132.

Castell, D. O. (1989). Dysphagia: A general approach to the patient. In D. W. Gelfand (Ed.), *Dysphagia: Diagnosis and treatment* (1st ed., pp. 3–9). New York: Igaku-Shoin.

Chen, Y. M., Gelfand, D. W., Ott, D. J., & Wu, W. C. (1985). Barrett esophagus as an extension of severe esophagitis: Analysis of radiologic signs in 29 cases, *American Journal of Roentgenology, 145,* 275–281.

Chernin, M. M., Amberg, J. R., Kogan, F. J., Morgan, T. R., & Sampliner, R. E. (1986). Efficacy of radiologic studies in the detection of Barrett's esophagus. *American Journal of Roentgenology, 147,* 257–260.

Cleall, J. F. (1965). Deglutition: A study of form and function. *American Journal of Orthodontics, 51*(8), 566–594.

Cohen, B. R., & Wolf, B. S. (1968). Cineradiographic and intraluminal pressure correlations in the pharynx and esophagus. In F. Code (Exec. Ed.) & H. Werner (Sec. Ed.), *Handbook of Physiology Vol IV. Section 6: Alimentary Canal* (pp. 1841–1860). Washington, DC: American Physiological Society.

Cook, I. J., Blumbergs, P., Cash, K., Graham, S., Jamieson, G. G., Hains, J. D., & Shearman, D. J. (1989). *Gastroenterology, 96*(5), A98.

Cook, I. J., Gabb, M., Panagopoulos, V., Jamieson, G. G., Hains, J. D., Dodds, W. J., Dent, J., & Shearman, D. J. (1989). *Gastroenterology, 96*(5), A98

Cordaro, M. A., & Sonies, B. C. (1993). An image processing scheme to quantitatively extract and validate hyoid bone motion based on real-time ultrasound recordings of swallowing. *IEEE Transactions on Biomedical Engineering, 40*(8), 941–944.

Dengel, G., Robbins, J., & Rosenbek, J. C. (1991). Image processing in swallowing and speech research. *Dysphagia, 6,* 30–39.

Dodds, W. J., Taylor, A. J., Stewart, E. T., Kern, M. K., Logemann, J. A., & Cook, I. J. (1989). Tipper and dipper types of oral swallows. *American Journal of Roentgenology, 153,* 1197–1199.

Donner, M. W., & Silbiger, M. L. (1966). Cinefluorographic analysis of pharyngeal swallowing in neuromuscular disorders. *The American Journal of the Medical Sciences, 251,* 600–614.

Dorland. (1985). *Dorland's illustrated medical dictionary* (27th ed.). Philadelphia: W. B. Saunders.

Ekberg, O. (1982). Defective closure of the laryngeal vestibule during deglutition. *Acta Otolaryngology, 93,* 309–317.

Ekberg, O., & Nylander, G. (1982). Cineradiography of the pharyngeal stage of deglutition in 250 patients with dysphagia. *British Journal of Radiology, 55,* 258–262.

Ekberg, O., & Sigurjonsson, V. (1982). Movement of the epiglottis during deglutition. *Gastrointestinal Radiology, 7,* 101–107.

Flores, T. C., Wood, B. G., Levine, H. L., Koegel, L., & Tucker, H. M. (1982). Factors in successful deglutition following supraglottic laryngeal surgery. *Annals of Otology, Rhinology, and Laryngology, 91,* 579–583.

Frager, D., Kotler, D. P., & Baer, J., (1994). Idiopathic esophageal ulceration in the acquired immunodeficiency syndrome: Radiologic reappraisal in 10 patients., *Abdominal Imaging, 19,* 2–5.

Hrycyshyn, A. W., & Basmajian, J. V. (1972). Electromyography of the oral stage of swallowing in man. *American Journal of Anatomy, 133,* 333–340.

Jacob, P., Kahrilas, P. J., Logemann, J. A., Shah, V., & Ha, T. (1989). Upper esophageal sphincter opening and modulation during swallowing. *Gastroenterology, 97,* 1469–1478.

Jones, B., Ravich, W. J., Donner, M. W., & Kramer, S. S (1985). Pharyngoesophageal interrelationships: Observations and working concepts, *Gastrointestinal Radiology, 10,* 225–233.

Kagel, M. C., & Leopold, N. A. (1992). Dysphagia in Huntington's disease: A 16-year retrospective. *Dysphagia, 7*(2), 106–114.

Kahrilas, P. J., Lin, S., Logemann, J. A., Ergun, G. A., & Facchini, F. (1993). Deglutitive tongue action: Volume accommodation and bolus propulsion. *Gastroenterology, 104,* 152–162.

Laccourreye, H., Laccourreye, O., Menard, M., Weinstein, G., & Brasnu, D. (1990). Supracricoid laryngectomy with cricohyoidepiglottopexy: A partial laryngeal procedure for glottic carcinoma. *Annals of Otology Rhinology and Laryngology, 99,* 421–426.

Lambert, J. R., Tepperman, P. S., Jimenez, J., & Newman, A. (1981). Cervical spine disease and dysphagia. *American Journal of Gastroenterology, 76,* 35–40.

Levine, M. S., Dillon, E. C., Saul, S. H., & Laufer, I. (1986). Early esophageal cancer, *American Journal of Roentgenology, 146,* 507–512.

Levine, M. S. (1988). Barrett's esophagus: A radiologic diagnosis? *American Journal of Roentgenology, 151,* 433–438.

Levine, M. S., Herman, J. B., & Furth, E. E. (1995). Barrett's esophagus and esophageal adenocarcinoma: The scope of the problem. *Abdominal Imaging 20,* 291–298.

Liedberg, B., & Owall, B. (1991). Masticatory ability in experimentally induced xerostomia. *Dysphagia, 6,* 211–213.

Linden, P., Kuhlemeier, K., & Patterson, C. (1993). The probability of correctly predicting subglottic penetration from clinical observations. *Dysphagia, 8*(3), 170–179.

Logemann, J. A. (1983). *Evaluation and treatment of swallowing disorders*. San Diego: College-Hill Press.

Logemann, J. A. (1993). *Manual for the videofluorographic study of Swallowing* (2nd ed.). Austin, TX: Pro-Ed.

Logemann, J. A., Kahrilas, P. J., Begelman, J., Dodds, W. J., & Pauloski, B. R. (1989). Interactive computer program for biomechanical analysis of videoradiographic studies of swallowing. *American Journal of Roentgenology, 153*, 277–280.

Logemann, J. A., Sisson, G. A., & Wheeler, R. (1980). The team approach to rehabilitation of surgically treated oral cancer patients. In *Proceedings of the National Forum on Cancer Rehabilitation*, Williamsburg, VA:

Mansson, I., & Sandberg, N. (1975). Salivary stimulus and swallowing reflex in man. *Acta Otolaryngologica, 79*, 445–450.

Mehran, A., Richards, D., Dent, J., Waterfall, W. E., & Stevenson, G. W. (1989). The effect of glucagon on esophageal peristalsis and clearance. *Gastrointestinal Radiology, 14*, 100–102.

Mendl, K., McKay, J. M., & Tanner, C. H. (1960). Intramural diverticulosis of the esophagus and Rokitansky-Aschoff sinuses in the gall-bladder. *British Journal of Radiology, 33*, 496–501.

Mitros, F. A. (1988). *Atlas of gastrointestinal pathology* (Chap 2, p. 2.2). Philadelphia, Lippincott

Mosher, H. P. (1927). X-ray study of movements of the tongue, epiglottis and hyoid bone in swallowing, followed by a discussion of difficulty in swallowing caused by retropharyngeal diverticulum, postcricoid webs and exostoses of cervical vertebrae. *Laryngoscope, 37*(4), 235–262.

Meyers, C., Durkin, M. G., & Love, L. (1975). Radiographic findings in herpetic esophagitis. *Radiology 119*, 21–22.

Ott, D. J., & Gelfand, D. W. (1978). Esophageal stricture secondary to candidiasis. *Gastrointestinal Radiology, 2*, 323–325.

Otto, D. J., Chen, Y. M., & Gelfand, D. W. (1989). Effect of hiatal hernia, reflux esophagitis, and glucagon on the quality of double contrast esophagogram. *Gastrointestinal Radiology, 14*, 97–99.

Perlman, A. L., Booth, B. M., & Grayhack, J. P. (1994). Videofluoroscopic predictors of aspiration in patients with oropharyngeal dysphagia. *Dysphagia, 9*, 90–95.

Perlman, A. L., Grayhack, J. P., & Booth, B. M. (1992). The relationship of vallecular residue to oral involvement, reduced hyoid elevation, and epiglottic function. *Journal of Speech and Hearing Research, 35*, 734–741.

Perlman, A. L., & VanDaele, D. J. (1993). Simultaneous videoendoscopic and ultrasound measures of swallowing. *Journal of Medical Speech-Language Pathology, 1*(4), 223–232.

Perlman, A. L., VanDaele, D. J., & Otterbacher, M. (1995). Quantitative assessment of hyoid bone displacement from video images during swallowing. *Journal of Speech and Hearing Research, 38*, 579–585.

Rademaker, A. W., Logemann, J. A., Pauloski, B. R., Bowman, J. B., Lazarus, C. L., Sisson, G. A., Milianti, F. J., Graner, D., Cook, B. S., Collins, S. L., Stein, D. W., Beery, Q. C., Johnson, J. T., & Baker, T. M. (1993). Recovery of postoperative swallowing in patients undergoing partial laryngectomy. *Head and Neck, 15*, 325–334.

Rosenbek, J. C., Wertz, R. T., & Darley, F. L. (1973). Oral sensation and perception in apraxia of speech and aphasia. *Journal of Speech and Hearing Research, 16*, 22–36.

Semenkovich, J. W., Balfe, D. M., Weyman, P. J., Heiken, J. P. & Lee, J. K. T., (1985). Barium pharyngography: Comparison of single and double contrast. *American Journal of Roentgenology, 144*, 715–720.

Sharon, P., Greene, M. L., & Rachmilewitz, D. (1978). Esophageal involvement in bullous pemphigoid. *Gastrointestinal Endoscopy, 24*, 122–123.

Shortsleeve, M. J. & Levine, M. S. (1992). Herpes esophagitis in otherwise healthy patients: Clinical and radiographic findings. *Radiology, 182*, 859–861.

Sitzmann, J. V. (1990). Nutritional support of the dysphagic patient: Methods, risks, and complications of therapy. *Journal of Parenteral and Enteral Nutrition, 14*(1), 60–63.

Schneider, R. (1976). Tuberculous esophagitis. *Gastrointestinal Radiology, 1*, 143–145.

Schuford, W. H., Sybers, R. G., Gordon, I. J., Baron, M. G., & Carson, G. C. (1986). Circumflex retroesophageal right aortic arch simulating mediastinal tumor or dissecting aneurysm, *American Journal of Roentgenology, 146*, 491–496.

Sonies, B., Ship, J., & Baum, B. (1989). Relationship between saliva production and oropharyngeal swallow in healthy, different-aged adults. *Dysphagia, 4*, 85–89.

Splaingard, M. L., Hutchins, B., Sulton, L. D., & Chaundhuri, G. (1988). Aspiration in rehabilitation patients: Videofluoroscopy vs bedside clinical assessment. *Archives of Physical Medicine and Rehabilitation, 69*, 637–640.

Stroudley, J., & Walsh, M. (1991). Radiological assessment of dysphagia in Parkinson's disease. *The British Journal of Radiology, 64*, 890–893.

Taylor, A. J., Dodds, W. J., & Steward, E.T. (1991). Pharynx: Value of oblique projections for radiographic examination, *Radiology, 178*, 59–61.

Teixidor, H. S., Honig, C. L., Norsoph, E., Albert, S., Mouradian, J. A., & Whalen, J. P. (1987). Cytomegalovirus infection of the alimentary canal: Radiologic findings with pathologic correlation. *Radiology, 163*, 317–323.

Thompson, J. K., Koehler, R. E., & Richter, J. E. (1994). Detection of gastroesophageal reflux: Value of barium studies compared with 24-hr pH monitoring. *American Journal of Roentgenology, 162,* 621–626.

Tracy, J. F., Logemann, J. A., Kahrilas, P. J., Jacob, P., Kobara, M., & Krugler, C. (1989). Preliminary observations on the effects of age on oropharyngeal deglutition. *Dysphagia, 4,* 90–94.

Valadka, A. B., Kubal, W. S., & Smith, M. M. (1995). Updated management strategy for patients with cervical osteophytic dysphagia. *Dysphagia, 10,* 167–171.

VanDaele, D. J., Perlman, A. L., & Cassell, M. (1995). Contributions of the lateral hyoepiglottic ligaments to the mechanism of epiglottic downfolding. *Journal of Anatomy, 186,* 1–15.

Wall, S. D., & Jones, B. (1992). Gastrointestinal tract in the immunocompromised host: Opportunistic infections and other complications. *Radiology, 185,* 327–335.

Weaver, G. A. (1979). Upper esophageal web due to a ring formed by a squamocolumnar junction with ectopic gastric mucosa (another explanation of the Paterson-Kelly, Plummer-Vinson syndrome). *Digestive Diseases and Sciences, 24,* 959–963.

Weinstein, G., Perlman, A., & Jones, D. (1990). *Analysis of phonation and deglutition following supracricoid laryngectomy.* Paper presented to the American Academy of Otolaryngology—Head and Neck Surgery, San Francisco.

Wilcox, C. M., & Schwartz, D. A. (1992). A pilot study of oral corticosteroid therapy of idiopathic esophageal ulcerations associated with human immunideficiency virus infection. *American Journal of Medicine, 93,* 131–133.

Williams, S. M., May, C., Krause, D. W., & Harned, R. K. (1987). Symptomatic congenital ectopic gastric mucosa in the upper esophagus. *American Journal of Roentgenology, 148,* 147–148.

Yoshinaka, H., Shimazu, H., Fukumoto, T., & Baba, M. (1991). Superficial esophageal carcinoma: A clinicopathological review of 59 cases. *The American Journal of Gastroenterology, 86,* 1413–1418.

Zerhouni, E. A., Bosma, J. F., & Donner, M. W. (1987). Relationship of cervical spine disorders to dysphagia. *Dysphagia, 1,* 129–144.

7

Examination of the Pharynx and Larynx and Endoscopic Examination of Pharyngeal Swallowing

Susan E. Langmore and Timothy M. McCulloch

The purpose of this chapter is to discuss the techniques of pharyngeal and laryngeal physical examination including the FEES[SM],[1] or Fiberoptic Endoscopic Evaluation of Swallowing, procedure in the assessment of patients with swallowing complaints (Langmore, Schatz, & Olsen, 1988). The authors will also define the role of FEES[SM] relative to other techniques of swallow evaluation. The examination as we describe it in this chapter begins with the standard examination of the oral cavity, nasopharynx, oropharynx, hypopharynx, and larynx utilizing direct visualization and hand mirrors, then proceeds to the endoscopic examination of structure and function, and ends with a direct assessment of swallowing itself.

The diagnostic approach to the patient with swallowing complaints is going to vary greatly from situation to situation. However, if the complaints involve the oral and/or pharyngeal phase of swallowing, useful information will come from an examination of the structure and function of the upper aerodigestive tract. Oftentimes the cause of the dysphagia will be obvious from the medical history, in which case the examination is not used to establish a medical diagnosis but to document and confirm the diagnosis as well as describe the pathophysiology. The examination sets the stage for treatment recommendations and follow-up planning. Treatment plans are oftentimes formulated after consultation with a variety of involved clinicians, the patient, and family members. Good documentation of the physical findings and results of therapeutic interventions will be helpful in the conference setting. Videotape recordings of the examination and still photos or illustrations of pathology are exceptionally helpful.

---

[1]FEES[SM] is a service mark of Susan E. Langmore, Ph.D.

THE EXAMINATION OF THE ORAL CAVITY, PHARYNX AND LARYNX (NONENDOSCOPIC)

A complete physical examination of patients with oropharyngeal dysphagia is often essential for making diagnostic and treatment decisions. Also, significant diagnostic information is obtained through the patient history. This has been outlined in other chapters, and needs to be emphasized here. Before the examination a complete patient history is required. Many patients will be examined in a clinical setting sitting in an exam chair. However, with the use of a headlight, the exam can be easily carried out at the patient's bedside.

Equipment and Patient Preparation

The equipment required to complete this examination is fairly minimal (Table 7–1). The primary need is the light source to illuminate the oral cavity and pharynx. Traditionally a head mirror is used to reflect light from a primary source placed behind the patients head (Figure 7–1). A headlight may be used but has the disadvantage of providing divergent light that cannot be directly focused on the areas of interest.

To carry out this examination the patient needs to be in a sitting position; this is best done using an adjustable examination chair in a clinic setting. The patient may be examined while sitting up in bed; however, this usually requires that the examiner stand, which is a suboptimal examining position.

TABLE 7–1. Equipment Required for Basic Head and Neck Examination.

Examination gloves

Tongue blades

Gauze sponge

Light source (headlight or mirror and external source)

Laryngeal mirrors

Mirror warmer or defogging agent

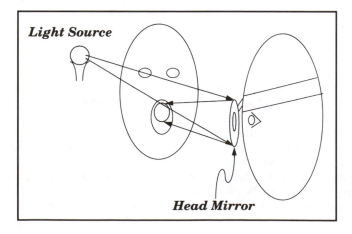

Figure 7–1. The path of light between light source, clinician and patient, when using a head mirror.

The Examination Technique

The patient examination should begin with a general assessment of the patient's condition, for example, is the patient awake, alert, and ambulatory or bedridden and dyspneic? Conversation with the patient may also identify a dysarthria, for example, nasal, breathy, harsh, or slurred speech which may be the sign of a nervous system or neuromuscular disorder.

Oral Cavity and Oropharynx

The directed examination begins at the oral cavity. The general rule is that all mucosal surfaces should be examined and all abnormalities documented. The role of the clinician is to determine abnormalities along the course of the bolus path which starts at the oral commissure. Important elements of the oral cavity exam include testing sensation along the distribution of the mental and lingual nerves as well as testing for facial and hypoglossal nerve function by evaluating strength of lip closure and tongue motion. The oral cavity itself should be evaluated for appropriate saliva production, the condition of the natural teeth, and/or appropriate fit and use of dentures or partials. Evidence of tongue fasciculations, atrophy, or weakness may point toward cranial nerve abnormalities.

Silent tongue-base lesions may became evident with palpation of the tongue. Tongue palpation is done with a gloved finger placed in the oral cavity. Slowly moving from anterior to posterior decreases the risk of gagging the patient. Bimanual palpation is possible by placing the second hand under the patients chin and neck. The tongue base may be palpated only briefly in the neurologically intact patient, as the gag reflex will be stimulated.

Tonsillar pillar sensation and function of the palate elevators can be checked during the oral cavity exam by a gentle palpation with a tongue depressor and mirror while asking the patient to phonate. Superior pharyngeal constrictor muscle contraction can be seen in some patients along the posterior pharyngeal wall during a gentle gag. As a general rule sensation is not tested directly until the final stage of the examination as the patient may become overly sensitive making visualization difficult (Figure 7–2).

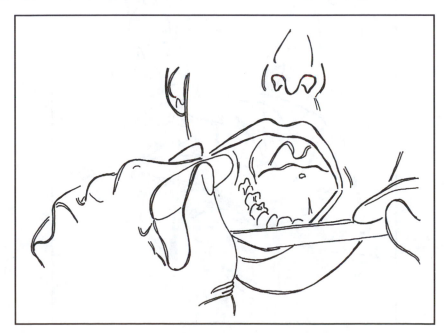

Figure 7–2. The oral cavity examination.

Pharynx and Larynx

Once the oral cavity has been examined, the hypopharynx and larynx can be evaluated. This examination requires hand-held mirrors and a head mirror or headlight. The hand-held mirrors allow well-illuminated visualization of the tongue base, pyriform sinuses, and larynx, providing panoramic views of these structures. Attempts should be made to examine patients with a mirror before proceeding to the flexible laryngoscope. In general this is felt to be a difficult examination to master and patients will vary with regard to tolerance of the procedure.

The mirror examination begins by positioning the patient such that the posterior pharynx is in view and well illuminated. The patients tongue tip is grasped with a gauze sponge, using the examiners nondominant hand and gently retracted from the mouth. The mirror is warmed and then placed in the oropharynx at the level of the uvula, providing a reflected view of the hypopharynx and tongue base (Figure 7–3). The patient is then asked to produce a gentle phonation, "ee," which brings the larynx into view. Abnormalities to be inspected include vocal fold paralysis, pyriform sinus and supraglottic masses, or lesions and inflammation from infection or gastroesophageal reflux. Vocal fold paralysis can be found in patients without voice complaints. Poor palate and tongue control, severely depressed gag reflex, and pyriform sinus pooling are often seen in a patient after a stroke. Once this portion of the exam has been completed, progression to flexible nasopharyngoscopy is appropriate.

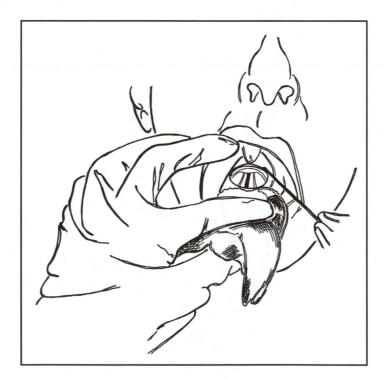

Figure 7–3. The hand–held mirror examination.

THE FLEXIBLE ENDOSCOPIC EXAMINATION

Equipment and Patient Preparation

The minimal equipment requirements are a flexible nasopharyngolaryngoscope and a portable light source. While this equipment is sufficient for the static part of the exam, it is not adequate for the dynamic portion because the pharyngeal swallow occurs rapidly and much information will be missed. Therefore, we highly recommend a chip camera, videotape recorder, and monitor. Some clinicians have added a video timer and video printer to this package. All of the equipment needs to fit on a cart that can be rolled to the bedside or be stationed in the clinic where outpatients are seen for the exam. In the latter case, a good examining chair that adjusts in height and provides a head rest is recommended. Figure 7–4 illustrates the components of the fiberoptic scope, the connection to a light source, and the various controls. In Figure 7–5, an entire FEES[SM] set-up is shown, mounted on a cart. Table 7–2 lists the complete equipment needs for a flexible endoscopic examination.

The scope is prepared by adjusting the brightness of the light source, checking

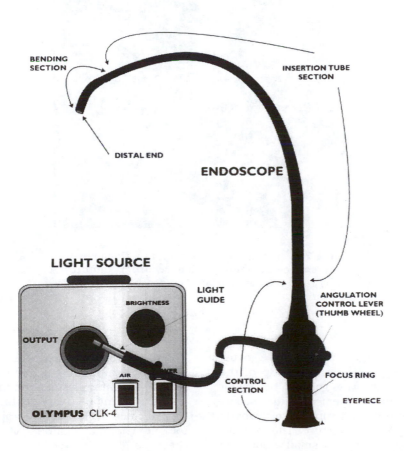

Figure 7–4. The components of a flexible nasopharyngolaryngoscope and light source.

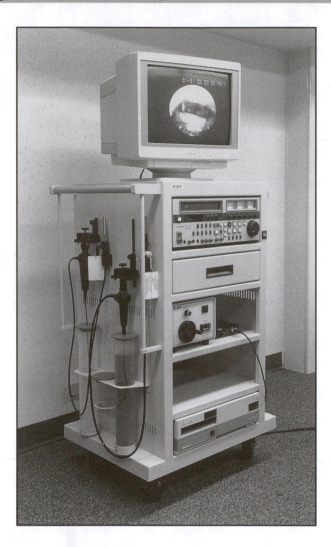

Figure 7–5. A complete FEES^{SM} set-up with endoscope, light source, camera, video recorder, monitor, timer/frame counter, and video printer. (Courtesy of Kay Elemetrics.)

the image clarity by adjusting the focus, and checking the lens at the tip of the scope. If the camera is going to be used it is attached to the eyepiece of the scope, white balanced, and rotated to properly orient the projected picture. The examiner may want to apply a small amount of defogging agent to the lens and a small amount of lubricant to the distal region of the scope (viscous lidocaine or Surgilube).

Prior to inserting the endoscope, a non-fiberoptic examination of the nasal cavity is done, and if no lesions are identified, a small amount of decongestant and/or topical anesthesia may be applied (Pontocaine 1% or Lidocaine 2%). The anesthesia is given in the form of a viscous solution delivered by a cotton-tipped applicator or gauze pad to the nares which will be entered. A brief period of time is

TABLE 7–2. List of equipment needed for a flexible endoscopic examination.

Flexible fiberoptic nasopharyngolaryngoscope
3.6-mm diameter or smaller for infants, 26 cm working length, 85 degree field of view, and angulation of 130 degrees /130 degrees up/down.)

Endoscopic video camera
Light-weight; attached to the endoscope.

Light source
Halogen tends to reflect light differently and results in a slightly bluish picture. Xenon reflects more accurately and is preferred but is considerably more expensive.

Videotape recorder
Super-VHS will give greater resolution. It is important to purchase a unit that can still a single frame without flicker or tracking problems. It is also important to acquire a deck capable of frame-by-frame advance during slow playback mode. There are light weight units available which are very portable.

Color monitor
We recommend a 13-inch color monitor or larger because the larger the monitor the better the view during the examination. Do not purchase a consumer grade TV set. It is suggested that you purchase a video monitor that has BNC cable connectors on the rear panel.

Time character generator
This unit will generate the date and frame number or milliseconds on the screen.

Video printer
Provides the user with the ability to print stilled images from the screen. This may be an essential component for those needing graphic documentation for reimbursement.

---

allowed for the topical agents to work, generally 5 minutes. This method of delivering anesthesia maintains sensation in the pharynx, which is critical for normal swallowing function. Afferent neural signals carried from tactile and chemoreceptors beneath the mucosa are vital for triggering a normal threshold for the motor response of swallowing.

Endoscopic Examination Technique

As with the direct and mirror examinations, no structure visualized should be ignored. The flexible scope allows visualization of portions of the nasal cavity, the entire nasopharynx, the oropharynx, the larynx, and hypopharynx. This does not include any portion of the esophagus or significant portions of the trachea.

Assessment of Structures

The examination begins by positioning the tip of the scope in the patient's nasal vestibule and then visualizing the anterior nasal anatomy through the scope (Figure 7–6). Both nasal passages are briefly examined and then the scope is passed through the nasal passage identified as most widely patent. For patient comfort, the ideal location for scope passage is along the floor of the nose, between the septum and the inferior turbinate. Occasionally, it is necessary to pass the scope above the inferior turbinate and below the middle turbinate. This area is more sensitive and therefore less tolerated by patients. The nasal cavity is a common site to manifest signs of infection and allergy (rhinosinusitis, viral papilloma, allergic edema, and nasal polyposis). When the scope has passed the turbinates, the velum and other structures comprising the nasopharynx will be visible (Figure 7–7). The nasopharynx is assessed for adenoid enlargement, cysts, ulcers, and masses.

The first view of the oropharynx occurs as the scope is rotated down just behind the soft palate as the patient breathes

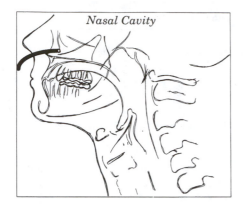

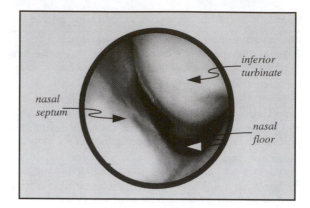

Figure 7–6. Anterior nasal cavity. (Left) location of endoscope, (right) endoscopic view.

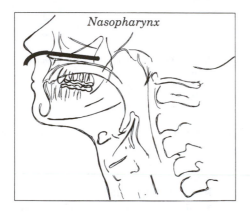

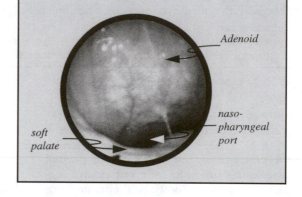

Figure 7–7. Endoscopic view of nasopharynx. velum to the bottom. Nasopharyngeal sphinc-ter slightly open. (Left) location of endoscope, (right) endoscopic view.

quietly through the nose. This allows for close visualization of the tongue base, the palatine tonsils, and the posterior pharyngeal wall. Advancing the scope further, the entire hypopharynx should be examined carefully, as silent tumors of the oro- and hypopharynx are often found in the tongue base, tonsils, epiglottis, posterior pharynx, and pyriform sinuses (Figure 7–8).

The endoscope is then advanced to a point within the laryngeal vestibule as shown in Figure 7–9, where a detailed inspection of the larynx can be made. The laryngeal surface of the epiglottis, true and false vocal folds, and aryepiglottic folds are all examined. Any evidence of mucosal lesions, edema, erythema, or gross asymmetry should be documented. The pyriform sinuses should be viewed by rotating the scope slightly to the right and left. If the patient is asked to blow out his cheeks, the pyriform sinuses will be expanded, improving the view of mucosal surfaces. The esophageal inlet is not visualized with a flexible nasopharyngoscope. The posterior hypopharynx, however, should be viewed. During all parts of the examination, the status of the mucosa is of great importance; one looks not only for

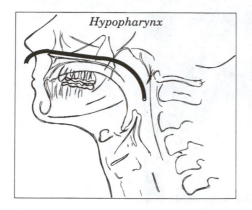

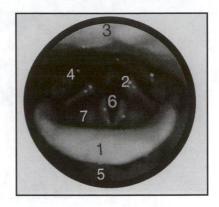

Figure 7–8. The hypopharynx. (Left) location of endoscope, (right) endoscopic view. 1, epiglottis; 2, arytenoid;, 3, posterior pharyngeal wall; 4, pyriform sinus; 5, base of tongue; 6, subglottic shelf; 7, false vocal fold.

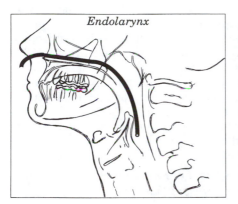

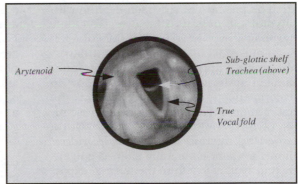

Figure 7–9. The endolarynx. View of true vocal folds, false vocal folds, arytenoids, and subglottic shelf containing the thyroid and cricoid cartilages and cartilaginous edge of the cricoid cartilage. (Left) location of endoscope, (right) endoscopic view.

mucosal lesions but also, edema, atrophy, erythema, excessive secretions, or dryness.

Although this portion of the endoscopic examination does not assess swallowing directly, it gives the examiner important information about the patient's anatomy that may directly impact his or her ability to swallow. Anatomic abnormalities caused by congenital defects, intubation trauma, radiation therapy, neurologic insult, or surgical resection can be a primary cause of dysphagia. For example, an edematous epiglottis and/or arytenoids will not be as mobile or as sensitive as normal structures and, during swallowing, they may not be able to move sufficiently to cover the glottis and protect the airway (see Figure 7–10).

While abnormal anatomy is an obvious cause of dysphagia, it is also true that normal variations in anatomy may be a secondary cause of dysphagia. In a healthy state, people can function adequately with almost any variant of nor-

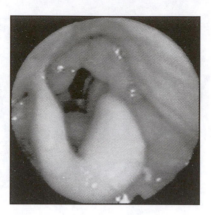

Figure 7–10. Edematous laryngeal structures.

mal. In a compromised state, however, such as poststroke, a person dealing with physiologic deficits that directly cause dysphagia may have further difficulties if he or she must also deal with an unfavorable, albeit normal, anatomy. This anatomical state may cause the swallow to decompensate sooner than if he or she had a more favorable anatomy. An example of this would be an epiglottis with a curled tip, resting on the tongue, rather than the more commonly shaped epiglottis that rests away from the tongue, exposing the vallecular recesses (see Figure 7–11). In a normal state, a person with this anatomy would unconsciously learn to trigger the pharyngeal swallow *before* the bolus reached the epiglottis, which in this case would function like a trough, directing the bolus into the laryngeal vestibule and down to the anterior commissure. After neurologic damage, this same person with dysphagia may have difficulty initiating the swallow and be unable to prevent spillage of the bolus into the hypopharynx. Because of the shape of the epiglottis, a minor amount of spillage that would pool in the valleculae in most persons would result in frequent laryngeal penetration and aspiration in this unfortunate person.

Another common example of a patient with altered anatomy is the patient who is treated for cancer of the epiglottis with a supraglottic laryngectomy. This procedure will significantly modify laryngopharyngeal anatomy postoperatively. This greatly increases the patient's risk for aspiration during the postoperative period and, in some cases, for extended periods of time after surgery. Figure 7–12 shows a typical example of anatomy after supraglottic laryngectomy.

Assessment of Pharyngeal and Laryngeal Function

The goal of this portion of the endoscopic examination is to assess the physiologic functioning of the muscle groups used in swallowing. While many of the tasks are indirect, that is, they do not look directly at swallowing, they reveal underlying competence of the muscle groups of interest, and therefore, are useful for understanding a particular pattern of dysphagia.

When the endoscope is within the nasal cavity, soft palate function can be briefly evaluated by having the patient phonate, whistle, or dry swallow. A dry swallow (or bolus swallow), when seen spontaneously or performed on request, should result in maximal elevation of the velum. At the velopharyngeal port, contribution of lateral and posterior pharyngeal wall movement to this sphincteric closure can also be assessed.

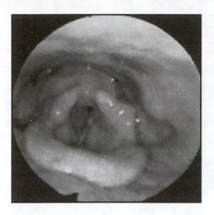

Figure 7–11. Curled-tip epiglottis, obliterating much of the vallecular space.

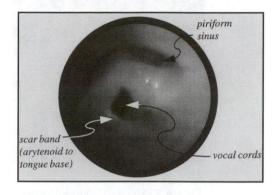

Figure 7–12. Anatomy after supraglottic laryngectomy

Once the endoscope is passed to the oropharynx, the examiner has a view of all the pharyngeal and laryngeal structures involved in swallowing. This vantage point is ideal for observing tongue base movement and symmetry with a repetitive speech task such as *kuh-kuh-kuh* vs. *kee-kee-kee*. An assessment of middle and inferior pharyngeal constrictor movement, necessary for pharyngeal-clearance of the bolus, can be elicited by asking the patient to produce a high-pitched, very tight *ee* or by grunting with much effort (Bastian, 1993).

By lowering the endoscope to a point within the laryngeal vestibule, the examiner can assess laryngeal function in greater detail, especially for respiration and airway protection, which are directly related to swallowing. Laryngeal activity during respiration is observed for symmetry, range, and rate of movement. Just before and during inhalation, the vocal folds and arytenoids open slightly, while during exhalation, the glottis narrows. Exaggerated movement is sometimes seen in neurologic disease or pulmonary disease. A rapid breathing rate, especially common in chronic obstructive pulmonary disease, is a possible predictor of difficulty in coordinating breathing and swallowing, especially as the patient becomes fatigued.

Maximal vocal fold abduction (a function of the posterior cricoarytenoid muscle) can be elicited by asking the patient to sniff or inhale deeply. Maximal vocal fold adduction (most other intrinsic muscles) will be seen by having the patient hold the breath, clear the throat, cough, or vocalize. The examiner should look for movement of the true and false vocal folds as well as observe the extent of arytenoid medial and anterior movement. During swallowing, it is critical that the glottis be closed and an impression of the adequacy and briskness of the closure is gained from observing movements during these non-swallowing tasks. It is sometimes possible to assess this movement at the onset of a swallow, but before maximum closure is attained, the view is usually blocked.

Normal breath-holding does not always result in vocal fold adduction, even in normals. By asking the patient to hold the breath tightly, at the level of the throat, or to bear down as if having a bowel movement (the Valsalva maneuver), he or she may produce more effective adductory vocal fold movements and should recruit additional ventricular fold contraction, arytenoid medial/anterior movement, and bulging of the petiole of the epiglottis. Figure 7–13 shows two views of normal breath-holding: in the left photo, the true vocal folds are

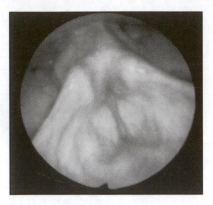 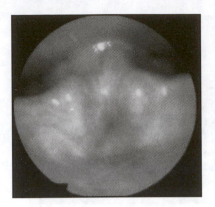

Figure 7–13. (Left) normal breath–holding, with true vocal folds adducted. (Right) tight breath-holding, with true and false vocal folds adducted, arytenoids contacting medially and tilted anteriorly, and petiole of epiglottis bulging.

adducted, whereas in the right, the breath is being held tightly, producing adduction of both the true and false folds and greater excursion of the arytenoids.

Sustained breath-holding with vocal fold adduction can be assessed by asking the patient to hold the breath to the count of 7 or to sustain phonation for several seconds. If the patient has difficulty sustaining breath-holding, the examiner may anticipate a problem during swallowing if the patient needs to protect the airway for several seconds before the swallow or after the swallow.

Asymmetry of movement should also be noted during these tasks and the examiner should look for subtle clues of undiagnosed vocal fold paresis or paralysis. Incomplete movement of the affected vocal fold will reveal recurrent laryngeal nerve damage. This can occur following surgical procedures in the skull base, neck, or chest (secondary to masses or malignancy), from trauma anywhere along the course of the vagus nerve, or post-cerebral vascular accident (Figure 7–14).

Superior laryngeal nerve damage may be revealed most easily during phonation tasks. When the patient glides upward in pitch, the posterior commissure will cant or tilt to the affected side. Pharyngeal and laryngeal sensation on the affected side will also be depressed, and this will impair swallowing as well.

More generalized neurologic damage, including upper motor neuron involvement, will manifest as a generalized weakness on the affected side. The vocal folds may move asymmetrically and the epiglottis may tilt to one side.

The physiologic assessment of pharyngeal/laryngeal competence can reveal many abnormal findings that will help to explain problems the patient may encounter when swallowing food and liquid. For example, vocal fold paresis or paralysis will reduce glottic closure, which in turn affects swallowing pressure gradients, airway protection and cough. Tasks the patient is asked to perform during this part of the exam can also reveal strengths and weaknesses relevant to the consideration of behavioral techniques designed to improve the swallow. For example, if the patient has difficulty producing or sustaining good airway closure, the "supraglottic" swallow technique may not be an effective maneuver for the patient to try to utilize, even if this is the indicated technique for his or her swallowing deficit.

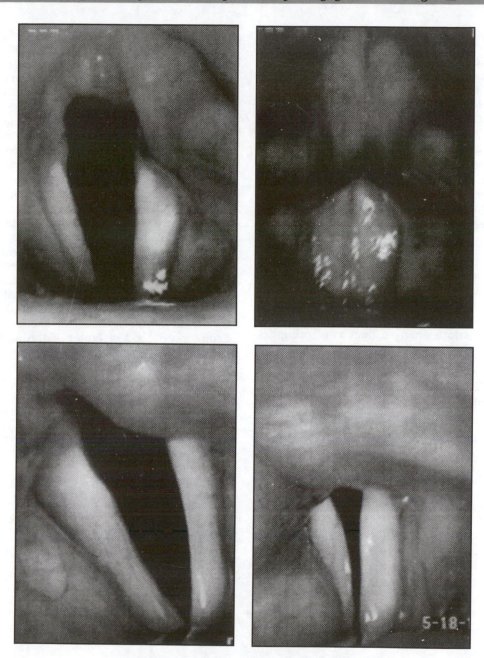

Figure 7–14. Vocal fold paralysis due to recurrent laryngeal nerve damage. (Top left) open, (Right) with phonation compensated with complete closure. (Bottom left) open, (right) with phonation, incomplete closure.

Assessment of Secretions and Sensation

The presence of excess secretions in the valleculae and/or pyriforms, within the laryngeal vestibule, or passing beneath the glottis are important clues to a dysfunctional swallow. When this is found, concerns about aspiration should be raised. The significance of retained secretions in the hypopharynx as a predictor of aspiration of a food bolus was demonstrated by Murray, Langmore, Ginsberg, and Dostie (1996). These investigators developed a secretions retention rating scale as follows:

0—Normal rating. No visible secretions anywhere in the hypopharynx or some transient bubbles visible in the valleculae and pyriform sinuses. The secretions are not bilateral or deeply pooled.

1—Any secretions evident in the channels surrounding the laryngeal vestibule, including the pyriform or vallecular recesses, that are bilaterally or deeply pooled. This rating is also used when the amount of pooled secretions changed from a "0" rating to a "1" rating over a period of time.

2—Any secretions that changed from a "1" rating to a "3" rating during the observation period.

3—Most severe rating. Any secretions seen in the area defined as the laryngeal vestibule. Pulmonary secretions are included if they are not cleared by swallowing or coughing by the close of the observation segment.

In Figure 7–15, an example of excess secretions that would be rated as "3" is illustrated.

In this study by Murray and colleagues, 47 patients with a variety of medical diagnoses and 17 normal controls were given a FEES^SM exam, which included an assessment of standing secretions. Table 7–3 shows the secretions rating given to the hospitalized patients and the percentage who subsequently aspirated food or liquid in the later part of the examination. As can be seen, the probability of food or liquid aspiration increased significantly as the secretions rating increased. (Fisher's exact test $p < .001$). Thus, the finding of excess secretions that are not readily cleared should serve as a red flag for the examiner, signaling the likelihood of aspiration of food or liquid. If the patient cannot tolerate aspiration, the examiner may decide not to present any boluses other than ice chips or a small sip of ice water. In addition to noting their presence, the examiner should note the patient's reaction to any excess secretions, his or her ability to clear the secretions with dry swallows or throat clearing, and the frequency of spontaneous swallowing.

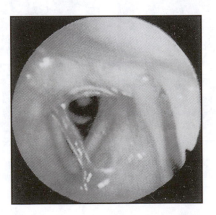

Figure 7–15. Excess secretions in the laryngeal vestibule, some passing below the glottis. Score of 3 (see text)

TABLE 7–3. Scaled Secretions Ratings and Aspiration of Food or Liquid.

Secretions Rating	Number of Subjects With Rating	Number Who Aspirated
0	14	3 (21%)
1	15	8 (53%)
2	5	5 (100%)
3	13	13 (100%)

Source: Adapted from The Significance of Accumulated Oropharyngeal Secretions and Swallowing Frequency in Predicting Aspiration by J. Murray, S. E. Langmore, S. Ginsburg, & A. Dostie, 1995. *Dysphagia..*

Pharyngeal/laryngeal sensation can be indirectly assessed throughout this examination from various behaviors displayed by the patient. For example, whenever the endoscope accidentally touches a struc-ture, the patient should feel this stimulation. Absence of response to the presence of the endoscope and/or absence of response to excess secretions in the laryngeal vestibule also suggest hypoasthesia. Later in the examination, when food and liquid are presented, the patient's response to residue, penetration, or aspiration are also clues to the intactness of sensation. It is important to realize that sensation can be impaired for several reasons, many of which are poorly understood or difficult to isolate. Peripheral nerve involvement of the glossopharyngeal (CN IX) or superior laryngeal (CN X) nerves can directly impair sensation. More commonly, with the nonsurgical patient, the hypoasthesia seems due to reduced cortical or thalamic appreciation of sensation in this region, or may be due to neural accommodation to an habitual stimulus in the region. Aging has also been found to increase sensory thresholds and lengthen response time to a sensory stimulus. For example, the threshold for eliciting the protective laryngeal response of the larynx (adductory response) to chemical stimulation is elevated in the elderly (Pontoppidan & Beecher, 1960). Also, the volume of water needed to elicit a pharyngeal swallow is elevated in the elderly (Shaker et al., 1994).

Sensation can be directly assessed by lightly touching the pharyngeal walls, the base of tongue, or the epiglottis with the tip of the scope. Because this part of the exam can be uncomfortable for the patient who is fully sensate, it may be prudent to postpone sensory testing until the end of the entire FEES[SM] exam, just before removing the endoscope.

Assessment of Swallowing of Food and Liquid

For many years, clinicians have inferred swallowing ability from their findings on a traditional endoscopic exam. For example, if laryngeal airway protection is impaired, the physician will often assume that swallowing is also compromised. With the examination we describe here, these assumptions can be directly tested in the same examination by delivering food and liquid and observing swallowing function. The delivery of food and liquid is unique to the FEES[SM] swallowing evaluation. This portion calls upon the expertise of the examiner in the area of dysphagia to identify abnormal findings, to interpret the abnormal findings in terms of previously displayed anatomic and physiologic problems, and to apply the appropriate dietary or behavioral changes directly, as problems are identified, in an attempt to reduce aspiration or make the swallow more efficient.

EXAMINATION TECHNIQUE. The protocol for this part of the exam will vary with the needs of the patient. Usually, several different food and liquid consistencies are given to the patient to determine which consistencies are safe to swallow without aspirating, spilling, or leaving excess residue. A representative sample of a thin liquid, pureed, and soft solid food are often tried, followed by particular foods or liquids that are reported to give the patient trouble. The beauty of this procedure is that any real food or liquid can be given, as opposed to barium-laced food or liquid used in the fluoroscopy examination. Bolus sizes should be given in measured amounts so that the safest and most effective bolus size can be determined. If excess secretions were observed in the previous part of the exam, the examiner may decide to approach this part of the examination more conservatively, since aspiration is a strong possibility. With such patients, we recommend preceding any food presentations with ice chips, which if aspirated in small amounts, are not harmful. If these are aspirated consistently, the examiner will probably not proceed to any other consistency.

One goal of the FEES^{SM} exam is to simulate the patient's natural eating environment as much as possible. The examiner should position the patient in whatever posture is typical of his or her feeding environment and then alter this only if it appears to be important for improving the safety of the swallow. It is usually easiest to have a partner feed the patient, as the endoscopist will be occupied with the image from the endoscope.

As soon as swallowing abnormalities are noted, the examiner should make appropriate alterations in the protocol. Although the abnormal findings may ultimately require surgical management (i.e., vocal fold medialization, palatal adhesion), they are more frequently treated with behavioral therapy. These techniques are tried during the assessment procedure itself to determine whether they reduce aspiration and/or improve bolus clearance; if so, they may be implemented as part of the management program.

Many therapeutic alterations can be tried during the FEES^{SM} examination. For example, if a patient spills material into the hypopharynx before initiating the swallow and this material overflows into the laryngeal vestibule, the clinician might alter the bolus consistency or bolus size to determine the effect on the spillage. Alternatively, the clinician may have the patient try a postural change such as chin tuck or head rotation to see if these reduce the tendency of the material to spill. Finally, the clinician might want to assess the effect of various swallowing maneuvers on this abnormal pattern. In this particular case, purposeful breath-holding prior to swallowing might be taught, with the patient turned to face the monitor so that he or she can receive biofeedback regarding the ability to produce quick, effective vocal fold adduction. In a biofeedback mode, the patient might also learn to increase his or her awareness of the spillage sensation by visualizing the spillage event on the monitor and subsequently learning to reduce or eliminate it. This may take a few sessions, but fortunately, the FEES^{SM} procedure can be repeated on a limitless basis to monitor improvement or provide additional therapy.

Before the endoscope is removed and the exam ends, a brief assessment of sensory function should be done if the patient has not reacted to the presence of the endoscope in the hypopharynx and/or has not reacted immediately to aspiration, penetration, or residue by coughing or clearing the throat, and so on. If sensation is normal, the patient will not tolerate a direct probe with the endoscope and will respond by swallowing, coughing, or gagging.

FINDINGS IN THE NORMAL SWALLOW. An endoscopic view of a normal swallow is fairly uninteresting since the bolus may not be seen in the hypopharynx prior to the swallow and there is no residue of material after the swallow. In addition, approximately .09 sec after hyoid elevation begins, white-out of the view will occur for approximately .66 sec, as the lingual, velar, and/or pharyngeal tissues squeeze against the tip of the endoscope and reflect the light. If the endoscope is positioned in the posterior nares during the swallow, velar elevation can be seen. Furthermore, when the scope is positioned within the endolarynx, glottic closure can be visualized at the onset of the swallow (true vocal fold adduction and arytenoid medial and anterior motion) until the view is obliterated.

FINDINGS IN THE ABNORMAL SWALLOW. Abnormal swallowing, on the other hand, will be evidenced by a number of interesting findings. Some of the most common salient abnormal findings are spillage before the swallow, residue after the swallow, laryngeal penetration, and tracheal aspiration.

The most common abnormal finding reported for patients with neurogenic dysphagia is spillage or leakage of the bolus into the pharynx prior to the swallow. This pattern is usually due to a delayed initiation of the swallow. (Horner, Buoyer, Alberts, & Helms, 1991; Horner, Massey, Riski, Lathrop, & Chase, 1988; Veis & Logemann, 1985). On fluoroscopy, swallow initiation is evidenced by laryngeal/pharyngeal elevation, whereas on endoscopy, it is

indicated by epiglottal retroversion and white-out. In normal individuals, the swallow is always triggered before the bolus spills too far, that is, before it spills into the laryngeal vestibule. With endoscopy, the examiner can visually follow the bolus before the swallow occurs as material flows down the base of the tongue and around the laryngeal vestibule. If the spillage is excessive, the bolus may penetrate the borders of the laryngeal vestibule and possibly be aspirated. During a FEES[SM] exam, the examiner should note the vulnerable point of entry into the vestibule, typically over the epiglottis, over the interarytenoid space, or over the aryepiglottic folds where the pharyngo-epiglottic band lies. The clinician should also note the status of airway protection, that is, whether the glottis is open or closed as the material approaches the glottis. This information is not available fluoroscopically and has important therapeutic implications for the examiner. As will be discussed in a later chapter, altering head posture may redirect bolus flow and make the swallow safer.

In Figure 7–16, two examples of liquid spillage are shown. In the first photo, the fluid has spilled to the pyriforms and, as

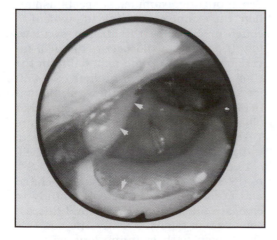 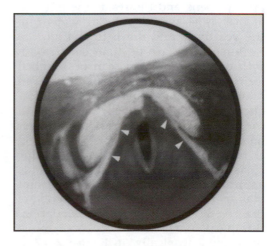

Figure 7–16. Liquid spillage to the pyriforms and on the aryepiglottic folds. (Left) with vocal folds closed and protecting the airway; (right) with vocal folds open, not protecting the airway (image computer-enhanced to improve contrast).

can be seen, the airway is protected by adducted vocal folds. In the second photo, a similar amount of spillage has occurred, but the glottis is open. If the liquid overflows the rim of the vestibule, this patient will likely aspirate.

Residue of material after the swallow is also a very common finding (Horner et al., 1988; Horner et al., 1991; Veis & Logemann, 1985) and suggests a problem with bolus propulsion or clearance. Bolus propulsion forces such as tongue base contact with the pharyngeal wall, pharyngeal constrictor movement, and laryngeal elevation are generally better visualized fluoroscopically. In a FEES[SM] exam, these movements are not directly viewed during swallowing and must be inferred from the previous muscle testing portion of the exam. The onset of hyoid-laryngeal elevation can be inferred from the first phase of epiglottal retroversion and by sudden enlargement of the larynx, but this cannot be quantified. Nonetheless, the result of impaired bolus propulsion forces is residue left in the hypopharynx after the swallow, and this *can* be visualized endoscopically, with much better ability to localize the residue than is possible fluoroscopically. In addition, aspiration of the residue can be observed, either immediately after the swallow as the patient's airway opens and the residue is inhaled, or over time as the material seeps into the vestibule and down to the glottis. Because there are no time constraints with this exam, residue can be watched for a period of several seconds or even minutes to see if it builds up with subsequent bolus presentations, and also how the patient reacts to the residue, whether he or she produces multiple swallows in an attempt to clear it, whether the residue spills into the vestibule, and whether it is aspirated. Because fluoroscopy cannot maintain a view for a prolonged period of time or detect inhalation or exhalation, this particular event is captured much better endoscopically. In Figure 7–17, a view of residue as seen endoscopically is depicted. In this examination, a significant amount of residue of bread and cheese

has remained in the valleculae and a lesser amount throughout the hypopharynx after the swallow.

Laryngeal penetration and tracheal aspiration can be viewed directly unless the event occurs during the period of whiteout. Most events of aspiration will be viewed directly, simply because aspiration is more likely to occur before or after the swallow (Horner et al., 1988; Horner et al., 1991; Veis & Logemann, 1985) and the view is available endoscopically during these periods. Only when laryngeal function is directly impaired by damage to the vagus nerve (e.g., due to a brainstem stroke or surgical complications) is aspiration more likely to occur *during* the swallow (Veis & Logemann, 1985). In these patients, the examiner should be prepared for this possibility after directly testing laryngeal competence earlier in the examination. Of course, with all patients, the examiner must be astute for any signs suggesting aspiration has occurred during the swallow and period of white-out. Usually, this is revealed by residue of material either in the endolarynx, on the folds themselves, or on the subglottic shelf. As a matter of routine, the examiner should pass the endoscope down to view the glottis closely for evidence of aspiration after each swallow. If there is no visual evidence but the examiner suspects aspiration, the examiner can ask the patient to cough or clear the throat after swallowing. If aspiration did occur, this will invariably bring up some material from the trachea. Finally, the examiner can wait for several seconds and then ask the patient to cough again, just to ensure that all aspiration has been detected. In Figure 7–18, aspiration of pureed food is seen, with material resting on the subglottic shelf.

To directly evaluate sensitivity of FEES[SM] to detect aspiration, Langmore, Schatz, and Olson (1991) undertook a study to compare findings of FEES[SM] and fluoroscopy examinations. Twenty-one subjects were given both examinations within a 48-hour period. Their taped studies were scored for presence or absence of salient findings (spillage, residue, penetration,

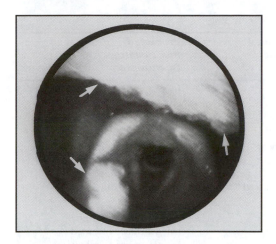

Figure 7–17. Residue of bread and cheese, visible on laryngeal surface of epiglottis on patient's right and along posterior pharyngeal wall (image computer-enhanced to improve contrast).

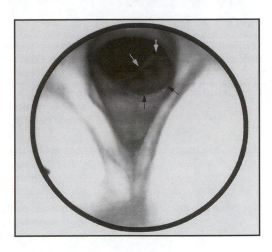

Figure 7–18. Aspiration of pureed food. Residue visible on the subglottic shelf and anterior commissure (image computer-enhanced to improve contrast).

aspiration). Good agreement was found, especially for the finding of aspiration (90% agreement). Sensitivity of FEES[SM] was .88 or greater for all parameters, and specificity was .92 for detection of aspiration and somewhat lower for the other parameters. Thus, the high sensitivity of FEES[SM] for detecting aspiration was confirmed.

Miller, Willging, Strife, and Rudolph (1994) reported on the use of FEES[SM] to assess swallowing in infants and young children, from age 4 months to 6 years. They compared events that were detected by FEES[SM] and by fluoroscopy using a similar protocol as that described by Langmore (1986). Results of the two procedures were similar, with identical findings for aspiration. The authors concluded that there is good agreement between fluoroscopy and FEES[SM] in children

Synthesis of Findings

The astute clinician will approach the FEES[SM] examination much like any diagnostic puzzle, with discovery of abnormal findings leading to predictions that are then confirmed with further testing. One

goal of the examination is to determine the underlying anatomic and physiologic deficits that can explain the nature of the dysphagia and relate to the patient's clinical symptoms. Table 7–4 lists some of the possible relations between clinical symptoms, nonswallowing endoscopic findings, and predicted and possible endoscopic findings for swallowing function.

Several levels of interpretation are possible from a FEES[SM] examination. One can simply identify the salient findings (aspiration, residue, etc.) directly and diagnose dysphagia. However, by relating the salient swallowing findings to the results of the earlier portions of the patient exam and by bringing a knowledge of normal and abnormal swallowing to the examination, an experienced clinician will be able to interpret the findings with regard to the underlying anatomic and physiologic causes. For example, if material spills to the pyriforms after the tongue has stopped its characteristic oral preparatory movements, but before the swallow begins, the examiner's first impression will be spillage, giving evidence of dysphagia. Going one step further, the examiner would interpret

TABLE 7–4. Clinical symptoms and possible endoscopic findings

Clinical Symptom or Patient Complaint	Predicted Anatomic and/or Physiologic Dysfunction	Predicted Swallowing Dysfunction
Hypernasal voice	Incomplete velopharyngeal (v/ph) closure	Incomplete v/ph closure during the swallow; nasal reflux; v/ph residue after the swallow
Hoarse, breathy voice	Incomplete true vocal cord (TVF) adduction; true paralysis of TVF with open glottis; bowed TVFs	Penetration, aspiration before or during the swallow; ineffective cough/clearing
Wet voice quality	Secretions pooling in laryngeal vestibule and being aspirated	Aspiration of food, liquid; residue after the swallow; reduced frequency of swallow
Lack of awareness or reaction to wet voice	No spontaneous clearing of secretions; impaired sensitivity when probed	Reduced awareness or reaction to spillage, penetration, aspiration, or residue
Reduced pitch range	Deviation of posterior commissure; TVF bowed or has inferior displacement; impaired sensitivity when tested	Reduced sensitivity to residue or aspiration to level of glottis
Rapid respiratory rate	Cannot sustain TVF adduction more than a few seconds	No airway protection during spillage; aspiration before, during, or after swallowing, especially with fatigue
Weak cough	Incompetent larynx; inadequate TVF adduction/TVF paralysis; poor sustained breath-holding	Aspiration during swallow; ineffective clearance if aspirates
Complains of food/liquid going wrong way; coughs immediately after swallowing	Incompetent larynx and/or generalized weakness	Aspiration with good sensitivity; spillage before the swallow; residue in vestibule aspirated on inhalation after the swallow
No complaint, but coughs several seconds after swallowing	Reduced sensation to touch of endoscope	Aspiration, with reduced sensitivity; esophageal-pharyngeal reflux
Complains that food sticks in throat	Obstruction, exam; pharyngeal mass or normal pharyngeal good sensation when tested	Incomplete bolus clearance with residue; or normal pharyngeal swallow
Complains of food backing up into throat after the swallow.	Posterior glottic erythema or edema; pyriform secretions; or normal pharyngeal exam.	Esophageal or gastric reflux

this spillage as signifying a delayed initiation of the swallow due to slowed or reduced neural processing somewhere along the swallowing pathway (peripheral and cortical afferent input to the brainstem swallowing center, brain-stem processing of information, efferent transmission along the motor pathway to the appropriate muscles). An astute clinician would then probe to see whether impaired sensation was a causative factor by noting the patient's response to aspiration, residue, or standing secretions in the endolarynx, and possibly by directly testing sensation within the hypopharynx.

Indications and Contraindications for Endoscopy

Indications and Relative Role of FEES

As in other areas of medicine, there is a choice of procedures to select to assess a suspected problem of pharyngeal dysphagia. The most common procedure used currently to evaluate oropharyngeal dysphagia is the fluoroscopic procedure known by various names, including modified barium swallow, videofluoroscopy of swallowing, or the cookie swallow. This procedure was formalized several years ago by Logemann (1986) and has been shown to be sensitive to various swallowing dysfunctions.

The relative merits of the fluoroscopic and endoscopic exam have been debated in the literature (Kidder, T., Langmore, S. and Martin, B, 1994; Langmore, S. & Logemann, J., 1991). Each procedure is valuable and that the decision of which one (or, perhaps, neither) is indicated should be based on many factors, including availability, cost, patient symptoms, and sensitivity of each procedure to the nature of the problem. Sometimes the decision to use endoscopy is based solely on practical, logistic reasons, as, for example, when the patient needs a bedside examination or when an examination is needed that day, or that hour. The practical and logistic reasons for choosing the FEES[SM] exam are outlined in Table 7–5. Other times, both exams are accessible and the examiner must predict which procedure will be more useful clinically. In Table 7–6, the FEES[SM] exam and videofluoroscopy are compared regarding their ability to evaluate the important clinical findings

TABLE 7–5. Practical indications for a FEES[SM] Exam.

Patient is bedridden or extremely weak.

Patient has contractures, is in pain, or has decubitus ulcers.

Patient is quadriplegic and/or has neck halo.

Nursing staff would need to accompany patient.

Patient is in ICU; on monitors, ventilator, multiple tubes.

Patient is demented, confused, fearful.

Need exam that day.

Need repeat exam to assess change (e.g., possible diet change).

Want therapeutic tool for biofeedback or to assess effectiveness of postural maneuver.

Want to assess swallowing potential without needing to give food or liquid orally; risk of aspiration is great.

Concern about excess radiation exposure, especially for young patients.

Concern about cost of fluoroscopy.

Concern about strain on patient if he must be transported to another facility.

Source: Adapted from Indications and Techniques of Endoscopy in Evaluation of Cervical Dysphagia: Comparison with Radiographic Techniques by T. M. Kidder, S. E. Langmore, & B. J. W. Martin, 1994. *Dysphagia, 9,* 256–261.

TABLE 7–6. Clinical findings revealed from endoscopy and fluoroscopy.

Clinical findings better revealed endoscopically:

Airway closure achieved by true vocal fold adduction, false vocal fold adduction, arytenoid medial and anterior movement.

Mobility of arytenoids.

Amount and location of secretions.

Frequency of spontaneous swallowing.

Pharyngeal/laryngeal sensitivity.

Residue buildup.

Aspiration before the swallow.

Aspiration after the swallow.

Coordination of bolus flow and airway protection.

Coordination of breathing and swallowing.

Ability to adduct TVFs to produce supraglottic swallow maneuver.

Ability to sustain adduction of TVFs for several seconds.

Fatigue over a meal, possibly leading to aspiration.

Altered anatomy contributing to dysphagia.

Effectiveness of postural change to alter anatomy and path of bolus flow.

Clinical findings revealed better fluoroscopically:

Tongue control and manipulation of the bolus.

Tongue contact to posterior pharyngeal wall.

Hyoid and laryngeal elevation.

Cricopharyngeal opening.

Airway closure at level of arytenoid to epiglottal contact.

Epiglottic retroversion.

Esophageal clearance.

Aspiration during the swallow.

Ability to produce Mendelsohn maneuver.

Source: Adapted from Indications and Techniques of Endoscopy in Evaluation of Cervical Dysphagia: Comparison with Radiographic Techniques by T. M. Kidder, S. E. Langmore, & B. J. W. Martin, 1994. *Dysphagia, 9*, 256–261.

for dysphagia. Sometimes, if both tools are available, they will both be used for the diagnostic workup.

When used to assess swallowing function, both the fluoroscopy and endoscopy examinations have identical outcomes; that is, both can identify a dysphagia and both purport to explain the pattern of dysphagia. The fluoroscopy examination provides a more comprehensive view of the oral, pharyngeal, and esophageal structures, whereas the endoscopic exam provides a more detailed view of the pharyngeal and laryngeal structures. The strengths of the videofluoroscopy exam are its ability to image the entire swallow event, to evaluate soft tissue and bony motion, and to image events occurring in the oral cavity and at the level of the cricopharyngeus and below. The clinical strengths of the FEES[SM] procedure are its ability to evaluate laryngeal competence and to assess airway closure at the initiation of the swallow or for a therapeutic maneuver, its ability to accurately localize retained materials after the swallow, its ability to relate anatomy to disordered swallowing, and its ability to observe events over a prolonged period of time. Both exams can be used to guide recommendations regarding safety of oral feeding, the appropriate diet for the patient, and the ability of the patient to benefit from various postural or swallowing maneuvers. The advantages of the FEES[SM] for treatment are its availability, its repeatability, and the potential for using it as a biofeedback tool.

If both exams are available and the patient has a previously undiagnosed dysphagia, the fluoroscopy exam may be the procedure of choice for the initial diagnostic study, with the FEES[SM] used for follow-up examinations. If, however, the patient is medically compromised or unstable, a FEES[SM] may be the better initial examination so that a more conservative approach can be taken in assessing the patient's ability to receive any food or liquid by mouth.

Contraindications and Risks of the Endoscopic Examination

There are several well-known risks of endoscopy, which should occur very rarely, if ever, in the hands of an experienced and competent endoscopist. These include the following: nose bleed (epistaxis), mucosal injury, gagging, allergic reaction to the topical anesthesia, laryngospasm, and vasovagal response.

If the endoscopist is careful, all of these risks can be minimized or prevented and patients at risk for these complications can be identified beforehand. Since the examiner has a view at all times, any nose bleed or mucosal injury should be minimal. Gagging is typically a problem with oral (rigid) endoscopy, but not with flexible endoscopy. If the topical anesthesia used for the exam is lidocaine hydrochloride 2% viscous solution and if it is restricted to the nares of the patient, an allergic reaction should rarely occur. If it does, a local reaction would be the most likely outcome (Eyre & Nally, 1971).

In the literature, laryngospasm is reported most often as a postoperative complication when general anesthesia has been used and the patient is being extubated (Staffel, 1991) or by a sudden inflow of refluxed gastric contents (Bortolotti, 1989). Aspiration of food or liquid might also trigger laryngospasm. Patients who have a history of significant aspiration, patients who require supplemental oxygen, and patients with acute mental status depression may be at increased risk if they are functioning on the edge of an "adequate" respiratory status and cannot tolerate the minor laryngo-pulmonary trauma caused by the endoscope, the aspiration that may occur during the exam, or the possible reflux that swallowing may induce. Examinations done with these patients should be done in a highly controlled setting with appropriate equipment and medical personnel standing by.

Finally, vasovagal response, commonly manifested as fainting, is a fairly common event but, on rare occasions, can be dangerous. Vasovagal response can be triggered by a wide range of stimuli or maneuvers, including a Valsalva maneuver (Arnold, Dyer, Gould, Hohberger, & Low, 1991), coughing or defecation, nausea and vomiting, swallowing, or mechanical stimulation of the upper airway with instrumentation (Waddel, 1989). The majority of persons who experience vasovagal responses have a history of fainting under stressful conditions or when hungry, hot, and tired (Kelly, 1991; Kleinknecht, Lenz, Ford, & DeBerard, 1990) and do not suffer any ill effects from this event. Nonetheless, the examiner is well advised to inquire about a history of fainting and to monitor the patient for signs of anxiety; a calm, reassuring manner goes a long way in preventing vasovagal responses in the majority of patients. Patients in whom a vasovagal response can be serious are those with an acute cardiac condition predisposing them to bradycardia or cardiac dysrhythmia (Fitzpatrick, et al., 1991; Van Lieshout, Weiling, Karemaker, & Eckberg, 1991). If they faint, these patients are at some risk of incurring further cardiac damage and should therefore be monitored carefully during the exam. If blood pressure and heart rate/rhythm are monitored as well as the patient's level of anxiety, an impending vasovagal response can usually be identified and prevented. If it does occur, the patient should be positioned in a head down, feet up position. The availability of supplemental oxygen is also recommended. Patients with acute cardiac conditions would need further attention.

In the hospital setting, medical help is always available should any complication arise. In the intensive care unit, where complications are most likely to occur, the patients are already being constantly monitored. In the nursing home setting, however, where many dysphagic patients reside, there is not such a sophisticated back-up system available. For the clinician in this setting, a registered nurse should be present for the exam, perhaps serving as the feeder and assessing the patient for any adverse reactions (monitoring blood pressure or pulse if indicated). Although physicians are not always available in nursing homes, the FEES^SM examination, as described in this chapter, is a very safe procedure.

The unlikely possibility of encountering an adverse reaction with a flexible endoscopic exam needs to be balanced against the daily risks faced by our patients with dysphagia, especially those in institutions. The complications from aspirating are well documented, are much more likely to occur, and are far more serious than any complication that may result from the examination. Better patient care is the best justification for doing FEES^SM and for bringing endoscopy into settings outside the hospital.

SUMMARY

A comprehensive examination of the patient with oropharyngeal dysphagia is essential to diagnosis and treatment planning. Multiple medical disciplines are oftentimes involved in the patient assessment, each with their own expertise. However, in many cases, a complete head and neck examination and a dynamic examination of the swallow are necessary parts of diagnosis and treatment planning. Today, one of the primary tools for evaluation and treatment is the flexible endoscope. Flexible endoscopy is a well-established tool, but it has only recently been applied to the assessment of pharyngeal dysphagia.

As new procedures and techniques for assessing oropharyngeal dysphagia emerge, it is incumbent on the practicing clinician to evaluate their efficacy. Cost savings, timely and efficient service, accurate and sensitive recording, and effective and informative results are some of the factors that need to be considered when assessing a new procedure. FEES^SM is not a replacement for the more comprehensive videofluoroscopy procedure, but it is a better choice for some patients, in some settings, and for revealing certain clinical findings. FEES^SM has expanded and improved our ability to assess and treat patients with dysphagia in a variety of settings.

Acknowledgment: The authors wish to acknowledge Mr. Joseph T. Murray who assisted in the production of figures for this chapter.

MULTIPLE CHOICE QUESTIONS

1. When anesthetizing the patient prior to inserting a flexible endoscope for a FEES^SM exam
   a. it is recommended that only the nares be anesthetized because the taste of the topical anesthesia can be unpleasant and may alter the taste of the food that follows.
   b. a general anesthesia is not necessary, but a sedative may be advisable for agitated patients
   c. it is critical that only the nares be anesthetized so that thresholds for activation of chemo and tactile receptors in the pharynx or larynx are not depressed
   d. a spray consisting of a mixture of anesthesia and decongestant should be squirted into the chosen nostril

e. it is necessary to wait 2 minutes for the anesthesia to take effect

2. Assessment of anatomy in the fiberoptic swallowing examination
   a. is done because it can directly affect swallowing function
   b. may detect a Zenker's diverticulum
   c. is no different from the standard examination done in every otolaryngological examination
   d. is done only with patients referred to otolaryngology.
   e. includes assessment of oral, pharyngeal, and esophageal structures

3. The dynamic examination of pharyngeal/laryngeal activity
   a. is done to reveal problems the patient may be having with phonation
   b. is done with EGG (electroglottography)
   c. can reveal superior laryngeal nerve damage if the affected vocal fold does not adduct for breathholding
   d. can reveal pharyngeal constrictor weakness if there is no visible contraction during breath holding
   e. may reveal inadequate laryngeal closure that could account for aspiration of food and liquid

4. Excess secretions in the laryngeal vestibule are often associated with
   a. hypersalivation
   b. hyposalivation
   c. depressed gag reflex
   d. increased frequency of swallowing
   e. aspiration of food and liquid

5. In the FEES examination, excess residue in the hypopharynx after the swallow
   a. suggests a delayed initiation of the swallow
   b. suggests a weak swallow or obstruction
   c. may fall into the vestibule and be aspirated as the person exhales after the swallow
   d. is not easily seen endoscopically
   e. is normal in the elderly.

REFERENCES

Arnold, R. W., Dyer, J. A., Gould, A. B., Hohberger, G. G., & Low, P. A. (1991). Sensitivity to vasovagal maneuvers in normal children and adults. *Mayo Clinic Proceedings, 66*, 797-804.

Bastian, R. W. (1993). The videoendoscopic swallowing study: An alternative and partner to the videofluoroscopic swallowing study. *Dysphagia, 8*, 359-367.

Bortolotti, M. (1989). Laryngospasm and reflex central apnea caused by aspiration of refluxed gastric contents in adults. *Gut, 30*, 233-238

Eyre, J., & Nally, F. F. (1971). Nasal test for hypersensitivity Including a positive reaction to lignocaine. *The Lancet, 1*, 264-265.

Fitzpatrick, A., Theodrakis, G., Vardas, P., Kenny, R. A., Travill, C. M., Ingram, A., & Sutton, R. (1991). The incidence of malignant vasovagal syndrome in patients with recurrent syncope. *European Heart Journal, 12*, 389-394.

Horner, J., Massey, E. W., Riski, J. E., Lathrop, D. L., & Chase, K. N. (1988). Aspiration following stroke: Clinical correlates and outcome. *Neurology, 38*, 1359-1362.

Horner, J., Buoyer, F. G., Alberts, M. J., & Helms, M. J., (1991). Dysphagia following brain-stem stroke: clinical correlates and outcome. *Archives of Neurology, 48*, 1170-1173.

Kelly, T. J. (1991). Mechanics and treatment of vasovagal syncope. *Patient Care, 62*, 216-218.

Kidder, T. M., Langmore, S. E., & Martin, B. J. W. (1994). Indications and techniques of endoscopy in evaluation of cervical dysphagia: Comparison with radiographic techniques *Dysphagia, 9*, 256-261.

Kleinknecht, R. A., Lenz, J., Ford, G., & DeBerard, S. (1990). Types and correlates of blood/injury-related vasovagal syncope. *Behavioral Research Therapy, 28*, 289-295.

Langmore, S. E., Schatz, K., & Olsen, N. (1988). Fiberoptic endoscopic examination of swallowing safety: A new procedure. *Dysphagia, 2*, 216-219.

Langmore, S. E., Schatz, K., & Olsen, N (1991). Endoscopic and videofluoroscopic evaluations of swallowing and aspiration. *Annals of Otorhinolaryngology, 100*, 678-681.

Langmore, S. E. & Logemann, J. A. (1991) After the clinical bedside swallowing examination: What next? *American Journal of Speech-Language Pathology, 1*, 13-20.

Logemann, J. A. (1986). *Manual for the videofluorographic study of swallowing.* San Diego, CA: College-Hill Press.

Miller, C. K., Willging, J. P., Strife, J. L., Rudolph, C. D. (1994). Fiberoptic endoscopic examination of swallowing in infants and children with feeding disorders. *Dysphagia, 9*, 266.

Murray, J., Langmore, S. E., Ginsberg, S., & Dostie, A. (1996). The significance of accumulated oropharyngeal secretions and swallowing frequency in predicting aspiration. *Dysphagia., 11*, 99–103.

Pontoppidan, H., & Beecher, H.D. (1960). Progressive loss of protective reflexes in the airway with the advance of age. *Journal of the American Medical Association, 174*, 2209–2213.

Sawashima M., & Hirose H. (1968). New laryngoscopic technique by use of fiberoptics. *Journal of the Acoustical Society of America. 43*, 168–169.

Shaker, R., Ren, J., Zamir, Z., Sarna, A., Liu, J., & Zhumei, S. (1994). Effect of aging, position, and temperature on the threshold volume triggering pharyngeal swallows. *Gastroenterology, 107*, 396–402.

Staffel, G. J. (1991). The prevention of postoperative stridor and laryngospasm with topical lidocaine. *Archives of Otolaryngology—Head and Neck Surgery, 117*, 1123–1128.

Van Lieshout, J. J., Weiling, W., Karemaker, J. M., & Eckberg, D. L. (1991). The vasovagal response. *Clinical Science, 81*, 575–586.

Veis, S. J., & Logemann, J. A. (1985). Swallowing disorders in persons with cerebrovascular accidents. *Archives of Physical Medicine and Rehabilitation, 66*, 372–375.

Waddel, S. (1989). Vasovagal syncope. *Critical Care Nurse, 9*, 35–43.

8

Diagnostic Methods to Evaluate Swallowing Other Than Barium Contrast

Bruce P. Brown and Barbara C. Sonies

CHARACTERISTICS OF THE IDEAL METHOD FOR IMAGING SWALLOWING

To obtain the most useful and valid representation of swallowing a diagnostic test should

1. Depict soft tissues, air, fluid-filled cavities, and surrounding bone
2. Produce clear images of functional changes in multiple planes and real time
3. Allow viewing of the entire swallow
4. Be noninvasive and risk-free
5. Detect and quantify aspiration
6. Allow objective and repeatable measurements
7. Estimate prognosis and treatment potential.

No one imaging technique fully satisfies all of these criteria. Videofluoroscopic imaging is the diagnostic standard for evaluation of swallowing. This is because it is readily available, easy to interpret, and has a dynamic, video-based format. However, it has

limitations. Implicit in any radiographic evaluation is prolonged radiographic exposure, thus limiting its usefulness in repeated studies. Videofluoroscopy does not clearly delineate soft tissues; it best visualizes facial and cranial bones, teeth, and soft tissue-air interfaces of the oral cavity. In addition, such studies are not quantitative and require use of unphysiologic radiopaque contrast material.

Esophageal manometry is a common adjunct to fluoroscopy especially in cases of suspected motility disorders. However, this procedure may alter normal patterns of motility because of the need for placement of a manometric tube. Furthermore, pressure measurements do not display structures and are only one component of the physiology of the swallow.

Additional techniques can be used to evaluate portions of the oropharynx and esophagus that may be ill-defined with standard methods. These include ultrasound, scintigraphy, computed tomography (CT) and magnetic resonance imaging (MRI). This chapter will discuss each of these techniques and relate the usefulness of the procedures to the above-stated characteristics.

ULTRASOUND EVALUATION OF SWALLOWING

Principles of Ultrasound Imaging

In ultrasound imaging a small transducer capable of sending and receiving high frequency (2–10 MHz) sound waves is placed in contact with the skin overlying the deep soft tissue structure to be imaged. In the sending mode, the transducer sends short bursts of sound into the tissues. It then switches to receiving mode, where it listens for the return of the sound from reflective interfaces such as the borders between fascia and muscle. As the pulse returns, it appears as a bright dot along a scan line on the videodisplay screen. The brightness of this dot is proportional to the ability of the tissues imaged to reflect sound. The position of the dot on the scan line depends on the length of time taken for the sound to return to its source.

As the transmitted ultrasound energy is rapidly driven across the tissues, with thousands of reflections returning, the dots form a pattern representing the soft tissue structures beneath the transducer. Tissues with many strong reflected echoes, such as fibrous interfaces between organs appear as bright, while those that reflect a moderate amount of sound such as muscle appear less bright, and clear liquids which reflect almost no sound, appear black. Thus, one tissue can be differentiated from another. Sound at these frequencies is completely reflected by bone and air. With no sound reaching the area of interest, there is no image, and a black area or "shadow" is displayed (Rumack, Wilson, & Charboneau, 1991).

With each sweep of the scan line, these brights and darks are frozen in a computer matrix to form a static image of the structures being scanned. This matrix is then rapidly updated to produce a real-time display of the motion of the organ examined.

Thus, ultrasound affords a way of rapidly, safely, and cheaply evaluating soft tissue structures of the oropharynx and their movements in real time.

Technique for Ultrasound Evaluation of Swallowing

Real-time ultrasound imaging has gained prominence in medical imaging in cardiology, oncology, and obstetrics. It was applied to the assessment of the oropharynx for speech and swallowing in the 1980s (Shawker, Hall, Gerber, & Leighton, 1981; Shawker, Sonies, Stone, & Baum, 1983; Sonies, Baum, & Shawker, 1984; Sonies, Stone, & Shawker, 1984). Because the oral cavity is mostly soft tissue (floor muscles, tongue, and palate) and is surrounded by air and demarcated by bones, the soft tissue anatomy of the tongue and floor of the mouth are easily imaged in real time with ultrasound. The surface of the tongue is clearly imaged as well as the various intrinsic lingual muscles, fascia, glands, and muscles that support the tongue in the floor of the mouth. Images can be obtained in the sagittal, coronal, and transverse planes by rotation of the transducer without moving the patient. Ultrasound is portable and can be moved to the bedside or used in the office or clinic. In addition to videotape documentation of the real-time events, static images can be printed out in hard-copy format.

Advantages of Ultrasound for Swallowing Studies

Ultrasound is noninvasive and harmless; its primary feature is the ability to image soft-tissue structures that cannot be clearly delineated using videofluorography. Because it overcomes the risks of radiation exposure on still x-rays and videofluoroscopy, ultrasound can be used repeatedly and for extended durations. Thus, ultrasound provides a valuable tool to assess the oral preparatory and oropharyngeal phases of swallowing. Images are collected in multiple planes in real time. These can be frozen for immediate inspection, digitized and enlarged for specific examination of the fine details of soft tissue structures, and stored on videotape for later evaluation (Sonies 1991a, 1991b). Audio recording of the study as well as timing and frame data can be displayed and recorded on the videotape at the time of the study. The patient is able to be studied in an upright seated position or lying down. Infants or children can be held in the examiner's lap. Since contrast material is not required, dry saliva swallows can be examined without aspiration risk. Any amount or type of solid or liquid food can be imaged during swallowing. This ability to study a more normal diet is an advantage for many persons with an aversion to the taste or texture of barium contrast material needed for radiographic studies.

The Clinical Ultrasound Examination of Swallowing

Initiation of normal swallowing movement results from the coordination of a series of complex movements of the soft tissue structures of the oral and hypopharyngeal cavities. Hyoid motion is the fulcrum of activity of the tongue, epiglottis, and larynx and assists in the opening of the upper esophageal sphincter. Because ultrasound is able to clearly track hyoid motion in real time, it is an ideal instrument to determine hyoid elevation time during the swallow. To accomplish this, the patient is scanned upright or supine with the transducer held against the skin of the underside of the jaw or upper anterior neck. From this position, sound is transmitted upward through the soft tissues of the floor of the mouth and tongue to view motion and activity of the swallow in sagittal, coronal, or axial planes.

In the oral preparatory and oral-transport phases of the swallow, the tongue deforms and transports the bolus posteriorly into the pharynx. These volitional motions require the coordinated movements of the major tongue muscle (genioglossus) and muscles of the floor of the mouth (geniohy-

oid, mylohyoid, digastric), which can be viewed directly with ultrasound. Compensatory motions of these muscles can be visualized, and decompensation can be studied by increasing the bolus size and noting abnormal movement. Linear measurements can be made directly on the screen to quantify displacement of the tongue, hyoid, or other soft tissue.

The operator usually scans in the mid-coronal or mid-sagittal planes so that the ultrasound image includes the center of the tongue. This clearly visualizes bolus-holding and central grooving during the oral phase of the swallow (Maniere-Ezvan, Dural, & Darnauff, 1993; Shawker, Sonies, & Stone, 1984). In the coronal view, the genioglossus muscle forms a small central triangular mass that contracts during swallowing. The lateral muscles that compose the tongue are also visualized in the coronal view (Figure 8–1). Any unusual or asymmetric motion, tremors, or fasiculations can be clearly seen and are helpful in evaluating the physiology of compensatory muscle motions.

Bolus size can vary depending on the age and condition of the patient. The standard bolus is size 7 cc to 10 cc for liquids but smaller amounts of 3 cc to 5 cc may be given to stimulate a swallow in patients with neurologic disease. In these patients, if poor tongue control and impaired oral transmit are observed, the likelihood of pharyngeal pooling and laryngeal penetration is increased. Larger bolus sizes of 15 cc to 20 cc can be given to selected patients, without advanced neurologic or cognitive conditions, to determine how a larger bolus is partitioned. Any natural food can be given to study the effect of postural changes or therapeutic maneuvers. Ultrasound images clearly display the lingual surface changes that occur as the bolus is contained, transported, and altered by tongue–palate contact.

While the coronal view is most suited to examine abnormalities or asymmetries in tongue-bolus containment during oral preparation, midline sagittal scanning of the tongue may be easier to interpret, as

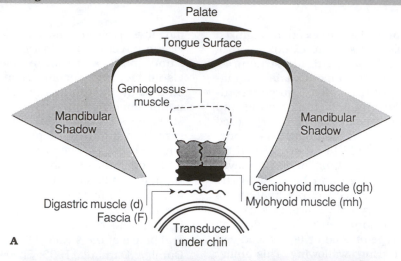

A

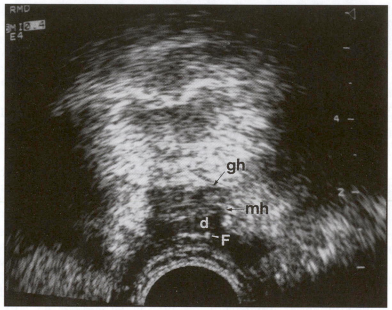

B

Figure 8–1. Coronal scan of the blade of the tongue. **A.** Schematic diagram. **B.** Scan. At the top of the image is the surface of the tongue seen as a white band. The geniohyoid (gh), mylohyoid (mh), and diagastric (d) floor muscles appear at the bottom of the scan. The digastric muscle is sometimes seen as separated by a bright midline septum. The tongue itself is separated from the floor muscles by a fascial border (F).

the entire surface of the tongue from tip to dorsum is visible (Figure 8–2). Bolus propulsion and transfer over the lingual surface of the tongue can be visualized throughout the oropharyngeal swallow.

Simultaneous motions of the tongue and the hyoid bone are also evident. Since ultrasound does not pass through bone, the position of the hyoid is represented by a triangular echo-free region, or shadow,

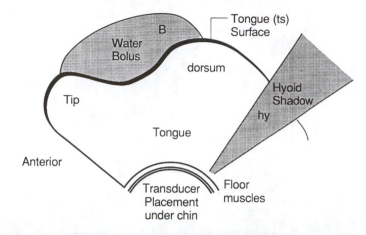

A

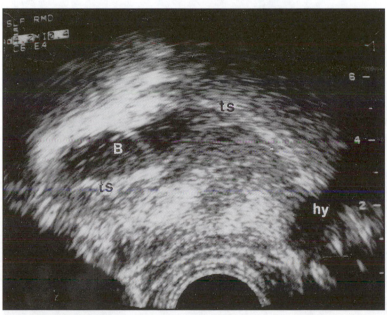

B

Figure 8–2. Midline sagittal view of the tongue. **A.** Schematic diagram. **B.** Scan. Anterior is on the left of the image. The tongue surface (ts) is seen as a bright white curved region reaching from anterior to posterior until the hyoid shadow appears as a black triangular wedge (hy). The tongue tip and dorsum are against the palate with the bolus in a central groove (B).

that appears posteriorly at the base of the tongue. The floor of the mouth muscles that attach to the hyoid (mylohyoid and geniohyoid) can be seen when using a high-resolution, 5-MHz linear transducer

(Figure 8–3). Soon after the start of a swallow, the hyoid shadow moves anteriorly and superiorly, remains forward for a brief moment, then quickly moves backward to its original resting position when the pha-

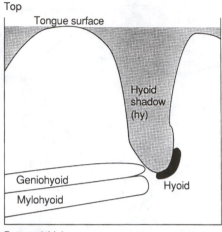

A

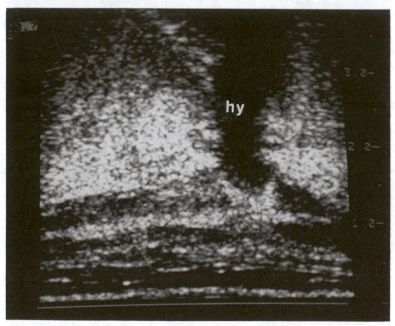

B

Figure 8–3. Midline sagittal expanded view of hyoid area using a 5 MHz linear transducer. **A.** Schematic diagram. **B.** Scan. Positioned posteriorly and caudally, the hyoid wedge (hy) is clearly seen along with its muscular attachments.

ryngeal phase of swallowing is completed, and the bolus is in the esophagus. The floor of the mouth muscles contract to elevate the hyoid and assist in relaxation/opening of the cricopharyngeal muscle (Figure 8–4). When the bolus enters the upper esophagus, the hyoid has moved back to it original resting position. The surface of the tongue will be

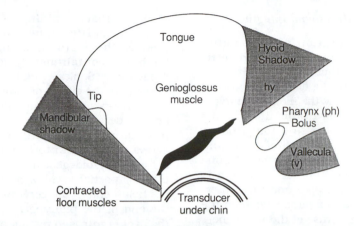

A

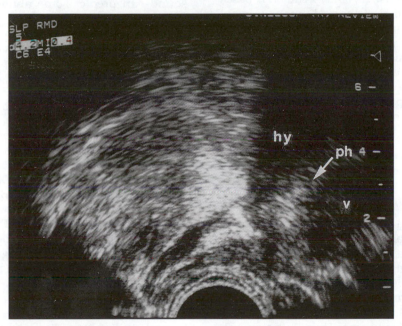

B

Figure 8–4. Midline sagittal scan during a swallow. **A.** Schematic diagram. **B.** Scan. The hyoid (hy) is at its maximum anterior-rostral displacement, and the tongue is retracted and elevated posteriorly as the bolus has entered the pharynx (ph). The second triangular wedge is the valleculae (v) and the shadow cast by the epiglottis. The bolus appears as a bright oval as it passes the tongue base into the pharynx.

visualized again at the end of the swallow. This rapid swallow sequence occurs in approximately 1 sec (Sonies, Parent, Morrish, & Baum, 1988). The duration of the entire oropharyngeal swallow can be directly measured by using the time code on the ultrasound monitor or the videotape record.

Limitations of Ultrasound Imaging

The primary limitation of ultrasound imaging is that it cannot be used to determine directly whether aspiration has occurred, as the imaging field of view is not broad enough to view the mouth, pharynx, and esophagus simultaneously. Since ultrasound does not pass through bones or air, soft tissues lying directly behind areas such as the larynx or hyoid bone cannot be imaged. Another limitation is that the quality of images and their interpretation depends to a large degree on the experience and expertise of the ultrasonographer. Because this interpretation is based on observation of the real-time movement and coordination of the soft tissues in the oropharynx and hypopharynx, rather than the traditional bony landmarks of the more commonly used methods, the ultrasound examiner needs to be very familiar with the relationships and interactions of the oropharyngeal musculature.

Applications of Ultrasound in the Evaluation of Swallowing

Clinical Applications

Ultrasound systems are compact, portable, and easy to use at the bedside, allowing evaluation of even fragile or infirm patients. The strength of ultrasound imaging is that it can clearly visualize in real time the interrelated motion and coordination of the soft tissues that shape and propel the food bolus. Thus, it is an excellent technique to measure the timing of oral transit and the oral pharyngeal swallow. With its excellent resolution of the surface of the tongue, ultrasound is best employed to evaluate the oral preparatory and oral phases of the swallow. Such things as the relationship of tongue tip motion to the initiation of the swallow, abnormal compensatory motions, and decompensation of muscle groups, as well as tongue blade or dorsum activity during bolus transfer can easily be assessed.

Because ultrasound is harmless when used for prolonged periods, it is effective in biofeedback training of oral feeding patterns and teaching patients how to produce the appropriate lingual gestures for bolus containment and propulsion (Shawker & Sonies, 1985). It can be used to evaluate the effects of indirect and direct oral sensory motor stimulation techniques and to determine if thermal application has stimulated a swallow. Ultrasound allows the clinician to determine whether a tongue–hyoid gesture leads to a complete or partial swallow gesture. Because the bolus enters the cervical esophagus at the end of the pharyngeal swallow when the hyoid returns to resting position, ultrasound can predict some abnormal pharyngeal phase activity.

The safety, mobility, and noninvasive features of ultrasound have made it useful in studying the sucking patterns of preterm infants and following the development of the swallow in infants and developmentally delayed children who are receiving treatment. (Bosma, Hepburn, Josell, & Baker, 1990; Bu'Lock, Woolridge, & Baum, 1990; Smith, Ehrenberg, Nowak, & Franken, 1985; Sonies, 1991a; Sonies, 1991b; Weber, Woolridge, & Baum, 1986). Ultrasound should be considered a primary technique to study children with disorders such as cerebral palsy (Casas, McPherson, & Kenny, 1995), who are poor feeders and require frequent monitoring during the course of treatment for swallowing difficulty.

Research Applications

Several studies have employed ultrasound to investigate the durational components of the oropharyngeal swallow and have shown that differences occur based on age and gender (Sonies, Parent, et al., 1988). Elderly individuals, especially females over age 55, have been found to produce extra tongue–hyoid gestures and take longer to complete oropharyngeal swallows. With the addition of physiologic monitors, laryngeal elevation movements have been timed in relation to tongue activity during swallowing (Shawker, Sonies, Hall, & Baum, 1984). Movement patterns of tongue–hyoid activity during swallowing have been studied using pellets affixed to the tongue (Stone & Shawker, 1986). A study using fiberoptic endoscopy simultaneously with ultrasound imaging of swallowing has clarified the temporal relationships between laryngeal and hyoid activity (Perlman & Van Daele, 1993).

Ultrasound has been used to examine the swallowing of individuals with hyposalivation (Caruso, Sonies, Fox, & Atkinson, 1989; Sonies, Schipp, & Baum, 1989) and in patients with bulimia (Roberts, Tylenda, Sonies, & Elin, 1989). Casas, Kenny, and McPherson (1994) combined ultrasound and plethysmography to evaluate swallowing of milk and cookies in children with cerebral palsy. As patients can be studied repeatedly, the effects of dysphagia treatment, thermal application and oral retaining can be evaluated (Sonies, 1991a, 1991b). By scanning with a linear transducer in the transverse plane, the larynx can be visualized and laryngeal adduction, laryngeal elevation, and epiglottal lowering can be imaged (Hamlet, 1980; Sonies 1991a, 1991b) (Figures 8–5 and 8–6). This method for imaging the larynx is also useful for evaluating the effect of masses and tumors on the structures needed to swallow (Balough, Fruhwald, Neuhold, Wicke, & Firbas, 1986; Gritzmann, Traxler, Grasl, & Pavelka, 1989; Kaneko et al., 1988; Raghavendra et al., 1987).

Future of Ultrasound Evaluation of Swallowing

Ultrasound imaging has the potential to extend our ability to image the esophagogastric junction, visualize hiatal hernias, and evaluate patients with complaints of reflux esophagitis (Aliotta et al., 1995). Because images can be acquired in various planes, ultrasound may have potential in three-dimensional reconstruction of the oropharynx. Although currently used to assess blood flow, Doppler ultrasound has shown initial promise in evaluating the motion of the hyoid bone and transport of the bolus through the pharynx and esophagus during swallowing (Nilsson, Ekberg, & Hindfelt, 1995; Sonies & Wang, 1994).

SCINTIGRAPHIC EVALUATION OF SWALLOWING

Principles of Scintigraphic Imaging

Radionuclides are isotopes of certain elements, such as Technetium 99m, which have unstable nuclei. The nucleus of these elements seeks stability by emitting small amounts of radiation at a known rate. If such an isotope is placed in front of a sheet of thallium-activated sodium iodide crystal (a gamma camera), the small amount of radiation emitted will produce a pulse of fluorescent light that can be precisely located on the face of the crystal. When these radionuclides are taken orally or injected intravenously, and the patient is placed in front of the gamma camera, images of the organs containing them can be recorded. Over time, a quantitative picture of radionuclide transit and metabolism within that organ can be shown as a plot of radioactivity versus time (time-activity curve) (Mettler & Guiberteau, 1991).

Scintigraphic studies of swallowing employ external monitoring of liquid or solid foods labeled using the gamma camera. Such methods allow quantitative evaluation of transit of food, under physiologic conditions, with patients in any body position for prolonged periods. To date, both oropharyngeal and esophageal transit have been studied.

Oropharyngeal and Esophageal Transit Studies

Espinola (1986) and Muz, Mathog, Rosen, Miller, and Borrero (1987) have developed radionuclide methods for studying oropharyngeal transit and aspiration. In these and other studies, (Hamlet, Muz, Patterson, & Jones 1989; Holt et al., 1990), the oral cavity, pharynx, hypopharynx, and the upper esophagus are delineated as separate regions of interest by placing small external cobalt markers on the lip, chin, angle of the mandible, cricoid cartilage, and sternal notch. Holt et al. (1990) observed the transit of small amounts (2 mCi) of Technetium 99m in 10 ml of water ingested as a single swallow. Rapid

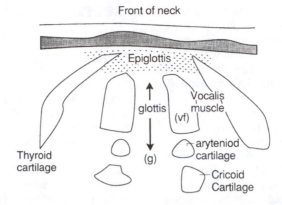

Front of neck

Epiglottis

glottis

Vocalis
muscle
(vf)

Thyroid
cartilage

(g)

aryteniod
cartilage

Cricoid
Cartilage

A

B

Figure 8–5. Transverse view of the larynx using 5–MHz linear transducer. **A.** Schematic diagram. **B.** Scan. Vocal folds (vf) are beginning to adduct to close the glottis (g) at the instant the swallow begins.

acquisitions (.05 sec/frame) of lateral images of the swallow were stored in computer memory. Subsequently, time–activity curves for each region of interest were drawn for each swallow. Transit times and rates of transfer between regions of interest were calculated in normal controls and in patients with neuromuscular disorders with and without dysphagia.

There were significant delays in the bolus transit times between mouth and esophagus in patients with and without dysphagia compared to healthy volunteers. However, such studies have not been closely controlled for differences in patient age and sex and their role in clinical decision making has yet to be delineated.

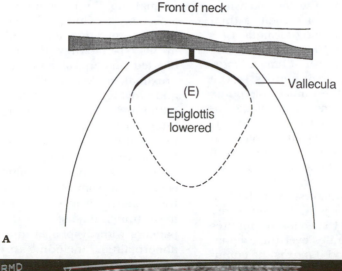

A

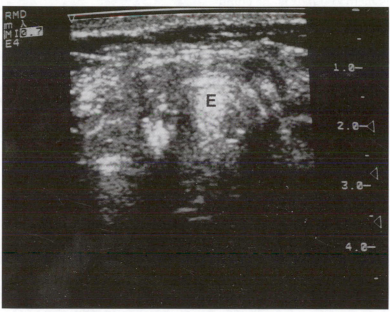

B

Figure 8–6. Transverse view of the larynx later in the same swallow when the epiglottis has lowered to protect the airway. The glottis is no longer visible.

Esophageal Transit Studies

Kazem (1972) and, later, Tolin, Malmud, Reilley, and Fisher (1979) and Russell et al. (1981) used scintigraphic techniques for measuring the time of bolus transit in the esophagus. To study transit after a single swallow, fasted patients lie supine under the gamma camera for imaging of the entire esophagus including the proximal stomach during ingestion of 150–300 µCi of Technetium 99m sulfur colloid mixed with 10–15 ml of water taken in a single swallow. Rate of transit is then computed by the following formula: $Ct = (Emax - Et/Emax) \times 100$, where Ct is the percent esophageal transit at time t; $Emax$, the maximal number of counts in the esophagus; and Et the number of counts in the esophagus at time t. Percentage esophageal transit is measured at 1 sec intervals for the first 15 sec after maximal esophageal activity is achieved. In normal volunteers, 90% of the activity traverses the esophagus after 15 sec.

To study serial swallows, after the first swallow, the subject is instructed to dry swallow once every 15 sec for 10 minutes while imaging continues over the esophagus. With this method, $Emax$ is the cumulative activity in the esophagus during the first 15 sec.

Using methods similar to these, Tolin et al. (1979) showed that patients with achalasia, diffuse esophageal spasm, scleroderma, and symptomatic reflux esophagitis had prolonged esophageal transit times compared to asymptomatic normal subjects. In addition, some patients with symptomatic gastroesophageal reflux with normal motility by manometry had prolonged serial scintigraphic clearances.

To improve time and spatial resolution in this type of study, Russell et al. (1981) divided imaging of bolus swallows into proximal, middle, and distal esophagus and proximal stomach regions of interest. With rapid acquisition of images at 0.4-sec intervals for each region of interest, the resultant time-activity curves quantitatively represented the progression of the bolus through the esophagus. Using these methods, normal controls had bolus transit to the stomach in less than 15 sec, with a mean transit time of 7.7 ± 1.7 sec. Fifteen patients with dysphagia and manometric abnormalities, including three with only tertiary contractions, all had abnormal transit studies. More importantly, 9 of 14 patients with dysphagia and normal manometry had abnormal scintigraphic studies. Although anatomic detail was poorly shown, the patterns of transit in these studies were specific enough in some cases to allow distinction between delayed transit produced by such disorders as achalasia and diffuse esophageal spasm (Figure 8–7).

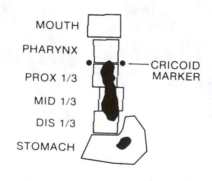

MOUTH

PHARYNX

PROX 1/3

MID 1/3

DIS 1/3

STOMACH

CRICOID MARKER

A

Figure 8–7. A. single scintigraphic image taken from normal swallowing sequence demonstrating regions of interest monitored by computer. **B.** Radionuclide esophageal transit study from a normal volunteer. Note the sequential peaks in proximal, middle, and distal esophagus, indicating smooth passage of the bolus in an aboral direction, with prompt complete entry into the stomach. **C.** Transit study from patient with achalasia. There is poor progression of bolus beyond the midsegment at 30 s. This is an adynamic pattern. Note that only a small amount of radioactivity enters the stomach. **D.** Transit study from patient with diffuse esophageal spasm. Note multiple peaks of activity representing disorganized bolus transit. Some of the bolus, how-

(continued)

NORMAL

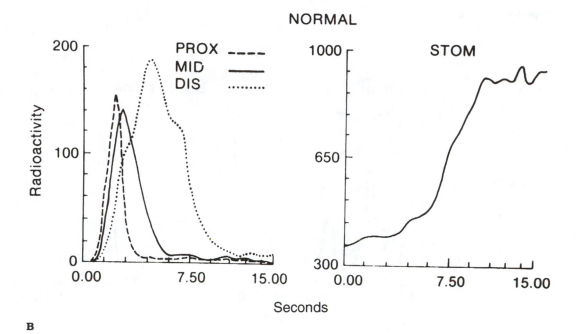

B

Achalasia

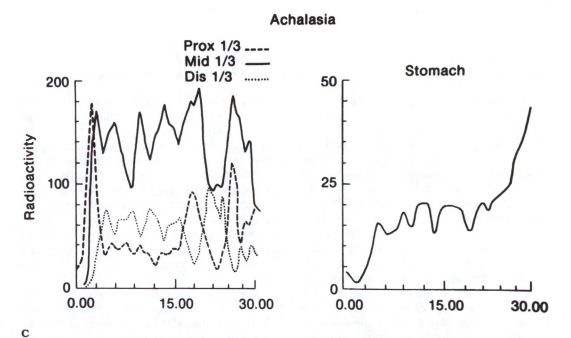

C

Figure 8–7. *(continued)* ever, reaches the stomach within the 30 s time period. (*Note*. From Radionuclide Transit: A Sensitive Screening Test for Esophageal Dysfunction, by C. O. H. Russell, L. D. Hill, E.R. Holmes III, D. A. Hull, R Gannon, and C.E. Pope II, 1981. *Gastroenterology, 80*, p. 887. Copyright 1981 by the American Gastroenterological Association. Reprinted with permission.) *(continued)*

Figure 8–7. *(continued)*

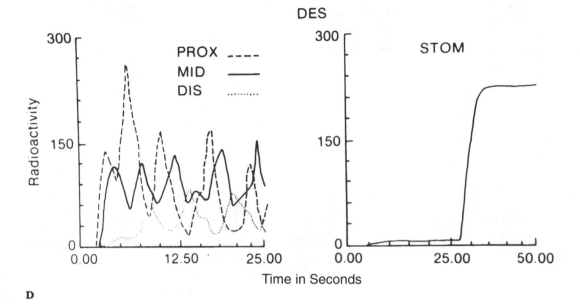

D

Limitations of Scintigraphic Studies

Although radionuclide methods provide excellent sensitivity in detecting motility disorders of the esophagus, their use has been limited in practice because of their inability to present adequate anatomic detail. Given that most patients who are ultimately diagnosed with disordered esophageal motility present with dysphagia, it is important that the esophagus be evaluated for anatomic narrowing as the cause for such symptoms. Even though radiographic studies may be less sensitive for motility problems, they allow detection of mechanical obstruction as well as motility disorders in a single examination. For this reason, radiography remains the primary modality for evaluation of most symptomatic esophageal disorders. If there is a role for scintigraphy, it may lie in the evaluation of patients with subtle or intermittent symptoms. Other possible uses include evaluation and quantitation of gastrointestinal reflux and aspiration.

Evaluation of Gastroesophageal Reflux

Fisher, Malmud, Roberts, and Lobis (1976) performed some of the earliest studies to quantitate gastroesophageal reflux. In these and minor variations of these studies, Technetium 99m sulfur colloid mixed with 300 cc of water is ingested. Subsequent scintigraphic views of the gastroesophageal junction are performed as incremental increases in abdominal pressures are produced by an abdominal binder. A reflux index (RI) or percentage reflux is then computed according to the formula: $RI = E1 - EB/G \times 100$ where $E1$ = esophageal counts, EB = esophageal background counts, and G = the maximal gastric counts (Figure 8–8). By these methods, the best separation between controls and symptomatic patients was at a 100-mmHg pressure gradient between the stomach and the lower esophagus. The mean reflux indices at this pressure were $11.8 \pm 7.1\%$ in those with symptoms and $2.2 \pm 0.8\%$ in controls. Significant

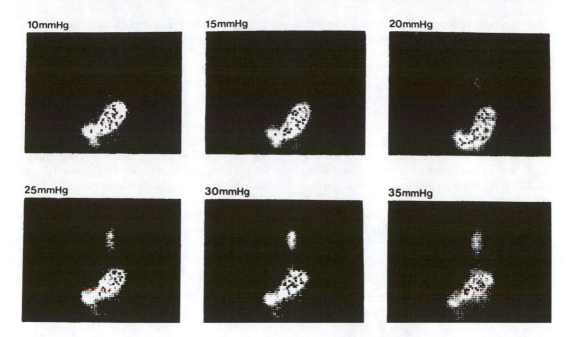

Figure 8–8. Serial gastroesophageal scinti-scans in a patient with reflux as intrabdominal pressure is increased. Note that at 15 mmHg and below no radiolabeled marker projects above the outline of the gastric fundus. However, at 20 mmHg and above radiolabel projects above the gastric contour, indicating gastroesophageal reflux. (*Note.* From Gastro-esophageal (GE) Scintiscanning to Detect and Quantitate GE Reflux, by R. S. Fisher, L. S. Malmud, G. S. Roberts, and I. F. Lobis, 1976. *Gastroenterology, 70,* p. 301. Copyright 1976 by the American Gastroenterological Association. Reprinted with permission.)

reflux occurred in 90% of patients with symptoms and only 10% of controls. Fluoroscopic demonstration of reflux, positive Bernstein test, and lower esophageal sphincter pressure <15 mmHg were the next most sensitive tests and were seen in 50, 63, and 77% of patients, respectively.

Scintigraphic Evaluation of Aspiration

Although cineradiography with barium contrast remains the most commonly used examination for the presence or absence of aspiration, scintigraphic methods for evaluation of aspiration offer several unique advantages. Unlike conventional radiographic contrast studies, scintigraphy allows monitoring for aspiration over long periods of time at a reduced radiation dose.

Muz et al. (1987) have estimated that the total body radiation dose for a standard cineradiographic swallowing study is approximately 3.5 centiGy, whereas a study of the same area using scintigraphy would require only an estimated .043 centiGy. However, the advantage with the most potential is the ability to quantify the amount of aspiration and to track its clearance from the lung over time.

Reich et al. (1977) was one of the first to suggest that radionuclide scanning of the lungs after ingesting Technetium 99m sulfur colloid could detect pulmonary aspiration. Humphries et al. (1987) and Muz, Mathog, Hamlet, Davis, and Kling, et al. (1991) studied pulmonary aspiration with techniques adapted from Russell and colleagues' (1981) scintigraphic methods for evaluation of esophageal function. They compared cinefluoroscopy and scintigraphy in patients who had head and neck cancer, neurologic disorders, and complaints of dysphagia. As in Russell's studies of esophageal function, the oropharynx, esophagus, and stomach were observed as separate regions of interest so that real-time transit studies could be performed. Swallows were observed with patients upright in front of a gamma camera during ingestion of Technetium 99m sulfur colloid in 20 cc of water. The swallow was continuously recorded and stored on computer at ingestion and for 6 sec thereafter. Ten minutes after ingestion, additional static

images in anterior and right anterior oblique projections were done to include the lungs. Percentage of aspirated material (PA) was then computed according to the formula $PA = RA \times 100/RT$, where RA was the counts in the region of aspiration, and RT the total counts (Figure 8–9). This and other studies have subsequently suggested that scintigraphy is limited in demonstrating the presence and anatomic mechanism for penetration above the vocal folds (Silver, Van Nostrand, Kuhlemeier, & Siebens, 1991), but imaging the chest, may be useful in detecting aspiration below the folds and in quantitating the extent and clear-

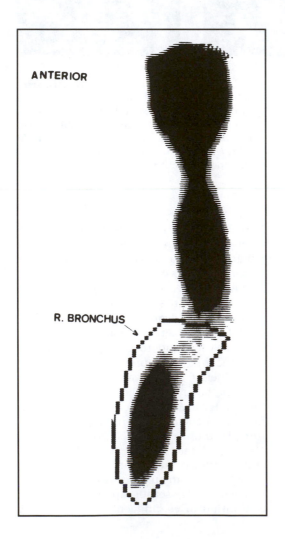

Figure 8–9. Static image 10 min after ingestion shows 16% of total dose aspirated into the right mainstem bronchus. (*Note.* From Detection and Quantification of Laryngotracheopulmonary Aspiration with Scintigraphy, by J. Muz, R. H. Mathog, R. Rosen, P. R. Miller, and G. Borrero, 1987. *Laryngoscope, 90,* p. 1180. Copyright 1987 by The American Laryngological, Rhinological, and Otological Society. Reprinted with permission.)

ance of aspirated material over time (Muz et al., 1987; Muz, Mathog, Nelson, & Jones, 1989; Muz, Hamlet, Mathog, & Farris, 1994; Reich et al., 1977; Silver et al., 1991).

Radionuclides have also been used to detect aspiration in children using what has been called a milk scan. Heyman, Kirkpatrick, Winter, and Treves (1979) studied 39 children for reflux and aspiration by mixing 5 µCi/ml of Technetium 99m sulfur colloid in 30–200 cc of the milk or other liquid ingested. Using 2-hour delayed images, he found two children with pulmonary aspiration, which was not apparent on barium contrast examination. Boonyaprapa, Alderson, Garfinkel, Chipps, and Wagner, (1980) applied similar methods to study children referred for recurrent pulmonary disease and correlated their findings with barium contrast studies. In these 20 selected cases, they imaged the lungs at 5 min, 4 hours, and the morning after ingestion and found 5 with aspiration. In the 15 who had contrast gastrointestinal studies, the 2 patients with aspiration on GI studies, as well 1 patient with a normal GI study, showed pulmonary aspiration on nuclear medicine scanning.

McVeagh, Howman-Giles, and Kemp (1987) used rapid-sequence early imaging of swallowing with follow-up scans at 2 hours and the next morning in 120 children referred for gastroesophageal reflux, pulmonary symptoms, or near-miss sudden infant death syndrome. Of these patients, 96 also had barium studies. They found the incidence of aspiration to be 5, 23, and 20% respectively. In comparing the radionuclide scan with barium contrast examinations in 96 of these patients, of the 19 who had aspiration on radionuclide scanning, 15 had no aspiration seen on barium exam. On the other hand, of the 9 showing aspiration on barium studies, 5 showed no aspiration on radionuclide scanning. With these data, the authors suggest that the radionuclide milk scan is more sensitive than barium. However, because each type of study excels in detecting aspiration in different phases of the swallow, it is probably more accurate to say that they are complementary studies, each looking at a different part of the swallow for aspiration.

In an attempt to evaluate whether infants may be silently aspirating their oral secretions, Heyman and Respondek (1989) developed what has been termed a radionuclide salivagram. These studies attempt to increase the sensitivity for aspiration by using a small volume (0.1–0.3 ml saline) with relatively high concentrations of tracer (200–300 µCi of Technetium 99m sulfur colloid), which is placed on the tongue as the child lies supine above the gamma camera. Subsequent images are taken at 1-minute intervals for 1 hour. In their first 27 patients, they found 7 positive for aspiration. Three of these had milk studies that were negative. Subsequent studies by Levin, Colon, DiPalma, and Fitzpatrick (1993) have shown similar results; however, no rigorous comparisons have been made between the milk scan and the salivagram.

A few investigators have begun to use radionuclide scanning to investigate the features of the pathophysiology of aspiration. Silver and Van Nostrand (1994) studied patients who had aspirated up to 25% of what was ingested, with follow-up scans at 3 and 6 hours. In all cases, the aspirated material was almost completely cleared at 3 hours.

Limitations of Scintigraphic Studies of Aspiration

Although promising, there are few rigorous studies of the clinical utility of the scintigraphic technique. Comparisons with the current standard of fluoroscopy are incomplete, because scintigraphic and fluoroscopic examinations have not always been performed concurrently (Silver & Von Nostrand, 1991). Although scintigraphy holds the promise of being able to document the ability of patients to clear aspirated material (Silver & Van Nostrand 1994), it needs to be shown that the apparent disappearance of radionuclide is not just dispersal into the periphery of the lung to a degree that the gamma camera can no longer detect it. Some studies have begun investigating the need to correct values for tissue attenuation (Hamlet, Choi, Kumpuris, Holliday, & Stachler, 1994). Additional studies with these techniques documenting the absolute value of the volume aspirated versus the time to clearance and the rate of clearance of different types of material aspirated (e.g., liquid vs. paste vs. solid) need to be done in a wide variety of patient groups.

Future Investigation of Scintigraphic Evaluation of Aspiration

With the realization that hypopharyngeal incoordination and weakness, distal esophageal disease, and gastroesophageal reflux can be associated with silent pulmonary aspiration and that such aspiration may be associated with acute and possibly chronic lung disease (Padhy et al., 1990; Silver & Van Nostrand, 1994); studies that merely document presence or absence of aspiration are no longer sufficient. We must now attempt to determine how much aspiration is significant, what are the mechanisms of clearance of aspirated contents, and which of these mechanisms are faulty in patients who eventually develop lung disease from chronic aspiration. Thus, prospective, long-term controlled investigations that combine the use of precise anatomic studies such as cineradiography with quantitative scintigraphy and measurement of lung function are needed to tell us what is significant aspiration in populations at risk.

COMPUTED TOMOGRAPHY

Conventional Static Computed Tomographic Scanning

In conventional CT scanners, an x-ray tube is mechanically rotated around the patient, allowing density measurements of anatomic structures along many radii of the scan circle. These density measurements are then reconstructed by a computer into an axial image of the structures in question. This technique has been most commonly used to evaluate the possibility that a swallowing disorder or complaint of dysphagia may be produced by aberrant anatomy such as vascular rings or evolving masses arising from within or surrounding the oropharynx, the esophagus, or upper abdomen. With suspicions of such lesions, the patient lies supine in the scanner after ingesting oral contrast during injection of intravenous iodinated contrast. With traditional scan protocols, axial cuts anywhere from 1 to 10 mm thick are obtained over a period of 5–10 min, and these static scans are reviewed for anatomic abnormalities that may explain the patient's complaint (Figure 8–10).

Ultrafast CT Scanning

To create an image in conventional CT scanning, the x-ray tube must rotate once around the patient. For this reason, even the fastest of these scanners has a scan time of at least 1 sec. Because total oropharyngeal transit time is less than 1 sec, evaluation of swallowing with standard CT imaging has been limited to evaluation of static anatomy.

More recently, ultrafast computed tomography has been used to produce rapid, high-quality axial images of the oropharynx. Using this method, an electron beam is electrically driven to scan tungsten targets that surround the subject. This eliminates the need for mechanical motion of the x-ray tube and produces a fan of x-rays that pass through the patient and onto a curvilinear array of detectors (Figure 8–11).

Ergun, Kahrilas, Lin, Logemann, and Harig (1993) have used these scanning techniques to visualize the oropharyngeal phases of swallowing in normal subjects. Serial axial scans 8-mm thick were taken simultaneously from up to 8 different levels at 17 images per second. Thus, scanning an 8-cm length of the oropharynx, they were able to reconstruct a real-time picture of normal swallowing. In this way, they found that large-volume boluses are moved primarily by motion of the anterior

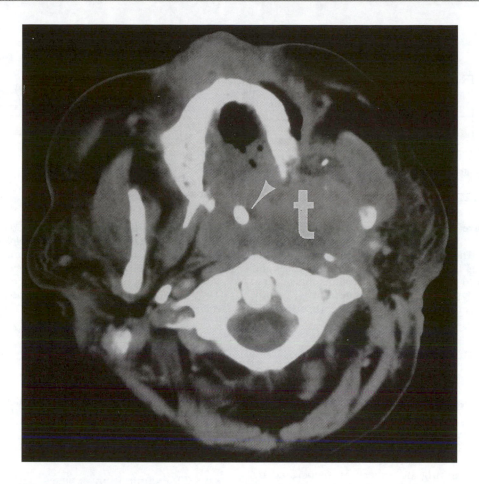

Figure 8–10. Axial computed tomographic view through the hypopharynx in patient with a large squamous cell cancer (t), which involves the nasopharyngeal, retropharyngeal, and paravertebral areas on the left. Note that part of the left mandible has been resected. A nasogastric tube marks the course of the esophagus (white arrow head).

pharyngeal surfaces, particularly the base of the tongue, and that smaller volume boluses are moved primarily by contraction of the posterior pharyngeal wall. They also noted a significant, obligatory bolus of air was swallowed with ingestion of liquid contrast and that the liquid swallowed tended to gather around the periphery of the bolus while the air remained in the center (Figure 8–12).

Lin, Chen, Kahrilas and Hertz (1994) used combined biplane fluoroscopy and ultrafast-

CT techniques to produce an anatomically precise, three-dimensional, real-time model of a normal oropharyngeal swallow, which can be viewed interactively on a computer screen. This interaction allows study of the motion and anatomic configuration of any of the structures involved in swallowing. As complex as gut motility is, in the future, it will require elegant, innovative techniques such as these to advance the study of the physiology and pathophysiology of swallowing and gut motility in general.

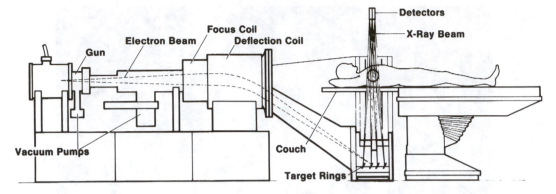

Figure 8–11. Longitudinal section through the ultrafast computerized tomography scanner. The electron beam originates at the gun and is accelerated toward the target rings and bent in its path by a focus coil. As this beam is rapidly rotated, a thin column of x-rays are projected in an axial plane through the patient's body. (*Note.* From *Ultrafast Computed Tomography in Cardiac Imaging: Principles and Practice* (p. 7), by William Stanford and John Rumberger 1992, Mount Kisco, New York: Futura Publishing Company, Inc. Copyright 1992 by Futura Publishing Company, Inc. Adapted with permission.)

Helical (Spiral) CT techniques

With conventional static and fast scanning techniques, each image is constructed from an electron beam that travels in the axial plane. Contiguous slices are generated by interrupting the scanning, advancing the patient through the gantry, and obtaining another slice. A new generation of CT scanners produces scans by having the patient move at a constant rate through the bore of the scanner while the scanning tube is rotated around the patient. This produces a continuous spiral "slicing" of the volume scanned, which is uninterrupted in space. The data sets gathered are continuous, volumetric representations of the area scanned. Even if they have been gathered at 10-mm intervals between peaks of the spiral, they can be postprocessed to any thickness along any plane desired. Such data are well suited for three-dimensional rendering of complex spaces such as the oropharynx, gastroesophageal junction, or stomach. In addition, such data sets require only seconds to gather (e.g., one breath hold) to scan the entire chest. This produces images with virtually no distortion from breathing artifact.

Limitations of CT

Any CT examination exposes patients to ionizing radiation. Because of the reduced scan time and the narrow width of the x-ray beam, the ultrafast and helical scanners pose no significant increase in the radiation exposure compared to conventional CT. Evaluation of swallowing by any computed tomography method must be done with the patient supine, although the ultrafast scanner will allow the patient's head to be elevated up to 25°.

At present, with large amounts of data, computer reconstruction times can be lengthy, but as three-dimensional computer reconstruction hardware and software become faster, more widely available, and easier to use, such data reconstruction will be quickly and easily rendered for viewing in any plane. Because of anatomic variations between patients, the lack of consistent landmarks for choosing scanning levels can

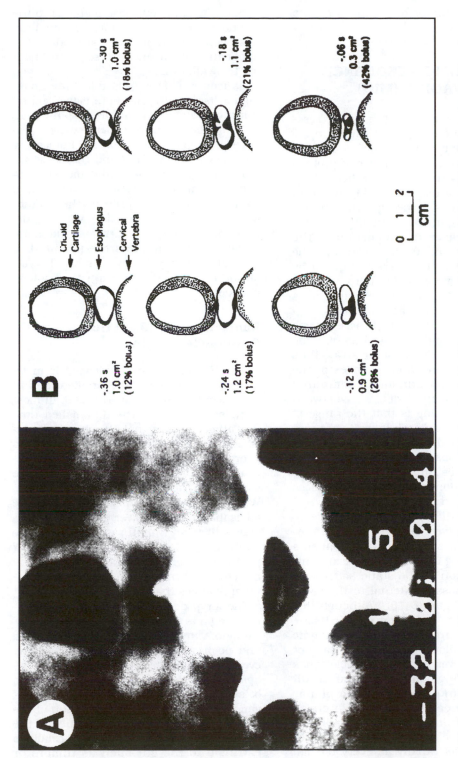

Figure 8–12. Representative axial view (A) an from one subject at the level of the upper esophageal sphincter 0.18 s before closure. Line drawings (B) show sequential views of sphincter from 0.36 to .06 s prior to complete upper esophageal sphincter closure. Listed also is the percentage of the total sphincter cross-sectional area occupied by the liquid contrast bolus. Note how the sphincter is tightly confined between the cricoid cartilage and the cervical vertebra. The bolus is distributed around the perimeter of the opened sphincter and mixed with a substantial quantity of air. Air = white, bolus = black in the accompanying line drawing. (*Note.* From Shape, Volume, and Content of the Deglutitive Pharyngeal Chamber Imaged by Ultrafast Computerized Tomography, by G. A. Ergun, P. J. Kahrilas, S. Lin, J. A. Logemann, and J. M. Harig, 1993, *Gastroenterology, 105,* p. 1396. Copyright 1993 by the American Gastroenterological Association. Reprinted with permission.)

produce difficulties in comparing data among patients.

MAGNETIC RESONANCE IMAGING (MRI)

To create an image using magnetic resonance, the patient is placed supine in the bore of a large magnet. When the magnet is turned on, a small number of protons in the various tissues of the body align with the strong magnetic field produced. As the magnet is turned off, the protons fall out of alignment. In doing so, they emit radio waves in proportion to the number of protons in each tissue and the degree to which they were perturbed by the magnetic field. This energy can be detected by a radio receiver coil just as used in tuning into a radio station.

The origin and strength of these signals can be located and displayed as differing shades of gray in a computer array, thus producing cross-sectional images of the body in a format similar to computed tomography. The main difference between MR and CT imaging is that the range of these shades from black to white are representations of differences in the perturbation of protons within the body rather than differences attenuation to an x-ray beam. In addition, with MR imaging slices can be displayed in any plane.

Because until recently magnetic resonance images have required several minutes to obtain, such imaging of patients with swallowing disorders has been limited to evaluation of the static soft tissue anatomy of masses external to the swallowing path (Figure 8–13) . Although this allows excellent definition of soft tissue anatomy for surgical planning, dynamic viewing of swallowing mechanics was not possible. However, evolving technology has enabled the development of ultrafast MR imaging techniques using echo-planar pulse sequences techniques such as MBEST (modulus blipped echo-planar single pulse technique), which can produce images as rapidly as every 64 ms. Stehling et al. (1989) and Evans et al.

(1994) have applied these methods to the evaluation of gastric emptying, but little has been written or demonstrated on the application of magnetic resonance imaging to swallowing.

Gauger et al. (1993) used fast MR imaging to display swallowing in eight healthy volunteers using an optimized spin-density TurboFLASH pulse sequence, which produced a temporal resolution of 3 frames/sec and showed midsagittal and coronal views of normal swallowing, with demonstration of movement of soft tissue, the tongue, and palate. Although at present these cine-MR presentations are crude, with rapidly evolving techniques, ultrafast magnetic resonance imaging has the potential to evaluate the physiology of normal swallowing in selected patients with swallowing complaints.

Limitations of Magnetic Resonance Imaging

Fast MR scanning of swallowing is in its infancy. At present, the applications of these techniques are experimental. In most of these sequences, the diminished time for gathering the signal also means diminished signal intensity for each image and poorer definition of soft tissues. In addition, MR imaging requires subjects to swallow in the supine or prone position. While the horizontal orientation may be advisable to study lower esophageal peristalsis, it is an unnatural position for the study of upper esophageal function. Other problems include artifacts induced by movement, chemical shift artifact, and dental appliances that degrade image detail.

The long, deep bore of most MRI scanner magnets may produce patient claustrophobia and problems with monitoring and positioning disabled patients. However, even with these imperfections, development of MR imaging to allow evaluation of swallowing would be a significant advance, allowing not only evaluation of the complex motion of the soft tissues of the head, neck, and chest, but abnormalities extrinsic to the gut such as tumors or vascular malformations.

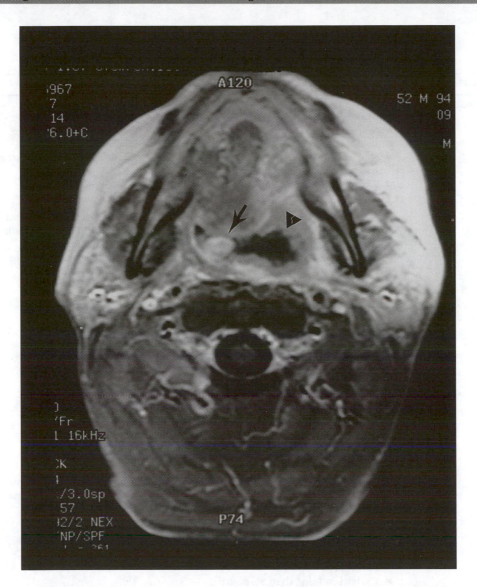

Figure 8–13. A T1 weighted spin-echo MRI image of the same patient as in Figure 8–10. The examination was done after tissue enhancement with injection of intravenous MRI contrast agent gadolinium-DTPA (diethylenetriaminepentaacetate). Note the low signal in the center of the tumor (black arrowhead). This was aspirated and found to be a necrotic portion of a squamous cell carcinoma. The course of the esophagus through the image plane is denoted by the black arrow.

SUMMARY

Although video fluoroscopy and manometry still remain the most widely used methods for evaluation of swallowing, we have attempted to place in perspective several alternative methods of diagnosing swallowing disorders. A summary of these methods, their strengths, and weaknesses is presented in Table 8–1.

Table 8–1. Summary of Imaging Methods.

Method	Strengths	Weaknesses
Ultrasound	■ Real-time evaluation of soft tissue movement ■ No radiation; repeatable ■ Well tolerated by patients ■ Can examine patient at bedside in any body position ■ Excellent for timing events	■ Limited field of view ■ Operator-dependent ■ Image degraded by bone and air ■ Cannot visualize aspiration
Scintigraphy	■ Quantitative ■ Allows examination for prolonged periods, (e.g., overnight) ■ Potential for study of pathophysiology of lung disease due to aspiration	■ Poor anatomic definition obviates determination of mechanism of abnormality ■ Poor detection of small amounts of aspiration in upper airway ■ Patient must remain motionless for exam
Standard CT	■ Excellent resolution between bone, air, soft tissues; good for showing masses or abnormalities extrinsic to GI tract that may produce dysphagia	■ Poor definition of intraluminal pathology ■ Difficult to conceptualize anatomy of scanned area as a whole ■ Not real time ■ Uses ionizing radiation ■ Patient must lie horizontally in gantry; may be claustrophobic
Ultrafast CT	■ As with standard CT ■ Can show rapid movement in a cine mode ■ Eliminates most motion artifact	■ As with standard CT ■ Not generally available ■ Long reconstruction times because of the many images
Helical CT	■ As with standard CT ■ Gives true volumetric data set; can reconstruct accurate representations of complex volumes ■ Faster scanning than standard CT; but slower than ultrafast CT (15–30 seconds to do chest)	■ As with standard CT ■ Still not real time
MR	■ Potential for depicting soft tissue component of swallow ■ No ionizing radiation	■ Many artifacts to be dealt with: metal from dental work, motion artifact on some pulse sequences, chemical shift on fast sequences ■ Claustrophobia may be significant problem ■ Patient must be examined supine ■ Cannot use with some metal clips in brain, pacemakers

MULTIPLE CHOICE QUESTIONS

1. Which of the following is/are true statements in regard to using ultrasound in the evaluation of swallowing?
   a. Ultrasound can directly visualize the movement of the muscles of the tongue.
   b. Ultrasound can evaluate the movements of the oropharyngeal muscles in any plane.
   c. The sound energy used in ultrasound imaging is harmless and allows repeated, extended evaluations.
   d. Ultrasound is able to "see through" the bony structures of the oral cavity.

2. Which of the following is/are true statements in regard to using radionuclide scintigraphy in the evaluation of swallowing?
   a. It produces excellent anatomic detail of the oral cavity, hypopharynx, and esophagus.
   b. It allows quantitative evaluation of the time course of the bolus through the esophagus.
   c. It gives a quantitative picture of aspiration into the bronchi.
   d. It is sensitive for evaluation of aspiration in the portion of the airway just below the vocal folds.

3. Which of the following is/are true in regard to the use of CT examination in the evaluation of swallowing?
   a. CT is often used to look for lesions producing dysphagia that originate outside the esophagus.
   b. CT is the primary modality for evaluating for tumor or lesions that originate from inside the esophagus.
   c. Helical CT scanning and ultrafast CT scanning both allow scanning times fast enough to freeze the motion of the oropharynx and hypopharynx.
   d. Because ultrafast CT scans are done rapidly, there is less radiation risk than with standard CT.

REFERENCES

Aliotta, A., Rapaccini, G., Pompili, M., Grattagliano, A., Cedrone, A., Trombino, C., DeLuca, F., & De Vitis, I. (1995). Ultrasonographic signs of sliding gastric hiatal hernia and their prospective evaluation. *Journal of Ultrasound in Medicine,14,* 457–461.

Balough, B., Fruhwald, F., Neuhold, A., Wicke, L., & Firbas, W. (1986). Sonography of the tongue and floor of the mouth. *Anatomischer Anzeiger, 161,* 249–258.

Boonyaprapa, S., Alderson, P. O., Garfinkel, D. J., Chipps, B. E., & Wagner, H. N. Jr., (1980). Detection of pulmonary aspiration in infants and children with respiratory disease: Concise communication. *Journal of Nuclear Medicine, 21,* 314–318.

Bosma, J., Hepburn, L., Josell, S., & Baker, K. (1990). Ultrasound demonstration of tongue motions during suckle feeding. *Developmental Medicine and Child Neurology, 32,* 223–229.

Bu'Lock, F., Woolridge, M., & Baum, J. (1990). Development of coordination of sucking, swallowing and breathing: Ultrasound study of term and preterm infants. *Developmental Medicine and Child Neurology, 32,* 669–678.

Casas, M., Kenny, D., & McPherson, K. (1994). Swallowing ventilation interactions during oral swallow in normal children and children with cerebral palsy. *Dysphagia, 9,* 40–46.

Casas, M., McPherson, K., & Kenny, D. (1995). Durational aspects of oral swallowing in neurologically normal children and children with cerebal palsy: An ultrasound investigation. *Dysphagia, 10*(3), 155–159.

Caruso, A., Sonies, B., Fox, P., & Atkinson, J. (1989). Objective measures of swallowing in patients with primary Sjögrens syndrome. *Dysphagia, 4*(2), 101–105.

Ergun, G. A., Kahrilas, P. J., Lin, S., Logemann, J. A., & Harig, J. M. (1993). Shape, volume, and content of the deglutitive pharyngeal chamber imaged by ultrafast computerized tomography. *Gastroenterology, 105,* 1396–1403.

Espinola, D. (1986). Radionuclide evaluation of pulmonary aspiration: Four birds with one stone—esophageal transit, gastroesophageal reflux, gastric emptying, and bronchopulmonary aspiration. *Dysphagia, 1,* 101–104.

Evans, D. F., Lamont, G., Stehling, M. K., Blamire, A. M., Gibbs, P., Coxon, R., Hardcastle, J. D., & Mansfield, P. (1993). Prolonged monitoring of the upper gastrointestinal tract using echo planar magnetic resonance imaging. *Gut, 34*, 848–852.

Fisher, R. S., Malmud, L. S., Roberts, G. S., & Lobis, I. F. (1976). Gastroesophageal (GE) scintiscanning to detect and quantitate GE reflux. *Gastroenterology, 70*, 301–308.

Gauger, J., Crary, M. A., Burton, S. S., Stoupis, C., Ros, P. R., & Mao, J. (1993). Dynamic MR Evaluation of biomechanics during swallowing with an optimized turboFLASH sequence. *Radiology, 189*(P), 427.

Gould, R. G. (1992). Principles of ultrafast computed tomography: Historical aspects, mechanism of action, and scanner characteristics. In W. Stanford & J. A. Rumberger (Eds.), *Ultrafast computed tomography in cardiac imaging: Principles and practice* (pp. 1–15). Mount Kisco NY: Futura.

Gritzman, N., Traxler, M., Grasl, M., & Pavelka, R. (1989). Advanced laryngeal cancer: Sonographic assessment. *Radiology, 171*, 171–175.

Hamlet, S. (1980). Ultrasonic measurement of larynx height and vocal fold vibratory pattern. *Journal of the Acoustical Society of America, 68*(1), 121–124.

Hamlet, S., Choi J., Kumpuris, T., Holliday, J., & Stachler, R. (1994). Quantifying aspiration in scintigraphic deglutition testing: Tissue attenuation effects. *Journal of Nuclear Medicine, 35*, 1007–1013.

Hamlet, S., Muz, J., Patterson, R., & Jones, L. (1989). Pharyngeal transit time: Assessment with videofluoroscopic and scintigraphic techniques. *Dysphagia, 4*, 4–7.

Heyman, S., Kirkpatrick, J. A., Winter, H. S., & Treves, S. (1979). An improved radionuclide method for the diagnosis of gastroesophageal reflux and aspiration in children (milk scan). *Radiology, 131*, 479–482.

Heyman, S., & Respondek, M. (1989). Detection of pulmonary aspiration in children by radionuclide "salivagram." *Journal of Nuclear Medicine, 30*, 697–699.

Holt, S., Miron, S. D., Diaz, M. C., Shields, R., Ingraham, D., & Bellon E. M. (1990). Scintigraphic measurement of oropharyngeal transit in man. *Digestive Diseases and Sciences, 35*, 1198–1204.

Humphries, B., Mathog, R., Miller, P., Rosen, R., Muz, J., & Nelson, R. (1987). Videofluoroscopic and scintigraphic analysis of dysphagia in the head and neck cancer patient. *Laryngoscope, 97*, 25–32.

Kaneko, T., Numata, T., Haruhiko, S., Hino, T., Komatsu, K. & Masuda, T. (1988). Newly developed ultrasound laryngographic equipment and its clinical application in voice physiology. In O. Fujimura (Ed.), *Voice production mechanism and function* (Chap. 24). New York: Raven Press.

Kazem I. (1972). A new scintigraphic technique for the study of the esophagus. *American Journal of Roentgenology. Radiation Therapy and Nuclear Medicine, 115*, 681–688.

Levin, K., Colon, A., DiPalma, J., & Fitzpatrick, S. (1993). Using the radionuclide salivagram to detect pulmonary aspiration and esophageal dysmotility. *Clinical Nuclear Medicine, 18*(2), 110–114.

Lin, S., Chen, J., Kahrilas, P. J., & Hertz, P. (1994). Three-dimensional animation of the oropharyngeal swallow. *Radiology, 193*(P), 446.

Maniere–Ezvan, A., Dural, J., & Darnault, P. (1993). Ultrasonic assessment of the anatomy and function of the tongue. *Surgical Radiologic Anatomy, 15*, 55–61.

McVeagh, P., Howman-Giles, R., & Kemp, A. (1987). Pulmonary aspiration studied by radionuclide milk scanning and barium swallow roentgenography. *American Journal of Diseases of Childhood, 141*, 917–921.

Mettler, F. R., & Guiberteau, M. J. (1991) *Essentials of nuclear medicine* (3rd ed.) Philadelphia: W. B. Saunders.

Muz, J., Hamlet, S., Mathog, R., & Farris, R. (1994). Scintigraphic assessment of aspiration in head and neck cancer patients with tracheostomy. *Head and Neck, 16*, 17–20.

Muz, J., Mathog, R. H., Hamlet, S. L., Davis, L. P., & Kling, G. A. (1991). Objective assessment of swallowing function in head and neck cancer patients. *Head and Neck, 13*, 33–39.

Muz, J., Mathog, R. H., Miller, P. R., Rosen, R., & Borrero, G. (1987). Detection and quantification of laryngotracheopulmonary aspiration with scintigraphy. *Laryngoscope, 97*, 1180–1185.

Muz, J., Mathog, R.H., Nelson, R., & Jones Jr., L.A. (1989). Aspiration in patients with head and neck cancer and tracheostomy. *American Journal of Otolaryngology, 10*, 282–286.

Nilsson, H., Ekberg, O., & Hindfelt, B. (1995). Oral function test for monitoring suction and swallowing in the neurologic patient. *Dysphagia, 10*, 93–100.

Padhy, A. K., Gopinath, P. G., Sharma, S. K., Prasad, A. K., Arora, N. K., Tiwari, D. C., Gupta, K., & Chetty, A. (1990). Radionuclide detection of gastroesophageal reflux in children suffering from recurrent lower respiratory tract infection. *Indian Journal of Pediatrics, 57*, 517–525.

Perlman, A., & Van Daele, D. (1993) Simultaneous videoendoscopic and ultrasound measures of swallowing. *Journal of Medical Speech-Language Pathology, 1*(4), 223–232.

Raghavendra, B., Horri, S., Reede, D., Rumancik, W., Persky, M., & Bergeron, T. (1987). Sonographic anatomy of the larynx with particular reference to the vocal cords. *Journal of Ultrasound in Medicine, 6,* 225–230.

Reich, S. B., Earley, W.G., Ravin, T. H., Goodman, M., Spector, S., & Stein, M R. (1977). Evaluation of gastropulmonary aspiration by a radioactive technique. *Journal of Nuclear Medicine, 18,* 1079–1081.

Roberts, M., Tylenda, C., Sonies, B., & Elin, R. (1989). Dysphagia in bulimia nervosa. *Dysphagia, 4,* 106–111.

Rumack, C. M., Wilson, S. R., & Charboneau, J. W. (1991). *Diagnostic ultrasound.* St. Louis: Mosby.

Russell, C .O. H., Hill, L. D., Holmes, E. R., III, Hull, D. A., Gannon, R., & Pope, C. E., II. (1981). Radionuclide transit: A sensitive screening test for esophageal dysfunction. *Gastroenterology, 80,* 887–892.

Shawker. T., & Sonies, B. (1985). Ultrasound biofeedback for speech training. Investigative *Radiology, 20,* 90–93.

Shawker, T., Sonies, B., Hall, T., & Baum B. (1984). Ultrasound analysis of tongue, hyoid and larynx activity during swallow. *Investigative Radiology, 19,* 82–86.

Shawker, T., Sonies, B., & Stone, M. (1984). Soft tissue anatomy of the tongue and floor of the mouth: An ultrasound demonstration. *Brain and Language, 21,* 335–350.

Shawker, T., Sonies, B., Stone, M., & Baum, B. (1983). Real-time ultrasound visualization of tongue movement during swallowing. *Journal of Clinical Ultrasound, 11,* 485–489.

Silver, K. H., & Van Nostrand, D. (1992). Scintigraphic detection of salivary aspiration: Description of a new diagnostic technique and case reports. *Dysphagia, 7,* 45–49.

Silver, K. H., & Van Nostrand, D. (1994). The use of scintigraphy in the management of patients with pulmonary aspiration. *Dysphagia, 9,* 107–115.

Silver, K. H., Van Nostrand, D., Kuhlemeier, K. V., & Siebens, A. A. (1991). Scintigraphy for the detection and quantification of subglottic aspiration: Preliminary observations. *Archives of Physical Medicine and Rehabilitation, 72,* 902–910.

Smith, W., Erenberg, A., Nowak, A., & Franken, E. (1985). Physiology of sucking in the normal term infant using real time ultrasound. *Radiology, 156,* 379–381.

Sonies, B. (1991a). Instrumental procedures for dysphagia diagnosis. *Seminars in Speech and Language, 12,* 185–198.

Sonies, B. (1991b). Ultrasound imaging and swallowing. In M. Donner, & B. Jones (Eds.), *Normal and abnormal swallowing* (Chap. 8). New York: Springer–Verlag.

Sonies, B., Baum, B., & Shawker, T. (1984). Tongue motion in the elderly: Initial in situ observations. *Journal of Gerontology, 39*(3), 279–283.

Sonies, B., Parent, L., Morrish, K., & Baum, B. (1988). Durational aspects of the oral–pharyngeal swallow in normal adults. *Dysphagia, 3*(1), 637–648.

Sonies, B., Schipp, J., & Baum, B. (1989). Relationship between saliva production and oral swallow in healthy, different aged adults. *Dysphagia, 4*(2), 85–89.

Sonies, B., Shawker, T., Hall, T., Gerber, L., & Leighton, S. (1981). Ultrasonic visualization of tongue motion during speech. *Journal of the Acoustical Society of America, 70*(3), 693–696.

Sonies, B., Stone, M., & Shawker, T. (1984). Speech and swallowing in the elderly. *Journal of Gerontology, 3,* 115–123.

Sonies, B., & Wang, C. (1994). *Ultrasound Doppler spectral analysis of hyoid bone movement during swallow: A preliminary study.* Presented at Dysphagia Research Society, Tysons, Virginia.

Stanford, W., & Rumberger, J. (Eds.). (1992). *Ultrafast computed tomography in cardiac imaging: Principles and practice.* New York: Futura.

Stehling, M. K., Evans, D. F., Lamont, G., Ordidge, R. J., Howseman, A. M., Chapman, B., Coxon, R., Mansfield, P., Hardcastle, J. D., & Coupland, R. E. (1989). Gastrointestinal tract: Dynamic MR studies with echo-planar imaging. *Radiology, 171,* 41–46.

Stone, M., & Shawker, T. (1986). An ultrasound examination of tongue movement during swallowing. *Dysphagia, 1,* 78–83.

Tolin, R. D., Malmud, L. S., Reilley, J., & Fisher, R. S. (1979). Esophageal scintigraphy to quantitate esophageal transit (quantitation of esophageal transit). *Gastroenterology, 76,* 1402–1408.

Weber, F., Woolridge, M., & Baum, J. (1986). An ultrasonographic study of the organization of sucking and swallowing by newborn infants. *Developmental Medicine and Child Neurology, 28,* 19–24.

9

Electromyography in the Functional and Diagnostic Testing of Deglutition

Donald S. Cooper and Adrienne L. Perlman

Electromyography (EMG) records electrical phenomena associated with the first stage of the sequence of physiological events that link muscle excitation with muscle contraction (Aidley, 1989). The technique of electromyography may be applied to a given muscle to assess suspected pathology of nerve and/or muscle, to specify and quantify muscle activity during particular movements, or as part of basic studies in nerve and muscle physiology. An EMG system may consist of separate components or of an integrated system. It will minimally include electrode inputs, a physiological preamplifier, oftentimes separate amplifier and filter stages, signal display, speaker, and recording device (Figure 9–1). The anti-aliasing filter may be a separate unit; or with a computer, this same function can be carried out by using a sampling rate sufficient to prevent aliasing, followed by digital low pass filtering.

ORIENTATION TO ELECTROMYOGRAPHY

An initial orientation to fundamental EMG concepts can be found in the first part of Goodgold and Eberstein's (1983) introduction to electrodiagnosis. Johnson (1988) provides a transition from fundamental EMG studies to the clinic, while more systematic treatises such as those of Kimura (1989), Brown (1984), and Brown and Bolton (1993) provide deeper orientation to the role of electromyography in electrodiagnosis. The kinesiologic aspect of electromyography is surveyed as a part of Basmajian and De Luca's (1985) overview of EMG, which joins the engineer's technical insights of De Luca to Basmajian's viewpoint from functional anatomy and kinesiology. On a concrete hands-on level, the manual of EMG technique in the context of physiological experimentation by Loeb and Gans (1986) is an indispensable resource. Historically, EMG has been less frequently applied in the cranial nerve area than in the spinal nerve area, but many important considerations for EMG of the head and neck have been recently addressed by Luschei and Finnegan (1995).

The present chapter will review the underlying principles of electromyography, basic techniques for electromyographic recording, and swallowing-related

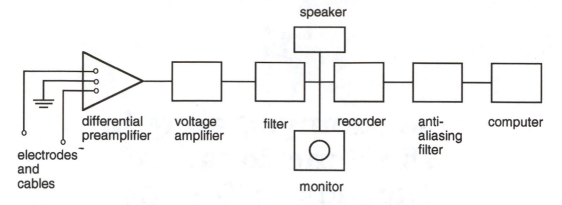

Figure 9–1. An EMG system may consist of separate components or of an integrated system, but will minimally include electrode inputs and cables, a physiological preamplifier and sometimes separate amplifier and filter stages, and signal display and recording devices.

research on EMG of those oral, pharyngeal, and laryngeal areas which, besides other functions, subserve the basic mechanisms of deglutition.

Motor Unit Physiology and Character

Differences of structural, biochemical, and physiological detail exist between large limb muscles and those of the head and neck (e.g., see Blitzer, Brin, Fahn & Harris, 1992; Cooper, Partridge, & Alipour-Haghighi, 1993; Goldberg, 1990; Luschei & Goldberg, 1981; Zealear, 1979). These specializations are expressed primarily on the level of the character of motor units.

Nearly half a century passed between the initial formulation of the concept of the *motor unit* and the substantial clarification of its anatomic and physiological aspects. Notions formulated in C. S. Sherrington's laboratory during the 1920s (Eccles & Gibson, 1979) crystallized in a classic definition of the motor unit: "The axone of a nerve-cell together with all the muscle-fibres which it innervates by its numerous divisions is a single functional unit called the 'motor unit'" (Creed, Denny-Brown, Eccles, Liddell, & Sherrington, 1932, p. 6). The muscular section of this structure is referred to as a muscle unit.

Because the muscle fibers of a given motor unit are essentially homogeneous in regard to the type of fibers that compose it (Kugelberg, 1981), characterization of a type of muscle fiber also characterizes a type of motor unit. Three main types of muscle fiber, and thus three main types of motor unit, are found in adult humans; details of classification are debated. The primary histochemical classification is based in practice on tissue reaction to staining for myosin ATPase with preincubation at various pHs (usually pH 9.4, 4.6, 4.3, but with minor variations). By combining this classification with one based on muscle fiber color (redness indicates a concentration of myoglobin associated with a strong oxidative metabolism) and physiological properties (contraction speed and fatigue resistance), three basic types of adult skeletal muscle are observed: *type 1* or slow red fatigue-resistant fibers, *type 2A* or fast red fatigue-resistant fibers, and *type 2B* or fast white fatiguable fibers. Details of the histochemical and histologic classifications (Table 9–1) may be found in a variety of sources from the readable clinical manual of muscle biopsy by Dubowitz (1985), and the text on muscle disease of Walton, Karpati, and Hilton-Jones (1994), to the encyclopedic treatise on myology

TABLE 9–1. Classification of Adult Human Skeletal Muscle Fibers

Histochemical Type	Contraction Speed	Fatigue Resistance	Color	Metabolism
1	Slow twitch	Fatigue resistant	Red	Oxidative
2A	Fast twitch	Fatigue resistant	Red	Oxidative-glycolytic
2B	Fast twitch	Fatigue sensitive	White	Glycolytic

Note. For details see sources listed in text.

edited by A. Engel and Franzini-Armstrong (1994). Important reviews of motor unit characteristics include Brown (1984), Buchthal and Schmalbruch (1980), Burke (1981), Clamann (1981), Close (1972), Gollnick and Saltin (1989), Henneman (1980a, 1980b), Henneman and Mendell (1981), Lewis (1981), and Németh (1990). Desmedt has focused on basic motor unit concepts in two important symposia (1973, 1981); they are also the main topic of a more recent collection edited by Binder and Mendell (1990).

Considering the cross-section of a muscle, the muscle fibers of a given motor unit are scattered among other fibers often of different muscle fiber types; depending on anatomic detail, muscle fibers from as many as 20 motor units may overlap in the space of a single motor unit. For this reason a characteristic checkerboard pattern of muscle fibers in the transverse muscle section is observed after staining for myosin ATPase. Local continuity of a number of fibers of the same type (fiber type grouping) is often a sign of local denervation followed by reinnervation of those fibers (Dubowitz, 1985), although sometimes clumping of fibers of a given type occurs as one aspect of functional specialization of one region of a muscle. The number of motor units in a muscle, and motor unit cross-sectional area, may vary considerably and constitute part of the functional specialization of a given muscle (Kugelberg, 1981).

Activation of Motor Units

Activation of the lower motor neuron cell body (e.g., in voluntary or reflex acti-

vation) and/or axon (e.g., in indirect stimulation by application of a stimulating electrode to the motor nerve) of a given motor unit results in the quasisimultaneous electrical activation first of the motor nerve fibers and then of the muscle fibers composing the muscle unit, with a fine-scale and slightly variable temporal scatter of these firings, which is termed *action potential jitter*. This is one focus of the technique of single muscle fiber electromyography (SFEMG), which has special importance in the investigation of neuromuscular transmission (Oh, 1988).

The results of motor nerve activation depend in detail on the length and integrity of nerve fibers innervating muscle fibers, and the condition of myoneural junctions, as well as on the condition of the muscle innervated. For this reason EMG is an important clinical tool in the assessment of these physiological subsystems (e.g., Brown, 1984; Brown & Bolton, 1993; Kimura, 1989; Notermans, 1984; Oh, 1988, 1993).

RECORDING ELECTRODES AND ELECTRODE ARRAYS

A number of excellent overviews of the basic phenomena of action potential generation and the general neural context of electromyography are available, at various levels of biophysical and mathematical sophistication (e.g., Aidley, 1989; Brazier, 1977; Cole, 1972; Hodgkin, 1964; Kandel & Schwartz, 1991; Katz, 1966; Partridge & Partridge, 1993; Plonsey, 1969; Stein, 1980; Stevens, 1966;). Although the generation of action potentials in nerve and in skeletal muscle are basically similar, there are differences of detail between them, readably surveyed by Junge (1992). One difference that impinges on EMG measurements is that because of the greater capacitance of the muscle membrane which results from the presence of its internal tubular network, propagation of the action potential in muscle fibers is appreciably slower than is observed in nerve fibers, even considering their diameters (Adrian, 1983; Costantin, 1977).

Other important differences arise from the size and geometry of the tissues studied with respect to the electrodes. Nerve fibers course in small bundles of fibers separated and insulated from one another by connective tissue, and electrodes may be laid on the nerve surface, inserted into a nerve bundle, inserted into single fibers, or form cylinders with respect to the nerve, and so on. Thus it is possible to record a whole nerve action potential summing the electrical effects of the activity of all these fibers, or to use microelectrodes to record from smaller structures including single fibers. However, muscles are characteristically large with respect to electrode size, so that intramuscular electrodes sample muscle activity selectively from small portions of the muscle studied. Surface electrodes placed on the skin over the muscle are not discriminating as to the source of the potentials recorded. In some cases surface electrodes may make possible important spatial and temporal analyses of action potential propagation (e.g., Emerson & Zahalak, 1981). Surface electrodes are often used in the submental region to identify the onset and duration of activity from this region, including the mylohyoid, geniohyoid, and anterior belly of the digastric muscles, during swallowing.

Differential Recording

The signal reaching the amplifier from a given electrode is the average of all of the electrical activity sensed in the immediate region of the electrode at a given moment. However, the bipolar electrode configuration and differential amplifier together emphasize electrical activity that occurs within a limited tissue volume. The differential recording arrangement was developed almost simultaneously by Jan Tönnies, a German electrical engineer and neurophysiologist (Jung, 1975), and by the British neurophysiologist B. H. C. Matthews (1934), as a procedure to eliminate large interfering signals from electroencephalographic (EEG) recordings in the microvolt range by subtracting the signal seen at one electrode from that seen by the other with the same ground reference. As a result, the remaining signal shows only voltage differences between the signals seen at a given moment at the two electrodes (Figure 9–2). Since interference signals are almost identical at both electrodes, they are sometimes referred to as *common mode signals*; identical elements of the signals seen at the two differential electrodes are eliminated from the output signal by this procedure.

When differential recording is applied to muscle, its effect depends on geometric considerations which are commonly overlooked. Let us consider the case in which differential electrodes are inserted in a muscle with the interelectrode axis perpendicular to the course of muscle fibers. In this case, the output signal is the difference between the simultaneous signals from partly overlapping groups of motor units, and no mathematical operation on this signal can reconstruct the original signals. When the signals seen at pairs of EMG derivations spaced across the muscle are compared, their agreement increases not only with proximity, but also with the level of muscle effort (Hogan & Mann, 1980), and with the degree of muscle fatigue (Person & Mishin, 1964). However, if both electrodes are on the same side of the motor end-plate region and the differential electrodes are inserted so that the interelectrode axis is parallel to the course of the muscle fibers, the electrodes monitor the activity of largely identical sets of muscle fibers at two longitudinally sepa-

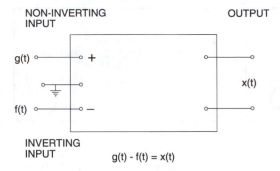

Figure 9-2. The output of the differential amplifier is the voltage difference between the signal inputs from the electrodes, subjected to successive amplification and filtering.

rated regions (Cooper & Folkins, 1985). In this case the original signals seen by each of the two electrodes are distinguished only by a time delay (Parker & Scott, 1973), and can be approximately reconstructed by integration of the output signal with respect to time. Because a given muscle action potential passes the two electrodes at different times, the system executes a continuous differencing of the signal. The filtering effect of the amplifier on the action potential will depend not only on the am-plifier's internal electronics, but also on the average velocity and direction of propagation of the action potential and on the longitudinal distance by which the electrodes are separated. If the interelectrode axis is parallel to the muscle fibers but the electrodes are inserted at equal distances from the end-plate region on opposite sides of it, connected so that the matching potentials seen by the electrodes have the same polarity, the differential amplifier output will cancel out myopotentials that match at the two electrodes. The differential amplifier's output signal has been the subject of important physiological interpretations that are not possible (or at least not justified) if the geometry of the interelectrode axis is ignored (Lindström & Petersén, 1983).

In practice, detailed information regarding the location of motor end-plates or the muscle fiber course may not be avail-

able, and with some techniques the angle of the interelectrode axis relative to the muscle fiber course is not or cannot be controlled. This is the case in using the Basmajian and Stecko arrangement in which two fine wire electrodes are inserted inside the same hypodermic needle (Basmajian, 1973; Basmajian & Stecko, 1962), which is common in studies of swallowing and speech production. Even with these limitations, EMG data can still provide important indications as to the identity of active muscles, character of muscle excitation (e.g., single motor units, summation of motor unit activity, interference pattern), and the time course and gradation of muscle excitation. However, in any given case it is necessary to consider whether the electrode configuration used corresponds to that which is assumed in the detailed interpretation of the resulting data. If, for instance, interpretation of the EMG signal will be in terms of a power spectrum model that assumes that the interelectrode axis is parallel to the muscle fibers (Lindström & Petersén, 1983), an electrode insertion procedure must be used in which this axis is controlled.

Electrodes and Myopotential Scaling

Above we emphasized the implications of electrode configuration. Now let us consider the characteristics of the individual electrode. Electrodes for muscle are subdivided on the basis of their physical construction, most commonly as intramuscular electrodes constructed of fine wire, or hypodermiclike needles, or as surface electrodes of metal on which a conductive gel is applied between cleansed and slightly abraded skin and the electrode (Figure 9–3). Depending on the task at hand, special adaptations are sometimes required: For instance, Perlman, Luschei, and DuMond (1989) described their use of a plastic sheath applied to the insertion needle in order to limit the depth of insertion of hooked wire electrodes into the

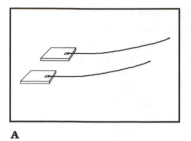
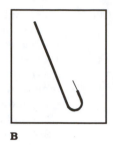
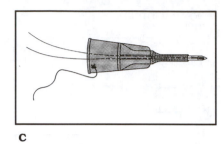

A   B   C

Figure 9–3. EMG electrode types applied in studies of deglutition: (*left*) surface electrode; (*middle*) hooked fine wire electrodes; (*right*) hooked fine wire electrodes inside hypodermic needle for purpose of insertion. Note the sheath on the needle for control of the depth of insertion into thin muscle tissue.

thin superior constrictor muscle of the pharynx. Details on electrode construction and effects are provided in standard clinical sources (Brown, 1984; Kimura, 1989) and in various manuals on electrophysiological research techniques (Bureš, Petraň, & Zachar, 1967; Loeb & Gans, 1986). There is a thought-provoking literature in which recording electrodes are considered more or less analytically; particularly useful are extensive treatments by Cobbold (1974); Ferris (1974); Geddes (1971); Miller and Harrison (1974), especially the chapters by Gatzke and Waring; Geddes and Baker (1989) and by Neuman (1978a). The technical considerations of electroencephalography (EEG) overlap to a considerable degree with those of electromyography, so that the electromyographer may often profit from technical studies of EEG (e.g., Cooper, Osselton, & Shaw, 1980) and technical chapters in the large handbooks of EEG. Where dedicated equipment for EMG is not available, the possibility of application of evoked potential equipment for EMG or intraoperative monitoring (Møller, 1988), for example, should not be overlooked, if its functional characteristics (e.g., frequency response and gain) are appropriate.

In clinical EMG manuals, detailed reference to the expected range of amplitude (usually measured as peak-to-peak voltage in this context) of EMG potentials can often be found (e.g., Liveson & Ma, 1992). However, the amplitude of these poten-

tials depends not only on the physiological phenomena in question, but also on the structure and arrangement of the electrodes employed, and on the subsequent signal processing. The validity of reference to any published standards of EMG signal amplitude is dependent on the substantial functional identity of the structure and arrangement of electrodes employed in the reference study and in the procedures to which it is compared. Therefore clinicians and investigators will likely find it necessary to develop standards relative to the electrodes, equipment, and procedures in use in a given laboratory. For many purposes, reference to the temporal pattern of EMG activity observed will be more informative than absolute signal amplitude.

Frequency Domain Considerations

It is worthwhile to dwell briefly on the frequency filter effect of the differential amplifier in the longitudinal electrode configuration. It can be shown on the basis of a general model first established on the basis of surface electrodes (Kadefors, 1973; Lindström & Magnusson, 1977), which can be extended to fine wire electrodes (Parker & Scott, 1973), that longitudinally arranged bipolar electrodes with the interelectrode axis parallel to the muscle fibers used with a differential amplifier constitute a special type of high-pass filter.

With this configuration, dips in the output signal spectrum occur at a frequency (and its integral multiples), which depends in a simple manner on the mean propagation velocity of the muscle action potentials and the interelectrode distance. The peak of spectral energy in the electromyogram is found at lower frequencies for the surface electromyogram than for the intramuscular signal because of the low-pass filter characteristics of the tissue through which the potentials are conducted from their sources to the electrodes (Gath & Stålberg, 1977; Lindström & Petersén, 1983). In both cases, however, the lowest-frequency dip occurs in the middle of a region of high EMG spectral energy. Thus, as Hogan and Mann (1980) have pointed out, to observe the EMG signal without this spectral dip, one would want to decrease interelectrode distance in order to move the dip out to a frequency beyond 1000 Hz, below which falls the main mass of energy in the electromyogram.

However, this increase in signal bandwidth is obtained at the expense of a decrease in signal amplitude as the electrodes are brought closer (Brown, 1984; Emerson & Zahalak, 1980; Parker & Scott, 1973). With consistent execution of such a signal-based strategy for design of the electrode array and corresponding signal analysis, it becomes possible to derive from the electromyogram information that relates to such physiological and anatomic factors as muscle fatigue, the width of the innervation zone, muscle action potential propagation velocity, and related basic and clinical information (Brown, 1984; Lindström & Magnusson, 1977; Lindström & Petersén, 1983).

SUMMATION AND ANALYSIS OF ACTION POTENTIALS

When sensed by a single-ended amplifier, the muscle action potential seen at a single electrode may be considered with some simplification as a single spike of voltage (strictly, an extracellular potential has three phases). The output of a differential amplifier monitoring the same event through electrodes displaced longitudinally along the muscle as described above is approximately the first time derivative of the above signal; since its value approximately corresponds to the slope of the monopolar signal, it is a roughly biphasic spike with both negative and positive components. This description holds good for the case of single spikes or spike trains from motor units, or a single simultaneous firing of all of the motor units in a muscle, such as results from the indirect stimulation of the muscle through its motor nerve.

Part of the signal sensed by the electrode is relayed by immediate contact of the recording electrode with active muscle tissue, and part of it is conducted to the electrodes through tissue from active muscle tissue spatially removed from the electrodes, a phenomenon known as *volume conduction* (Gath & Stålberg, 1977, 1978; Plonsey, 1969). The significance of volume conduction should not be underestimated, because where monopolar EMG techniques are applied in recording from a small muscle (as is common in the head and neck), part of the electrical activity observed may be conducted passively from an adjacent muscle.

For this reason the application of single-ended or monopolar recording in small muscles such as those of the larynx does not provide the precise localization of signal source that is supplied by differential recording. For instance, it has been demonstrated that electrical activity in denervated thyroarytenoid muscle may be observed with a monopolar technique, because of potentials supplied by the cricothyroid muscle through volume conduction (Dedo & Dunker, 1966; Dedo & Hall, 1969; Dedo & Ogura, 1965). Alternative strategies for making EMG derivations more selective, such as decreasing the size of the electrode recording surface or high-pass filtering the EMG signal at 200–500 Hz, are discussed by Brown (1984).

Since muscle fibers from many motor units occur within the cross-sectional area of any one motor unit (Kugelberg, 1981), as increasing numbers of motor units are recruited, their activity will summate (Figure 9–4). Effects and details of such summation depend partly on the microanatomy and distribution of motor units of the muscles involved, which is often unstudied for muscles of the head and neck involved in swallowing. While the activity of a single motor unit will be represented by an approximately periodic series or train of myopotentials (single spikes, or sometimes repeating small groups of spikes known as polyphasic potentials) of ap-

proximately identical shape and size, trains representing activity of motor units firing at different rates gradually summate into a complex pattern known as an interference pattern. For practical purposes this is an irreversible process; much ingenuity has gone into attempts to analyze the interference pattern into the activity of single motor units that are summated in it, with some success for summation patterns representing the activity of a small number of units. Consequently the char-

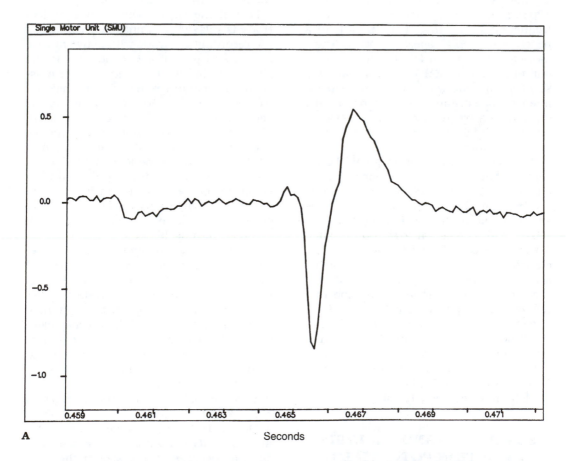

A   Seconds

Figure 9–4. The rate of motor unit firing and recruitment of additional motor units determine the complexity of the EMG signal. **A.** A single motor unit action potential (duration expanded) from the thyroarytenoid muscle of a normal adult subject. **B.** A train of single motor unit action potentials from the thyroarytenoid muscle of a normal adult subject.

C. Gross EMG activity (interference pattern) from the thyroarytenoid muscle during a 10-ml water swallow of a normal adult subject. Note the quiet period well into the swallow; this was not uncommon EMG behavior from the thyroarytenoid muscle during swallowing. (From Perlman, 1993).

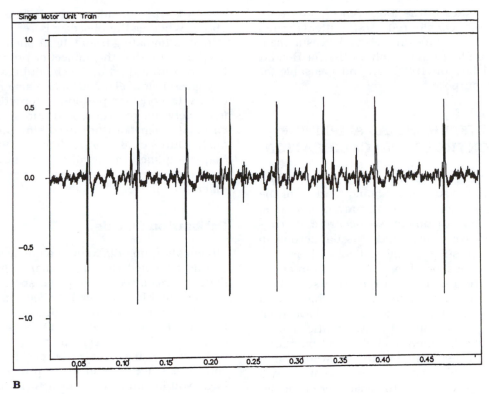

B

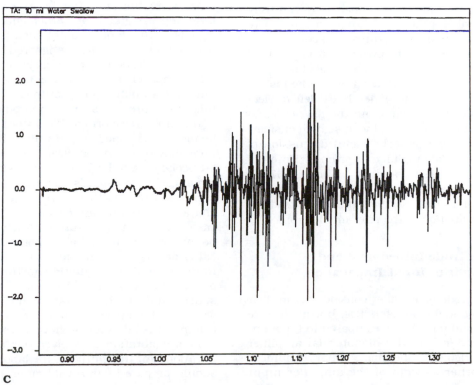

C

acteristics of the interference pattern are usually considered in statistical terms. Treatises on the analysis and measurement of random data, such as that of Bendat and Piersol (1986), are indispensable for this purpose.

DIFFERENTIAL AMPLIFIER CONTROLS AND CALIBRATION

The user of a given complex of electromyographic equipment should start from the assumption that, until proven otherwise, a given instrument is inaccurate, its controls are faulty, and it is dangerous to human subjects and patients. This is not an accusation of manufacturers but an indication of the equipment user's responsibility to experimental subjects and patients. Thus it is necessary to have available the results of a systematic instrument calibration, including not only individual instruments but the system as a whole. However, the present remarks will bear especially on the character of the differential amplifier, which is deceptively complex quite apart from its relation to the anatomic structures studied.

For the present purposes it is practical to consider not circuitry details but signal relations; circuitry lying under the instrument cover is in general best left to electronics technicians, but the user can and must be able to deal with signal considerations. Particularly useful discussion of differential amplifiers is given by Horowitz and Hill (1989) and by Neuman (1978b). The appendix by Seaba and Walker to Kimura's treatise (1989) provides a readable introduction to the relevant electronics.

Electrode Impedance and Amplifier Input Impedance

Electrode types differ considerably in their functional characteristics, but must have a small impedance compared to the input impedance of the biopotential amplifier (Goodgold & Eberstein, 1983). A number of other aspects of the amplifier input

must also be considered (Loeb & Gans, 1986). Whether the observer is recording from or stimulating tissue, he or she must keep in mind that the subject or preparation constitutes part of the circuit between any given pair of electrodes. It is also necessary to consider possible interactions (e.g., between recording and stimulating circuits) when both are used simultaneously (Bureš et al., 1967; Kimura, 1989). Some amplifiers have controls to switch their circuitry from single-ended mode to differential mode.

Calibration Signals

When calibrating differential amplifiers, it should be noted that only small signals (for how small, see the amplifier specifications) should be presented to their inputs; this may require use of a specialized attenuator to reduce the level of the signal output of a function generator. For some applications, it may also be possible to connnect some type of input protection (e.g., voltage-limiting diodes) to prevent damage to the amplifier by excessively large input signals, but other effects on signals of the application of such protective devices should not be ignored. Input signal amplitude is a necessary consideration when checking the accuracy of the different amplifier gain settings. During this procedure, the accurate reproduction of the input waveform at the output must be monitored, since output voltage limitations may result in waveform clipping.

Special care must be taken in using internal calibration signals built into the system to verify that they have the claimed characteristics and are consistent; in the case of some manufacturers, it may even be exceptional that a calibration pulse is either accurate or consistently maintained from one pulse production to the next one, so that an external calibration signal source and standard may be indispensable. For both research and clinical applications, it is advisable to have a record of system calibration on a given day or application. For this purpose, the laboratory should prepare its own calibration protocol, or incorporate a standardized calibration protocol in data collection software.

Frequency Response

The response of a measurement system to dynamically varying input signals depends on its frequency response (Doebelin, 1983; Oliver & Cage, 1971; Rosa, 1990; Sydenham, 1982, 1983). Thus a standard measurement required for the differential amplifier is the indication of the ratio of the amplitude of the input to the output signals as a function of frequency. A frequency response may be measured for a given input channel by shorting the other input to ground, connecting a small-voltage arbitrary signal to the input, and measuring the output signal. A common procedure is to sweep the frequency of a sinusoidal signal of constant amplitude across the frequency range of interest, in which case the amplification factor G may be obtained as the ratio of the amplitude (voltage) of the output signal to that of the input as a function of frequency, often stated in dB. Thus

$$G(f) = A_{out}(f) / A_{in}$$

or

$$G(f)_{dB} = 20 \log_{10}(A_{out}(f) / A_{in})$$

As a measured quantity, *gain* is often plotted as a function of frequency. Various alternative procedures exist that require more complex mathematical considerations: For instance, use of transient input signals such as a voltage step may render unnecessary some equipment used in sinusoidal frequency response measurement.

Common Mode Rejection Ratio

The quantification of the degree of elimination of interfering signals by the differential amplifier is central to its evaluation (Oliver & Cage 1971). Since the elimination of common mode voltages in the signals to the amplifier inputs is never complete, a quantity is formed as the ratio of signal gain when a given signal is fed to a single input with the other one shorted to ground (differential gain, DG), and the gain when the same signal is fed to both inputs (common mode gain, CMG). The resulting ratio is known as the common mode rejection ratio (CMRR)

$$CMRR = DG/CMG$$

and may be stated in dB:

$$CMRR_{dB} = 20 \log_{10} DG/CMG$$

Since the gain is a function of frequency, so must common mode rejection be frequency-dependent. Most commonly, however, some frequency or range of frequency values over which the variation is limited is chosen as the basis of the determination of CMRR, and a single value of CMRR is stated. A common range of CMRR of adequate differential amplifiers at frequencies in the range of the rapid firing rate of motor units (50–60 Hz and higher) is about 80 dB or 10,000 to 1 or better.

System Noise

Some types of noise originate at the electrodes and are determined by the selection or application of electrodes (Geddes 1972; Geddes & Baker 1989). Other types of noise are added to the input signals as they pass through the EMG system. A standard approach to the measurement of such added noise is to connect the input to the component considered to ground (i.e., short-circuit the input) and observe the amplitude of the voltage output. In general, the wider the system's bandwidth, the greater will be the system noise, so it is customary to specify it with reference to a signal bandwidth of interest. Since the EMG power spectrum has little energy in it above 2000 Hz (Basmajian, Clifford, McLeod, & Nunnally, 1975), a bandwidth of 3000 Hz might be considered ample.

System Bandwidth

Bandwidth is specified by the settings of low-pass and high-pass filters on the amplifier. The effect of such a filter is defined by specifying that the amplitude or power of a signal which has a reference value in frequency regions relatively unaffected by the filter (the pass-band) is reduced to at least the indicated degree in other frequency regions. Reference points for the transition between the pass-band of a filter and regions with substantial loss of signal amplitude are sometimes specified as half-amplitude (6 dB down) points, but more commonly as half-power (3 dB down) points. Ordinarily a high-pass filter setting at 30 Hz, for example, may be recommended in order to eliminate any effects of movement artifact, as observed in some EMG recordings where large slow baseline voltage shifts are found (Basmajian et al., 1975). A low-pass filter setting that passes energies below 2000 Hz unattenuated will ordinarily be ample for raw EMG, since energy at frequencies above this range will only add noise to the signal.

60 Hz and Other Interference Signals

The problem of 60 Hz interfering signals in the EMG amplifier output may be partly eliminated by switching a 60 Hz band-reject or notch filter into the system; higher multiples of 60 Hz may be present and require a more elaborate notch filter. Since 60 Hz falls within the high range of the firing frequency of motor units, a better approach is to eliminate the interfering signal to the extent possible; large 60 Hz components may indicate a defective electrode configuration, connection, or insertion. Sometimes it is necessary to use or construct a small shielded and grounded room or cage in order to eliminate interference signals. A conventional audiological booth may suffice, although its grounding system must be checked; occasionally it may be found that a booth has not been connected to the building ground.

Grounding and Safety Considerations

Special care may be required in adapting research equipment to clinical surroundings or human subjects. For instance, for subject safety, optical coupling may be required on differential amplifiers, and computer-based equipment not certified for medical use may have enough current leakage to set off operating room alarms even in experimental suites.

At this point it is worthwhile to recall general considerations of grounding practice in instrumentation systems (Morrison, 1986), which acquire particular importance in electrophysiology, especially when stimulators are applied (Bureš et al., 1967). A general rule is that multiple grounds in an instrument system should be avoided, and the best ground available should be sought, which will not necessarily be that in the grounded power receptacle (Mleczko, 1972). Some buildings for scientific research are constructed with a special laboratory ground system running to every laboratory. Where optical or other types of isolation are built into medical or research equipment, however, an earth ground to the subject is not used, because it would defeat the purpose of the isolators. Inquiries to local technicians are in order, and so are measurements of continuity and impedance relations of supposed ground systems. Since both validity of measurement results and subject safety (e.g., Kimura, 1989; Roth, Teltscher, & Kane, 1975) are in question, this area requires both careful thinking and the willingness to consult available technical expertise.

SIGNAL RECORDING AND PROCESSING

Recording Systems

The modern practitioner is likely to record EMG data digitally, either with a digital tape recorder or directly into the computer. In either case a signal-to-noise ratio of up to twice that previously available on magnetic tape recorders can be obtained. Bandwidth and signal duration are limited only by practical needs and available equipment. Detailed principles of analog to digital conversion of electrical signals are not obvious, and we mention only a few of many works in this area (Garrett, 1981; Horowitz & Hill, 1989; Magrab & Blomquist, 1971; VanDoren, 1982;). Two principal considerations will intrude on the user's attention.

Signal Bandwidth and Data Sampling Rate

Given that the experimenter or clinician has some notion of the signal bandwidth necessary for given data, in order to reproduce these data correctly, it is necessary to record data points sampled at rates at least twice, and better at several times, the sampling frequency that corresponds to the upper bound of the signal bandwidth. This is necessary to avoid aliasing, in which energy from spectral regions higher than the signal is folded into the signal bandwidth. Thus if we assume that EMG has a spectral bandwidth from DC to 2000 Hz, a sampling rate of 4,000 samples per second for raw EMG is marginally adequate, while one of 10,000–12,000 samples per second is good. If the data have been subjected to analog low-pass filtering, their bandwidth will be narrower and the necessary sampling rate will be slower. For very detailed analysis of the EMG waveform, for which a signal frequency range of up to 10 KHz may be considered, sampling rates as high as 50 KHz have been used (Desmedt, 1983). It will often be advantageous to low-pass filter the data before they are digitized; such specialized filters (anti-aliasing filters) are intended to remove energy at frequencies that are not part of the signal of interest to avoid the production of artifacts in some signal processing such as spectral analysis.

Signal Dynamic Range

A second principal consideration is the expected range of signal amplitude. Any digitization system has a measurable level of background noise and a specifiable (sometimes adjustable) range of ampli-

tude within which its reproduction of signal amplitude will be linear. Optimal signal reproduction depends on using this signal range so that the signal is as large as possible relative to the system noise. If the input signal is known to exceed the available signal range, or only uses a small part of the available range, it is advantageous to use an attenuator or conditioning amplifier to adjust signal amplitude or DC offset for purposes of digitization, so that the full range of the analog to digital converter is used to best advantage. Later the signal amplitude or DC level can be corrected digitally where this is necessary. In some systems, special buffer amplifiers between successive analog signal-processing stages may be required because of specialized input or output impedance characteristics of some item of equipment. In some cases, simple insertion of a parallel or series resistance into the circuit may suffice, but such considerations of impedance-matching are ignored at the risk of acquiring unusable data.

Data Analysis

Although the investigator can carry out extensive EMG data analysis on an analog level, such analysis can almost always be done more precisely on a digital level. The flexibility and range of digital analysis is virtually infinite, and data access is much more rapid than in working from magnetic tape. Limitations and details of analysis depend not only on whether the available computing facility, signal-processing package, or locally developed computer programs can carry out a given mathematical procedure, but also on the interpretability and relevance of the results (e.g., Stålberg & Young, 1981). For instance, although a power spectrum can be calculated for any EMG data, its interpretability in particular physiological senses depends on the choice of the original configuration of the electrodes, as discussed earlier.

If the objective of the analysis is to relate the EMG data to the level of muscle mechanical output, then it is usual to take the absolute (full-wave rectified) values of the data and subject them to some low-pass filter or averaging procedure, or to derive the running root mean square (rms) value (Basmajian et al., 1975; De Luca, 1979; De Luca & van Dyk, 1975) although this relation of EMG to force is straightforward only in isometric conditions. Since, as noted above, the absolute scale of EMG voltages depends partly on the character of electrodes and other factors, it is common to establish relative and linear scaling of the EMG, using some external criterion to establish a maximum and minimum for the EMG signal range. The value of such scaling is decreased by the fact that changes of muscle length may produce changes of the scaling of EMG signals apart from changes of the level of muscle excitation, as discussed by Cooper and Folkins (1985), but in practice such effects are usually ignored. The link between the signals recorded by EMG and the mechanical output of muscle is complex (Bouisset, 1973; Perry & Bekey, 1981), and there is reason to expect that eventually other measurements will make possible a more direct measurement of the mechanical output of muscle, complementary to EMG which is a measure of muscle excitation (Cooper, Pinczower, & Rice, 1993).

At this point, some acquaintance with the concepts of time series analysis becomes indispensable; readable introductions with various orientations are available (e.g., Chatfield, 1975), as well as more advanced treatises. The introductory book of Basmajian and colleagues (1975) on analog and digital EMG signal processing, although dated in minor regards, provides a valuable initial orientation. More advanced treatises on bioelectric signal analysis are often based on EEG data (e.g., Glaser & Ruchkin, 1976, and the major collective EEG treatises), but are still often useful for EMG. Desmedt has edited two fundamental and accessible symposia on the computer-aided analysis of EMG signals (1983, 1989). In application to clinical problems, related concepts may often be found under the heading of clinical neurophysiology (e.g., Stålberg & Young, 1981).

EMG STUDY OF SWALLOWING

As stated earlier, the EMG signal is the cumulative result of the filter effects of a number of successive stages. Figures 9–5a through 9–5k (Figure 9–5) recapitulate the process of generation, and of analog and digital processing of myoelectric signals. The original signal, considered as the extracellular potential seen by a monopolar electrode in the vicinity of an excitable fiber, is proportional to the second derivative with respect to time of the transmembrane potential (Geddes, 1972). The detailed shape of the myopotential (*a*) depends on the physiological condition of the muscle. Every myopotential that reaches any electrode has been damped (attenuated and low-pass filtered) by the tissues through which it has passed (*b*) Details of motor unit recruitment vary, for example, as a result of fatigue and contraction level. Myopotentials from the muscle fibers in a given motor unit sum in a spectrum with the shape of a low-pass filter function while the greater the number of active motor units summing in an EMG pattern, the greater will be the representation of low-frequency energy from distant signal sources (*c*) (Lindström & Petersén, 1983).

The structure and application of electrodes determine their intrinsic impedance and filter characteristics (*d*), while in differential recording the geometry of electrode arrangement relative to the muscle fibers and motor end plates partly determines the filter effect of the differential amplifier (*e*). The electrical properties of the electrodes, electrode cables, and amplifier input impedance interact; the capacitance of electrode cables and amplifier input sum and low-pass filter the EMG signal (*f*) (Goodgold & Eberstein, 1983). The output signal from the first stage of the preamplifier is simply the voltage difference between the simultaneous input signals (*g*). Subsequent stages (*h*) may amplify (*B* in h) this difference signal, and filter (designated by the symbols *h(t) in h) to eliminate interference components and signal baseline shifts. Extraneous signal components at frequencies higher than

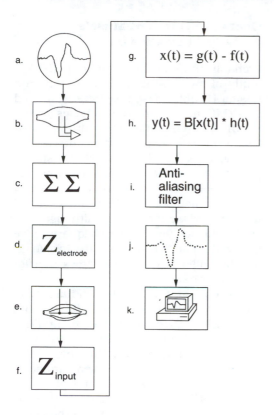

$$x(t) = g(t) - f(t)$$

$$y(t) = B[x(t)] * h(t)$$

Anti-aliasing filter

b. An EMG potential from a given motor unit (MUAP) is damped by its passage from the signal source through tissue to the electrode. **c.** Summation of MUAPs in the interference pattern alters the spectrum, as do physiological factors, like fatigue. **d.** The electrical impedance and filter effects of electrodes depend on their physical structure, experimental preparation, and details of electrode application. Surface electrodes have a low-pass filter effect. **e.** The geometric arrangement of electrodes relative to the course of muscle fibers and motor end plates partly determines the filter effect of the differential amplifier on the EMG signals. **f.** The capacitance of electrodes and electrode cables adds to the amplifier input capacitance; together they exert a low-pass filter effect on the EMG signal. **g.** The output of the difference stage of the differential amplifier is the voltage difference between the two input signals as a function of time. **h.** The differential amplifier usually has optional 60-Hz band-reject characteristics, and adjustable high-pass and low-pass filter stages. **i.** The output of the differential amplifier is usually subjected to low-pass anti-alias filtering to remove higher frequency spectral components not part of the signal of interest, which at the rate of digitization used could result in computational artifacts. **j.** The sampling rate of digitization of analog data, nature of the converter, system dynamic range and resolution, and other specifications limit bandwidth and determine the precision with which the data can be analyzed or reconstructed. **k.** In the computer, EMG signals may be stored, rescaled, analyzed in relation to other physiological information, subjected to time series analysis of various types, plotted for display, and so on.

Figure 9–5. The character of the EMG signal is the cumulative result of the filter effects of a number of successive stages. **a.** The shape of the muscle action potential reflects slower changing factors related to the condition of the muscle as well as rapid changes in the membrane potential associated with muscle action.

the myoelectric signal are removed by anti-aliasing filters (*i*) before analog to digital conversion, or, if sampling is sufficiently rapid, by subsequent digital filtering. The recording and digitatization systems (*j*) impose their own limits on the data observed and must be controlled to optimize data quality. The analysis and interpretation (*k*) of the resulting myoelectric signal depend on detailed and systematic consideration of its generation, character, and processing as a signal.

Now we turn to the application of electromyography specifically to the assessment of the physiological systems that

underlie swallowing. Most of the early study of the muscles of the human larynx and pharynx were performed because of researchers' interest in speech science and otolaryngology (Faaborg-Andersen, 1957, 1965; Fritzell, 1963, 1969; Gay, Hirose, Strome, & Sawashima,1972; Haglund, 1973; Hirano, Ohala & Vennard, 1969; Hirose, 1971; Kawasaki, Ogura, & Takenouchi, 1964; Minifie, Abbs, Tarlow, and Kwaterski, 1974; Sawashima, Funasaka, & Totsuk, 1958). Today, EMG is used as a diagnostic tool by otolaryngologists to assess the viability of muscles of the head and neck and the change in muscle function resulting from surgical or behavioral treatment (e.g., Lovelace, Blitzer, & Ludlow, 1992). Speech and swallowing scientists continue to use EMG for improved understanding of muscle function during specific phonation tasks (Hirano, 1981) and during deglutition (Palmer, Tippett, & Wolf, 1991; Perlman et al., 1989; Perlman, Palmer, McCulloch, & VanDaele, in preparation). And, of course, experiments on the muscles of the oral cavity and pharynx during speech and swallowing are found in the dental literature. Naturally, EMG is used by other clinicians and researchers in areas such as neurology and physical medicine and re-habilitation; many times the clinician in these disciplines uses electromyography for differential diagnosis. However, the scope of this portion of our chapter is limited to electromyography of the head and neck as it relates to swallowing.

Electromyographic research using animal models as well as human subjects has contributed to our present knowledge of deglutition. At times the study was not performed for the purposes of understanding deglutition, but swallowing data were presented along with other information, for example, respiratory data. Most swallowing studies using human subjects have concentrated on the actions of a single muscle or just a few muscle pairs, rather than on the dynamic relationships between various muscles. A good review of the literature relating to electromyographic activity of muscles of the oral cavity, larynx, and pharynx was presented by Basmajian and DeLuca (1985). The muscles discussed in their review can often serve three major purposes, respiration, deglutition, and communication, and their review includes all three aspects of muscle function. Studies performed specifically to study deglutition constitute only a few among those reported by the two investigators. Of course, since the publication of that material in 1985, additional studies have been reported in the literature.

Overall Patterns of Muscle Activity in Swallowing

Probably the most frequently cited EMG study of swallowing is that of Doty and Bosma (1956). These researchers studied the EMG activity of the muscles of the mouth, pharynx, and larynx during swallowing in cats, dogs, and monkeys. The investigators found a relatively consistent pattern of activity, and no effects on the sequence of muscle activation were found when the methods by which the swallows were evoked were changed. Although that study did not provide much quantitative information on the swallow, the investigation by Miller (1972) did address that issue somewhat.

Subsequent investigators (Filaretov & Filimonova, 1969; Kawasaki et al., 1964; Sumi, 1964) have found that the findings of Doty and Bosma held up in in other mammalian species. In the dog, Miller (1972) found activity in several muscles of the soft palate, tongue, and pharynx, begins 0–40 ms after the onset of mylohyoid EMG activity. Other muscles then contract with latencies ranging from 40 to 360 ms. The duration of EMG activity of the individual muscles studied ranged from 250 to 500 ms, and the total duration of the swallow from first onset to last offset was generally in the range of 700 to 900 ms.

In a study similar to that of Doty and Bosma (1956), Kawasaki et al. (1964) studied 34 dogs where bipolar hooked wire electrodes were inserted into a series of muscles, including submental, pharyngeal, laryngeal, esophageal, and respiratory muscles. They too found a coordinated pattern of activity between the groups of muscles. Interestingly, they reported that in the fully conscious animal, deglutition occurred during inspiration in 94% of the swallows. This disagrees with reports on human swallowing (Selley, Ellis, Flack, Bayliss, & Pearce, 1994; Smith, Wolkove, Colacone, & Kreisman, 1989), where swallowing is almost exclusively seen on expiration.

The finding of a consistent pattern of contraction in spite of muscle ablation has been replicated by Maeyama (1975). In his study of anesthetized dogs, Maeyama also concluded that the geniohyoid and the thyrohyoid muscles play the most important role in laryngeal elevation. Other muscles that contribute to laryngeal elevation include the mylohyoid and stylohyoid, as well as other suprahyoid muscles.

In Perlman's laboratory simultaneous electromyographic recordings were performed on humans as they swallowed. The subjects each had submental bipolar surface electrodes and three pairs of bipolar hooked-wire electrodes. The hooked wire electrodes were inserted in the superior pharyngeal constrictor muscle, which served as the muscle from which time zero was calculated, and in two other muscles. Different subjects had different insertions of the remaining two pairs of electrodes. Along with the superior pharyngeal constrictor and submental muscle complex, the muscles studied included thyroarytenoid, interarytenoid, and cricopharyngeus. At the time of the writing of this chapter, the data have been analyzed and the paper is being prepared for publication (Perlman et al., in preparation). Figure 9–6 shows the raw data from the superior pharyngeal constrictor, thyroarytenoid, interarytenoid, and submental muscles during a 5-ml bolus swallow of a young adult male. Notice the silent segment in the thyroarytenoid muscle that occurs after the submental complex and the superior pharyngeal constrictors have begun contracting; this was often observed in the thyroarytenoid muscles of our subjects.

For this individual during this swallow, the onset of EMG of the submental com-

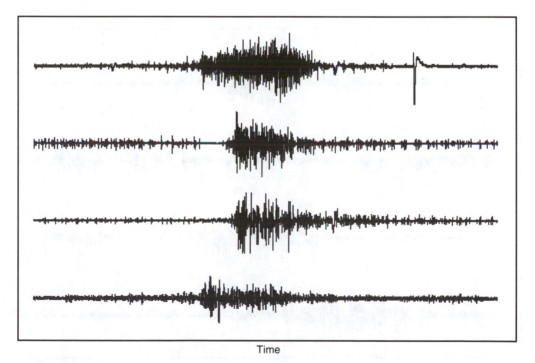

Time

Figure 9–6. Simultaneous EMG activity, from top to bottom, the superior pharyngeal constrictor, thyroarytenoid, interarytenoid, and submental muscles during a 5 ml bolus swallow from a normal subject.

plex was 24 ms following the onset of EMG activity of the superior pharyngeal constrictor. The thyroarytenoid began to contract 155 ms and the interarytenoid began to contract 190 ms following the onset of EMG activity of the superior pharyngeal constrictor muscle.

Figure 9–7 shows the EMG activity in the submental, thyroarytenoid, cricopharyngeus, and superior pharyngeal constrictor during a dry swallow, also from a young adult male. Again, notice the quiet segment in the thyroarytenoid muscle after the swallow has begun. Additionally, as would be expected, the EMG activity in the cricopharyngeus ceases as the muscle relaxes in preparation for passage of saliva. In this example, the superior pharyngeal constrictor begins to contract about 179 ms after the submental complex. The cricopharyngeus ceases activity 123 ms after the the superior pharyngeal constrictor has begun to contract, and the thy-

roarytenoid begins to contract 155 ms after the superior pharyngeal constrictor. The duration of the silent segment was 190 ms.

When the RMS values were calculated for the muscles that were studied, it was apparent that they are more active during swallowing than during the two other tasks that the subjects performed: those tasks were speech production and a Valsalva maneuver. This finding from all muscles studied in that investigation was compatible with the findings of Perlman et al. (1989) in their study of EMG activity from the superior pharyngeal constrictor during a series of tasks including swallowing.

Lingual and Sublingual Activity in Swallowing

Bole (1965) published an early study on the use of wire electrodes in the study of

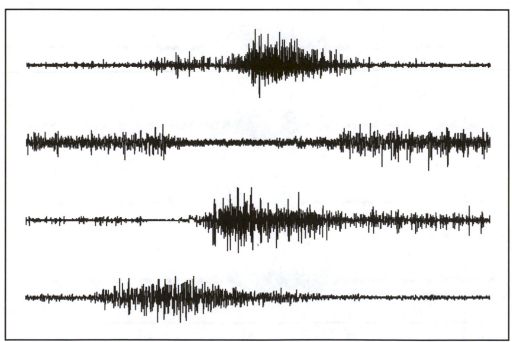

Time

Figure 9–7. Simultaneous EMG activity, from top to bottom, the superior pharyngeal constrictor, cricopharyngeus, thyroarytenoid, and submental muscles during a dry swallow from a normal subject.

the human tongue. In his study of the genioglossus muscle, he found that during swallowing there were usually two or more bursts of activity; the bursts reportedly appeared at the onset of the swallow and after the substance had left the tongue. Several different patterns of tongue movement were evident during the swallow. Cunningham and Basmajian (1969) also studied the tongue and found differences in the swallowing pattern within subjects as well as between subjects. They reported that the duration of tongue EMG was greater during saliva swallows than during water bolus swallows; furthermore, a period of active inhibition was evident just prior to the burst of activity.

Additional work by Basmajian and colleagues found that during a swallow, the onset of activity from the anterior belly of the digastric, geniohyoid, mylohyoid, and genioglossus muscles of adults varied within a subject as well as between subjects. However, individuals were more likely to have a given pattern from which they sometimes varied (Hrycyshyn & Basmajian, 1972; Vitti et al., 1975). The anterior belly of the digastric muscle was not involved in swallowing in approximately one fourth of the 20 subjects studied by Hrycyshyn and Basmajian (1972). They also found that the duration of EMG activity from the genioglossus and geniohyoid muscles increased with the viscosity of the bolus. Electromyographic activity of the intrinsic and extrinsic muscles of the human tongue (Sauerland & Mitchell, 1975) has revealed that when a person shifts from a sitting to a supine position, the EMG activity in the genioglossus increases considerably, but other tongue muscles do not increase their activity. This increase in activity is not eliminated when the mucosa is anesthetized. Since the genioglossus is the muscle that protrudes the tongue, it has a role in respiration; therefore, it is important that this muscle move forward in order to keep the airway open for respiration. The genioglossus is active during both phases of respiration, but particularly during inspiration. Other tongue muscles examined in that study did not show activity related to respiration. The genioglossus does play a part in deglutition, in that during oral preparation the tongue moves anteriorly to the alveolar ridge for the swallow, and protrudes beyond that point for licking such as that associated with eating an ice cream cone or a sucker.

Submandibular Muscles

The variability in the order of firing of the submental muscles that has been observed within as well as between subjects supports the acceptability of the use of surface electrodes in the submandibular region for recording of these muscles. The use of surface electrodes results in the recording from any or all of these muscles during the oral and pharyngeal stages of swallowing. Submental surface electrodes are commonly used as a method of identifying the onset of the swallow (Martin, Logemann, Shaker, & Dodds, 1994; Reimer-Neils, Logemann, & Larson, 1994; Schultz, Perlman, & VanDaele, 1994; Takada, Miyawaki, & Tatsuta, 1994).

Jaw Muscles

The temporalis and masseter muscles were studied in ten children ranging from 8 years to 15 years of age (Ahlgren, 1967). Ahlgren reported that during the closing phase of mastication both muscles contracted isotonically, during the closed phase they contracted isometrically, and during the opening phase of mastication, the muscles were not active. Approximately 75% of the EMG activity occurred during the closing phase, and therefore only 25% occurred during the closed phase of chewing. A silent period occurred at the beginning of the closed phase, which the investigator interpreted as serving as a protective mechanism for the teeth.

The temporalis muscle was also investigated by Vitti (1971). He used needle electrodes with 57 adults. Each temporalis muscle had three insertions, anterior, medial, and posterior. The subjects fell into three groups depending on their individual dentition. He reported that the muscle was always inactive when the jaw was protruded from the position of maximum retraction; and, in the retraction of the jaw from rest position, the posterior portion was active in all groups, but the middle portion was active only in the subjects with complete and normal dentition.

The muscles of mastication were studied in some depth by Møller (1966, 1974, 1976). Using human subjects, he reported on the medial and lateral pterygoid, anterior and posterior digastric, orbicularis oris, mylohyoid, temporalis, and masseter muscles during various levels of contraction and during chewing. He reported that the muscles perform a vigorous chewing action for about one third of a second, and that for most subjects, the amount of activity in the anterior temporalis, masseter, and medial pterygoid muscles was at approximately 50% of their maximal level. The muscles responsible for jaw opening during mastication were activated in the sequence of mylohyoid, digastric, and lateral pterygoid. The medial pterygoid muscles were the first of the elevators to show active EMG on closing.

Subjects for another study of mastication were 15 children who chewed hard and soft jellies especially prepared for that study (Takada et al., 1994). Wire electrodes had been placed in the posterior portion of the temporalis muscle and in the inferior orbicularis oris muscle. The investigators studied the effects of viscosity on mastication with particular attention to the lateral jaw movements and temporalis activity. They found that the closing phase was longer when the subjects chewed the hard jelly, but the opening and intercuspal portions of mastication remained the same. Furthermore, the velocities of jaw closing were slower with the hard jelly, and the temporalis muscle displayed EMG timing differences related to viscosity.

Oral and Buccal Muscles

When bipolar hooked-wired electrodes were inserted into the superior pharyn-

geal constrictor, buccinator, and inferior and superior orbicularis oris muscles (Perkins, Blanton, & Biggs, 1977), it was found that swallowing was the only function in which there appeared a consistently sequential pattern of muscle activity. Furthermore, as would be expected, it was reported that the orbicularis oris and buccinator muscles showed greater EMG activity during the oral preparatory phase than during the pharyngeal phase. Twelve of the 14 subjects studied in this experiment showed greater activity of those muscles when swallowing peanuts than when swallowing water. Eleven subjects showed onset of EMG activity from the buccinator before the orbicularis oris. Durations of muscle EMG activity averaged 0.54 sec for the buccinator, 0.44 sec for the orbicularis oris, and 0.80 sec for the superior pharyngeal constrictor. Simultaneous activity was approximately 0.18 sec in duration.

Palatal and Pharyngeal Muscles

Some of the work on palatal muscles has been performed by specialists in cleft palate speech. However, when studying the cleft palate population, it was often necessary to have a control group of normal subjects; and so the data from some of those studies are of use to the researcher who is interested in swallowing. Such was the work presented by Trigos, Ysunza, Vargas, and Vazquez, (1988). Because the primary purpose of their study was to examine the effectiveness of a particular surgical procedure on phonation, their results can only partially be applied to the study of swallowing. However, after performing an EMG study of the palatopharyngeus muscle, they concluded that the major role of the palatopharyngeus muscle is in swallowing. Additionally, they stated that the muscle should be considered a palatal depressor and principal antagonist of the levator veli palatini. This statement may appear somewhat confusing, since the velum elevates significantly during the swallow. However, it is possible that during the swallow, the levator muscle contracts to elevate the pharynx and that the palatoglossus relaxes somewhat at that time. Obviously, there is need for further study of the relationships between EMG activity of the palatopharyngeus and the levator veli palatini muscles during swallow before conclusions can be drawn.

Basmajian and Dutta (1961) studied the levator veli palatini and the superior, medial, and inferior constrictors in ten young normal adults. Although the investigators used bipolar needle electrodes, which may have had an effect on structural movement during swallowing, the results were very interesting. They reported that the levator veli palatini showed a low level of activity during sucking and while holding a liquid bolus in the mouth, but the constrictors were not active during these activities. During swallowing, the levator was active for about 300 ms, and the three constrictors were active for an average of 492 ms. The muscles relaxed completely at the end of the swallow. Because the investigators were unable to make these measures simultaneously, there was no information on the overlap of constrictor muscle function; such information is important to those who are presently researching the pharyngeal stage of the swallow. The same investigators (Basmajian & Dutta, 1961) performed a study on these muscles with rabbits; in that investigation, simultaneous measurements were performed.

Using bipolar hooked wire electrodes, the superior pharyngeal constrictor muscles were studied by Perlman et al. (1989). Their subjects performed a variety of tasks, and the duration and extent of EMG activity for each task was calculated. They found that swallowing produced significantly higher EMG amplitudes than did any of the other tasks. Gagging, also a reflexive task, had the second highest amplitude, which was an average of 63% of that obtained by swallowing. The mean duration of the superior pharyngeal constrictor muscle activity during the swallow was 0.8 s, which was the same as that reported by Perkins et al. (1976). The next greatest level of EMG activity occurred during production of a modified Valsalva maneuver, which involved prolonged, tight velar closure. This study has been cited as a rationale for use of the modified Valsalva maneuver or hard [k] sound as a method of reducing the likelihood of disuse atrophy in patients with pharyngeal weakness or paralysis.

Some activity in the superior pharyngeal constrictor has also been reported during expiration, although the muscle was reportedly nonfunctional during inspiration (Hairston & Sauerland, 1981). In a pioneer study of the laryngeal muscles (Nakamura, Uyeda, & Sonoda, 1958), the abductor muscle (posterior cricoarytenoid) was active during inspiration and all the other muscles were active during expiration except for the thyroarytenoid muscle, which was quiet throughout both inspiration and expiration. Given subsequent advances in technique, the findings regarding thyroarytenoid muscle function require modification. From indirect laryngoscopic views as well as from endoscopic observation of the larynx during respiration, mild adduction of the vocal folds is visible during expiration. Laryngeal activity during respiration has been discussed by Kirchner (1986). Because of the relative ease with which the superior pharyngeal constrictor can be accessed, electromyographic assessment of that muscle is a reasonable procedure to consider when paralysis is suspected. Figures 9–8a and 9–8b show the rectified EMG from the superior pharyngeal constrictor muscle of an individual with normal muscle function and a patient who had pharyngeal paralysis poststroke.

Muscles of the Lower Pharynx

A recent study by Ertekin et al. (1995) investigated the relationship between the direction of laryngeal motion, measured with a piezoelectric sensor, and surface submental and needle electrode cricopharyngeal electromyography. The article provided some interesting information regarding their findings on the relationships between laryngeal motion and cricopharyngeal relaxation. The investigators found

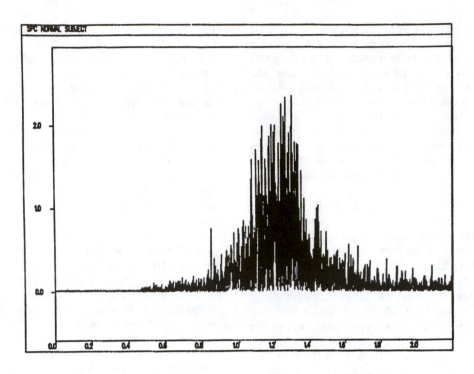

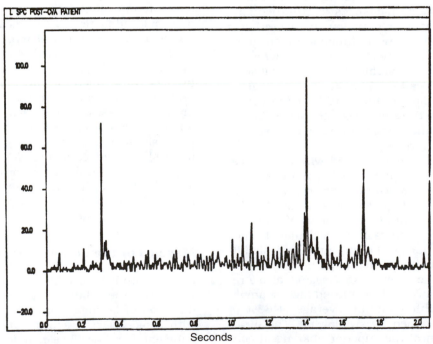

Figure 9–8. (*Top*) rectified EMG from the superior pharyngeal constrictor muscle of an adult with a normal swallow. (*Bottom*) rectified EMG from the superior pharyngeal constrictor muscle of an adult who had suffered a stroke. The EMG confirms the diagnosis of pharyngeal paralysis. (From Perlman, 1993).

that changes in both bolus type and volume resulted in a change in each of the measurements they were obtaining. Unfortunately, the results did not show a linear change that could be easily interpreted.

In an earlier study, the inferior pharyngeal constrictor and cricopharyngeus muscles were studied in patients who were in surgery and had been lightly anesthetized in preparation for a total laryngectomy (Shipp, Deatsch, & Robertson, 1970). The muscles of interest were studied as soon as they could be visualized and before any major surgical alterations had occurred. The muscles were then studied later in surgery after the laryngectomy, and again up to 3 years postsurgery. The investigators found that early in surgery there was a typical pattern characterized by a single large burst of activity from the inferior pharyngeal constrictor, very closely followed by a drop in the level of cricopharyngeus activity. After laryngectomy, both muscles showed dramatic changes in activity patterns, and the altered pattern remained over a period of years.

In another study in which patients were anesthetized for an esophagoscopy, hooked wire electrodes were placed in the upper esophageal sphincter and into the hypopharynx (van Overbeek, Wit, Paping, & Segenhout, 1985). Approximately 2 hours after the patients were fully awake, simultaneous manometry and EMG were recorded during swallowing. The authors reported that electrical activity was present in the UES, but that the activity abruptly stopped during the swallow, and at the same time the UES pressure reached its minimum. A low level of hypopharyngeal activity was also present at rest, and this activity increased with the swallow at the same time that the UES activity disappeared.

In a study of the effectiveness of different types of electrodes for recording myoelectric activity, Palmer, Tanaka, and Siebens (1989) found that, in the pharynx, bipolar suction electrodes work as well as bipolar hooked wire electrodes. Two other papers (Palmer, 1989; Tanaka, Palmer, & Siebens, 1986) described their bipolar suction electrodes and their application in more detail.

As discussed in the first portion of this chapter, in the area of the head and neck it is important to use bipolar rather than monopolar electrodes, whether suction or wire, for EMG observations. With monopolar electrodes it is possible to record volume-conducted activity from muscles other than those in which the electrodes are inserted.

In an early electromyographic experiment, Storey (1968) studied the effects of various stimuli in triggering the pharyngeal stage of swallowing in decerebrate cats. He found that, among a wide selection of mechanical, chemical, and thermal stimuli, the most effective stimuli for triggering a swallow when applied by dropper to the laryngeal surface of the epiglottis, the glottis, and the internal surface of the larynx, were water, a 20% solution of ethyl alcohol and water, and an isotonic sucrose solution. Isotonic saline solutions evoked swallowing less effectively than did water.

An interesting report by Rowe, Miller, Chierici, and Clendenning (1984) discussed the finding of functional fiber components within the pharyngeal constrictor muscles. In their study of six rhesus monkeys, a series of bipolar wire electrodes was inserted in a rostrocaudal line in the pharynx. During deglutition, the investigators found variability in successive swallowing patterns, but normally the palatopharyngeus and superior pharyngeal constrictor would discharge simultaneously. The rostral and caudal regions of the middle pharyngeal constrictor fired 100 to 150 ms after the upper muscles. Of particular interest was the discovery that although most of the fibers of the pharyngeal constrictors were recruited during swallowing, certain regions of each of the three constrictors never discharged during swallowing. The authors concluded that a degree of regional functional specialization of muscle fibers is present in each of the three constrictors of the monkey; this hypothesis has not been tested in humans.

Another animal study (Lang, Dantas, Cook, & Dodds, 1991) found that the peak upper esophageal pressure zone was closely associated with the site of the EMG electrodes attached to the cricopharyngeus muscle. Furthermore, the cricopharyngeus muscle in dogs relaxed approximately 200 ms before the upper esophageal sphincter opened as seen on simultaneous videofluoroscopy, and about 100 ms before the pressure values demonstrated that the muscle was relaxing. Superior movement of the thyrohyoid complex occurred in close association to that of the upper esophageal sphincter relaxation; however, the anterior movement of the hyoid and larynx almost always occurred just before the opening of the sphincter. In the dog model, the temporal pattern of cricopharyngeal relaxation and tonicity were not affected by changing the bolus volume.

Perspectives for Future EMG Applications in Swallowing Studies

Although a number of different types of electrodes have been used to deal with the various structures involved in the complex physiological patterns of swallowing, the general perspective of the EMG aspect of such research has rarely gone far beyond a descriptive kinesiologic viewpoint. Modern electromyography has developed many fascinating approaches to examine such questions as the indicators of muscle fatigue, the distribution of the motor end plates, and the like, on the basis of electrophysiological data, as well as applications in a more traditional context of motor control. Even when the descriptive task of the mapping of temporal sequences of myoelectric activity in swallowing has reached a much more precise level of detail than is available at present, electromyography will continue to play an important role in the analysis and assessment of swallowing behaviors in the laboratory and in the clinic.

MULTIPLE CHOICE QUESTIONS

Complete the following sentences.

1. Changing a monopolar to a bipolar electrode arrangement when recording EMG from a muscle:
   a. has no effect on the output signal.
   b. means that the output signal from the differential amplifier is a multiple of the difference between the signal measured between one input and the neutral electrode, and the signal measured between the other input and the neutral electrode.
   c. has an effect on the output signal which depends on the relation between the interelectrode axis and the direction of the muscle fibers.
   d. all of the above
   e. b. and c.

2. The bandwidth of the EMG output signal recorded from the differential amplifier depends on
   a. the frequency setting of the anti-aliasing filter through which it is fed to the computer or recording device.
   b. the distance between the intramuscular electrodes, when the axis between them is parallel to the muscle fibers.
   c. the power spectrum of the EMG signal
   d. whether the electrodes used are surface, needle, or wire electrodes
   e. all of the above

3. The amplitude of an unprocessed EMG interference pattern output by the differential amplifier, by itself,
   a. is linearly related to the force produced by the muscle under all conditions.
   b. is a good indicator of the health and innervation of the muscle.
   c. can be interpreted physiologically without other information.
   d. must be converted to absolute values and averaged over short periods in order to bear a linear relation to muscle force under isometric conditions.
   e. is unaffected by change of muscle length.

4. The amplitude of the interfering electrocardiogram signal seen in the EMG signal when recording EMG from a given skeletal muscle
   a. depends on the choice of a bipolar or monopolar electrode array.
   b. depends on the common mode rejection of the differential amplifier.
   c. depends on the level of contractile activity of the muscle from which EMG is being recorded.
   d. a and b
   e. a. b. and c.

5. If the level of interfering signals (e.g. 60 Hz) in the EMG output signal from the differential amplifier suddenly increases, the best solution is to
   a. switch in a 60 Hz band-reject filter on the differential amplifier.
   b. get rid of the source of the 60 Hz interference (e.g., turn off fluorescent lights).
   c. check the integrity and placement of all EMG electrodes and their connections.
   d. switch from differential to monopolar operation.
   e. check the integrity and placement of the neutral electrode and its connections.

6. When recording electromyographic activity from the muscles of the pharynx or larynx, movement artifacts and interfering signals can best be avoided by use of
   a. unipolar surface electrodes
   b. bipolar surface electrodes
   c. unipolar intramuscular needle electrodes
   d. bipolar intramuscular needle electrodes
   e. unipolar intramuscular hooked wire electrodes
   f. bipolar intramuscular hooked wire electrodes

REFERENCES

Adrian, R. H. (1983). Electrical properties of striated muscle. In L. D. Peachey (Ed.), Skeletal muscle (pp. 275–300). (*Handbook of physiology*. Section 10). Bethesda, MD: American Physiological Society.

Ahlgren, J. (1967). Kinesiology of the mandible. *Acta Odontologica Scandinavica, 25*, 593–611.

Aidley, D. J. (1989). *The physiology of excitable cells* (3rd ed.). Cambridge, UK: Cambridge University Press.

Basmajian, J. V., Clifford, H. C., McLeod, W. D., & Nunnally, H. N.(1975). *Computers in electromyography*. Boston: Butterworths.

Basmajian, J. V. & Dutta, C. (1961). Electromyography of the pharyngeal constrictors and levator veli palatini in man. *Anatomical Records, 139*, 561–563.

Basmajian, J. V. (1973). Electrodes and electrode connectors. In J. E. Desmedt (Ed.), *New developments in electromyography and clinical neurophysiology* (Vol.1, pp. 502–510). Basel: Karger.

Basmajian, J. V. & DeLuca, C. (1985). *Muscles alive. Their functions revealed by electromyography* (pp. 378–434). Baltimore: Williams & Wilkins.

Basmajian, J. V., & Stecko, G. A.(1962). A new bipolar indwelling electrode for electromyography. *Journal of Applied Physiology, 17*, 849.

Bendat, J. S., & Piersol, A. G. (1986). *Random data: Analysis and measurement procedures*. New York: Wiley-Interscience.

Binder, M. D., & Mendell, L. M. (Eds.). (1990). *The segmental motor system*. New York: Oxford University Press.

Blitzer, A., Brin, M. F., Fahn, S., & Harris, K. S. (1992). *Neurologic disorders of the larynx*. New York: Thieme.

Bole, C. T. (1965). *Electromyographic kinesiology of the genioglossus muscles in man*. Unpublished master's thesis, Ohio State University, Columbus.

Bouisset, S. (1973). EMG and muscle force in normal motor activities. In J. E. Desmedt (Ed.), *New developments in electromyography and clinical neurophysiology* (Vol. 1, pp. 547–583). Basel: Karger.

Brazier, M. A. B. (1977). *Electrical activity of the nervous system* (4th ed.). Baltimore: Williams & Wilkins.

Brown, W. F. (1984). *The physiological and technical basis of electromyography*. Boston: Butterworth.

Brown, W. F., & Bolton, C. F. (1993). *Clinical electromyography* (2nd ed.). Boston: Butterworth.

Buchthal, F., & Schmalbruch, H. (1980). Motor unit of mammalian muscle. *Physiological Reviews, 60*(1), 90–142.

Bureš, J., Petráň, M., & Zachar, J. (1967). *Electro-physiological methods in biological research*. New York: Academic Press.

Burke, R. E. (1981). Motor units: Anatomy, physiology, and functional organization. In V. B. Brooks (Ed.), *Motor control* (pp. 345–422). (*Handbook of physiology.* Section 1, Vol. II, Pt. 1.) Bethesda MD: American Physiological Society.

Chatfield, C. (1975). *The analysis of time series: Theory and practice.* London: Chapman and Hall.

Clamann, H. P. (1981). Motor units and their activity during movement. In A. L. Towe & E. S. Luschei (Eds.), *Handbook of behavioral neurology* (Vol. 5, pp. 69–92). New York: Plenum Press.

Close, R. (1972). Dynamic properties of mammalian skeletal muscles. *Physiological Reviews, 52,* 129–197.

Cobbold, R. S. C. (1974). *Transducers for biomedical measurements* (pp. 412–475). New York: Wiley.

Cole, K. C. (1972). *Membranes, ions, and impulses.* Berkeley, CA: University of California Press.

Cooper, D. S., & Folkins, J. W. (1985). Comparison of electromyographic signals from different electrode placements in the palatoglossus muscle. *Journal of the Acoustical Society of America, 78*(5), 1530–1540.

Cooper, D. S., Partridge, L. D., & Alipour-Haghighi, F. (1993). Muscle energetics, vocal efficiency, and laryngeal biomechanics. In I. R. Titze (Ed.), *Vocal fold physiology* (pp. 37–92). San Diego: Singular Publishing Group.

Cooper, D. S., Pinczower, E., & Rice, D. H. (1993). Thyroarytenoid intramuscular pressures. *Annals of Otology Rhinology and Laryngology, 102*(3), 167–175.

Cooper, R., Osselton, J. W., & Shaw, J. C. (1980). *EEG technology* (3rd ed.). Boston: Butterworth.

Costantin, L. L. (1977). Activation in striated muscle. In J. M. Brookhart & V. B. Mountcastle (Eds.), *The nervous system* (pp. 215–259). (Handbook of Physiology. Sect. 1, Vol. 1, pt. 1, chap. 7). Bethesda, MD: American Physiological Society.

Creed, R. S., Denny-Brown, D., Eccles, J. C., Liddell, E. G. T., & Sherrington, C. S. (1932). *Reflex activity of the spinal cord.* Oxford: Clarendon Press.

Cunningham, D. P., & Basmajian, J. V. (1969). Electromyography of genioglossus and geniohyoid muscles during deglutition. *Anatomical Records, 165,* 401–410.

Dedo, H. H., & Ogura, J. H. (1965). Vocal cord electromyography in the dog. *Laryngoscope, 75*(2), 201–211.

Dedo, H. H., & Dunker, E. (1966). The volume conduction of motor unit potentials. *Electroencephalography and Clinical Neurophysiology. 20,* 608–613.

Dedo, H. H., & Hall, W. N. (1969). Electrodes in laryngeal electromyography. *Annals of Otology Rhinology and Laryngology, 78,* 172–181.

De Luca, C. J. (1979). Physiology and mathematics of myoelectric signals. *IEEE Transactions on Biomedical Engineering, 26*(6), 313–325.

De Luca, C. J., & van Dyk, R. J.(1975). Derivation of some parameters of myoelectric signals recorded during sustained constant force isometric contractions. *Biophysical Journal, 15,* 1167–1180.

Desmedt, J. E. (Ed.). (1973). *New developments in electromyography and clinical neurophysiology* (Vol. 1). Basel: Karger.

Desmedt, J. E. (Ed.). (1981). *Motor unit types, recruitment and plasticity in health and disease.* Basel: Karger.

Desmedt, J. E. (Ed.). (1983). *Computer-aided electromyography.* Basel: Karger.

Desmedt, J. E. (Ed.). (1989). *Computer-aided electromyography and expert systems.* New York: Elsevier.

Doebelin, E. O. (1983). *Measurement systems* (3rd ed.). New York: McGraw-Hill.

Doty, R. W., & Bosma, J. F. (1956). An electromyographic analysis of reflex deglutition. *Journal of Neurophysiology, 19,* 44–60.

Dubowitz, V. (1985). *Muscle biopsy: A practical approach.* London: Bailliere Tindall.

Eccles, J. C., & Gibson, W. C. (1979). *Sherrington: His life and thought.* New York: Springer International.

Emerson, N. D., & Zahalak, G. I. (1981). Longitudinal electrode arrays for electromyography. *Medical and Biological Engineering and Computing, 19,* 504–506.

Engel, A., & Franzini-Armstrong, C. (1994). *Myology* (Vols. I, II, 2nd ed.) New York: McGraw-Hill.

Ertekin, C., Pehlivan, M., Aydogdu, I, Ertas, M., Uludag, Burhanettin, Celebi, G., Colakoglu, Z., Sagduyu, A., & Yuceyar, N. (1995). An electrophysiological investigation of deglutition in man. *Muscle and Nerve, 18,* 1177–1186.

Faaborg-Andersen, K. A. (1957). Electromyographic investigation of intrinsic laryngeal muscles in humans. *Acta Physiologica Scandinavica, 41*(suppl. 140), 1–148.

Faaborg-Andersen, K. A. (1965). Electromyography of laryngeal muscles in humans. Technics and results. *Aktuelle Probleme der Phoniatrie* (Vol. 3.). Basel: Karger.

Ferris, C. D. (1974). *Introduction to bioelectrodes.* New York: Plenum Press.

Filaretov, A. A., & Filimonova, A. B. (1969). O propriotseptsii glotatel'nykh myshts. [On proprioception in the muscles of deglutition.] *Fiziol Zh. SSSR Sechenov, 55,* 552–557.

Fritzell, B. (1963). An electromyographic study of the movements of the soft palate in speech. *Folia Phoniatrica, 15,* 307–311.

Fritzell, B. (1969). The velopharyngeal muscles in speech. *Acta Otolaryngologica* (Göteborg), *250* (Suppl.), 1–81.

Garrett, P. H. (1981). *Analog I/O design.* Reston, VA: Reston Publishing.

Gath, I., & Stålberg, E. (1977). On the volume conduction in human skeletal muscle: in situ measurements. *Electroencephalography and Clinical Neurophysiology, 43,* 106–110.

Gath, I., & Stalberg, E. (1978). The calculated radial decline of the extra-cellular action potential compared with in situ measurements of the human brachial biceps. *Electroencephalography and Clinical Neurophysiology, 44,* 547–552.

Gatzke, R. D. (1974). The electrode: A measurement systems viewpoint. In H. A. Miller & D. C. Harrison (Eds.), *Biomedical electrode technology: Theory and practice* (pp. 99–116). New York: Academic Press.

Gay, T., Hirose, H., Strome, M., & Sawashima, M. (1972). Electromyography of the intrinsic laryngeal muscles during phonation. *Annals of Otology, Rhinology, and Laryngology, 81,* 401–409.

Geddes, L. A. (1972). *Electrodes and the measurement of bioelectric events.* New York: Wiley-Interscience.

Geddes, L. A., & Baker, L. E. (1989). *Principles of applied biomedical instrumentation* (3rd ed.). New York: Wiley-Interscience.

Glaser, E. M., & Ruchkin, D. S. (1976). *Principles of neurobiological signal analysis.* New York: Academic Press.

Goldberg, S. J. (1990). Mechanical properties of extraocular motor units. In M. D. Binder & L. M. Mendell (Eds.), *The segmental motor system* (pp. 222–238). New York: Oxford University Press.

Gollnick, P., & Saltin, B. (1989). Skeletal muscle physiology. In C. C. Teitz (Ed.), *Scientific foundations of sports medicine* (pp. 185–241). Philadelphia: Decker.

Goodgold, J., & Eberstein, A. (1983). *Electrodiagnosis of neuromuscular diseases* (3rd ed.). Baltimore: Williams & Wilkins.

Haglund, S. (1973). The normal electromyogram in human cricothyroid muscle. *Acta Otolaryngologica Scandinavica, 75,* 448–453.

Hairston, L. E., & Sauerland, E. K. (1981). Electromyography of the human pharynx: Discharge patterns of the superior pharyngeal constrictor during respiration. *Electromyography and Clinical Neurophysiology, 21,* 299–306.

Henneman, E. (1980a). Skeletal muscle. In V. B. Mountcastle (Ed.), *Medical physiology* (Vol. I, pp. 674–702). St. Louis: C. V. Mosby.

Henneman, E. (1980b). Organization of the motoneuron pool. The size principle. In V. B. Mountcastle (Ed.), *Medical physiology* (Vol. I, pp. 718–741). St. Louis: C. V. Mosby.

Henneman, E., & Mendell, L. M. (1981): Functional organization of the motoneuron pool and its inputs. In V. B. Brooks (Ed.), *Motor control.* (*Handbook of physiology.* Section 1: Vol. II Pt 1, pp. 423–507). Bethesda, MD: American Physiological Society.

Hirano, M. (1981). *Clinical examination of voice.* New York, Springer-Verlag.

Hirano, M., Ohala, J., & Vennard, W. (1969). The function of laryngeal muscles in regulating fundamental frequency and intensity. *Journal of Speech and Hearing Research, 12,* 616–628.

Hirose, H. (1971). Electromyography of the articulatory muscles: Current instrumentation and technique. *Haskins Laboratories Status Report on Speech Research,* SR 25/26, 73–86.

Hodgkin, A. L. (1964). *The conduction of the nervous impulse.* Liverpool: Liverpool University Press.

Hogan, N., & Mann, R. W. (1980). Myoelectric signal processing: Optimal estimation applied to electromyography—Part II: Experimental demonstration of optimal myoprocessor performance. *IEEE Transactions on Biomedical Engineering, BME-27*(7), 396–410.

Horowitz P., & Hill, W. (1989). *The art of electronics* (2nd ed.). Cambridge, UK: Cambridge University Press.

Hrycyshyn, A. W., & Basmajian, J. V. (1972). Electromyography of the oral stage of swallowing in man. *American Journal of Anatomy, 133,* 333–340.

Johnson, E. (Eds.). (1988). *Practical electromyography* (2nd ed.). Baltimore: Williams & Wilkins.

Jung, R. (1975). Some European neuroscientists: A personal tribute. In F. G. Worden, J. P. Swazey, & G. Adelman (Eds.), *The neurosciences: Paths of discovery* (pp. 476–511). Cambridge, MA: MIT Press.

Junge, D. (1992). *Nerve and muscle excitation* (3rd ed.). Sunderland, MA: Sinauer Associates.

Kadefors, R. (1973). Myo-electric signal processing as an estimation problem. In J. E. Desmedt (Ed.), *New developments in electromyography and clinical neurophysiology* (Vol. 1, pp. 519–532). Basel: Karger.

Kandel, E. R., & Schwartz, J. H. (1991). *Principles of neural science* (3rd ed.). East Norwalk, CT: Appleton and Lange.

Katz, B. (1966). *Nerve, muscle, and synapse.* New York: McGraw Hill.

Kawasaki, M., Ogura, J. H., & Takenouchi, S. (1964). Neurophysiologic observations of normal deglutition I. Its relationship to the respiratory cycle. *Laryngoscope, 74,* 1747–1765.

Kimura, J. (1989). *Electrodiagnosis in diseases of nerve and muscle: Principles and practice* (2nd ed.). Philadelphia: F. A. Davis.

Kirchner, J. A.. (1986). *Pressman and Kelemen's physiology of the larynx* (3rd ed.). Washington, DC: American Acadamy of Otolaryngology—Head and Neck Surgery.

Kugelberg, E. (1981). The motor unit: Morphology and function. In J. E. Desmedt (Ed.), *Motor unit types, recruitment and plasticity in health and disease* (pp. 1–16). Basel: Karger.

Lang, I. M., Dantas, R. O., Cook, I. J., & Dodds, W. J. (1991). Videoradiographic, manometric, and electromyographic analysis of canine upper esophageal sphincter. *American Journal of Physiology, 260*, G911-G919.

Lewis, D. M. (1981). Motor units in mammalian skeletal muscle. In A. L. Towe & E. S. Luschei (Eds.), *Handbook of behavioral neurology* (Vol. 5, pp. 1–67). New York: Plenum Press.

Lindström, L., & Magnusson, R. I. (1977). Interpretation of myoelectric power spectra: A model and its application. *Proceedings of the IEEE, 65*(5), 653–662.

Lindström, L., & Petersén, I. (1983). Power spectrum analysis of EMG signals and its applications. In J. E. Desmedt (Ed.), *Computer-aided electromyography* (pp. 1–51). Basel: Karger.

Liveson, J. A., & Ma, D. M. (1992). *Laboratory reference for clinical neurophysiology*. Philadelphia: F. A. Davis.

Loeb, G. E., & Gans, C. (1986). *Electromyography for experimentalists*. Chicago: University of Chicago Press.

Lovelace, R. E., Blitzer, A., & Ludlow, C. L. (1992). Clinical laryngeal electromyography. In A. Blitzer, M. F. Brin, S. Fahn, C. T. Sasaki, & K. S. Harris (Eds.), *Neurologic disorders of the larynx* (pp. 66–81). New York: Thieme.

Luschei, E., & Finnegan, E. (1995). Electromyographic techniques for the assessment of motor speech disorders. In I. Tietze (Ed.), *NCVS status and progress report* (pp. 157–174) Iowa City: National Center for Voice and Speech.

Luschei, E. S., & Goldberg, L. J. (1981). Neural mechanisms of mandibular control: Mastication and voluntary biting. In V. B. Brooks (Ed.), *Motor control.* (*Handbook of physiology*, Section 1: Vol. II, Pt 2, pp. 1237–1274). Bethesda MD: American Physiological Society.

Maeyama, T. (1975). Experimental investigations of the function of the intrinsic and extrinsic laryngeal muscles during deglutition, especially for elevation of the larynx. *Otologia (Fukuoka), 21*, 787–807.

Magrab, E. B., & Blomquist, D. S. (1971). *The measurement of time-varying phenomena*. New York: Wiley-Interscience.

Martin, B., Logemann, J., Shaker, R., & Dodds, W, (1994). Coordination between respiration and swallowing. *Journal of Applied Physiology, 76*, 714–723.

Matthews, B. H. C. (1934). A special purpose amplifier. *Journal of Physiology, 81*, 28P–29P.

Miller, A. J. (1972). Significance of sensory inflow to the swallowing reflex. *Brain Research, 43*, 147–159.

Miller, H. A., & Harrison, D. C. (1974). *Biomedical electrode technology: Theory and practice*. New York: Academic Press.

Minifie, F. C., Abbs, J. H., Tarlow, A., & Kwaterski, M. (1974). EMG activity within the pharynx during speech production. *Journal of Speech and Hearing Research, 17*, 497–504.

Mleczko, E. L. (1972). Instruments in systems. In C. F. Coombs (Ed.), *Basic electronic instrument handbook* (Chap. 18). New York: McGraw-Hill.

Moller, A. R. (1988). *Evoked potentials in intraoperative monitoring*. Baltimore: Williams & Wilkins.

Møller, E. (1966). The chewing apparatus. An electromyographic study of the action of the muscles of mastication and its correlation to facial morphology. *Acta Physiologica Scandinavica, 69*(Suppl. 280).

Møller, E. (1974). Action of the muscles of mastication. In Y. Kawamura (Ed.), *Frontiers of oral physiology* (Vol. 1, pp. 121–158). Basel: Karger.

Møller, E. (1976). Human muscle patterns. In B. J. Sessle & A. G. Hannam (Eds.), *Mastication and swallowing* (pp. 128–141). Toronto: University of Toronto Press.

Morrison, R. (1986). *Grounding and shielding techniques in instrumentation* (3rd ed.). New York: John Wiley.

Nakamura, F., Uyeda, Y., & Sonoda, Y. (1958). Electromyographic study on respiratory movements of the intrinsic laryngeal muscles. *Laryngoscope, 68*, 109–119.

Németh, P. M. (1990). Metabolic fiber types and influences on their transformation. In M. D. Binder & L. M. Mendell (Eds.), *The segmental motor system* (pp. 258–277). New York: Oxford University Press.

Neuman, M. R. (1978a). Biopotential electrodes. In J. G. Webster (Ed.), *Medical instrumentation: Application and design* (pp. 215–272). Boston: Houghton Mifflin.

Neuman, M. R. (1978b). Biopotential amplifiers. In J. G. Webster (Ed.), *Medical instrumentation: Application and design* (pp. 273–335). Boston: Houghton Mifflin.

Notermans, S. L. H. (Ed.). (1984). *Current practice of clinical electromyography*. New York: Elsevier.

Oh, S. J. (1988). *Electromyography: Neuromuscular transmission studies*. Baltimore: Williams & Wilkins.

Oh, S. J. (1993). *Clinical electromyography. Nerve conduction studies* (2nd ed.). Baltimore: Williams & Wilkins.

Oliver, B. M., & Cage, J. M. (Eds.). (1971). *Electronic measurements and instrumentation*, New York: McGraw Hill.

Palmer, J. B. (1989). Electromyography of the muscles of oropharyngeal swallowing. *Dysphagia, 93*, 192–198.

Palmer, J. B., Tanaka, E., & Siebens, A. A. (1989). Electromyography of the pharyngeal musculature: technical considerations. *Archives of Physical Medicine and Rehabilitation, 70*(4), 283–287.

Palmer, J. B., Tippett, D., & Wolf, J. (1991). Synchronous positive and negative myoclonus due to pontine hemorrhage. *Muscle and Nerve, 14*, 124–132.

Parker, P. A., & Scott, R. N. (1973). Statistics of the myoelectric signal from monopolar and bipolar electrodes. *Medical and Biological Engineering, 11,* 591–596.

Partridge, Lloyd D., & Partridge, L. Donald (1993). *The nervous system: Its function and its interaction with the world.* [Bradford Book.] Cambridge MA: MIT Press.

Perkins, R. E., Blanton, P. L., & Biggs, N. L. (1976). Electromyographic analysis of the buccinator mechanism in human beings. *Journal of Dental Research, 56*(7), 783–794.

Perlman, A. L., Luschei, E. S., & DuMond, C. E. (1989) Electrical activity from the superior pharyngeal constrictor during reflexive and nonreflexive tasks. *Journal of Speech and Hearing Research, 32,* 749–754.

Perlman, A. L. (1993)., Electromyography and the study of oropharyngeal swallowing, *Dysphagia, 8,* 4, 351–355.

Perlman, A. L., Palmer, P. M., McCulloch, T. M., & VanDaele, D. S. (1996). Temporal relationships of select oral, pharyngeal, and laryngeal muscles. Manuscript in preparation.

Perry, J., & Bekey, G. A. (1981). EMG-force relationships in skeletal muscle. *Critical Reviews of Biomedical Engineering, 7,* 1–22.

Person, R. S., & Mishin, L. N. (1964). Auto- and cross-correlation analysis of the electrical activity of muscles. *Medical Electronics and Biological Engineering, 2,* 155–159.

Plonsey, R. (1969). *Bioelectric phenomena.* New York: McGraw-Hill.

Reimers-Neils, L., Logemann, J., & Larson, C. (1994). Viscosity effects on EMG activity in normal swallow. *Dysphagia, 9,* 101–106.

Rosa, A. (1990). Electromagnetics and circuits. In B. D. Tapley (Ed.), *Eshbach's handbook of engineering fundamentals* (pp. 11–1 to 11–131). New York: Wiley-Interscience.

Roth, H. H., Teltscher, E. S., & Kane, I. M. (1975). *Electrical safety in health care facilities.* New York: Academic Press.

Rowe, L. D., Miller, A. J., Chierici, G., & Clendenning, D. (1984). Adaptation in the function of pharyngeal constrictor muscles. *Otolaryngology—Head and Neck Surgery, 92,* 392–401.

Sauerland, E. K., & Mitchell, S. P. (1975). Electromyographic activity of intrinsic and extrinsic muscles of the human tongue. *Texas Reports on Biology and Medicine, 33*(3), 445–455.

Sawashima, M., Sata, M., Funasaka, S., & Totsuk, G. (1958). Electromyographic study of the human larynx and its clinical application. *Journal of Otolaryngology of Japan, 61,* 1357–1364.

Schultz, J., Perlman, A. L., & VanDaele, D. J. (1994). Laryngeal movement, oropharyngeal pressure, and submental muscle contraction during swallowing. *Archives of Physical Medicine and Rehabilitation, 75,* 183–189.

Selley, W. G., Ellis, R. E., Flack, F. C., Bayliss, C. R., & Pearce, V. R. (1994). The synchronization of respiration and swallow sounds with videofluoroscopy during swallowing. *Dysphagia, 9,* 162–167.

Shipp, T., Deatsch, W. W., & Roberston, K. (1970). Pharyngoesophageal muscle activity during swallowing in man. *Laryngoscope, 80,* 1–16.

Smith, J., Wolkove, N., Colacone, A., & Kreisman, H. (1989). Coordination of eating, drinking, and breathing in adults. *Chest, 96*(3), 578–582.

Stålberg, E., & Young, R. R. (1981). *Clinical neurophysiology.* Boston: Butterworth.

Stein, R. B. (1980). *Nerve and muscle.* New York: Plenum Press.

Stevens, C. F. (1966). *Neurophysiology: A primer.* New York: John Wiley.

Storey, A. T. (1968). Laryngeal initiation of swallowing. *Experimental Neurology, 20,* 359–365.

Sumi, T. (1964). Neuronal mechanisms in swallowing. Archiv für die gesamte *Physiologie, 278,* 467–477.

Sydenham, P. H. (Ed.). (1982, 1983). *Handbook of measurement science.* (Vols. 1, 2). Chichester, UK: Wiley-Interscience.

Takada, K., Miyawaki, S., & Tatsuta, M. (1994). The effects of food consistency on jaw movement and posterior temporalis and inferior orbicularis oris muscle activities during chewing in children. *Archives of Oral Biology, 39,* 793–805.

Takada, E., Palmer, J. B., & Siebens, A. A. (1986). Bipolar suction electrodes for pharyngeal electromyography. *Dysphagia, 1,* 39–40.

Trigos, I., Ysunza, A., Vargas, D., & Vazquez, M. D. C. (1988). The San Venero Roselli pharyngoplasty: An electromyographic study of the palatopharyngeus muscle. *Cleft Palate Journal, 25,* 385–388.

VanDoren, A. (1982). *Data acquisition systems.* Reston, VA: Reston Publishing.

van Overbeek, J. J. M., Wit, H. P., Paping, R. H. L., & Segenhout, H. M. (1985). Simultaneous manometry and electromyography in the pharyngoesophageal segment. *Laryngoscope, 95,* 582–584.

Vitti, M. (1971). Electromyographic analysis of the musculus temporalis in basic movements of the jaw. *Electromyography, 11,* 389–403.

Vitti, M., Basmajian, J. V., Ouelette, P. L., Mitchell, D. L., Eastman, W. P., & Seaborn, R. D. (1975). Electromyographic investigations of the tongue and circumoral muscular sling with fine-wire electrodes. *Journal of Dental Research, 54,* 844–849.

Walton, J., Karpati, G., & Hilton-Jones, D. (1994). *Disorders of voluntary muscle* (6th ed.). Edinburgh: Churchill-Livingstone.

Waring, W. (1974). Observing signals from nerve and muscle. In H. A. Miller & D. C. Harrison (Eds.), *Biomedical electrode technology: Theory and practice* (pp. 215–260). New York: Academic Press.

Zealear, D. L. (1979). *Specialization of laryngeal motor units for their functions.* Unpublished doctoral dissertation, University of California, San Francisco.

10

Esophagoscopy and Tests of Esophageal Function

Edy Soffer, Joseph A. Murray, and Konrad Schulze-Delrieu

Barium contrast examination is commonly used to assess esophageal structure and function (see also chapter 6). This chapter discusses the techniques, indications, contraindications, and modifications of esophagoscopy. The diagnostic advantages of direct mucosal inspection and sampling of tissue for histologic, cytologic, and microbial processing will be stressed. Dilatation of the esophagus, as is often performed in combination with esophagoscopy, will be presented as the major treatment of dysphagia for benign or malignant esophageal strictures.

Esophageal manometry is a functional test whose values and limitations need to be clearly understood. This chapter will present criteria for its performance and its interpretation. Similarly, indications, test performance, and interpretation of esophageal pH recording are given.

ENDOSCOPY IN THE DIAGNOSIS AND TREATMENT OF ESOPHAGEAL DISEASE

In endoscopy, the inside of the esophagus is inspected by the introduction of light through optical systems. Optical systems consist of serial reflectors and lenses (as in conventional rigid esophagoscopy), of fiberoptic bundles, or of digital imaging devices. (See below for technical details and specific advantages of various systems.)

In clinical practice, inspection of the esophagus is typically included in the endoscopic examination of several adjacent structures. It may be performed as part of a panendoscopy of mucosal structures in the head and neck, which focuses on pharyngeal and laryngeal structures. It may be performed as part of an esophagogastroduodenoscopy, which assesses the duodenum and stomach as well as the esophagus for inflammatory, structural, or neoplastic lesions. Endoscopic examination provides precise information on appearance, location, distribution, and extent of mucosal disease. Biopsies and brushings can be obtained for histologic, cytologic, and microbial studies. Samples serve to identify Barrett's metaplasia (replacement of squamous by columnar epithelium), dysplasia (occurrence of premalignant changes), and neoplasia (tumor formation), or fungal or viral infections (Baehr & McDonald, 1994). If the esophagus is strictured, forceful stretching (bougineage or other dilatation) can be undertaken at the time of esophagoscopy to relieve the mechanical obstruction and the dysphagia resulting from it.

Indications

Endoscopic examination is called for when inflammatory, infectious, or neoplastic disease of the esophagus is suspected. This applies to virtually all instances of dysphagia and odynophagia, especially if they are progressive, accompanied by systemic symptoms like weight loss (see also Chapters 5 and 13). Occasionally esophagoscopy may be performed to determine an esophageal cause for chest pain. Esophagoscopy is helpful to grade the severity of gastroesophageal reflux by determining the extent of inflammatory (i.e, erosive esophagitis), metaplastic (Barrett's) mucosa or structural changes (esophageal shortening or stricturing). Documentation of the absence of esophageal lesions provides reassurance and may help the patient avoid unnecessary operations (Kobayaski & Kasugai, 1974).

Endoscopic examination with biopsy, cytology, and dilatation is indicated when barium studies reveal strictures. These include the smooth functional (bird's beaklike) stricture at the gastroesophageal junction typical of achalasia (see Chapter 6). Tumors may cause an achalasialike syndrome (see Chapter 13). Careful endoscopic examination may reveal a tumor that is amenable to resection with potential cure.

Endoscopic brushings and samples for viral and fungal cultures can diagnose opportunistic esophageal infections. Opportunistic infections leading to odynophagia are common in immunosuppressed patients, particularly those with AIDS, the acquired immunodeficiency syndrome (Baehr & McDonald, 1994). (See Chapter 13.)

Esophageal dilatation relieves dysphagia caused by strictures and often alleviates dysphagia even if no discrete esophageal stenosis is documented radiographically or endoscopically (Ebert, Ouyang, Wright, & Cohen, 1983). Barium contrast esophagography is superior to endoscopy in the detection of webs or strictures at the esophageal inlet and in the cervical esophagus. These segments are poorly visualized during intubation and lesions in them may be ablated during instrument insertion. Contrast radiography is a safer test to identify large pharyngeal diverticula, and can more readily identify extrinsic lesions impinging on the esophageal lumen such as osteophytes, vascular structures, mediastinal tumors, or intramural tumors (leiomyomas, or lung cancers with invasion into the esophagus).

Bolus Impaction

Endoscopic removal of foreign bodies is needed when other measures (sedatives, spasmolytics, carbonated beverages) to relieve an esophageal bolus impaction have failed. Removal should be completed within hours to avoid aspiration or esophageal perforation. (Schwartz & Polsky, 1975). Impactions at the upper esophageal sphincter (UES) or in the cervical esophagus are best handled by rigid esophagoscopy using airway intubation and general anesthesia. Boluses in the thoracic and abdominal segments of the esophagus can be dislodged under conscious sedation. Digestible boluses are advanced into the stomach if possible. Others are broken apart and extracted. The airway is protected during extraction by passing the endoscope through an overtube placed through the pharynx into the esophagus.

Technical Aspects of Endoscopy

Equipment

Flexible instruments have revolutionized endoscopy because they allow for complete inspection of the esophagus, stomach, and duodenum. The risk of perforation is reduced by the small diameter and suppleness of the instruments. Patient discomfort is minimal and conscious sedation sufficient.

Thousands of ultra thin glass fibers in its core transmit the image from the tip to the eyepiece of the fiberoptic instrument. A handle next to the eyepiece has controls to direct the tip, nozzles for air insuflation and water injection, and a suction channel (see Chapter 7 for figure and technical details). The esophageal lumen is cleared of secretions and mucus through suction and then fully inflated for complete inspection of the esophageal surface. The suction channel is used to pass biopsy forceps, brushes, balloon dilators, and other accessories into the lumen to obtain diagnostic samples or to treat specific lesions. In videoendoscopy the image is generated electronically and projected on to a screen. Video systems are less prone to damage by torquing and bending the instrument than fiberoptic systems. The procedure is easily followed by many observers, can be transmitted to distant sites, or videotaped and stored for documentation and review.

Conduct of the Endoscopic Study

Patients are prepared by application of local anesthetic to the pharynx to suppress the gag reflex and conscious sedation is achieved by parenteral administration of a benzodiazepine derivative (diazepam or midazolam). The procedure is preferably done with the patient in the left lateral position so that any gastric contents collect in the fundus. An assistant suctions the oropharynx to minimize aspiration. Monitoring of oxygen saturation, blood pressure, and pulse is thought to enhance the safety of the procedure.

The tip of the scope is slid over the base of the tongue into the hypopharynx. Advancement of the scope through the pharynx and placement into the left (or occasionally the right) pyriform sinuses can be guided by the examiner's fingers in the patient's mouth. The tip of the scope is advanced with mild pressure as the patient opens the esophageal inlet on order to swallow. Intubation under direct visualization is a simple alternative to guided intubation. Visual control is the preferable approach when the pharyngeal anatomy is distorted by tumor, prior surgery, or diverticulum and avoids the risk of the endoscopist being bitten. As the scope advances towards the hypopharynx, the semilunar-shaped epiglottis is seen first, then the larynx, the vocal cords, and arytenoid carti-

lages, (For the endoscopic aspects of the hypopharynx see Chapter 7, Figures 7–12, 7–3.) The esophageal inlet is located posteriorly and distal to the arytenoid cartilages; the access to the inlet widens on bending the head forward. The inlet is closed at rest by contraction of the cricopharyngeus muscle, but opens briefly with swallowing as the muscle relaxes and the inlet is pulled forward during laryngeal ascent.

The Normal Esophagus

The esophageal inlet is a narrow slit which at rest is closed by the upper esophageal sphincter formed by the cricopharyngeal muscle. It is located 15–20 cm from the incisors. Upon swallowing, the UES opens briefly and the tip of the instrument pops into the cervical esophagus. The esophagus at rest is a tube whose walls are collapsed forming longitudinal mucosal folds. Air insufflation readily opens the lumen, which should be empty except for some mucous residue. The mucosal surface is smooth, white-grayish, and glistening. It is covered by squamous epithelium, which differs from the columnar cell mucosa of the stomach, which is reddish and forms areae gastricae and fleshy rugae (serpiginous folds). The junction between the two types of mucosa is called the *squamocolumnar junction* (SCJ), the ora serrata, or the Z line (Figure 10–1). This is located at the distal end of the lower esophageal sphincter (LES) approximately 40 cm from the incisors, within or slightly distal to the diaphragmatic hiatus (Schatzki, 1963). Curvature of the distal esophagus to the left and closure of gastroesophageal junction combine to keep the gastric lumen out of view during moderate insufflation of the esophagus.

Endoscopic Features of Acute and Chronic Esophageal Injury

Injury of the esophageal mucosa leads to accelerated loss of cells from the top of the epithelium, and loss of all cell layers constitutes an erosion. There are vascular congestion, edema, and cellular infiltrates in the lamina propria. Inflammation involving the submucosa and muscular layers shortens and narrows the esophagus (Shirazi, Schulze-Delrieu, Custer-Hagen, Brown, & Ren, 1989) and leads to formation of esophageal strictures. After severe injury squamous mucosa may be replaced by columnar or metaplastic epithelium.

Mild acute esophageal inflammation is suggested if endoscopy reveals erythema and edema with blurring of the SCJ and of its delicate vascular pattern. Chronic esophageal inflammation leading to epithelial hyperplasia is suggested by granularity, opaque plaques, or linear erythema and friability of the esophageal mucosa (Kobayaski & Kasugai, 1974). These changes are notoriously difficult to assess by endoscopy alone and require histologic examination of biopsies to confirm acid reflux-related damage.

Discrete lesions like erosions, islands of Barrett's metaplasia, or strictures constitute definite endoscopic evidence for acute and chronic esophageal lesions. Erosions (Figure 10–2) should be judged for their acuteness (yellow-white exudate suggests acute damage) and for the extent of the esophageal surface they involve. A salmon pink discoloration of the mucosa is suggestive of Barrett's metaplasia, wherein the normally squamous mucosa has been replaced with columnar epithelium. Metaplasia should be judged for its longitudinal and circumferential extent and for the coexistence of inflammatory (erosions) or potentially neoplastic changes (nodules or other surface abnormalities) in it.

Severe chronic inflammation leads to formation of scars with collagen deposition in submucosal layers (Patterson et al., 1983; Schatzki, 1963; Spechler et al., 1983). Confluent lesions that encircle the esophagus are particularly likely to form strictures (Figure 10-3). True peptic ulcerations that form craters and penetrate the esophageal wall are rare and occur only at the junction of squamous and metaplastic epithelium. Barrett's metaplasia is frequently found in association with strictures, and particularly those in the mid

and upper esophagus (Spechler et al., 1983). Barium studies may be more sensitive in the diagnosis of esophageal strictures, specifically those wider than the diameter of the endoscope (Ott, Chen, Wu, & Gelfand, 1985).

Narrowed segments or strictures should be defined for their precise location, length and symmetry, ease of passage or dilatation, and inflammatory or neoplastic changes in them. Peptic strictures caused by gastroesophageal reflux disease (GERD) are short and concentric and located precisely at the squamocolumnar junction. If esophageal injury persists, the junction itself will likely be covered by exudate, and linear erosions may ascend from it. Lye strictures are often long, asymmetric, and bear no clear relation to mucosal boundaries. Neoplastic strictures are tortuous with irregular margins from ulcerations and tumor nodules. The functional stricture caused by the hypertensive LES of achalasia closes the lumen of the distal esophagus over several centimeters, but the mucosa is intact and there is no resistance to advancing the scope.

Endoscopic Grading of Esophagitis

Classifications serve to compare disease severity and to assess treatment effects. Observation of reflux lesions by endoscopy documents that the GERD has led to esophageal complications. Healing rates of esophagitis are inversely related to the severity of the disease under treatment, while the recurrence of disease after healing is directly related to its severity. Also, patients with higher grades of esophagitis require more potent therapy for complete healing (Sontag, 1990).

The Modified Savary-Miller Classification

The most commonly used method to grade the severity of esophageal injury is the classification proposed by Savary-Miller and later modified (Ollyo, Lang, Fontollet, & Monuier, 1993; Table 10–1). The main, difference between the various classifications is in the definition of grade I disease. Acceptance of erythema and other diffuse changes as grade I esophagitis increases the sensitivity of endoscopic testing for disease but, because of observer error and other problems, decreases its specificity (Behar & Biancani, 1993; Geboes et al., 1980; Ismail-Beigi, Horton, & Pope, 1970; Kobayaski & Kasugai, 1974; Schulze-Delrieu, Mitros, Shirazi; 1982).

Critique of Classification

This classification is sound in that it is based on easily identified endoscopic criteria and because it grades them according to current understanding of the natural history of reflux esophagitis. The classification assigns higher grades to lesions characteristic of chronic rather than of acute injury. Also, severity of disease is measured by confluence and circumferential but not by axial extent of lesions. The classification would assign a grade III to an acute esophagitis for erosions and exudate and a grade V for Barrett's regardless whether they involve the entire esophagus or only a couple of centimeters of the distal end. The classification has undergone no empiric testing for observer variability or its ability to prognosticate disease or treatment outcomes.

Barret's Metaplasia

In Barrett's metaplasia the normal squamous mucosa of the esophagus is replaced by columnar epithelium of different color and texture (Figure 10–3), Endoscopically, Barrett's epithelium is suspected when the squamocolumnar junction is by 2–3 cm or more proximally displaced into the tubular esophagus or when flame-shaped extensions or islands of columnar mucosa occur well above the SCJ. Barrett's mucosa is distinguished from the grayish white and smooth normal squamous mucosa by its salmon color and velvety surface.

In Barrett's columnar metaplasia the segment of esophagus which is lined by squamous epithelium has shortened, a condition also known as endobrachye-sophagus. Shortening of the muscular esophagus complicating esophagitis (Shirazi et al., 1989) manifests itself as a nonreducing hiatus hemia. Distinction of hiatus hernias and Barrett's esophagus is desirable because only the columnar epithelium of the latter has premalignant potential.

Hiatus Hernias and Schatzki's Rings

Hiatus hernia denotes a condition where a part of the stomach moves through a widened diaphragmatic hiatus and into the chest. On antegrade inspection a hiatus hernia is suspected when a patulous gastroesophageal junction flares into wide hernia sac several centimeters above the diaphragmatic hiatus. The sac narrows at the level of the diaphragm and is lined by gastric mucosal rugae. Inspection of the esophagogastric junction during a J-maneuver (inversion of the of tip of the scope) in the gastric fundus confirms the presence of a hernia (Figure 10-4). A normal junction is tightly closed around the scope, whereas with a hernia there is a wide gap between the scope and the walls of the junction. Recognition of a hiatus hernia is aided by location of the diaphragmatic hiatus, which descends and tightens upon inspiration or sniffing.

SCHATZKI'S RING. The upper border of hiatal hernias may be demarcated by a Schatzki's ring. The ring is a diaphragm-like membrane formed by the protrusion of the squamocolumnar junction into the lumen. Its core is constituted by lamina propria and bundles of mucosal muscle with a circumferential rather than a longitudinal orientation (Schatzki, 1963; Schatzki & Gary, 1953). Most rings narrow the esophageal lumen only negligibly (Figure 10–2). The classic presentation of rings with a luminal diameter of 13 mm or less is that of intermittent dysphagia, related to ingestion of poorly masticated, large boluses of solid food. (See also Chapters 5 and 13.) According to Schatzki, rings are not related to mucosal inflamma-

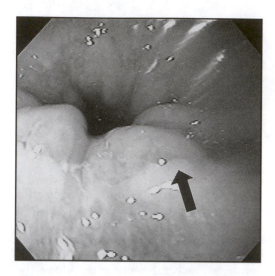

Figure 10-1. Typical appearance of the squamo-columnar junction showing the transition from the columnar epithelium of the stomach with its reddish color distally to the pale-appearing squamous epithelium of the esophagus proximally (arrow).

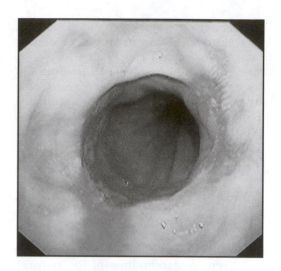

Figure 10-2. Grade II esophagitis with Schatzki's ring and hiatus hernia. Linear erosions are seen extending proximally from the squamo-columnar junction. A circular mucosa ring (Schatzki's) is seen at the border of the gastric and esophageal mucosa. Distal to the ring is a hiatus hernia, with the gastric fold extending upward to the squamo-columnar junction. These three findings typically occur together.

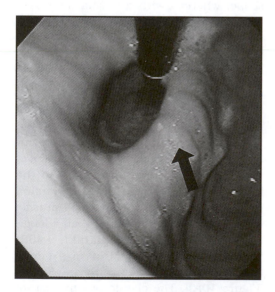

Figure 10-3. Barrett's metaplasia with stricture. The esophageal lumen is markedly narrowed (arrow) and tongues of reddish gastriclike mucosa, representing columnar metaplasia, are seen extending proximally into the pale, squamous esophageal mucosa.

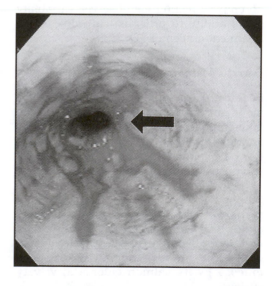

Figure 10-4. Hiatus hernia seen from the stomach by retroflexing the endoscope. The hernia sac sits above the diaphragmatic insertion (arrow).

TABLE 10–1. Endoscopic Grading of Esophagitis.

Grade I	Single, erosive, or exudative lesion, oval or linear, on only one longitudinal fold
Grade II	Nonencircling multiple erosions or exudative lesions on more than one longitudinal fold, with or without confluence (Figure 10–2)
Grade III	Encircling erosive or exudative lesions
Grade IV	Chronic lesions: ulcer(s), strictures(s), or short esophagus, isolated or associated with lesions of grades I, II, or III
Grade V	Islands, fingerlike formation or circumferential distribution of Barrett's epithelium isolated or associated with lesions of grades I through IV (Figure 10–3)

Source: Adapted from Ollyo et al. (1993). Savary's New Endoscopic Grading of Reflux-oesophagitis: A Simple Reproducible, Logical, Complete and Useful Classification. *Gastroenterology, 89, 89,* A100.

tion and do not change over time (Schatzki, 1963). Their relationship to GERD remains unclear.

With the lack of independent landmarks, impingement of the diaphragm on the distal hernia sac may be mistaken for the lower esophageal sphincter, and the normal gastric columnar epithelium lining the hernia sac mistaken for a Barrett's esophagus. Gastric mucosal folds extending to SCJ help in the distinction. A mucosal biopsy showing a specialized metaplastic columnar epithelium (foveolor epithelium with a viliform structure and goblet cells) is conclusive (Cameron, Ott, Payne, & 1985).

Additional features of esophagitis, particularly of esophagitis not related to GERD and histologic features, and of strictures will be discussed in Chapter 13

Esophageal Biopsy

Mucosal biopsies from the esophagus can be obtained with suction devices (like the Rubin tube) or with pinch biopsy forceps, introduced through the endoscope. Suction biopsy provides large mucosal samples that contain even the deep mucosal layer. They are easy to orient and the mucosal structure can be assessed comprehensively. However, suction biopsies require passage of an additional tube, and sampling specific sites is difficult. Therefore, esophageal mucosal samples are as a rule obtained during endoscopy as pinch biopsies.

Biopsies are mandatory for histologic proof of neoplasia, dysplasia, or Barrett's metaplasia. Biopsy also provides histologic samples for the recognition of infectious types of esophagitis.

Esophageal biopsy may document chronic reflux injury when endoscopic inspection reveals no discrete lesions of esophagitis. This may be particularly important in patients with unexplained dysphagia and chest pain. However, correlations between severity of reflux symptoms and histologic changes. (Kobayaski & Kasugai, 1974) are poor, and patients with healed esophagitis can have a symptomatic relapse without an endoscopic relapse; the converse may also occur. The histologic diagnosis of chronic reflux injury of the squamous epithelium is based on basal cell hyperplasia and increased relative height of the rete papillae, which the lamina propria forms. Vascular congestion, edema, and infiltration of the epithelium and lamina propia by granulocytes, especially eosinophilic ones, are also helpful observations for diagnosis (Behara & Sheehan, 1975; Geboes et al., 1980; 19 Ismail-Beigi et al., 1970; Schulze-Delrieu et al., 1982). If biopsies are small there may not be enough lamina propria to assess for acute inflammation; if they are poorly oriented, chronic restructuring of papillae may be impossible to assess. Histologic diagnosis is highly dependent on adequate sampling, as reflux lesions involve discrete areas of the esophagus.

Cytology

Brush cytology is used to collect a sample of cells from the surface of a lesion. It is a helpful adjunct to the biopsy in the diagnosis of malignancy and of fungal or viral infections.

Dilatation of Esophageal Strictures

Any narrowing of the esophageal lumen may compromise nutrition and pose the risk of *bolus impaction*. Dilatation is effective in eliminating the dysphagia associated with esophageal strictures. The endoscopic examination provides information on the location, diameter, length, and resistance offered by a stricture. If the stricture does not narrow the lumen severely and if virtually no pressure is needed to pass it, esophageal dilatation with the aid of mercury-filled rubber bougies is all that is needed. Tight and narrow strictures require use of more rigid dilators.

Techniques of Esophageal Dilatation

Commonly used rubber bougies have a tapered tip (Maloney type) or a rounded tip (Hurst type; Figure 10–5). Bougies are more than 60 cm long, and come in graded diameters from pencil thin to thicker than a thumb. The bougie is lubricated with warm water, and passed into the esophagus similarly to the intubation described for esophagoscopy. Minimal hand pressure is used. Sitting the patient up brings gravity into play. Use of soft, large rubber bougies is particularly helpful to break up esophageal webs and Schatzki's rings (Patterson et al., 1983) or to distend the esophagus in patients without discrete strictures but with a mechanical component to their dysphagia as encountered with many nonspecific motor disorders (i.e., bolus escape, tertiary contractions, high-amplitude esophageal contractions). In the past, patients prone to recurrent esophageal stricture formation were taught to dilate their own esophagus with bougies at regular intervals. Current medical and operative treatment for reflux has eliminated this need at least for peptic strictures. An almost addictive zeal to all-too-frequent self-bougineage is common in this setting.

To avoid esophageal perforation, dilatation of tight and resistant strictures is performed under visual control or over guidewires. Visual control and passage of guidewires may be achieved either through esophagoscopy or fluoroscopy. Through-the-endoscope balloon dilators are popular. (Figure 10–5). The collapsed balloon is passed through the suction channel of the endoscope and into the lumen of the stricture. It is then inflated under visual control to a specific pressure at which it will assume a predetermined diameter. Balloons of increasing diameter are used until the luminal width desired has been restored in the stricture. Alternatively, passage of rigid dilators combines axial with radial stretch of strictures. The endoscopist places a narrow guidewire through the stricture, removes the scope and then advances a metal (olive-shaped) or plastic Savary or Celestin dilator across the stricture. One starts with a diameter close to that estimated by endoscopy and by inserting gradually increased diameters. Full relief of symptoms of mechanical obstruction can be expected with diameters between 12 and 14 mm (corresponding to French sizes 36 to 42). With tight strictures, particularly those due to lye, dilatation is stepwise increased at successive sessions. With malignant strictures, repeated dilatations are needed to prevent reocclusion from tumor growth unless a stent can be placed into the stricture.

Complications of Endoscopy and Esophageal Dilatation

Upper gastrointestinal endoscopy is remarkably safe, with death reported in 1 in 10,000 during diagnostic procedure, and more likely to occur in the elderly, the acutely ill, and during an emergency procedure (Keeffe & Schrock, 1995). Perforation is the single most important complication of esophagoscopy. Other potential complications include aspiration, bleeding, allergic reaction to medications, oversedation and hypoxia (Keeffe & Schrock, 1995). The complication rate rises with therapeutic measures, with

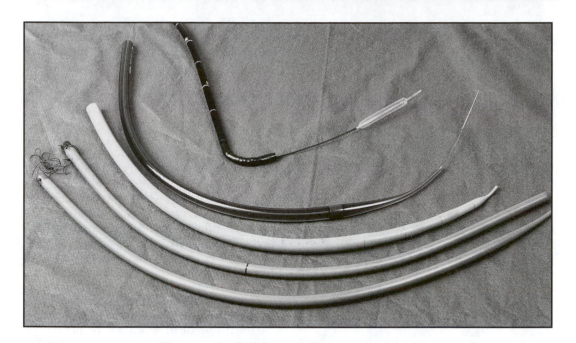

Figure 10–5. Photograph of the most common dilators. Shown from the top down: (1) Through-the-scope dilators can be passed thoughout the stricture under direct vision. The balloon is placed straddling the stricture and inflated to the desired pressure. (2) Savary-Gillard plastic dilator. This has a gradually tapered end and is advanced over a guide-wire. These dilators come in different sizes to achieve progressive dilatation. (3) The Celestin dilator is a rigid plastic dilator that is also passed over a guidewire. Its diameter increases stepwise from its tip. (4,5) There are two types of mercury weighted bougies. The Maloney type dilator has a tapered end and the Hurst type has a blunt end.

esophageal dilatation resulting in up to 0.4% perforations.

Meticulous technique of dilatation and prompt recognition and treatment of perforations are required. Crushing chest pain, particularly if persistent after no longer applying pressure to the dilator, dyspnea, or hypotension calls for immediate cessation of dilatation and patient resuscitation. Chest x-rays and abdominal films will detect mediastinal or subdiaphragmatic air. Subcutaneous emphysema takes longer to develop. If a contrast study confirms perforation, esophageal suction and operative closure of the perforation should be initiated.

Endoscopic reassessment of strictures determines whether dilatation was successful. Mucosal lacerations and modest bleeding are common, and no contraindication to biopsy after the dilatation or inspection of stomach and duodenum. However, the depth of lacerations is difficult to judge by endoscopic inspection alone. Contrast studies define sites and size of perforations and the risks posed by lesser complications like lacerations or intramural penetrations. That information may be valuable before resuming oral feeding in high risk dilatations. Hypaque studies are done for exploration, and are followed, in the absence of extravasation, by barium contrast examination.

Contraindications to endoscopy include an uncooperative or combative patient, particularly from delirium tremens; prior or impending perforation of the gastrointestinal tract; unstable cardiorespiratory function; severe coagulopathy; and meal ingestion within 3–4 hours prior to the study.

MANOMETRY

Unlike barium contrast and other imaging studies, esophageal manometry quantitates the contractile activity of the esophagus. By recording luminal pressures it informs on the presence, force, and the pattern of propagation of esophageal contractions, and on the resting tone and relaxation of the esophageal sphincters. Absence of sphincter relaxation and esophageal contractions allows a diagnosis of achalasia. Simultaneous high-pressure contractions suggest the diagnosis of diffuse esophageal spasm, a rare disease if classical manometric criteria are applied. Other manometric abnormalities occur in various diseases, including esophageal inflammation or tumors, and hence have no specific diagnostic value (Kahrilas, Clouse, & Hogan, 1994).

Technical Aspects of Manometry

Manometry uses catheters inside the esophagus to record its luminal pressures. Catheters are water-perfused and connected to a volume displacement transducer outside the body, or have built-in strain gauge transducers. Recording devices are either strip chart recorders of various types or analog to digital converters, connected to computers.

The Water-Perfused System

A pump perfuses bubble-free water through a multilumen manometric catheter bundle. Each lumen is connected to an external volume displacement pressure transducer. Impedance to water flow by an esophageal contraction raises the pressure in the channel and the external transducer. Accuracy of pressure recordings improved with the development of a low-compliance pneumohydraulic infusion pump (Arndorfer, Stef, Dodds, Linehan, & Hogan, 1977).

Catheters are typically made of polyvinyl, incorporating an assembly of separate capillary channels with a diameter of less than 1 mm each to minimize compliance. Catheters typically have 6–8 channels. A standard arrangement consists of four distal, radially oriented side holes located at the same level for detection of the asymmetrical LES pressure profile. Four proximal side holes, spaced 5 cm apart, span the entire length of the esophagus.

Fewer channels, or more closely spaced openings will require repositioning of the tube during the course of the study if the entire length of the esophagus is to be studied. Catheters with multiple channels, each functioning as a single point sensor, may not provide faithful recording of LES and UES pressure because of their 2–3 cm orad movement during swallowing and respiration. During such movement the point sensor may lose contact with the sphincter, with loss of pressure giving the false impression of sphincter relaxation.

The problem of dynamic recording of sphincter pressure was circumvented by the development of the *sleeve sensor*. The sleeve is formed by a 6-cm-long water-perfused cavity covered by a silicone membrane, and can detect pressure applied anywhere along its length. When incorporated into a catheter with an assembly of separate channels it allows dynamic recording of sphincter pressure and esophageal body simultaneously (Dent, 1976; Linehan, Dent, Dodds, & Hogan, 1985).

Intraluminal Strain Gauge System

Miniature strain gauge pressure transducers are incorporated into the catheter assembly and measure pressure directly inside the lumen. The probe can be connected to a polygraph, to a computer through an A-D converter, or to a small solid state recorder that stores the data in digital form while being carried by an ambulatory subject. Sleeve devices made of silicone, containing miniature transducers immersed in viscous fluid, have been recently developed for ambulatory recording of sphincteric function.

The perfused system is inexpensive, reliable, and durable. Its frequency responses do not accurately record the rapid pressure changes in the pharynx. Also, the system is not suitable for ambulatory studies. The intraluminal strain-gauge system has a much higher frequency response but is more expensive and fragile. Sleeve devices for ambulatory recording from sphincters have not been extensively tested.

The Conduct of Manometric Examination

Esophageal manometry (Kahrilas et al., 1994) is done while the subject is awake since cooperation is required. Subjects should fast for approximately 6 hours before the study and medications that can affect esophageal motility (anticholinergics, nitrates, calcium channel blockers, prokinetic agents) should be discontinued at least 24 hours before the test.

The probe can be inserted orally or nasally. The nasal route may be somewhat more uncomfortable during probe insertion, but it is better tolerated during the study. Local anesthetic, like viscous lidocaine, squirted into the nostril facilitates probe insertion.

When using the perfused catheter, side holes above or below the level of the external transducers will record pressures that are spuriously diminished or augmented, respectively, owing to hydrostatic changes. Consequently, most studies are performed with the patient in the supine position. Function of the pressure-sensing system can be confirmed by asking the patient to cough. The pressure in all sites should rise sharply, confirming proper functioning of the system. A pressure sensor taped to the submandibular area or a submental EMG electrode records swallowing. Pressure oscillations associated with respiration may be recorded with a flow-sensitive probe placed, at the nares or a pneumo belt wrapped around the chest. Once the subject is comfortable, the assessment of the three functional regions of the esophagus, the LES, the esophageal body, and the UES, can proceed.

The probe should be advanced initially so that the most distal sensor is at a distance of at least 50 cm from the nares (equivalent to 45 cm from the incisors).

Sensor location is assessed by observation of the pressure patterns produced by breathing. In the thoracic cavity inspiration generates a negative, and in the abdominal cavity a positive pressure deflection. An intragastric position of the probe is confirmed if a pressure raise is sustained during a deep breath or during abdominal compression. The point at which the polarity of the deflection switches from positive below the diaphragm to negative above the diaphragm is called the *pressure inversion point*, also called the *respiratory reversal point*. The respiratory reversal point corresponds to the level at which the phrenoesophageal ligament inserts in the wall of the distal esophagus. Normally this insertion occurs within the *diaphragmatic hiatus* and within the high-pressure zone generated by the LES as described below. With hiatus hernia there may be a double high-pressure zone.

Test Performance and Analysis

The three functional regions of the esophagus: the LES, the esophageal body, and the UES will be discussed separately.

The Lower Esophageal Sphincter

Variables measured are resting sphincter pressure and swallow-induced relaxation. LES pressure is assessed by a rapid pull-through (RPT) or stationary pull-through (SPT) technique. During RPT, the distal, circumferentially oriented side holes are pulled at a rate of 1–2 cm/s from the stomach and across the LES into the esophagus with the subject holding his or her breath at midexpiration. Paper speed of 2.5–5 mm/s is commonly used. The peak pressure above gastric baseline (which serves as the reference pressure for LES) is averaged for the number of side holes used and pulls made and presented as LES pressure. The RPT technique provides a fast and easy assessment of LES pressure and its location, but the movement of the catheter can induce contraction, resulting in abnormally high pressure, or alternatively, a low pressure, can be recorded if the patient swallows during the pull-through.

The SPT technique provides a more complete evaluation of LES function. With the distal side holes in the stomach the catheter is initially withdrawn 1 cm at a time. Respiration is not suspended. The first indication that the LES is encountered is by increased oscillations of base-line corresponding to respiratory effect (Figure 10–6, left). At this point the catheter is moved 0.5 cm at a time and held in each station for at least 1 min, and swallows of water (5 ml) can be given to assess LES relaxation (Figure 10–6 right).

With further withdrawing of the catheter one encounters the respiratory reversal point or the pressure inversion point. As

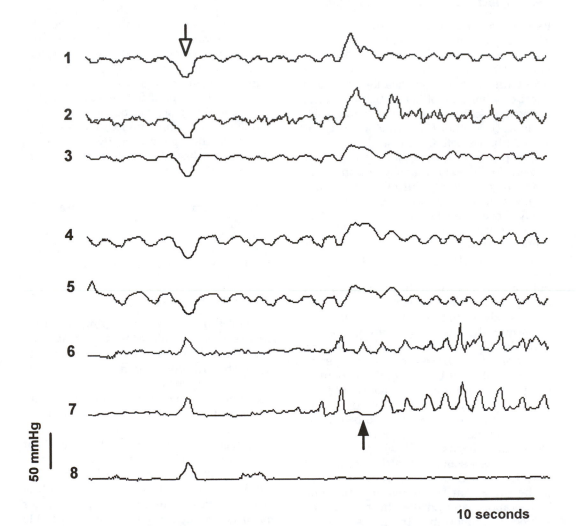

Figure 10–6. (Left) slow pull-through using the Dent sleeve. Channels 1 to 5 represent side-holes spaced 3 cm apart. Channel 7 represents the sleeve, while channels 6 and 8 represent side-holes just above and below the sleeve, correspondingly. The open arrow points to a deep breath with a downward deflection in channels 1–5, representing their position above the diaphragm, and upward deflection in channels 6–8 representing their position below the diaphragm. With continuous pull-through one observes the respiratory oscilllations indicating that the sleeve and the side-hole just above it have entered the high-pressure zone of the LES (closed arrow).

discussed above, pressures decrease above this point and increase below it during inspiration. It indicates that the sensors are above the diaphragm and in the thoracic cavity (Figure 10–7).

When using a sleeve device, the LES can first be localized by RPT. Approximately 2 cm of the sleeve are placed above the upper level of the LES to ensure its contact with the sleeve during swallowing. A continuous recording of 5–10 min is made and LES pressure is determined as the average of 1-min recordings. When determining LES pressure with SPT or with a sleeve device, the respiratory oscillations have to be taken into consideration. End-expiratory pressure provides sphincter pressure without diaphragmatic augmentation and is more widely used. When relaxation during swallowing is complete,

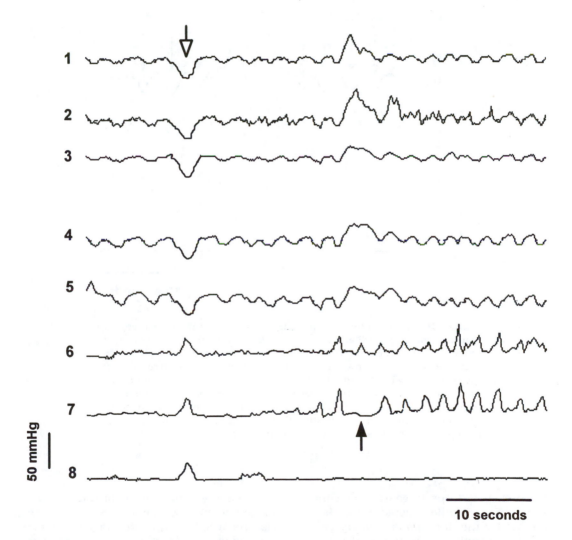

Figure 10–6. (Right) with further pulling there is a rise in pressure in the sleeve channel. After water swallow of 5 ml of water (ws) sequential contractions are observed in the body of the esophagus with a drop in pressure in the sleeve channel corresponding to LES relaxation (the interrupted line in channel 7 represents gastric baseline pressure). The most distal side hole (number 8) is still in the stomach.

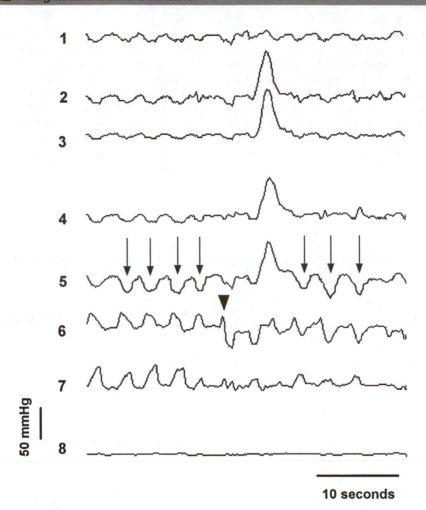

Figure 10–7. Manometric representation of the pressure inversion point. Respiratory oscillations in sensor 6, to the left of the arrowhead, show upward deflection with inspiration, while channel 5 shows the opposite, namely downward deflection with inspiration (arrows). This suggests that while channel 6 is still in the high pressure zone, it is below the diaphragm. With further pulling, the direction of the respiratory oscillations in sensor 6 become parallel to those of sensor 5 (to the right of the arrowhead), indicating that the side hole, while still in the high pressure zone, is now above the diaphragm.

LES pressure drops to gastric baseline. Normal LES relaxation should exceed 90% and last for the duration of primary peristalsis. Incomplete relaxation and a high baseline pressure (often exceeding 40 mmHg) are characteristics of a *hypertensive LES.*

Abdominal compression provides information about LES competence. A pressure rise recorded by the esophageal sensor concomitant with a rise in gastric pressure indicates a common cavity: an incompetent sphincter simply provides no pressure barrier between the lumina of the esophagus and stomach. Incompetence of the LES is rare and is typically associated with sphincter pressures below 10 mmHg and severe reflux esophagitis as in scleroderma. The LES is hypotensive or normotensive (generating pressures in the 10–30-mmHg range) in most cases of GERD. Normal values are in Table 10–2. Factors modulating LES are shown in Table 10–3.

Esophageal Body and Esophageal Peristalsis

The manometric variables measured are the amplitude, duration, and velocity of propagation of esophageal contractions. With the distal side holes, or sleeve, in the LES, the proximal ones will span the esophageal body. With the patient supine and the paper speed at 2.5 mm/s a series of swallows are recorded. Subjects are asked to swallow their own saliva (dry) or are given water (wet) swallows. Water boluses of 5 ml, at room temperature, are squirted gently to the dependent side of the mouth with the patient facing sideways, to avoid aspiration. Thirty seconds are allowed between swallows to avoid inhibition of peristalsis from rapid repetitive swallows. Wet swallows induce more consistent and vigorous peristaltic response than dry ones and should be analyzed separately. At least ten swallows of each type should be performed because abnormalities in peristaltic function or configuration of individual contractions can be intermittent (Dodds, Hogan, Reid, Stewart, & Arndorfer, 1973). Swallows of solid material (like bread) may increase the sensitivity of detection of motor abnormalities compared to liquid swallows. However,

experience is limited and no normal data are available (Howard, Maher, Pryde, & Heading, 1991). Because body position, volume, and consistency of the bolus swallowed all affect manometric variables, they should be standardized in each laboratory.

CONTACT AND CAVITY PRESSURES, BOLUS ESCAPE. Two types of pressure phenomena are recorded by manometry (Ren et al., 1991). Squeeze or contact pressures are generated by the compression forces at the site of the pressure sensor and are associated with occlusion of the port. Contact pressures are recorded as the contraction occludes a tubular segment forcefully. Contact pressures are generally of large amplitude and occur sequentially at different points of the esophagus. Pressures recorded from within the lumen of a fluid-filled cavity are known as *bolus, luminal,* or *cavity* pressures. Bolus pressures are generally of low amplitude and may be recorded by multiple sensors throughout the esophagus simultaneously (Lin, Brasseur, Pouderoux, & Kahrilas, 1995). During the course of a peristaltic contraction, the same sensor may record a two-phasic pressure wave, with the first phase corresponding to the arrival of the bolus and the second phase corresponding to the arrival of the contraction proper (Figure 10–8). For the contraction to advance the bolus, the squeeze pressure has to exceed the bolus pressure, typically by at least 30 mmHg. If the pressure in the bolus comes to equal or to exceed the squeeze pressure, the bolus is likely to reverse the direction of its flow. This phenomen is known as *bolus escape* on imag-

TABLE 10–2. Reference pressures for normal esophageal manometry.

	Amplitude (mmHg)	Duration (s)	Velocity (cm/s)	LES pressure (mmHg)
Wet swallows	99 ± 40	3.9 ± 0.9	3.5 ± 0.9	24.4 ± 10.1
Dry swallows	71 ± 28	4.1 ± 0.8	4.0 ± 0.3	

Note. Variables of distal esophageal contractions, and LES pressure in normal subjects; all values are represented as mean ± S.D. (Modified from Richter, J. E. Normal Values for Esophageal Manometry. In D. O. Castell and J. A. Castell, Eds., *Esophageal Motility Testing.* Norwalk, VA: Appleton & Lange, 1994, p. 84.)

TABLE 10–3. Factors that influence LES pressure.

	Increase	*Decrease*
Hormones	Gastrin	Secretin
	Motilin	Cholecystrokinin
	Substance P	Glucagon
	Galanin	Neurotensin
	Bombesin	Gastric inhibitory
	Somatostatin	polypeptide
		Vasoactive intestinal
		polypeptide
		Progesterone
Neural Agents	α-Andrenergic antagonists	β-Andrenergic agonists
	β-Andrenergic antagonists	α-Andrenergic antagonists
	Cholinergic agonists	Anticholinergic agents
Foods	Protein meals	Fat
		Chocolate
		Ethanol
		Peppermint
Others	Histamine	Nitric Oxide
	Antacids	Theophylline
	Metoclopramide	Caffeine
	Domperidone	Gastric acidification
	Met-enkephalin	Smoking
		Pregnancy
	Prostaglandin (F2a)	Prostaglandins (E_2, I_2)
	Coffee	Serotonin
		Merperidine, morphine
	Migrating motor complex	Dopamine
	Raised intra-abdominal pain	Calcium blocking agents
		Diazepam
		Barbiturates

Note. Adapted from Diamant, N. E. Physiology of the esophagus. In M. H. Sleisenger and J. S. Fordtran (Eds) *Gastrointestinal Diseases*, New York: W. B. Saunders, 1993.

ing and occurs, for instance, in front of an obstruction. The retrograde luminal flow occurring during bolus escape may be mistaken for retrograde peristalsis. *Retrograde peristalsis* implies that contrac-tions themselves move upstream in the esophagus as they do in the striated esophagus of ruminant animals (Lu, Schulze- Delrieu, Cram, Shirazi, & Raab, 1994).

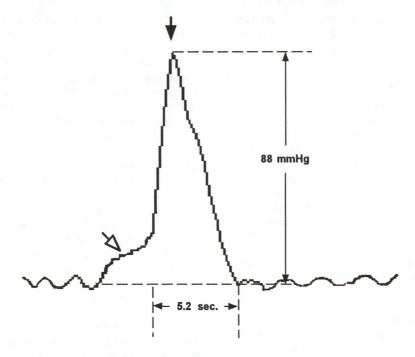

Figure 10–8. Contraction amplitude is measured from the esophageal baseline to the peak of the pressure wave, while the duration is measured from the point of initial upstroke of the pressure wave to the point of its return to baseline. Closed arrow indicates squeeze pressure; open arrow points to the bolus pressure.

Pressure amplitude is measured from mean intraesophageal pressure to peak pressure. Duration is calculated from initial upstroke to return to baseline (Figure 10–8). Velocity of propagation can be determined between two or more sensors. The time between the beginning of the upstroke of the contractions is simply divided by the distance between the sensors chosen. (Normal values for variables in Table 10–2.)

Esophageal contractions usually have a single peak but some double-peaked contractions may be considered a normal variant. Contractions are considered as abnormal multipeaked if having an amplitude of at least 10% of wave amplitude or are at least 1 s in duration (Clouse & Staiano, 1983). A contraction is considered *hypotensive* if its amplitude is below 30 mmHg. Contractions with this amplitude are associated with impaired bolus transport (Kahrilas, Dodds, & Hogan, 1988). *Hypertensive* contractions have amplitudes greater than 180 mmHg, but have no known association with bolus transit abnormalities (Massey, Dodds, Hogan, Brasseur, & Helm, 1991).

Peristalsis is considered abnormal when a swallow does not result in contractile activity, when the contraction propagates only through part of the length of the esophagus, or when simultaneous contractions are observed. These patterns are associated with abnormal fluid bolus emptying (Kahrilas et al., 1988). Artifacts can sometimes cause confusion. Exaggerated respiratory oscillations can give the impression of simultaneous contractions, which can be clarified by having the patient suspend respiration for 15–20 s. Pressure oscillations, at heart rate, may be recorded when a sensor overlies the aortic arch or the left atrium. Oscillations at a rate of

60/s and not corresponding to heart rate, represent electrical interference and usually disappear by adjusting probe position.

Upper Esophageal Sphincter

The sphincter length is 1–2 cm and is formed by the striated muscle of the cricopharyngeus. The UES high pressure zone is usually recorded 15–20 cm from the incisors. Like in the LES, there is radial resting asymmetry in pressure in the UES (Figure 10–9). The highest pressures are recorded in the antero-posterior planes (Winans, 1972). Manometric evaluation of UES function presents a number of difficulties. Intubation of the sphincter stimulates contraction, and lower resting pressures are obtained with stationary devices. The diameter of the catheters affects the pressures. Like the LES, the UES moves 2–3 cm orad with swallowing and therefore a sleeve device is more suitable to detect its true pressure changes. However, the rapid contraction rate of striated muscle exceeds the frequency response of perfused systems. Intraluminal transducers have the appropriate frequency response but are still subject to sensor displacement. Increased bolus pressures in the pharynx, weak pharyngeal contractions, and poor coordination between pharyngeal contractions and UES may explain some cases of pharygeal dysphagia (Ollson, Castell, Castell, & Ekberg, 1995).

Accurate recordings of sphincter pressures still fail to detect relevant abnormalities of UES function. Patients with dysphagia and Zenker's diverticula or cricopharyngeal bars have normal sphincteric relaxation in response to swallowing, but the cross section to which the UES opens is markedly reduced (Cook et al., 1992). This implies that the compliance of the UES is reduced. Bolus pressures above the noncompliant UES become abnormally high as long as oropharyngeal activity is preserved.

Provocative Tests

A variety of tests are in use, all intended to induce symptoms of esophageal origin, and specifically heartburn and chest pain. The oldest, the *Bernstein test*, employs acid perfusion to reproduce symptoms associated with reflux (Bernstein & Baker, 1958). Cholinomimetic agents like edrophonium (Richter, Hackshaw, Wu, & Castell, 1985) and esophageal balloon distension (Barish, Castell, & Richter, 1986) are used to evaluate patients with noncardiac chest pain. A way to evaluate the pathophysiology of dysphagia in patients with manometric findings of simultaneous or spontaneous contractions is the use of paired or multiple swallows at frequent intervals. This maneuver results in suppression of contractions in healthy subjects, but not in patients with dysphagia relating to simultaneous or spontaneous contractions. This implies a lack of inhibitory neuronal controls of esophageal smooth muscle activity (Behar & Biancani, 1993).

Inhibitory control of esophageal activity can also be demonstrated with an air-filled intraesophageal balloon, which induces a locally sustained contraction and high balloon pressure. In normal subjects swallowing first inhibits all pressures and then unleashes a pressure rebound. This inhibition is missing in some patients with chest pain and esophageal motor disorders (Sifrim, Janssens, & Vantrappen, 1994).

Impedance Planimetry

Assessment of the esophageal cross-section, in response to a distending pressure, enables determination of important biomechanical properties like wall tension and compliance. Impedance planimetry allows continuous measurement of the cross-sectional area of tubular organs while monitoring intraluminal pressure (Gregersen & Anderson, 1991). The system employs a probe with electrodes that are surrounded by a flaccid balloon that can be distended with conducting fluid. Passage of electrical current between the electrodes depends on the known conductivity of the fluid and the cross-sectional area of the balloon to be measured. With this technique the biomechanical properties of the human esophagus were defined (Orvar, Gregersen,

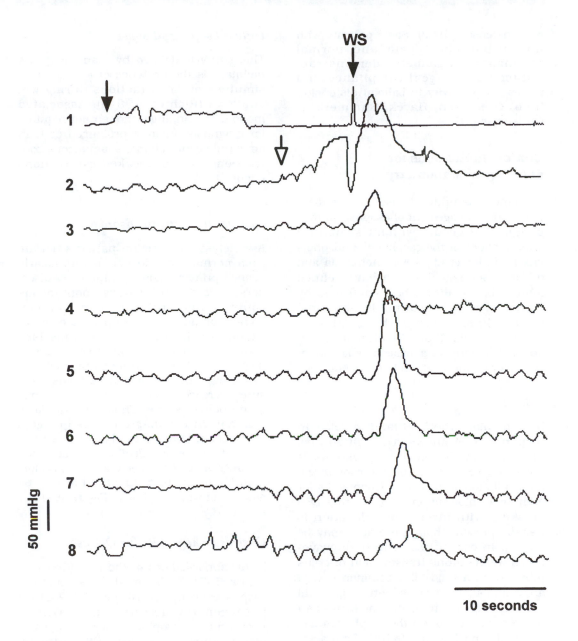

Figure 10–9. Pull-through showing the most proximal sensor (number 1) entering and leaving the high-pressure zone of the UES (arrow). With further pulling the second sensor (channel number 2) enters the high-pressure zone (open arrow). Swallow of 5 ml of water (ws) results in pharyngeal contractions and relaxation of UES, with subsequent sequential contractions of the esophageal body. Note the difference in pressures recorded by sensors 1 and 2 in the UES, representing the asymmetry of the sphincter.

& Christensen, 1993). Some patients with noncardiac chest pain and normal esophageal manometry demonstrate reduced esophageal compliance and increased reactivity to balloon distension (Rao, Gregersen, Hayek, Summers, & Christensen, 1994).

Clinical Indications for Esophageal Manometry

Manometry is primarily used in the diagnosis and management of esophageal dysphagia that occurs without structural abnormalities of the esophagus and pharynx (Kahrilas et al., 1994). Achalasia and diffuse esophageal spasm have defined motor abnormalities, best confirmed by manometry and resulting in abnormal bolus transit through the esophagus (Hewson et al., 1990). Treatments available particularly for achalasia make manometric evaluation helpful in these entities.

Achalasia

In achalasia, the LES fails to relax in response to swallows (a condition also known as *cardiospasm* or *hypertensive sphincter*; see above) and the esophageal body fails to contract. (See Chapter 13 for additional information.) High resting LES pressure with incomplete relaxation is usually present though pressure may be normal in early disease. Isobaric waveforms, representing transmission of bolus pressure in a fluid-filled common cavity, are common, and elevated intraesophageal pressure relative to gastric pressure can be seen, particularly if the esophagus has retained fluid (Figure 10–10). Manometry is often rendered difficult by curling of the catheter in the dilated esophagus. Position of sensors is assessed by identifying the expected sequence of pressure changes with swallowing and inspiration. Occasionally fluoroscopy may be needed to verify position and guidewire to advance the catheter through a tight sphincter into the stomach. The Dent sleeve, though, does not accommodate a guidewire.

Diffuse Esophageal Spasm

This entity is defined by manometry, its hallmark is the presence of at least 10% simultaneous contractions during wet swallows (Richter, 1994a). Associated manometric findings, though not required for diagnosis, include prolonged or high amplitude contractions, spontaneous contractions, or multipeaked contractions (Figure 10–11)

Nonspecific Motility Disorders

A variety of contraction patterns deviate from normal, but do not fit into clearly defined primary esophageal motility disorders. This group includes spontaneous contractions, prolonged contractions, high-amplitude or low-amplitude contractions, multipeaked contractions (see above), and nontransmitted contractions (Figure 10–12). Bolus transport abnormalities may present as increased bolus pressure, decreased squeeze pressure, or retrograde bolus escape. This is particularly common in esophagitis or esophageal obstruction. (Massey et al., 1991). A combined manometric-videofluoroscopic study is superior to manometry alone in abnormalities in bolus transport that can be associated with dysphagia (Figure 10–13).

Gastroesophageal Reflux Disease

Motor abnormalities of the LES (Cohen & Harris, 1971; Dodds et al., 1982) and the esophageal body (Kahrilas et al., 1986) are pathogenetic mechanisms of GERD. Recurrence of esophageal lesions is common in patients with low LES pressures. The primary LES abnormality associated with reflux episodes is that of transient LES relaxation, which occurs in the absence of swallowing. Hence, they have been called *inappropriate LES relaxations* (Dent et al., 1980). Hypotension and incompetence of the LES occur in GERD, but are not a prerequisite for it. Hypotensive contractions in the esophageal body are common in reflux esophagitis.

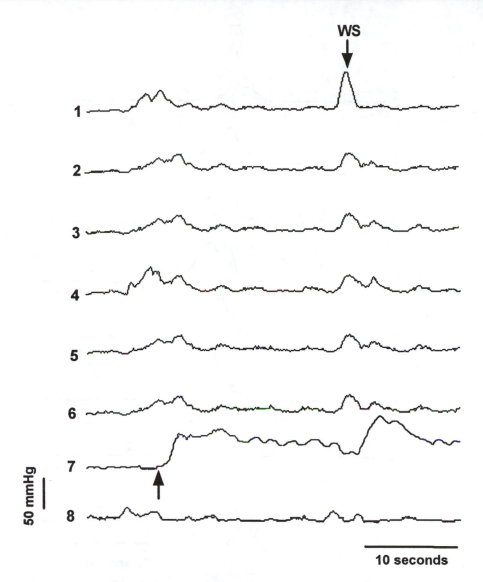

Figure 10–10. Achalasia. High LES pressure (sensor 7-arrow) with only partial relaxation in response to wet swallow (ws). Note adequate amplitude of contraction following the wet swallow in the proximal, striated muscle part of the esophagus (sensor 1), and the low amplitude, simultaneous pressure waves in the smooth muscle part of the esophagus (sensors 2–6), representing a common-cavity phenomena.

Documentation of abnormal esophageal motor by manometry becomes rarely a basis for therapeutic decisions (Johnston, Johnston, Collins, Collins, & Love, 1993). Assessment of disease severity by endoscopy is a more reliable tool in this regard. (Bell & Hunt, 1992). Manometry is routinely performed in the preoperative evaluation of patients considered for antireflux surgery. It has potential value in assessing the efficacy of the operation in restoring a high-pressure zone or predicting poor outcome when motor function of the esophageal body is severely impaired,

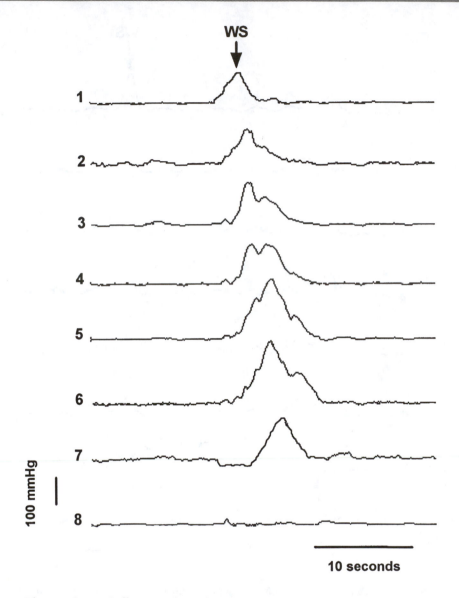

Figure 10–11. Diffuse esophageal spasm. Note the high-amplitude, simultaneous, and long duration contractions in response to wet swallow. (Note the change in the pressure scale as compared to the other graphs, so as not to lose the peak of the pressure waves.)

like in scleroderma. A partial rather than a 360° wrap, an alternative procedure with less potential for obstruction, or no operation may be indicated in these settings (Joelsson et al., 1982). The role of preoperative manometry remains controversial, though (Mughal, Bancie-wicz, Marples, 1990).

ESOPHAGEAL pH MONITORING

The esophagus is a transit organ that does not store, digest, or otherwise alter its contents. The stomach uses its mechanical activity and secretions to digest the food stored in it. Hydrochloric acid secreted by the stomach is highly corrosive, and expo-

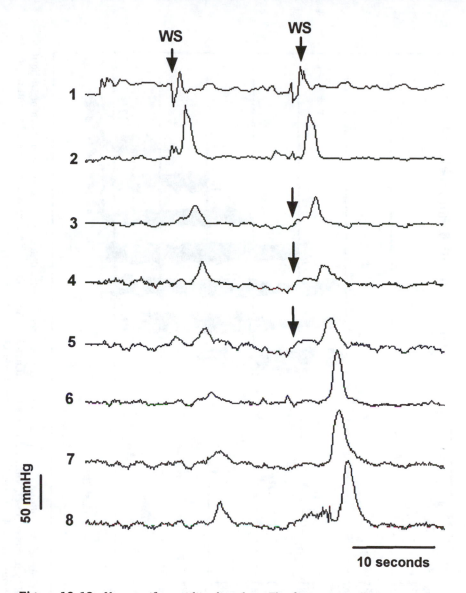

Figure 10–12. Nonspecific motility disorders. The first wet swallow produced a good response in the proximal esophagus but pressure waves with poor amplitude in the distal esophagus. The second swallow produced good response in the proximal esophagus, but poor response in the transition zone between the striated and the smooth muscle esophagus, with high intrabolus pressure in that area (arrows), with good response in the distal esophagus. This patient had GERD.

sure of the esophagus to acid causes lesions, especially of its mucosa. (See also Chapter 13.) Normally, the lower esophageal sphincter, an effective barrier to gastroesophageal reflux minimizes the exposure of the esophagus and, the oropharynx to gastric acid. Thus, records of the esophageal pH are an indirect measure of the competence of the barrier to gastroesophageal reflux and of the risk for its complications.

Ambulatory esophageal pH monitoring assesses reflux of acidic gastric contents under conditions of normal daily activity.

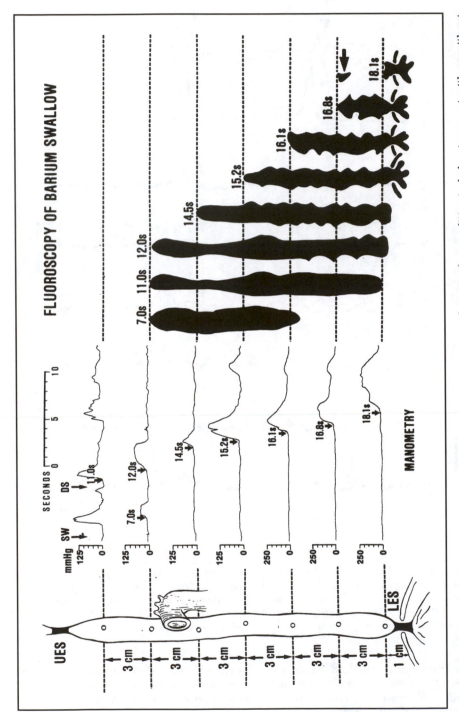

Figure 10–13. A tracing of combined videofluoroscopy and manometry showing abnormalities in bolus transport with or without nonpropagated contractions.(From Massey et al., Abnormal esophageal motility. An analysis of concurrent radiographic and manometric findings. *Gastroenterology, 101,* 344–54, 1991. Used with permission.)

It can provide an accurate recording of the pH at a point in the esophagus over a prolonged period of time, with a 24-h period having become a virtual standard. A pH value does not quantify the volume of the refluxate or any refluxate that has the same pH as the esophagus. It does not identify reflux of corrosives other than acid. While digestive enzymes like pepsin require acid to be activated, other compounds including bile salts and pancreatic enzymes may be active at neutral or even alkaline pH (see also below). To date, pH monitoring has been primarily tested in its predictive value for the occurence of reflux esophagitis. Techniques of the procedure and normative values derived for this indication are not necessarily applicable to other manifestations of GERD such as atypical chest pain.

Equipment

Prolonged esophageal pH monitoring is performed by placing an acid-sensitive probe in the lower esophagus, usually 5 cm above the manometrically defined LES. The esophageal pH (as detected by the probe) is recorded onto an attached portable electronic storage device. The record can be subsequently displayed or printed onto hard copy for inspection and analysis.

Probes

Two common types of pH-sensitive probes are in use: the glass electrode and the antimony electrode. These probes have some practical differences (Table 10–4). Glass electrodes are quite stable, have a broad range of pH detection, and can be used many hundreds of times. However, they are prone to breakage, expensive, and difficult to clean. Antimony probes are inexpensive, less vulnerable to breakage, but may be used only a limited number of times before being replaced. Both types of probes are prone to some pH drift and need to be carefully calibrated before and after each study. The antimony probe does not record accurately above a pH of 8. In

most situations this is unlikely to be of any practical significance.

Recording Systems

Some recording systems use a solid state recorder, some early models use a tape recorder, with different methods of compression of the data for storage. Apart from the size and weight of the recording device, reliability is a necessity in the recording device. The device should save the data even if its power supply fails.

The pH probe in the esophagus is part of an electrical circuit, which can be completed with an internal or, more commonly, a reference electrode placed on the skin of the thorax or upper abdomen. External reference electrodes are prone to dislocation. Careful skin preparation is necessary and high conductive electrode jelly is usually applied. The pad and wire need to be securely fixed to the skin. The patient must be instructed not to disturb the electrode. Probes with an internal reference electrode are expensive and prone to losing electrical contact with the esophageal wall.

Placement of the pH Probe

Accurate placement of the probe is essential for documentation of reflux. A site 5 cm above the LES is conventionally employed to avoid dipping of the probe into the stomach during esophageal shortening from swallowing. This location is thought to be distal enough to identify most significant episodes of reflux. Two probes placed at the same distance from the LES will reveal some discordant findings (Murphy, Yuan, & Castell, 1989)

One standard is to place the pH probe 5 cm above the upper border of the manometrically defined LES. Alternatively, one measures the distance from the incisor teeth to the squamocolumnar junction endoscopically. In the adult this measurement would place the probe 5 cm above the LES when introduced through the nostril. A less accurate method is the step-up pH method. The pH probe is advanced to where it detects a low acid pH of 1 and

TABLE 10–4. Differences between glass and antimony probes.

Glass	Antimony
Long lasting	<10 studies
Stable	Some drift
Expensive	Less expensive
Difficult to clean	Easy to clean
Wide pH range	Limited pH range (<8)
Fragile	Robust
Lower mean values	Higher mean values

then is withdrawn in a stepwise fashion until a step-up of the pH indicates passage into the esophagus. The probe is withdrawn another 5 cm to place it in the lower esophagus. With this method the probe may move out of acid long before passing the LES or conversely may never move out of acid when an incompetent LES levels to acidification of the esophagus may be acidified. Some probes incorporate a locator device, which is a single manometric sensor. A pull-through can locate the LES. Fluoroscopy placement is limited by coexistent hiatal hernias, which are not readily seen by fluoroscopy.

Interpretation

The entire record should be initially displayed, either on a computer screen or paper, and the profile of the pH visually inspected.

Esophageal Acidification From Episodes of Reflux and Other Mechanism

Abrupt drops in pH to a level below a pH of 4 (see Figure 10–14) indicate reflux of an acidic nature and are denoted as *reflux episodes*. The significance of a pH below 4 is that corrosives such as pepsin are not active unless the pH is below 4. Also, heartburn is relieved when the esophageal pH is brought above 4. After a reflux episode, the pH remains low for a variable time. It returns to baseline in a gradual, often stepwise fashion. Neutralization occurs as peristalsis and gravity clear refluxed acid back into the stomach. It is

enhanced by the buffering capacity of alkaline saliva or potentially of the ingested food. Unlike the acute drops in pH caused by reflux, esophageal obstruction from achalasia can lead to a gradual drop of pH (Figure 10–15). This intraesophageal acidification must be distinguished from reflux because of their different causes and treatments.

Computer Analysis and Correlation With Symptoms

Parameters that are typically processed include the frequency and the duration of reflux episodes, the total number of reflux episodes lasting more than 5 min, and the total or relative time of esophageal acidification. Data may be further broken down between times of meals, sleep, and other activity. The pH parameter that best correlates with esophageal lesions on endoscopic examination is the total time the pH is below 4. Table 10–5 provides the upper limits of normal data for ambulatory esophageal pH recordings. A pH profile within the range of this group of normal subjects does not exclude the possibility that reflux contributes to a disease manifestation nor does a pH profile outside this group of norms by itself constitute GERD or the need for reflux treatment.

Reflux Indices

The occurrence of classical reflux symptoms is a fairly reliable indicator of abnormal reflux. Reflux episodes remain often asymptomatic, even in patients with dam-

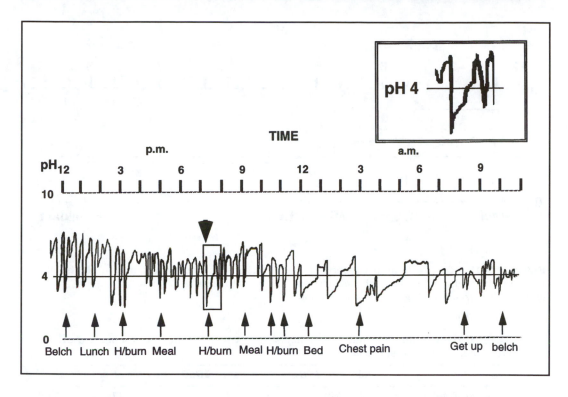

Figure 10–14. A 24-hour pH profile. A record from an individual with GERD. It illustrates the rapid drop in pH that occurs with reflux of acidic gastric contents into the esophagus (arrows indicate reflux events associated with symptoms).

aged esophageal mucosa. Problems occur when assessing the role of reflux in the absence of classical reflux symptoms or manifestations, for instance, individuals with chest pain. The demonstration of reflux does not by itself prove that it caused the chest pain, but the likelihood rises when episodes of pain and reflux coincide.

Several formulas have been devised to measure the degree of association between symptoms and reflux episodes. The first measure devised is the symptom index (SI):

$$SI = \frac{symptom\ association\ with\ GERD \times 100}{total\ number\ (\#)\ of\ symptoms} = \%$$

This measure does not take account of the number of reflux events not associated with pain. For example a patient who had 100 reflux events and a single episode of chest pain that coincided with a reflux episode would have a symptom index value of $1/1 \times 100 = 100\%$. To address this the reverse computation has been used, the so-called *symptoms sensitivity index* (SSI):

$$SSI = \frac{\#\ reflux\ episodes\ associated\ with\ symptoms \times 100}{\#\ reflux\ episodes} = \%$$

In the above example $1/100 \times 100 = 1\%$. Several attempts have been made to refine these two parameters. The symptom-association probability (Wuesten, Roelofs, Akkermans, Van Berge-Henegouwen, & Smout, 1994) was developed by using Fisher's exact test to test the likelihood that reflux episode and symptom were unrelated. The probability-generated P was subtracted from 1.0 and expressed as a percentage. This may be a J single test that might serve as a measure of the association. All of these measures are based on the premise that a reflux is likely to produce symptoms at any given time. Most

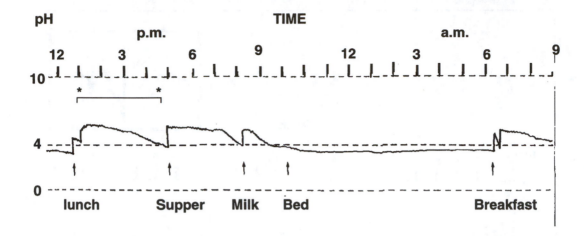

Figure 10–15. The 24-hour pH record of a patient with achalasia. Here, the pH drops gradully (∗—∗), suggesting in-site acidification rather than the abrupt drop in pH that occurs in reflux events.

TABLE 10–5. 95th percentile (upper limits) for 24-hour ambulatory esophageal pH recordings in normal subjects.

	Johnson, 1987[a]	DeMeester, 1989	Richter et al., 1992
Number of subjects	50*	50	110
% time pH < 4	3.4	4.45	5.78
Upright % time pH < 4	4.6	8.42	8.15
Supine % time pH < 4	3.2	3.45	3.45
Number of reflux episodes	31	46.90	46.00
Number of reflux episodes > 5 min	2	3.45	4.0
Duration of largest reflux episode	17	19.80	18.45

[a] All had prior normal endoscopy.

patients with many reflux events will have far fewer symptomatic episodes. These measures will really only be of help in individuals who have normal esophageal mucosa and atypical symptoms.

Indications for pH Monitoring

In the presence of classical symptoms of reflux and especially endoscopic features of erosive reflux esophagitis, little diagnostic, prognostic, or therapeutic benefits

are derived from pH monitoring. Current and potential uses for 24-hr pH monitoring include

1. to identify gastroesophageal reflux as a pathogenetic factor in patients without typical reflux symptoms and with chest pain not related to ischemic heart disease
2. to evaluate patients with dyspepsia and other gastrointestinal symptoms in the absence of other manifestations of GERD

3. to identify the role of reflux in respiratory symptoms including asthma and laryngitis
4. to assess the effectiveness of reflux control by medical or surgical therapy, particularly if reflux symptoms persist
5. to predict the necessity and timing of long-term antireflux therapy.

The poor correlation between results of 24-hr pH studies and the endoscopic documentation of esophagitis may be explained by prior treatment of the esophagitis, by factors such as mucosal resistance, or volume and composition of the refluxate. A particular problem is posed by so-called *alkaline reflux*. An increased pH correlates poorly with bile reflux as shown by pH and bile monitoring (Richter, 1994b). Probes detecting bilirubin in refluxate, utilizing a fiberoptic probe that detects the characteristic absorbence wavelength of bilirubin have been developed (Bilitec 2000). This probe has the ability to detect duodeno-gastroesophageal reflux even though it is often not alkaline in nature.

Special Applications and Methods

There have been several efforts looking at the effect of shortening the duration of pH study, examining a different location of the probe within the esophagus or even pharynx, and developing a probe that is sensitive to nonacidic refluxate.

While there is fairly good correlation between the quantity of reflux occurring in the 3 hours after a standardized meal and the daytime reflux in identifying gastroesophageal reflux in association with esophagitis, this is unlikely to be diagnostically of importance if one is studying patients with infrequent atypical symptomatology.

The placement of a pH probe in the upper esophagus or in the pharynx, in order to detect abnormal gastroesophageal pharyngeal reflux that may underlie reflux laryngitis or microaspiration, has been examined and may have some utility provided that it must be recognized that normal values must be established for upper esophageal or pharyngeal acid exposure, which may be quite different from normal ranges of lower esophageal acid exposure. Episodes of pharyngeal or upper esophageal reflux may be quite infrequent and may be missed by 24-hr recordings. Dual channel recordings may be helpful in delineating gastroesophageal-pharyngeal reflux events that predispose to a change of the upper aerodigestive tract or even aspiration of such refluxate. Esophageal pH measurements were equally well applied to infants both in the hospitalized and home settings and are usually well tolerated, even by preterm infants. It may be particularly useful in this population, as the child may be too young to relate typical symptoms of reflux. It may be particularly helpful in identifying reflux episodes associated with apnea events in infants.

SUMMARY

Esophagoscopy is a primary tool for the diagnosis, prognosis, and treatment of esophageal diseases. Endoscopic examination can often replace barium study as the first and only diagnostic test in all diseases that primarily involve the esophageal mucosa. GERD, for instance, is diagnosed once endoscopic examination demonstrates linear erosions in the distal esophagus in patients with chronic heartburn and regurgitation. Esophagoscopy is positively indicated if dysphagia is progressive or if radiographic studies suggest obstruction or structural lesions of the esophagus. Mucosal samples obtained by esophagoscopy and processed for histologic, cytologic, and microbial examination are primary tools to diagnose infectious (viral or fungal) causes of esophagitis or metaplastic, dysplastic, or neoplastic changes. Dilatation of esophageal strictures eliminates dysphagia from esophageal strictures and other forms of mechanical obstruction.

Esophageal manometry and pH profiles are not primarily diagnostic but rather functional tests. Manometry can complement or substitute for dynamic radiographic studies of the mechanical functions of the esophagus. Abnormal force and propagation of contractions can be quantified, and failure of adequate relaxation of the LES documented, but their cause typically has to be determined by other diagnostic tests. For example, a high-pressure zone may be generated by a sphincter, a stricture, or compression of the esophageal lumen from outside. Manometry provides no direct information about bolus transport, but has some predictive value for its effectiveness. Swallowing is associated with esophageal shortening and orad movement and this is not adequately assessed by manometry. Many diseases affect the distensiblity of the esophagus and thereby contribute to dysphagia and other symptoms. Esophageal distensibility can be assessed radiographically and by planimetry but not by manometry. The diagnostic value of manometry relates particularly to dysphagia in the absence of mucosal and other structural abnormalities of the esophagus.

Esophageal pH recording is a tool to record the frequency and severity of acid reflux over time. This is likely to be valuable where typical manifestations of GERD are absent and where prevention of reflux is important to treat pharyngitis, laryngitis, or asthma.

QUESTIONS

1. Peristalsis is considered abnormal when
   a. the lower esophageal sphincter does not relax with swallowing
   b. the swallow does not result in contractile activity
   c. contractions propagate only part of the length of the esophagus
   d. simultaneous contractions are observed
   e. the contractions are of abnormally low amplitude

2. Which of the following is consistent with achalasia?
   a. the upper esophageal sphincter does not relax with swallowing
   b. high amplitude, multipeaked, simultaneous contractions are seen in the striated muscle part of the esophagus
   c. aperistalsis in the distal part of the esophagus

3. The advantages of the sleeve device over single side holes for pressure recording are
   a. the sleeve has a better frequency response and so can better detect pharyngeal activity
   b. it maintains contact with the lower esophageal sphincter during swallowing
   c. it gives a pressure profile of both the esophagus and the stomach
   d. it is easier to insert, better tolerated by the patient, and more durable than standard perfused catheters

4. The pressure inversion point occurs as
   a. the pressure sensor moves out from the stomach and into the esophagus
   b. the pressure sensor moves from the abdominal cavity to the thoracic cavity
   c. the pressure sensor moves from the hiatus hernia and into the esophagus

5. 24-hr esophageal pH monitoring readily detects one of the following:
   a. acid
   b. radionuclide
   c. bile
   d. pH-neutral food

6. The most reliable means of placing a pH probe 5 cm above the LES is
   a. manometric localization of LES
   b. pH step on withdrawal of pH probe
   c. empiric placement of 35 cm
   d. endoscopic measurement of distance to LES

REFERENCES

Arndorfer, R. C., Stef, J. J., Dodds, W. J., Linehan, J. H., & Hogan, W. J. (1977). Improved infusion system for intraluminal esophageal manometry. *Gastroenterology, 73,* 23–27.

Baehr, P. H., & McDonald, G. B. (1994). Esophageal infections: Risk factors, presentation, diagnosis and treatment. *Gastroenterology, 106,* 509–532.

Barish, C. F., Castell, D. O., & Richter, J. E. (1986). Graded esophageal balloon distension, a new provocative test for noncardiac chest pain. *Digestive Diseases and Sciences, 31,* 1292-1298.

Behar, J., & Biancani, P. (1993). Pathogenesis of simultaneous esophageal contractions in patients with motility disorders. *Gastroenterology, 105,* 111–118

Behar, J., & Sheehan. (1975). Histologic abnorrnalities in reflux esophagitis. *Archives of Pathology, 99,* 387–391.

Bell, N. J. V., & Hunt, R. H. (1992). Role of gastric acid suppression in the treatment of gastroesophageal reflux disease. *Gut, 33,* 118–124.

Bernstein, L. M., & Baker, L. A. (1958). A clinical test for esophagitis. *Gastroenterology, 34,* 760–781.

Breumelhof, R., & Smout, A. J. P. M. (1990). The symptom sensitivity index: A valuable additional parameter in 24-hour intraoesophageal pH and pressure recordings vs provocation tests in the diagnosis of chest pain of oesophageal origin. *Gut, 31,* 738-744.

Cameron, A. J., Ott, B. J., & Payne, W. S. (1985). The incidence of adenocarcinoma in columnar-lined (Barrett's) esophagus. *New England Journal of Medicine, 313,* 857.

Clouse, R. E., & Staiano, A. (1983). Contraction abnormalities of the esophageal body in patients referred for manometry; a new approach to classification. *Digestive Diseases and Sciences, 28,* 784–791.

Cohen, S., & Harris, L. D. (1971). Does hiatus hernia affect competence of the gastroesophageal sphincter? *New England Journal of Medicine, 284,* 1053–1056.

Cook, I. J., Gabb, M., Panagopoulos, V., Jamieson, G. G., Dodds, W. J., Dent, J., & Shearman, D. J. (1992). Pharyngeal (Zenker's) diverticulum is a disorder of upper esophageal sphincter opening. *Gastroenterology, 103,* 1229–1235.

DeMeester, T. R. (1989). Prolonged oesophageal pH monitering. In NW Read (Ed.), *Gastrointestinal motility: Which test?* (pp. 41–52). Wrightson Biomedical.

Dent, J. (1976). A new technique for continuous sphincter pressure measurement. *Gastroenterology, 71,* 763-267.

Dent, J. A., Dodds, W. J., Friedman, R. H., Sekiguchi, T., Hogan, W. J., Arndorfer, R. C., & Petrie, D. J. (1980) Mechanisms of gastroesophageal reflux in recumbent subjects. *Journal of Clinical Investigation, 65,* 256–267.

Dodds, W. J., Dent, J., Hogan, W. J., Helm, J. F., Hauser, R., Patel, G. K., & Egide, M. S. (1982). Mechanisms of gastroesophageal reflux in patients with reflux esophagitis *New England Journal of Medicine, 307,* 1547–1552.

Dodds, W. J., Hogan, W. J., Reid, D. P., Stewart, E. T., & Arndorfer, R. C. (1973). A comparison between primary esophageal peristalsis following wet and dry swallows. *Journal of Applied Physiology, 35,* 851–857.

Ebert, E. c., Ouyang, Wright, S. H, & Cohen, S. (1983). Pneumatic dilatation in patients with symptomatic diffuse esophageal spasm and lower esophageal sphincter dysfunction, *Digestive Diseases and Science, 28,* 481.

Geboes, K., Desmet V., Vantrappen G., & Mebis, J. (1980). Vascular changes in the esophageal mucosa—An early histologic sign of esophagitis. *Gastrointestinal Endoscopy, 26,* 29–32.

Gregersen, H., & Andersen, M. B. (1991). Impedance measurement system for quantification of cross-sectional area in the gastrointestinal tract. *Medical and Biological Engineering, 29,* 108-110.

Heading, R. C. (1989). Epidemiology of oesophageal reflux disease *Scandinavian Journal of Gastroenterology, 24*(Suppl), 33–37.

Hewson, E. G., Ott, D. J., Dalton, C. B., Chen. Y. M., Wu, W. C., & Richter, J. E. (1990). Manometry and radiology, complementary studies in the assessment of esophageal motility disorders. *Gastroenterology, 98,* 26–632.

Hewson, E. G., Sinclair, J. W., Balton, C. B., & Richter, J. E. (1991) 24 hour esophageal pH monitoring: The most useful test for evaluating non-cardiac chest pain. *American Journal of Medicine, 90*(5), 76–583.

Howard, P. J., Maher, L., Pryde, A., & Heading, R. C. (1991). Systematic comparison of conventional oesophageal manometry with oesophageal motility while eating bread. *Gut, 32,* 64–1269.

Ismail-Beigi, F., Horton, P. F., & Pope, C. E., II (1970). Histological consequences of gastroesophageal reflux in man. *Gastroenterology, 58,* 163–174.

Jacob, P., Kahrilas, J., & Herzon, G. (1991). Proximal esophageal pH-metry in patients with 'reflux laryngitis.' *Gastroenteroloy, 100,* 305–310.

Joelsson, B. E., DeMeester, T. R., Skinner, D. B., Lafontaine, E., Waters, P. F., & O'Sullivan, G. C. (1982). The role of the esophageal body in the antireflux mechanism. *Surgery, 92,* 17–424.

Johnson, L. F., DeMeester, T. R., & Haggit, R. C. (1978). Esophageal epithelial response to gastroesophageal reflux. A quantitative study. *American Journal of Digestive Diseases, 23,* 498–509.

Johnsson, F., Joelsson, B., & Isberg, P. E. (1987). Ambulatory 24 hour intraesophageal pH-monitoring in the diagnosis of gastroesophageal reflux disease. *Gut, 28,* 1145–1150.

Johnston, P. W., Johnston, B. T., Collins, B. J., Collins, J. S. A. & Love, A. H. G. (1993). Audit of the role of oesophageal manometry in clinical practice. *Gut, 34,* 1158.

Kahrilas, P. J., Clouse, R. E., & Hogan, W. J. (1994). American Gastroenterological Association policy and position statement. *Gastroenterology, 107,* 1865–1994

Kahrilas, P. J., Dodds, W. J., & Hogan, W. J. (1988). The effect of peristaltic dysfunction on esophageal volume clearance. *Gastroenterology, 94,* 3–80.

Kahrilas, P. J., Dodds, W. J., Hogan, W. J., Kem, M., Arndorfer, R. C., & Reece, A. (1986). Peristaltic dysfunction in peptic esophagitis. *Gastroenterology, 91,* 897–904.

Keeffe, E. B., & Schrock, T. R. (1995). Complications of gastrointestinal endoscopy. In M. H. Sleisenger, & J. S. Fordtran (Eds), *Gastrointestinal diseases* (pp. 301–308) Philadelphia: W. B. Saunders.

Kobayaski, S., & Kasugai, T. (1974). Endoscopic and biopsy criteria for the diagnosis of esophagitis with a fiberoptic esophagoscope. *Digestive Diseases and Sciences, 19,* 345

Lin, S., Brasseur, J. G., Pouderoux, P., & Kahrilas, P. J. (1995). The phrenic ampulla: Distal esophagus or potential hiatal hemia? *American Journal of Physiology, 268,* (Gastrointest. liver physiol. 31) G32O–G327

Linehan, J. H., Dent, J., Dodds, W. J., & Hogan, W. J. (1985). Sleeve dence functions as a starling resistor to record sphincter pressure. *American Journal of Physiology, 248,* G251–255.

Lu, C. H., Schulze-Delrieu, K., Cram, M., Shirazi, S., & Raab, J. (1994). Dynamic imaging of the obstructed opossum esophagus. From altered load to altered contractility. *Digestive Diseases and Sciences, 39*(7), 1377–1388.

Massey, B. T., Dodds, W. J., Hogan, W. J., Brasseur, J. G., & Helm, J. F. (1991). Abnormal esophageal motility. An analysis of concurrent radiographic and manometric findings. *Gastroenterology, 101,* 344–354

Mattioli, S., Pilotti, V., Spangaro, M., Grigioni, W. F., Zannoli, R., Felice, V., Conci, A., & Gozzetti, G. (1989). Reliability of 24 hour home esophageal pH monitoring in diagnosis of gastroesophageal, reflux. *Digestive Diseases and Sciences, 34,* 71–78.

Mughal, M. M., Banciewicz, J., & Marples, M. (1990). Oesophageal manometry and pH recording does not predict the bad results of Nissen fundoplication. *British Journal of Surgery, 77,* 43–45.

Murphy, D. W., Yuan, Y., & Castell, D. O. (1989). Does the intraesophageal pH probe accurately detect acid reflux? Simultaneous recordings with two pH probes in humans, *Digestivse Diseases and Sciences, 34,* 649–656.

Ollson, R., Castell, J. A., Castell, D. O., & Ekberg, O. (1995). Solid-state computerized manometry improves diagnostic yield in pharyngeal dysphagia: Simultaneous videoradiography and manometry in dysphagia patients with normal barium swallows. *Abdominal Imaging, 20,* 230–235.

Ollyo, J. B., Lang, F., Fontollet, C. H., & Monnier, P. H. (1993). Savary's new endoscopic grading of reflux-oesophagitis: A simple, reproducible, logical, complete and useful classification. *Gastroenterology, 89,* A100.

Orvar, K. B., Gregersen, H., & Christensen, J. (1993). Biomechanical characteristics of the human esophagus. *Digestive Diseases and Sciences, 38,* 197–205.

Ott, D. J., Chen, Y. M., Wu, W. C., & Gelfand, D. W. (1985). Endoscopic sensitivity in the detection of esophageal strictures. *Journal of Clinical Gastroenterology, 7,* 121–125.

Patterson, D. J., Graham, D. Y., Smith, J. L., Schwartz, J. T., Alpert, E., Lanza, F. L., & Cain, J. D. (1983). Natural history of benign esophageal stricture treated by dilatation. *Gastroenterology, 85,* 346–350.

Rao, S., Gregerson, H., Hayek, B., Summers, R. W., & Christensen, J. (1996). Unexplained chest pain: The hypersensitive esophagus. *Annals of Internal Medicine, 124,* 950–958.

Ren, J., Dodds, W. J., Martin, C. J., Dantas, R. O., Mittal, R. K., Harrington, S. S., Kern, M. K., & Brasseur, J. D. (1991). Effect of increased intra-abdominal pressure on peristalsis in the feline esophagus. *American Journal of Physiology, 261,* G417–G425.

Richter, J. E. (1994a). Diffuse esophageal spasm. In D. O. Castell & J. A. Castell (Eds.), *Esophageal motility testing* (pp. 122–134). New York Appleton and Lange.

Richter, J. E. (1994b). Provocative tests in esophageal disease, *Frontiers in Gastrointestinal Research, 22,* 188–208.

Richter, J. E., Hackshaw, B. T., Wu, W. C., & Castell, D. O. (1985). Edrophonium: A useful provocative test for esophageal chest pain. *Annals of Internal Medicine, 103,* 14–21.

Richter, J. E., Bradley, L. A. . DeMeester T. R. & Wu W. C. (1992) Normal 24-hr ambulatory esophageal pH values; influence of study center, pH electrode, age and gender. *Digestive Diseases and Sciences, 37,* 849-856.

Schatzki, R. (1963). The lower esophageal ring. Long term follow-up of symptomatic and asymptomatic cases. *American Journal of Roentgenology, 90,* 805–810.

Schatzki, K., & Gary, J. E. (1953). Dysphagia due to a diaphragm-like localized narrowing in the lower esophagus ("lower esophageal ring") *American Journal of Roentgenology, 70,* 911–922.

Schulze-Delrieu, K., Mitros, F., & Shirazi, S. (1982). Inflammatory and structural changes in the opossum esophagus after resection of the cardia. *Gastroenterology, 82,* 76–283.

Schwartz, G. F., & Polsky, H S. (1975). Ingested foreign bodies of the gastrointestinal tract. *American Journal of Surgery, 42,* 236–238.

Shirazi, S., Schulze-Delrieu, K. Custer-Hagen, T., Brown, C. K., & Ren, J. (1989). Motility changes in the opossum esophagus from experimental esophagatus. *Digestive Diseases and Sciences, 34,* 1668–1676.

Sifrim, D., Janssens, J., & Vantrappen, G. (1994). Failing deglutitive inhibition in primary esophageal motility disorders. *Gastroenterology, 106,* 875–882.

Sontag, S. J. (1990). The medical management of reflux esophagitis: Role of antacids and acid inhibition. *Gastroenterology Clinics of North America, 19,* 683–712.

Spechler, S. J., Sperber, H. Doos, W. G., & Schimmel, E. M. (1983). The prevalence of Barrett's esophagus in patients with chronic peptic esophageal strictures. *Digestive Diseases and Sciences, 28,* 769–774

Weusten, B. L. A. M., Roelofs, J. M. M., Akkermans, L. M. A., Van Henegouwen, G. P., & Smout, A. J. P. M. (1994) The symptom-association probablity: An improved method for symptom analysis of 24-hour esophageal pH data. *Gastroenterology, 107,* 1741–1745.

Wiener, G. J., Richter, J. E., Copper, J. B., Wu, W. C., Castel, D. O. (1989). The Symptom Index: A clinically important parameter of ambulatory 24 hour esophageal pH monitoring. *American Journal of Gastroenterology, 83*(4), 358–361

Winans, C. S. (1972). The pharyngoesophageal closure mechanism: A manometric study. *Gastroenterology, 63,* 768–777.

11

Neurologic Diseases Affecting Oropharyngeal Swallowing

David W. Buchholz and JoAnne Robbins

The term *neurogenic dysphagia* refers to difficulty swallowing (or, more broadly, eating) as the result of neurologic disease or trauma. For the most part, the symptoms and complications that arise from neurogenic dysphagia are primarily due to sensorimotor dysfunction of the oral and pharyngeal phases of swallowing. More specifically, neurogenic dysfunction of the oral cavity and/or pharynx can disrupt the muscle actions that normally serve to deliver a bolus from the oral cavity into the esophagus without penetration into the nasopharynx or larynx and without retention in the mouth or pharynx. Some neurologic diseases impair esophageal as well as oropharyngeal function, but, in most instances, problems related to oropharyngeal dysphagia tend to be clinically predominant. This review will focus on the presentations, causes, evaluation, and management of neurogenic oropharyngeal dysphagia. Most cases of chronic oropharyngeal dysphagia are neurogenic, but oropharyngeal dysphagia may also result from structural problems such as postintubation edema, laryngeal webs, pharyngeal masses, and diverticulae (see Chapter 12).

CHARACTERISTIC PRESENTATIONS OF NEUROGENIC DYSPHAGIA

Neurogenic dysphagia may present in one of three ways. First, a patient with a known neurologic disease may have obvious symptoms or complications of dysphagia. The symptoms of neurogenic oropharyngeal dysphagia may include problems with chewing, difficulty initiating swallowing, nasal regurgitation, drooling, difficulty managing secretions, coughing or choking episodes during eating, and food sticking in the throat. Complications of neurogenic oropharyngeal dysphagia include dehydration, malnutrition, laryngospasm, bronchospasm, aspiration pneumonia, and asphyxia (Horner, Massey, & Brazer, 1988; Horner, Massey, Riski, Lathrop, & Chase, 1988; Martin, et al., 1994; Schmidt, Holas, Harvorson, & Reding, 1994; Teasell, Bach, & McRae, 1994). Neurogenic esophageal dysphagia may manifest as chest discomfort, food sticking in the chest, regurgitation, or heartburn or cause symptoms more pharyngeal or laryngeal in nature.

319

Second, a patient with a known neurologic disease may have substantial oropharyngeal dysfunction yet report only subtle clinical clues as to its presence. There are three essential reasons for this: (a) compensatory processes, (b) reduction of the laryngeal cough reflex, and (c) cognitive impairment.

Compensation for neurogenic dysphagia involves voluntary behavioral modifications and involuntary adjustments in oropharyngeal performance (Buchholz, Bosma, & Donner, 1985). Voluntary forms of compensation consist of alteration of dietary characteristics and eating methods. Especially when the onset of neurogenic dysphagia is gradual, patients may be relatively unaware of their adaptive changes in eating. It is important for the clinician to inquire specifically about elimination of difficult-to-swallow dietary items or development of habits such as cutting food into smaller pieces, chewing more thoroughly, washing down solids with liquids, double swallowing, throat clearing during meals, head turning or tilting while eating, and generally taking longer to finish a meal. Applying the detection of these historical clues to reveal the presence of neurogenic dysphagia is the first step in managing the problem proactively so as to put strategic measures in place that will facilitate avoidance of potentially catastrophic complications.

The process of involuntary compensation has not been well studied but seems to involve automatic adaptations in oropharyngeal motor performance in order to minimize the adverse functional consequences of a neurologic disease. Involuntary compensation in the setting of neurogenic dysphagia may represent the phenomenon of adaptive neuroplasticity, a process that is not well understood but probably also plays a role in, for example, recovery from stroke or traumatic brain injury (Bach-y-Rita, 1988; Cotman, 1985; Finger & Stein, 1982; Wolpaw, 1985).

Aside from the ways in which voluntary and involuntary compensation can reduce the apparent clinical evidence of neurogenic dysphagia, diminution of the laryngeal cough reflex is also a major factor in this regard. The consequence of a decreased laryngeal cough reflex is to allow laryngeal penetration or aspiration to occur silently (i.e., without provoking the normal response of coughing and choking) (Horner & Massey, 1988; Kahrilas, 1989; Linden, Kuhlemeier, & Patterson, 1993; Linden & Siebens, 1983). The laryngeal cough reflex may be diminished for several reasons. Some neurologic diseases affecting swallowing, such as brain stem stroke, can cause loss of laryngeal sensation and/or the motor response to invasive material as a direct result of the disease process itself. Even patients with pure motor disorders (such as motor neuron disease or myopathy) and oculopharyngeal muscular dystrophy may exhibit reduction of the laryngeal cough reflex. This may be because the reflex can become desensitized in response to chronic laryngeal stimulation (i.e., chronic aspiration), owing to damage of local sensory receptors or centrally mediated adaptation. Alternatively, the underlying motor disorder may compromise motor function of the components of the cough reflex (i.e., the larynx and the diaphragm). A host of other factors can impair the laryngeal cough reflex, including endotracheal intubation, tracheostomy, medications (e.g., sedatives and topical anesthetics), and decreased arousal (Bishop, Weymuller, & Fink, 1984; Cleaton-Jones, 1976; Greenberg, 1984; Hochman, Martin, & Devine, 1965; Huxley, Viroslav, Gray, & Pierce, 1978; Sasaki, Suzuki, Horiuchi, & Kirchner, 1977; Taylor & Towey, 1971).

The other reason why a patient with neurogenic dysphagia may report relatively few symptoms is cognitive impairment. Demented or mentally retarded individuals with dysphagia may have limited capacity to understand or communicate their difficulty swallowing. These barriers to the recognition of dysphagia can be overcome by carefully observing while the person eats, questioning the person's caregivers, and, above all, always keeping in mind that neurogenic dysphagia is often relatively silent.

The third way in which neurogenic dysphagia can present is in a patient with an underlying neurologic disease that is unrecognized but produces dysphagia as an initial or primary problem. In such cases, clinicians unfamiliar with neurogenic dysphagia often mistakenly consider esophageal or structural problems rather than oropharyngeal functional impairment. Clinicians should be able to recognize the symptoms indicative of oropharyngeal (hence, probably neurogenic) dysphagia, including the subtle clues related to voluntary compensation, and should further evaluate these symptoms by means of videofluorography of swallowing.

Videofluorography of a patient with neurogenic dysphagia usually demonstrates some combination of reduced or incoordinated oropharyngeal activity (evidenced by decreased or poorly timed excursion of oropharyngeal structures during swallowing), nasal regurgitation, retention of barium in the oral and/or pharyngeal recesses, decreased displacement of the epiglottis, hyoid bone, larynx and upper esophageal sphincter, and laryngeal penetration or aspiration (Bosma, 1953; Chen, Ott, Peele, & Gelfand, 1990; Chen, Peele, Donati, Oh, Donofri, & Gelfand, 1992; Donner, 1974; Jones & Donner, 1988; O'Connor & Ardran, 1976; Silbiger, Pikielney, & Donner, 1967; Stroudley & Walsh, 1991). Videofluorography of swallowing is sensitive in the detection of neurogenic oropharyngeal impairment but relatively nonspecific as to the responsible neurologic disease (Nilsson, Ekberg, Sjöberg, & Olsson, 1993). If videofluorographic findings suggest neurologic dysfunction but the specific cause is unclear, neurologic consultation is the next step toward defining the underlying problems.

Occasionally, what superficially appears to be neurogenic dysphagia turns out to have a psychogenic basis (Buchholz, Barofsky, Edwin, Jones, & Ravich, 1994). Such patients tend to be relatively young and otherwise physically healthy, and their symptoms of oropharyngeal dysphagia may fluctuate dramatically. These individuals are further clinically characterized by the absence of dysphonia or any other objective neurologic deficit, and neurologic investigation is negative. Videofluorographically, pharyngeal function is normal once initiated, but oral behavior is often distinctly peculiar. Patients with psychogenic dysphagia are frequently reluctant to initiate swallowing and may complain of their inability to do so even as the intactness of their oral ability is inadvertently revealed by videofluorographic observations of complex, coordinated, nonpropulsive oral and lingual activity. In the absence of any other evidence of neurologic disease, such oral struggle behavior, unaccompanied by oral leakage and followed by often delayed (due to oral struggling) but otherwise relatively normal pharyngeal performance, is suggestive of psychogenic dysphagia, although the importance of thoroughly searching for alternative diagnoses cannot be overemphasized.

CAUSES OF NEUROGENIC DYSPHAGIA

Neurologic diseases affecting swallowing do so by means of interruption of one or more of the steps in the complex neuromuscular pathways responsible for swallowing (see Chapters 2 and 3). These diseases include afflictions of the cerebral cortex, subcortical tracts, brain stem, cranial nerves, neuromuscular junction, and muscles. (Table 11–1).

Very few data reliably distinguish the characteristics of oropharyngeal dysphagia produced by any one of these diseases as compared to the others. In other words, current state of knowledge indicates that the clinical and videofluorographic features of dysphagia tend to overlap substantially among patients with, for example, stroke, head trauma, Parkinson's disease, motor neuron disease, multiple sclerosis, postpolio syndrome, and myopathy. The limited specificity may relate to variability of factors, including extent and severity of the

TABLE 11–1. Neurologic Disorders Causing Dysphagia.

Stroke

Head trauma

Cerebral palsy

Parkinson's disease and other movement and neurodegenerative disorders

Progressive supranuclear palsy

  Olivopontocerebellar atrophy

  Huntington's disease

  Wilson's disease

Torticollis

  Tardive dyskinesia

Alzheimer's disease and other dementias

Motor neuron disease (amyotrophic lateral sclerosis)

Guillain-Barré syndrome and other polyneuropathies

Neoplasms and other structural disorders

  Primary brain tumors

  Intrinsic and extrinsic brainstem tumors

  Base of skull tumors

  Syringobulbia

  Arnold-Chiari malformation

  Neoplastic meningitis

Multiple sclerosis

Postpolio syndrome

Infectious disorders

  Chronic infectious meningitis

  Syphilis and Lyme disease

  Diphtheria

  Botulism

  Viral encephalitis, including rabies

Myasthenia gravis

Myopathy

  Polymyositis, dermatomyositis, inclusion body myositis, and sarcoidosis

  Myotonic and oculopharyngeal muscular dystrophy

  Hyper- and hypothyroidism

  Cushing's syndrome

Iatrogenic conditions

  Medication side effects

  Postsurgical neurogenic dysphagia

    Neck surgery

    Posterior fossa surgery

    Irradiation of the head and neck

underlying disease, the characteristics of that disease in any given patient, and the premorbid characteristics of that patient's swallowing.

The relative nonspecificity of the clinical and videofluorographic features of neurogenic dysphagia is neither surprising nor unique to the problem of dysphagia, for a similar point could be raised regarding the difficulty of identifying the specific neurologic disease causing a weak leg based on the features of that limb alone. It is in the context of evaluating the entire patient that any specific diagnosis emerges, and this axiom applies as much to neurogenic dysphagia as to any other clinical problem.

On the other hand, certain findings in a weak leg—such as spasticity, hyperreflexia and an extensor plantar response—tell us that the problem is in the central rather than the peripheral nervous system, and the differential diagnosis is thereby narrowed. A similar analysis of the clinical features of neurogenic dysphagia may differentiate between the clinical syndromes of pseudobulbar palsy (indicative of neurologic disease above the brainstem nuclei) and bulbar palsy (indicative of disease anywhere from the brainstem nuclei to the muscles of swallowing). This is further discussed below (see Evaluation of Neurogenic Dysphagia later in the chapter).

At present, our ability to diagnose a specific neurologic disease affecting swallowing primarily depends not on our ability to recognize specific clinical or videofluorographic features of neurogenic dysphagia caused by that particular disease—because, for the most part, such unique features have not been sufficiently tested for generalization—but instead depends largely on our ability to evaluate the pattern of dysphagia in the context of other specific features of the underlying neurologic disease.

Stroke

Epidemiologic data are lacking regarding neurogenic dysphagia, but it is generally agreed that stroke is the most common single pathologic cause (Kuhlemeier,

1994). Approximately 500,000 new strokes occur annually in the United States, and one quarter to one half of strokes result in oropharyngeal dysphagia (1992 Heart and Stroke Facts, 1991; Chen et al., 1990; Groher & Bukatinan, 1986; Horner, Massey, & Brazer, 1988; Palmer & DuChane, 1991; Wade & Hewer, 1987). Dysphagia after stroke is a major cause of morbidity related to respiratory complications and malnutrition (Gresham, 1990; Gordon, Langton-Hewer, & Wade, 1987; Hewer & Wade, 1987; Horner, Massey, Riski et al., 1988; Veis & Logemann, 1985).

Hemorrhagic strokes are generally more devastating than ischemic strokes and therefore are more likely to cause dysphagia, but ischemic strokes have a several-fold higher incidence. Brainstem strokes are more likely to result in dysphagia than hemispheral strokes, but hemispheral strokes are much more common (Horner, Buoyer, Alberts, & Helms, 1991; Teasell et al., 1994).

Large hemispheral ischemic strokes most frequently are caused by either internal carotid artery atheroembolism or cardiac embolism. These strokes tend to involve the middle cerebral artery territory and are characterized by contralateral hemiparesis and, if the stroke is in the dominant (usually left) hemisphere, often also dysphasia. Although data are scant, large hemispheral strokes may produce oropharyngeal dysphagia by interrupting the ipsilateral corticobulbar pathway that connects the voluntary cortical control center for swallowing (in the inferior frontal region) with the bulbar (lower brain stem) nuclei that coordinate swallowing (Barer, 1989; Meadows, 1973).

Current evidence suggests that there may be differences between the consequences of left versus right hemispheral strokes on the oral and pharyngeal phases of swallowing. Left-sided lesions appear to predominately impair the oral phase, and right-sided strokes tend more to compromise pharyngeal function and result in aspiration (Logemann, et al., 1993; Robbins & Levine, 1988; Robbins, Levine,

Maser, Rosenbek, & Kempster, 1993; Teasell et al., 1994). Bilateral hemispheral strokes are associated with a higher incidence and greater severity of poststroke dysphagia (Celifarco, Gerard, Faegenburg, & Burakoff, 1990; Horner, Massey, & Brazer, 1988; Teasell et al., 1994).

Hemispheral strokes may also be small and deep, involving periventricular tracts and basal ganglia. These are often referred to as *lacunar* strokes and are presumed to be due to occlusion of penetrating arterioles by lipohyalinosis, a process associated with aging, hypertension, and diabetes mellitus. The corticobulbar tracts that pass through the anterior limb of the internal capsule near the ventricles are liable to be interrupted by lacunar strokes, often bilaterally. At present there is limited understanding of the relationship of nonspecific periventricular hyperintensities demonstrated by magnetic resonance imaging (MRI) in elderly individuals and the phenomenon of lacunar strokes (Buchholz, 1992; Levine, Robbins, & Maser, 1992). More specifically, it is unclear whether or not these periventricular hyperintensities represent multifocal or confluent small strokes and to what extent these phenomena may be responsible for either "normal" changes in oral and pharyngeal performance in healthy elderly subjects or clinically relevant findings among elderly patients with dysphagia symptoms (Alberts, Horner, Gray, & Brazer, 1992; Baum & Bodner, 1983; Borgstrom & Ekberg, 1988a; Buchholz, 1993; Robbins, Hamilton, Lof, & Kempster, 1992a; Robbins, Levine, Wood, Roecker, & Luschei, in press; Sonies, Tone, & Shawker, 1984; Tracy et al., 1989).

Brainstem strokes can result from either large or small vessel disease and often produce oropharyngeal dysphagia because of involvement of brainstem tracts and nuclei involved in control of swallowing, especially the corticobulbar tracts, the nuclei tracti solitarii, the nuclei ambigui in the medulla and the adjacent medullary "swallowing centers." Most brainstem strokes cause impairment of multiple other brainstem functions as

well, since the brain stem is densely packed with important tracts and nuclei (Horner et al., 1991). Occasionally brainstem stroke is extremely discrete and causes dysphagia as a sole or predominant finding. In these instances, MRI, despite its excellent spatial resolution, may fail to demonstrate a tiny brainstem stroke that has caused profound dysphagia (Buchholz, 1993).

When a patient has suffered a stroke, the clinical clues that may indicate substantial probability of poststroke dysphagia and risk of respiratory complications include dysphonia, overt difficulty managing secretions or food, abnormal gag reflex, and reduced level of consciousness (Alberts et al., 1992; Horner & Massey, 1988; Horner, Massey, & Brazer, 1988; Horner, Massey, Riski et al., 1988). Under these circumstances, patients should be evaluated with videofluorography prior to eating (which videofluorography may indicate to be too risky) and should be managed with swallowing therapy. It should be emphasized that correlation of the gag reflex and safe swallowing is weak, such that a normal gag reflex may coexist with profound neurogenic dysphagia, whereas an abnormal gag reflex may be found despite normal swallowing. Many normal individuals have an absent or relatively decreased gag reflex (Davies, Kidd, Stone, & MacMahon, 1995).

The diagnosis of stroke is based primarily on historical and physical examination evidence of abrupt onset of brain or brainstem dysfunction within a definable vascular territory. Confirmation and localization of the diagnosis are often aided by MRI, which may disclose additional, clinically silent strokes (which may add to the impact of an acute stroke in causing oropharyngeal dysphagia). Recognition of stroke-related dysphagia is important for several reasons. First, appropriate swallowing evaluation and management (including modification of both feeding method and medication intake) can be undertaken so as to avoid complications of dysphagia. Second, unnecessary diagnostic procedures such as esophagoscopy can be avoided. Third, acute stroke treatment such as control of blood pressure, hyperglycemia, and fever and use of thrombolytics or anticoagulants can be instituted. Fourth, preventive stroke management including risk factor reduction and antiplatelet medication can be recommended. Most patients suffering from poststroke dysphagia spontaneously improve over days to months, and optimal interim care can maximize their outcomes.

Head Trauma

Traumatic injury to the brain, brain stem, and/or cranial nerves may produce oropharyngeal dysphagia. Most of the principles regarding poststroke dysphagia pertain to posttraumatic dysphagia, including the potential for favorable outcome if dysphagia is properly evaluated and managed (Brown, Nordloh, & Donowitz, 1992; Dworkin & Nadal, 1991; Lazarus, 1989; Lazarus & Logemann, 1987; Tepid, Palmer, & Linden, 1987; Winstein, 1983; Ylvisaker & Logemann, 1986). Cognitive impairment secondary to stroke or head trauma can complicate swallowing therapy, although, in such instances, therapy efforts may be productively directed toward family members and staff who assist the patient with feeding (Hutchins, 1989; Mackay & Morgan, 1993).

Cerebral Palsy

Cerebral palsy (CP) is a general term that describes a syndrome in which neurologic symptoms result from damage to the developing brain (Pape & Wigglesworth, 1979). CP is estimated to involve 1.5 of 1000 live births in the United States, and, although the brain damage is not progressive, its effects are permanent (American Academy for Cerebral Palsy and Developmental Medicine, 1989; Blumberg, 1959). Most commonly, CP causes motor dysfunction such as spasticity, but problems with speech, swallowing, and breathing often occur.

Primitive reflexes of the normal infant such as suckle-swallowing, rooting, gag-

ging, and biting are essential for infant survival and are part of normal development (Dubner, Sessle, & Storey, 1978). However, the persistence of these and other primitive reflexes such as the asymmetrical tonic neck reflex can interfere with a CP patient's eating skills (Ogg, 1975; Ottenbacher, Bundy, & Short, 1983). Abnormal responses such as the bite reflex, suckle-swallow reflex, lack of tongue lateralization, instability of the lower jaw, and phasic biting can severely limit the individual's ability to chew, position, and swallow a food bolus safely (Casas, Kenny, & McPherson, 1994; Kenny et al., 1989; Mirrett, Riski, Glascott, & Johnson, 1994; Rogers, Arvedson, Buck, Smart, & Msall, 1994). Techniques designed to reduce abnormal muscle tone and to increase or decrease sensorimotor input may help to improve eating skills (Gisel, 1994; Morris, 1982). The individual with CP may require trunk, neck and head supports, customized utensils and related interventions to maximize function and facilitate independent, safe eating (Helfrich-Miller, Rector, & Straka, 1993).

Parkinson's Disease and Other Movement and Neurodegenerative Disorders

Parkinson's disease (PD) results from progressive neuronal degeneration of unknown cause involving multiple brainstem and subcortical areas, especially the dopamine-producing neurons of the substantia nigra in the midbrain. Impairment of both the oropharyngeal and esophageal phases of swallowing has been associated with PD (Croxson & Pye, 1988; Lieberman et al., 1980; Robbins, Logemann, & Kirshner, 1986; Schneider, Diamond, & Markham, 1985; Stroudley & Walsh, 1991). Dysphagia tends not to be an early or predominant symptom of PD, which instead is heralded by some combination of resting tremor, decreased and slowed limb movements, and characteristic gait impairment (slow, stooped, and shuffling). The limb difficulties, but less so oropharyngeal and esophageal dysphagia, can be alleviated by dopaminergic agonists, which unfortunately do not retard the gradual but relentless progression of PD (Bushmann, Dobmeyer, Leeker, & Perlmutter, 1989; Fuh, Lee, Wang, Wu, & Liu, 1995). Deprenyl, thought to function as an anti-oxidant, may help to delay further neuronal degeneration. Nonetheless, pneumonia related to recurrent, often silent aspiration is a leading cause of death in the latter stages of PD (Hoehn & Yahr, 1967).

Progressive supranuclear palsy is one of a number of "Parkinson's-plus" syndromes or multisystem atrophies that are characterized by even more widespread neuronal degeneration in multiple systems. Oral and pharyngeal dysfunction lead inevitably to dysphagia, although not as an initial symptom (Neumann, Reich, Buchholz, Purcell, & Jones, 1995; Sonies, 1992). Some of the other neurodegenerative disorders, such as *olivopontocerebellar atrophy*, are hereditary, but the mechanism of cell loss is obscure. Oropharyngeal dysphagia in these disorders is often more prominent and profound than in routine Parkinson's disease, and there is no substantially effective treatment to halt or reverse these conditions.

Huntington's disease is an autosomal dominant disorder characterized primarily by progressive psychiatric disturbance, dementia, and involuntary movements (chorea) with midlife onset. Dysphagia is a common accompaniment and often leads to terminal respiratory complications (Edmonds, 1966; Kagel & Leopold, 1992; Leopold & Kagel, 1985). Dopamine antagonists (neuroleptics) are sometimes used to control chorea in Huntington's disease, but they may result in sedation and other side effects. Swallowing therapy, specifically using compensatory techniques, has been of apparent benefit (Kagel & Leopold, 1992).

Wilson's disease is an inborn disorder of copper metabolism, which results in diffuse damage to the brain and liver. Neurologic problems include psychiatric disturbances, tremor, rigidity, dysarthria,

and dysphagia. Dysphagia associated with Wilson's disease may be both pharyngeal (Gulyas & Salazar-Grueso, 1988) and esophageal (Haggstrom & Hirschowitz, 1980). The diagnosis of Wilson's disease is based on its clinical features plus findings of Kayser-Fleischer corneal rings, elevated serum and urinary copper levels, and decreased serum ceruloplasmin. Wilson's disease is treatable with chelation therapy and is therefore a diagnosis that should not be overlooked.

Torticollis is involuntary turning of the head and neck to one side as a result of excessive, uncontrollable focal muscle contraction. Focal dystonias involving the region of the head and neck, such as torticollis, cause oropharyngeal dysphagia by either postural effects (compromise of the normal anatomic alignment of the swallowing apparatus) or direct neurogenic impairment (excessive contraction and incoordination of the muscles of the swallowing apparatus) (Horner, Riski, Ovelmen-Levitt, & Nashold, 1992; Horner, Riski, Weber, & Nashold, 1993; Kakigi, Shibasaki, Kuroda, Shin, & Oona, 1983; Logemann, 1988; Riski, Horner, & Nashold, 1990). This and other forms of dystonia and dyskinesia (involuntary movement disorders) are thought to arise from dysfunction of systems in the subcortex (basal ganglia) and/or brain stem that control muscle tone. These problems commonly have spontaneous onset but may be precipitated by dopamine antagonists, especially in the form of *tardive dyskinesia* involving the face, lips, and tongue after chronic neuroleptic exposure. Focal dystonias such as torticollis can be effectively controlled for several months at a time by means of chemodenervation, achieved by injecting botulinum toxin, which impairs neuromuscular transmission, into the overactive muscles.

Alzheimer's Disease and Other Dementias

Alzheimer's disease, the leading cause of dementia, does not significantly impair sensorimotor function, including that of the oral cavity and pharynx, until relatively late in its gradually progressive course (Horner, Alberts, Dawson, & Cook, 1994). Nonetheless, the global cognitive deterioration that results from Alzheimer's disease contributes greatly to eventual disability in independent eating (Volicer et al., 1989). Alzheimer's disease is characterized by diffuse loss of cortical, predominantly cholinergic, neurons. Although advances are rapidly being made in understanding its genetic and biochemical foundations, so far the treatment of Alzheimer's disease with drugs to enhance cholinergic function (such as tacrine) has proven only mildly beneficial.

There are many causes of dementia other than Alzheimer's disease, most commonly multiple strokes, but also, for example, sedating medications, depression, hypothyroidism, and vitamin B12 deficiency. Although there is as yet no practical clinical tool to positively diagnose Alzheimer's disease, thorough evaluation of dementia is mandatory in order to identify potentially treatable problems such as these. The workup of dementia should at least include blood counts, chemistry panel, thyroid screening, vitamin B12 level, serologic test for syphilis, computed tomographic (CT) or MR scanning of the brain, and neuropsychological testing in addition to careful clinical assessment.

The enormous and rising prevalence of Alzheimer's disease and other causes of dementia, related to the steadily increasing number of elderly individuals and the consequent loss of ability to self-feed and swallow among demented individuals pose a huge burden on caregivers. Gastrostomy may appear as an attractive option, but it is difficult to measure wisely the potential benefits in terms of decreased care demands, increased nutrition, and seemingly enhanced safety of feeding versus the potential detriment in terms of the potential for aspiration of refluxed material and loss of the pleasure of eating, which may be the major pleasure remaining for a patient with advanced Alzheimer's disease (Horner et al., 1994; Norbert, Norberg, & Bexell, 1980; Weir & Grostin, 1990).

Motor Neuron Disease

Motor neuron disease, also known as *amyotrophic lateral sclerosis,* causes degeneration of upper and lower motor neurons throughout the central nervous system. When the disease predominately involves lower motor neurons in the pons and medulla, the clinical syndrome of bulbar palsy results. This includes dysphagia and dysphonia or dysarthria accompanied by weakness, wasting, and fasciculation of affected muscles (Dworkin & Hartman, 1979; Lebo, Sang, & Norris, 1976; Meyer, Logemann, & Jubelt, 1985; Robbins, 1987; Smith, Mulder, & Code, 1957; Wilson, Bruce-Lockhart, & Johnson, 1990). Brainstem reflexes (jaw jerk and gag reflexes) tend to be reduced. When upper motor neurons of the corticobulbar tracts are primarily involved, the clinical syndrome of pseudobulbar palsy results. In this case, patients exhibit impaired voluntary function of the affected muscles, increased brainstem reflexes, and emotional lability.

The cause of motor neuron disease is unknown, but one popular theory implicates neurotoxicity related to excessive action of excitatory neurotransmitters such as glutamate. One study has suggested partial efficacy of an antiglutamate agent, riluzole, especially in cases of motor neuron disease with predominately bulbar problems (Bensimon, Lacomblez, & Meininger, 1994). Many other pathogenetic mechanisms and potential treatments are under investigation (Rowland, 1994). For now, the disease remains relentlessly progressive and ultimately fatal, usually within 5 years or fewer from the time of diagnosis. Diagnostic efforts should involve a diligent search for an alternative, treatable cause of the patient's condition. Positive test findings in motor neuron disease may include mild elevation of creatine kinase (creatine kinase, a muscle enzyme), diffuse acute and chronic denervation demonstrated by electromyography (EMG), and denervation evidenced by muscle biopsy.

Guillain-Barré Syndrome and Other Polyneuropathies

Immune-mediated demyelination (loss of the insulating material, myelin, around nerve fibers) of peripheral and cranial nerves in Guillain-Barré syndrome results in weakness and sensory loss that develop subacutely and vary in severity and distribution, sometimes profoundly affecting pharyngeal function. Patients usually recover spontaneously, but recovery is enhanced by treatment with plasmapheresis or intravenous immunoglobulin, and aggressive supportive care (often including gastrostomy and mechanical ventilation) is essential.

Neuropathies other than Guillain-Barré syndrome rarely cause oropharyngeal dysphagia, because neuropathic weakness is usually distal and therefore is unlikely to involve the muscles of the pharynx. Autonomic neuropathy, such as that related to diabetes mellitus, may lead to decreased smooth muscle activity in the gut, as a result of which esophageal hypomotility and dysphagia may occur. The effect of chronic, severe diabetes on pharyngeal function has not been studied.

Neoplasms and Other Structural Disorders

Primary brain tumors are associated with oropharyngeal dysphagia more frequently than has been generally recognized, even when the lesions are unilateral and supratentorial (Newton, Newton, Pearl, & Davidson, 1994).

Gliomas and other *intrinsic brain stem tumors* usually produce a variety of deficits, sometimes including oropharyngeal dysphagia, as a result of progressive invasion of brain stem nuclei and tracts (Frank, Schwartz, Epstein, & Beresford, 1989; Straube & Witt, 1990). *Extrinsic tumors* around the brain stem, such as meningiomas and acoustic neuromas, may compress the lower brain stem and/or cranial nerves and thereby cause dysphagia. *Base of skull tumors,* such as chordoma and nasopharyngeal carcino-

ma, can compress or invade cranial nerves and impair their function, often in association with local pain. The same is true of nonneoplastic structural disorders of and around the brain stem, including *syringobulbia,* in which there is congenital cavitation of the central brain stem, and *Arnold-Chiari malformation,* in which there is downward displacement and potential compression of the cerebellum and brain stem at the base of the skull (Achiron & Kuritzky, 1990; Bleck & Shannon, 1984; Fernandez, Leno, Commbarros, & Berciano, 1986; Massey, El Gammal, & Brooks, 1984). The diagnosis of neoplasms and other structural disorders of the brain stem and base of skull is usually made by MRI with enhancement, although CT scanning sometimes adds information regarding involvement of bony structures. Treatment of these conditions may involve surgery, radiation therapy and/or chemotherapy depending on the lesion and its location, and prognosis is similarly dependent on those factors.

Neoplastic meningitis typically arises from metastasis of adenocarcinoma, lymphoma, and other neoplasms. The usual presentation is multiple cranial nerve deficits, altered mental status, and headache. The cranial nerve deficits may include oropharyngeal dysphagia as a result of compression and infiltration of lower cranial nerves. Meningeal thickening and enhancement is often apparent by MRI, and cerebrospinal fluid examination with positive cytopathology is diagnostic. Despite treatment with radiation therapy and/or chemotherapy, the outcome is generally dismal.

Multiple Sclerosis

Central nervous system (CNS) demyelination in multiple sclerosis (MS) results from an immune-mediated attack that occurs for unclear reasons and typically produces fluctuating, multifocal CNS deficits. If the corticobulbar tracts or connections among lower brainstem nuclei are involved, dysphagia can result (Boucher & Hendrix, 1991; Daly, Code, & Anderson, 1962).

While motor impairment and variability of performance characterize dysphagia in MS, sensory changes including abnormal taste sensation have also been documented (Catalanotto et al., 1984). Multiple sclerosis is diagnosed based on a combination of clinical evidence (of CNS deficits that are multiple in space and time) and laboratory studies (MRI, cerebrospinal fluid examination looking especially for abnormal antibodies, and evoked potentials). Spontaneous remissions after symptomatic intervals of weeks to months are common, and therapeutic modulation of the immune system with high-dose corticosteroids or beta-interferon are potential treatments (Beck, Cleary, & Trobe, 1993; The IFNB Multiple Sclerosis Study Group, 1993).

Postpolio Syndrome

Acute paralytic poliomyelitis (APP) involves bulbar dysfunction, including dysphagia, in 10-15% or more of cases as a result of viral infection of brainstem lower motor neurons (Baker, Matzke, & Brown, 1950; Brahdy & Lenarsky, 1934). Today APP is rare, but approximately 20% of polio survivors complain of residual dysphagia (Bosma, 1953; Halstead, Wiechers, & Rossi, 1985; Lueck, Galligan, & Bosma, 1952). The term *postpolio syndrome* (PPS) refers to complaints of progressive fatigue, weakness, muscle wasting, and pain usually beginning several decades after APP (Speier, Owen, Knapp, & Canine, 1985). Many patients with PPS have readily identifiable and treatable causes of their progressive symptoms, such as orthopedic complications of chronic weakness, peripheral nerve entrapment, or depression. Some patients with PPS may suffer from progressive postpolio muscular atrophy (PPMA), which is thought to cause slowly progressive muscle wasting and weakness as a result of gradual disintegration of axon terminals of the motor neurons that survived acute paralytic poliomyelitis and have been chronically overextended for decades (Dalakas et al., 1986). There is controversy surrounding not only the clinical significance of PPMA in general but

also postpolio dysphagia complaints (Buchholz, 1987a; Buchholz, 1994b; Buchholz & Jones, 1991a, 1991b; Coelho & Ferrante, 1988; Ivanyi, Phoa, & de Visser, 1994; Jones, Buchholz, Ravich, & Donner, 1992; Sonies & Dalakas, 1991). There is no known treatment for PPMA. Any patient with bothersome postpolio dysphagia, especially if progressive, should be evaluated with videofluorography of swallowing in order to guide swallowing therapy and to search for coincident and potentially treatable structural and esophageal dysfunction (Buchholz & Marsh, 1986; Silbergleit, Waring, Sullivan, & Maynard, 1991).

Infectious Disorders

Chronic meningitis can result from multiple infectious causes such as fungi, mycobacteria, and parasites, and the clinical picture, including dysphagia related to lower cranial nerve involvement, is similar to that described for neoplastic meningitis. Spirochetal diseases including *syphilis* and *Lyme disease* may produce not only chronic meningitis but also parenchymal infection of the brain or brain stem, leading to dysphagia (Cook, 1953). Testing for these disorders includes serologic (antibody) studies and cerebrospinal fluid examination including cultures and antibody tests. *Diphtheria* is a bacterial infection of the throat that can produce acute lower cranial nerve dysfunction. *Botulism*, most often resulting from consumption of botulinum toxin produced by bacterial food contamination, causes generalized muscle weakness owing to impairment of neuromuscular transmission. *Viral encephalitis*, especially *rabies*, is sometimes associated with dysphagia (as a result of corticobulbar tract and brain stem viral infection) in addition to the characteristic features of headache, mental status abnormalities, and fever.

Myasthenia Gravis

Communication between nerve fibers and muscle membranes, which leads to muscle contraction, is accomplished at the neuromuscular junction by means of the release of acetylcholine from nerve terminals and its binding to receptors on muscle membranes, thereby triggering muscle action potentials. Myasthenia gravis results from the production of autoantibodies that bind to and degrade acetylcholine receptors, hence interfering with neuromuscular transmission and resulting in weakness, often in a distinctive pattern with progressive muscle fatigue brought about by sustained exertion. Common sites of involvement include the extraocular muscles (causing ptosis and diplopia), proximal limbs, and pharynx, tongue, and velum (producing dysphagia) (Carpenter, McDonald, & Howard, 1979; Edwards & Murray, 1957; Murray, 1962). Myasthenia gravis is diagnosed by a combination of clinical findings and ancillary evidence including the presence of antireceptor antibodies, decremental muscle response to repetitive nerve stimulation (an EMG technique), and positive response to anticholinesterase medication. Treatment includes not only anticholinesterases but also immunosuppressant medications (such as corticosteroids and others) and surgical removal of the thymus gland, which contains lymphocytes that produce the abnormal antibodies.

Myopathy

Myopathy (muscle disease) generally involves the proximal limbs but sometimes additionally or even selectively causes pharyngeal weakness. Inflammatory myopathies are immune-mediated and include *polymyositis, dermatomyositis, inclusion body myositis*, and *sarcoidosis* (Cunningham & Lowry, 1985; Darrow, Hoffman, Barnes, & Wiley, 1992; Dietz, Logemann, Sahgal, & Schmid, 1980; Hardy, Tulgan, Haidak, & Budnitz, 1967; Kagen, Hochman, & Strong, 1985; Metheny, 1978; Riminton, Chambers, Parkin, Pollock, & Donaldson, 1993; Vencovsky et al., 1988). Diagnostic findings include elevated creatine kinase, myopathic EMG findings with irritable

features, and muscle biopsy evidence of inflammatory cell inflammation and muscle fiber degeneration. Recognition of these disorders in cases of unexplained neurogenic dysphagia is especially important because of their potential reversibility with immunosuppressant therapy.

Noninflammatory myopathies associated with oropharyngeal dysphagia include late-onset muscular dystrophies such as *myotonic dystrophy* and *oculopharyngeal muscular dystrophy*, both of which are hereditary (Buckler, Pratter, Chad, & Smith, 1989; Casey & Aminoff, 1971; Dobrowski, Zajtchuk, LaPiana, & Hensley, 1986; Duranceau, Letendre, Clermont, Levesque, & Barbeau, 1978; Kiel, 1986; Swick, Werlin, Dodds, & Hogan, 1981). Diagnosis is established by clinical features, family history, and laboratory evidence (elevated creatine kinase and characteristic EMG and muscle biopsy results). Gene therapy may someday be available for these conditions.

It is important not to overlook myopathy associated with endocrine disturbances, especially *hyperthyroidism, hypothyroidism*, and *Cushing's syndrome* (related to corticosteroid excess, which may be exogenous or endogenous) (Branski et al., 1984). Thyroid screening should be a routine part of the workup of unexplained neurogenic dysphagia.

Iatrogenic Oropharyngeal Dysphagia

Oropharyngeal sensorimotor dysfunction can result from a variety of medication *side effects* and may exist independently or be superimposed on an underlying neurologic disease (Buchholz, 1995). In the latter case, even if the neurologic disease is itself untreatable, removal of medications that can exacerbate oropharyngeal dysphagia may be beneficial to the patient. Sedatives (e.g., benzodiazepines), antiseizure medications, and other CNS depressants can contribute to oropharyngeal dysphagia by decreasing arousal and directly suppressing brainstem function (Buchholz, Jones, Neumann, & Ravich,

1995; Wyllie, Wyllie, Cruse, Rothner, & Erenberg, 1986). Many medications result in myopathy, which can involve the pharynx, including corticosteroids, lipid-lowering agents, and colchicine (Kuncl & Wiggins, 1988). Neuromuscular transmission can be compromised by not only systemic medications such as aminoglycoside antibiotics but also local injection of botulinum toxin into neck muscles as treatment for torticollis and other focal dystonias in that area (Comella, Tanner, DeFoor-Hill, & Smith, 1992). Topical anesthetics applied to the base of tongue, pharynx, and larynx for procedures such as endoscopy can suppress the laryngeal cough reflex and promote silent dysphagia. Dopamine antagonists including neuroleptics, antiemetics, and metoclopramide are associated with drug-related movement disorders such as tardive dyskinesia, which preferentially involves the mouth (Craig & Richardson, 1982; Flaherty & Lahmeyer, 1978; Massengill & Nashold, 1969; McDanal, 1981; Menuck, 1981; Samie, Dannenhoffer, & Rozek, 1987). Many medications, such as tricyclic antidepressants and antihistamines, have anticholinergic effects that commonly result in decreased salivation and impaired bolus preparation (Hughes et al., 1987; Kaplan & Baum, 1993). Other drugs, including clonazepam, clozapine, and anticholinesterases may increase salivation and contribute to difficulty managing secretions in neurogenic oropharyngeal dysphagia (Bazemore, Tonkonogy, Ananth, & Colby, 1995).

Neurogenic oropharyngeal dysphagia has been reported to occur after a number of forms of *neck surgery,* including carotid endarterectomy, ventral rhizotomy for spasmodic torticollis, transhiatal esophagectomy, and anterior cervical fusion (Buchholz, Jones, & Ravich, 1993; Ekberg, Bergqvist, Takolander, Uddman, & Kitzing, 1989; Hambraeus, Ekberg, & Fletcher, 1987; Heitmiller & Jones, 1991; Hirano, Tanaka, Fujita, & Fujita, 1993; Hoehn & Yahr, 1967; Ong, Lam, Lam, & Wong, 1978). The common thread among these procedures is that they require trac-

tion and manipulation in the neck. It seems likely that in some cases pharyngeal dysfunction results from intraoperative disruption of connections of the pharyngeal nerve plexus to pharyngeal constrictor muscles. Depending on the degree of denervation, there may or may not be reinnervation and recovery. If this hypothesis is valid, other operative procedures around the neck may cause similar problems with dysphagia that are either unrecognized or mistakenly ascribed to factors such as intubation or postoperative edema. Of course, these factors and other surgical complications including hematoma may also contribute to transient postoperative dysphagia.

Posterior fossa surgery involving the brain stem, lower cranial nerves, and base of skull may also result in oropharyngeal dysphagia consequent to intraoperative manipulation or vascular compromise of the cranial nerves and brainstem structures responsible for swallowing (see Chapter 2). Patients undergoing these procedures should be managed cautiously in the postoperative setting, and any clinical hint of oropharyngeal impairment should lead to withholding of oral intake until the patient can be further evaluated with videofluorography of swallowing.

Irradiation of the head and neck as treatment for local cancer can produce either neurogenic dysphagia (as a result of radiation-induced nerve damage) or vascular and fibrotic changes that interfere with swallowing (Ekberg & Nylander, 1983). The latter situation, resulting in restricted movement of structures of the mouth and throat, may be difficult to distinguish from a neurogenic problem.

Age-Related Changes

Some studies have found, and others have not, evidence of changes in oropharyngeal performance in "normal" elderly subjects as well as symptomatic elderly individuals (Baum & Bodner, 1983; Borgstrom & Ekberg, 1988a, 1988b; Dejaeger, Pelemans, Bibau, & Ponette, 1994; Donner & Jones, 1991; Ekberg & Feinberg, 1991;

Ekberg & Nylander, 1982; Ekberg & Wahlgren, 1985; Feinberg & Ekberg, 1991; Feinberg, Ekberg, Segall, & Tully, 1992; Feinberg, Knebl, Tully, & Segall, 1990; Jaradeh, 1994; Logemann, 1990; Robbins, Hamilton, Lof, & Kempster, 1992a, 1992b; Robbins et al., 1995; Shaker & Lang, 1994; Sheth & Diner, 1988; Sonies, Stone, & Shawker, 1984; Tracy et al., 1989; Wood, Robbins, Roecker, Robin, & Luschei, 1994). Although changes have been reported in patterns of oral movement and bolus manipulation as well as in pharyngeal kinematics during swallowing by healthy older individuals, these people are asymptomatic for dysphagia and continue to eat full diets safely and with pleasure (Robbins et al., 1992b; Tracy et al., 1989). It appears that healthy aging affects swallowing differently than age-related neurologic diseases.

The notion of "presbypharynx" is presently unfounded and potentially dangerous. Oropharyngeal dysphagia in an elderly person is most likely related to his or her medical condition. In a generally weakened state as a result of concurrent illness, an aged individual may suffer decompensation of his or her oropharyngeal mechanism (i.e., dysphagia and its complications) even in the absence of a specific underlying neurologic disorder. Accordingly, the issue of safe and adequate nutritional intake should be considered in any elderly patient with superimposed systemic illness.

If an elderly person is dysphagic but not generally debilitated by systemic disease, the likely culprit is a neurologic disorder, not advanced age. The majority of neurologic disorders affecting swallowing have increased incidence with aging. The elderly patient with oropharyngeal dysphagia merits complete evaluation as to the specific cause.

EVALUATION OF NEUROGENIC DYSPHAGIA

As with any other clinical problem neurogenic dysphagia is best evaluated by tak-ing a thoughtful history and performing a careful physical examination (Buchholz, 1987b; Castell & Donner, 1987) (Table 11–2). Historical evidence of neurogenic dysphagia includes not only overt symptoms or complications of oropharyngeal dysphagia but also the subtle clues provided by behavioral alterations of eating (voluntary compensation). The temporal course of symptoms has considerable diagnostic power; stroke presents abruptly and usually resolves gradually, but motor neuron disease and myopathy are slowly progressive. Fluctuation of weakness over hours is consistent with myasthenia gravis, whereas symptomatic relapses and remissions over days to weeks is typical of multiple sclerosis.

The distinction between *bulbar palsy* and *pseudobulbar palsy* is a key step in the process of diagnosing a specific neurologic disease affecting swallowing. Both bulbar palsy and pseudobulbar palsy are clinical syndromes characterized by dysphagia, dysphonia, and/or dysarthria. Bulbar palsy is caused by neurologic disease involving the motor unit (i.e., including medullary lower motor neurons, cranial nerves, neuromuscular junctions, and muscles supplied by these neurons). Clinical features of bulbar palsy may include weakness, muscle atrophy, fasciculations, and decreased reflexes (jaw jerk and gag reflex). Examples of conditions producing bulbar palsy include brain stem stroke, Guillain-Barré syndrome, myasthenia gravis, and polymyositis.

Pseudobulbar palsy superficially resembles bulbar palsy (hence, the prefix *pseudo*), but it results from neurologic disease above the bulb (medulla). By history, patients may have difficulty initiating swallowing as a symptom of oral phase impairment due to interruption of the cerebral input necessary for this voluntary action. Examination tends to reveal an absence of the lower motor neuron features described above as part of bulbar palsy and, instead, the presence of increased reflexes as well as incoordination out of proportion to weakness.

TABLE 11-2. Evaluation of Neurogenic Dysphagia

History
  Symptoms and complications of dysphagia
  General medical history
  Neurologic history
Physical examination
  General examination
  Neurologic examination
Videofluoroscopy of swallowing
Neurologic consultation
Other consultations (as indicated by findings of the above)
  Otolaryngology
  Gastroenterology
  Surgery
  Swallowing therapy (speech-language pathology and others)
  Physical medicine and rehabilitation
  Nutrition
Blood studies[a]
  Complete blood counts
  Chemistry panel
  Creatine kinase
  Vitamin B12
  Thyroid screening
  Anti-acetylcholine receptor antibodies
  Serologic test for syphilis
  Lyme antibodies
Brain MRI with enhancement[a]
Electromyography, nerve conduction studies, and repetitive nerve stimulation[a]
Muscle biopsy[a]
CT of the skull base[a]
Cerebrospinal fluid examination[a]

[a] These studies may be indicated if the cause of neurogenic dysphagia is not otherwise apparent.

Pseudobulbar palsy is further characterized by discrepancy between voluntary functions, which tend to be impaired, and involuntary functions, which tend to be intact (because the intrinsic brainstem mechanisms necessary for these involuntary functions are intact in pseudobulbar palsy). For example, a patient with pseudobulbar palsy may show little if any elevation of the soft palate with attempted phonation, yet the palate rises well (some-times excessively) when the gag reflex is elicited or when swallowing is initiated.

Other features of pseudobulbar palsy include upper motor neuron signs in the limbs (spasticity, hyperreflexia, incoordination out of proportion to weakness, and extensor plantar responses), and emotional lability. Common causes of pseudobulbar palsy include bilateral hemispheral or subcortical strokes, traumatic brain injury, multiple sclerosis, and motor neuron disease (which, because it can involve both upper and lower motor neurons, often produces a mixture of pseudobulbar palsy and bulbar palsy).

Additional historical and examination findings may yield diagnostic patterns characteristic of stroke (e.g., hemiparesis), Parkinson's disease (bradykinesia and tremor), myopathy (proximal weakness), motor neuron disease (both upper and lower motor neuron signs), and many other neurologic diseases affecting swallowing. If a specific cause of neurogenic dysphagia is not apparent, neurologic consultation is advisable.

Videofluorography of swallowing is essential not only to document sensorimotor dysfunction of the oral cavity and pharynx but also to guide management decisions such as swallowing therapy and enteral tube feeding. Occasionally, videofluorography reveals a distinctive pattern of abnormality that is helpful in diagnosis of the underlying neurologic disease. Difficulty initiating swallowing (a form of swallowing apraxia) is characteristic of upper motor neuron dysfunction due to, for example, extensive bilateral strokes or multiple sclerosis. Patients with Parkinson's disease may exhibit lingual resting tremor upon attempts to initiate the swallow and/or reduced range of motion. Absence of the pharyngeal swallow response (i.e., failure of barium in the posterior oral cavity to trigger swallowing) indicates brainstem dysfunction. Asymmetric pharyngeal weakness suggests a unilateral lower motor neuron disorder of the brain stem or cranial nerves. Of note, unilateral medullary infarction (Wallenberg's syndrome) has been found to cause bilateral pharyngeal weakness, although often with ipsilateral predominance (Neumann, Buchholz, Jones, & Palmer, 1995; Newman et al., 1994), and impaired opening of the pharyngoesophageal segment (Robbins & Levine, 1993). As discussed earlier, psychogenic oropharyngeal dysphagia is characterized by videofluorographic demonstration of complex, nonpropulsive oral and lingual activity followed by normal pharyngeal function (Buchholz et al., 1994). It is hoped that further systematic studies using videofluorography will reveal specific diagnostic subtypes of neurogenic oropharyngeal (and perhaps esophageal) dysfunction, akin to patterns of dysarthria in terms of their reflection of underlying neuromuscular pathology.

Videofluorography of neurogenic dysphagia may also reveal accompanying nonneurologic problems that are independently treatable, such as esophageal dysmotility or an obstructive web or stricture (Buchholz & Marsh, 1986). Videofluoro-graphic findings may indicate a need for additional otolaryngologic or gastroenterologic studies. A note of caution is in order regarding anterior cervical osteophytes, demonstrated by videofluorography. These bone spurs, even when prominent, are infrequently the sole or primary cause of dysphagia (Zerhouni, Bosma, & Donner, 1987).

In cases of unexplained neurogenic dysphagia in which the underlying neurologic disease affecting swallowing is not apparent, further studies are indicated (Buchholz, 1994a) (Table 11–2). These include blood studies (complete blood counts, chemistry panel, creatine kinase, vitamin B12, thyroid screening, antiacetylcholine receptor antibodies, and, perhaps, serologic tests for syphilis and Lyme disease), brain MRI with enhancement, and EMG including nerve conduction studies and repetitive nerve stimulation. Depending on circumstances, CT of the base of the skull, cerebrospinal fluid examination, or muscle biopsy may be appropriate.

Dysphagia is often multifactorial, and, consequently, complete evaluation of dysphagia must often be multidisciplinary. Consultants from allied specialties including otolaryngology, gastroenterology, surgery, speech-language pathology, physical medicine and rehabilitation, and nutrition may play vital roles in correctly diagnosing and fully treating patients with neurogenic dysphagia.

MANAGEMENT OF NEUROGENIC DYSPHAGIA

Issues in the management of neurogenic dysphagia include:

1. determination of the safety and adequacy of eating (i.e., is a temporary enteral feeding tube or gastrostomy indicated?)
2. direct treatment of the neurologic disease affecting swallowing
3. avoidance of medications that can contribute to oropharyngeal dysphagia
4. treatment of coincident esophageal or structural problems
5. swallowing therapy
6. surgical management of dysphagia.

Issues two and three have been covered in this chapter, and issues one, four, five, and six are covered elsewhere (Chapters 12–16).

It is important not to overlook the psychological accompaniments of neurogenic dysphagia, especially anxiety, and depression, because these can often be effectively addressed even if the neurologic disease affecting swallowing cannot. Finally, the contribution of eating to quality of life in the face of neurologic disease should be considered carefully in treatment planning and implementation (Ely, Peters, Zweig, Elder, & Schneider, 1992; Emanuel, 1992; Olivares, Segovia, & Revuelta, 1974; Ouslander, Tymchuck, & Krynski, 1993).

MULTIPLE CHOICE QUESTIONS

1. Which of the following neurologic diseases is sometimes associated with the clinical syndrome of pseudobulbar palsy?
   a. myasthenia gravis
   b. polymyositis
   c. multiple sclerosis
   d. oculopharyngeal muscular dystrophy

2. Which of the following statements is false?
   a. Presbypharynx is a common cause of oropharyngeal dysphagia in the elderly.
   b. Benzodiazepines have been associated with oropharyngeal dysphagia without decreased level of arousal.
   c. MRI is superior to CT scanning in the evaluation of neurogenic dysphagia.
   d. Polyneuropathies do not often result in oropharyngeal dysphagia.

3. Which of the following statements regarding stroke and dysphagia is true?
   a. Brain stem stroke is less likely than hemispheral stroke to cause dysphagia.
   b. Brain stem stroke causing dysphagia may not be visualized by MRI.
   c. Left hemispheral stroke is more likely than right hemispheral stroke to cause pharyngeal dysphagia and aspiration.
   d. An increased gag reflex after a stroke indicates relatively greater risk of poststroke dysphagia and its complications.

4. Which of the following statements is false?
   a. Alzheimer's disease does not substantially impair pharyngeal function until relatively late in its course.
   b. Treatment of torticollis with injection of botulinum toxin may worsen dysphagia.
   c. Metoclopramide is an important cause of drug-induced movement disorders.
   d. Anterior cervical osteophytes are a common cause of oropharyngeal dysphagia.

REFERENCES

1992 Heart and Stroke Facts. (1991). Dallas: American Heart Association.

Achiron, A., & Kuritzky, A. (1990). Dysphagia as the sole manifestation of adult type I Arnold-Chiari malformation. *Neurology, 40*, 186–187.

Alberts, M. J., Horner, J., Gray, L., & Brazer, S. R. (1992). Aspiration after stroke: Lesion analysis by brain MRI. *Dysphagia, 7*, 170–173.

American Academy for Cerebral Palsy and Developmental Medicine. (1989). Statistical information. Richmond, VA.

Bach-y-Rita, P. (1988). Recovery of function: Theoretical considerations for brain injury rehabilitation. Baltimore: University Park Press.

Baker, A. B., Matzke, A., & Brown, J. R. (1950). Bulbar poliomyelitis: A study of medullary function. *Archives of Neurology and Psychiatry, 63,* 257–281.

Barer, D. H. (1989). The natural history and functional consequences of dysphagia after hemispheric stroke. *Journal of Neurology, Neurosurgery and Psychiatry, 52,* 236–241.

Baum, B. J., & Bodner, L. (1983). Aging and oral motor function: Evidence for altered performance among older persons. *Journal of Dental Research, 62,* 2–6.

Bazemore, P. H., Tonkonogy, J., Ananth, R., & Colby, J. (1995). Clozapine treatment and an unusual type of dysphagia. *Dysphagia, 10,* 62.

Beck, R. W., Cleary, P. A., & Trobe, J. D. (1993). The effect of corticosteroids for acute optic neuritis on the subsequent development of multiple sclerosis. *New England Journal of Medicine, 329,* 1764–1769.

Bensimon, G., Lacomblez, L., & Meininger, V. (1994). ALS/Riluzole Study Group: A controlled trial of riluzole in amyotrophic lateral sclerosis. *The New England Journal of Medicine, 330,* 585–591.

Bishop, M., Weymuller, E. A., & Fink, B. R. (1984). Laryngeal effects of prolonged intubation. *Anesthesia and Analgesia, 63,* 335–342.

Bleck, T. P., & Shannon, K. M. (1984). Disordered swallowing due to a syrinx: Correction by shunting. *Neurology, 34,* 1497–1498.

Blumberg, M. L. (1959). Respiration and speech in the cerebral palsied child. *American Journal Disabled Child, 89,* 48–53.

Borgstrom, P. S., & Ekberg, O. (1988a). Speed of peristalsis in pharyngeal constrictor musculature: Correlations to age. *Dysphagia, 2,* 140–144.

Borgstrom, P. S., & Ekberg, O. (1988b). Pharyngeal dysfunction in the elderly. *Journal of Medical Imaging, 2,* 74–81.

Bosma, J. F. (1953). Studies of the disabilities of the pharynx resultant from poliomyelitis. *Annals of Oto-Rhino-Laryngology, 64,* 529–547.

Boucher, R. M., & Hendrix, R. A. (1991). The otolaryngologic manifestations of multiple sclerosis. *Ear, Nose and Throat Journal, 70,* 224–233.

Brahdy, M. B., & Lenarsky, M. (1934). Difficulty swallowing in acute epidemic poliomyelitis. *Journal of the American Medical Association, 103,* 229–234.

Branski, D., Levy, J., Globus, M., Aviad, I., Keren, A., & Chowers, I. (1984). Dysphagia as a primary manifestation of hyperthyroidism. *Journal of Clinical Gastroenterology, 6,* 437–440.

Brown, G. E., Nordloh, S., & Donowitz, A. J. (1992). Systematic densensitization of oral hypersensitivity in a patient with a closed head injury. *Dysphagia, 7,* 138–141.

Buchholz, D. (1987a). Dysphagia in post-polio patients. In L. S. Halstead & D. O. Wiechers (Eds.). *Research and clinical aspects of the late effects of poliomyelitis.* New York: March of Dimes.

Buchholz, D. (1987b). Neurologic evaluation of dysphagia. *Dysphagia, 1,* 187–192.

Buchholz, D. (1992). Editorial. *Dysphagia, 7,* 148–149.

Buchholz, D. W. (1993). Clinically-probable brainstem stroke presenting primarily as dysphagia and nonvisualized by MRI. *Dysphagia, 8,* 235–238.

Buchholz, D. W. (1994a). Neurogenic dysphagia: What is the cause when the cause is not obvious? *Dysphagia, 9,* 245–255.

Buchholz, D. W. (1994b). Editorial: Postpolio dysphagia. *Dysphagia, 9,* 99–100.

Buchholz, D. W. (1995). Oropharyngeal dysphagia due to iatrogenic neurological dysfunction. *Dysphagia, 10,* 248–254.

Buchholz, D., Barofsky, I., Edwin, D., Jones, B., & Ravich, W. (1994). Psychogenic oropharyngeal dysphagia: Report of 26 cases. *Dysphagia, 9,* 267–268.

Buchholz, D. W., Bosma, J. F., & Donner, M. W. (1985). Adaptation, compensation and decompensation of the pharyngeal swallow. *Gastrointestinal Radiology, 10,* 235–239.

Buchholz, D., & Jones, B. (1991a). Dysphagia occurring after polio. *Dysphagia, 6,* 165–169.

Buchholz, D. W., & Jones, B. (1991b). Post-polio dysphagia: Alarm or caution? *Journal of Orthopedics, 14,* 1303–1305.

Buchholz, D., Jones, B., Neumann, S., & Ravich, W. (1995). Benzodiazepine-induced pharyngeal dysphagia: Report of two possible cases. *Dysphagia, 10,* 142.

Buchholz, D. W., Jones, B., & Ravich, W. J. (1993). Dysphagia following anterior cervical fusion. *Dysphagia, 8,* 390.

Buchholz, D. W., & Marsh, B. R. (1986). Multifactorial dysphagia: Looking for a second, treatable cause. *Dysphagia, 1,* 88–90.

Buckler, R. A., Pratter, M. R., Chad, D. A., & Smith T. W. (1989). Chronic cough as the presenting symptom of oculopharyngeal muscular dystrophy. *Chest, 95,* 921–922.

Bushmann, M., Dobmeyer, S. M., Leeker, L., & Perlmutter, J. S. (1989). Swallowing abnormalities and their response to treatment in Parkinson's disease. *Neurology, 39,* 1309–1314.

Carpenter, R., McDonald, T., & Howard, F. (1979). The otolaryngologic presentation of myasthenia gravis. *Laryngoscope, 89,* 922–928.

Casas, M. J., Kenny, D. J., & McPherson, K. A. (1994). Swallowing/ventilation interactions during oral swallow in normal children and children with cerebral palsy. *Dysphagia, 9,* 40–46.

Casey, E., & Aminoff, M. (1971). Dystrophica myotonia presenting with dysphagia. *British Medical Journal, 2*[suppl], 443.

Castell, D. O., & Donner, M. W. (1987). Evaluation of dysphagia: A careful history is crucial. *Dysphagia, 2,* 65–71.

Catalanotto, F. A., DoreDuffy, P., Donaldson, J., Testa, M., Peterson, M., & Ostrom, K. M. (1984). Quality specific taste changes in multiple sclerosis. *Annals of Neurology, 16,* 611–615.

Celifarco, A., Gerard, G., Faegenburg, D., & Burakoff, R. (1990). Dysphagia as the sole manifestation of bilateral strokes. *American Journal of Gastroenterology, 85,* 610–613.

Chen, M. Y., Ott, D. J., Peele, V. N., & Gelfand, D. W. (1990). Oropharynx in patients with cerebrovascular disease: Evaluation with videofluoroscopy. *Radiology, 176,* 641–643.

Chen, M. Y. M., Peele, V. N., Donati, D., Oh, D. J., Donofri, P. D., & Gelfand, D. W. (1992). Clinical and videofluoroscopic evaluation of swallowing in 41 patients with neurologic disease. *Gastrointestinal Radiology, 17,* 95–98.

Cleaton-Jones, P. (1976). The laryngeal-closure reflex and nitrous oxide analgesia. *Anesthesiology, 45,* 569–570.

Coelho, C. A., & Ferrante, R. (1988). Dysphagia in post-polio sequelae: Report of three cases. *Archives of Physical Medicine and Rehabilitation, 69,* 634–636.

Comella, C. L., Tanner, C. M., DeFoor-Hill, L., & Smith, C. (1992). Dysphagia after botulinum toxin injections for spasmodic torticollis. *Neurology, 42,* 1307–1310.

Cook, R. E. (1953). Progressive bulbar palsy due to syphilis. *American Journal of Syphilis, Gonorrhea and Venereal Diseases, 37,* 161–164.

Cotman, C. W. (1985). *Synaptic plasticity.* New York: Guilford Press.

Craig, T. J., & Richardson, M. A. (1982). Swallowing, tardive dyskinesia, and anticholinergics. *American Journal of Psychiatry, 139,* 1083.

Croxson, S. C. M., & Pye, I. (1988). Dysphagia as the presenting feature in Parkinson's disease. *Geriatric Medicine, 8,* 16.

Cunningham, J., & Lowry, L. (1985). Head and neck manifestations of dermatomyositis-poliomyositis. *Otolaryngology and Head and Neck Surgery, 93,* 673–677.

Dalakas, M. C., Elder, G., Hallett, M., Ravits, J., Baker, M., Papadopoulos, N., Albrecht, P., & Sever, J. (1986). A long-term follow-up study of patients with post-poliomyelitis neuromuscular symptoms. *New England Journal of Medicine, 314,* 959–963.

Daly, D. D., Code, C. F., & Anderson, H. A. (1962). Disturbances of swallowing and esophageal motility in patients with multiple sclerosis. *Neurology, 12,* 250–256.

Darrow, D. H., Hoffman, H. T., Barnes, G. J., & Wiley, C. A. (1992). Management of dysphagia in inclusion body myositis. *Archives of Otolaryngology and Head and Neck Surgery, 118,* 313–317.

Davies, A. E, Kidd, D., Stone, S.P, & MacMahon, J. (1995). Pharyngeal sensation and gag reflex in healthy subjects. *The Lancet, 345,* 487–488.

Dejaeger, E., Pelemans, W., Bibau, G., & Ponette, E. (1994). Manofluorographic analysis of swallowing in the elderly. *Dysphagia, 9,* 156–161.

Dietz, F., Logemann, J. A., Sahgal, V., & Schmid, F. R. (1980). Cricopharyngeal muscle dysfunction in the differential diagnosis of dysphagia in polymyositis. *Arthritis and Rheumatism, 23,* 491–495.

Dobrowski, J. M., Zajtchuk, J. T., LaPiana, F. G., & Hensley, S. D. (1986). Oculopharyngeal muscular dystrophy: Clinical and histopathological correlations. *Otolaryngology—Head and Neck Surgery, 95,* 131–141.

Donner, M. W. (1974). Swallowing mechanism and neuromuscular disorders. *Seminars in Roentgenology, 3,* 273–282.

Donner, M. W., & Jones, B. (1991). Aging and neurological disease. In B. Jones & M. W. Donner (Eds.), *Normal and abnormal swallowing: Imaging in diagnosis and therapy.* New York: Springer-Verlag.

Dubner, R., Sessle, B. J., & Storey, A. T. (Eds.), (1978). Mastication. In *The neural basis of oral and facial function* (pp. 311–345), New York: Plenum Press, 311–345.

Duranceau, C. A., Letendre, J., Clermont, R. J., Levesque, H. P., & Barbeau, A. (1978). Oropharyngeal dysphagia in patients with oculopharyngeal muscular dystrophy. *Canadian Journal of Surgery, 21,* 326–329.

Dworkin, J. P., & Hartman, D. E. (1979). Progressive speech deterioration and dysphagia in amyotrophic lateral sclerosis: Case report. *Archives of Physical Medicine and Rehabilitation, 60,* 423–425.

Dworkin, J. P., & Nadal, J. C. (1991). Nonsurgical treatment of drooling in a patient with closed head injury and severe dysarthria. *Dysphagia, 6,* 40–49.

Edmonds, C. (1966). Huntington's chorea, dysphagia and death. *Medical Journal of Australia, 53,* 273–274.

Edwards, J. W., & Murray, J. P. (1957). Barium swallow examination in myasthenia gravis. *British Journal of Radiology, 30,* 263–268.

Ekberg, O., Bergqvist, D., Takolander, R., Uddman, R., & Kitzing, P. (1989). Pharyngeal function after carotid endarterectomy. *Dysphagia, 4,* 151–154.

Ekberg, O., & Feinberg, M. J. (1991). Altered swallowing function in elderly patients with dysphagia: Radiographic findings in 56 patients. *American Journal of Roentgenology, 156*, 1181–1184.

Ekberg, O., & Nylander, G. (1982). Cineradiography of the pharyngeal stage of deglutition in 150 individuals without dysphagia. *British Journal of Radiology, 55*, 255–257.

Ekberg, O., & Nylander, G. (1983). Pharyngeal dysfunction after treatment for pharyngeal cancer with surgery and radiotherapy. *Gastrointestinal Radiology, 8*, 97–104.

Ekberg, O., & Wahlgren, L. (1985). Pharyngeal dysfunctions and their interrelationship in patients with dysphagia. *Acta Radiologica, 26*, 659–664.

Ely, J. W., Peters, P. G., Zweig, S., Elder, N., & Schneider, F. D. (1992). The physician's decision to use tube feeding: The role of the family, the living will and the Cruzan decision. *Journal of the American Geriatric Society, 40*, 471–475.

Emanuel, E. J. (1992). Securing patients' rights to refuse medical care: In praise of the Cruzan decision. *American Journal of Medicine, 92*, 307–312.

Feinberg, M. J., & Ekberg, O. (1991). Videofluoroscopy in elderly patients with aspiration: Importance of evaluating both oral and pharyngeal stages of deglutition. *American Journal of Roentgenology, 156*, 293–296.

Feinberg, M. J., Ekberg, O., Segall, L., & Tully, J. (1992). Deglutition in elderly patients with dementia: Findings of videofluorographic evaluation and impact on staging and management. *Radiology, 183*, 811–814.

Feinberg, M. J., Knebl, J. K., Tully, J., & Segall, L. (1990). Aspiration and the elderly. *Dysphagia, 5*, 61–71.

Fernandez, F., Leno, C., Commbarros, O., & Berciano, J. (1986). Cricopharyngeal dysfunction due to syringobulbia. *Neurology, 36*, 1635–1638.

Finger, S., & Stein, D. G. (1982). *Brain damage and recovery: Research and clinical perspectives.* New York: Academic Press.

Flaherty, J. A., & Lahmeyer, H. W. (1978). Laryngeal-pharyngeal dystonia as a possible cause of asphyxia with haloperidol treatment. *American Journal of Psychiatry, 135*, 1414–1415.

Frank, Y., Schwartz, S. B., Epstein, N. E., & Beresford, H. R. (1989). Chronic dysphagia, vomiting and gastroesophageal reflux as manifestations of a brainstem glioma: A case report. *Pediatric Neurosciences, 15*, 265–268.

Fuh, J.-L., Lee, R.-C., Wang, S.-J., Wu, Z.-A., & Liu, H.-C. (1995). Swallowing abnormalities in Parkinson's disease. *Neurology, 45*(suppl 4), A338–339.

Gisel, E. G. (1994). Oral-motor skills following sensorimotor intervention in the moderately eating-impaired child with cerebral palsy. *Dysphagia, 9*, 180–192.

Gordon, C., Langton-Hewer, R., & Wade, D. T. (1987). Dysphagia in acute stroke. *British Medical Journal, 295*, 411–414.

Greenberg, D. J. (1984). The incidence of aspiration in patients with tracheostomies. *Anesthesia and Analgesia, 63*, 1142.

Gresham, S. L. (1990). Clinical assessment and management of swallowing difficulties after stroke. *Medical Journal of Australia, 153*, 397–399.

Groher, M. E., & Bukatinan, R. (1986). The prevalence of swallowing disorders in two teaching hospitals. *Dysphagia, 1*, 3–6.

Gulyas, A. E., & Salazar-Grueso, E. F. (1988). Pharyngeal dysmotility in a patient with Wilson's disease. *Dysphagia, 2*, 230–234.

Haggstrom, G., & Hirschowitz, B. (1980). Disordered esophageal motility in Wilson's disease. *American Journal of Gastroenterology, 2*, 273–275.

Halstead, L. S., Wiechers, D. O., & Rossi, C. D. (1985). Late effects of poliomyelitis: A national survey. In L. S. Halstead & D. O. Wiechers (Eds.), *Late effects of poliomyelitis.* Miami: Symposia Foundation.

Hambraeus, G. M., Ekberg, O., & Fletcher, R. (1987). Pharyngeal dysfunction after total and subtotal oesophagectomy. *Acta Radiologica, 28*, 409–413.

Hardy, W. E., Tulgan, H., Haidak, G., & Budnitz, J. (1967). Sarcoidosis: A case presenting with dysphagia and dysphonia. *Annals of Internal Medicine, 66*, 353–357.

Heitmiller, R. F., & Jones B. (1991). Transient diminished airway protection following transhiatal esophagectomy. *American Journal of Surgery, 162*, 422–446.

Helfrich-Miller, K.R., Rector, K.L., & Straka, J.A. (1993). Dysphagia: Its treatment in the profoundly retarded patient with cerebral palsy. *Archives of Physical Medicine and Rehabilitation, 74*, 178–181.

Hewer, R. L., & Wade, D. J. (1987). Dysphagia in acute stroke. *British Medical Journal, 295*, 411–414.

Hirano, M., Tanaka, S., Fujita, M., & Fujita, H. (1993). Vocal cord paralysis caused by esophageal cancer surgery. *Annals of Otology, Rhinology and Laryngology, 102*, 182–185.

Hochman, R. A., Martin, J. T., & Devine, K. D. (1965). Anesthesia and the larynx. *Surgical Clinics of North America, 45*, 1031–1039.

Hoehn, M. M., & Yahr, M. (1967). Parkinsonism: Onset, progression and mortality. *Neurology, 17*, 427–442.

Horner, J., Alberts, M., Dawson, D., & Cook, G. (1994). Swallowing in Alzheimer's disease. *Alzheimer's Disease and Associated Disorders, 8*, 1–13.

Horner, J., Buoyer, F. G., Alberts, M. J., & Helms, M. J. (1991). Dysphagia following brain-stem stroke:

Clinical correlates and outcome. *Archives of Neurology, 48,* 1170–1173.

Horner, J., & Massey, E. W. (1988). Silent aspiration following stroke. *Neurology, 38,* 317–319.

Horner, J., Massey, E. W., & Brazer, S. R. (1988). Aspiration in bilateral stroke patients. *Neurology, 40,* 1686–1688.

Horner, J., Massey, E. W., Riski, J. E., Lathrop, D. L., & Chase, K. N. (1988). Aspiration following stroke: *Clinical correlates and outcome. Neurology, 38,* 1359–1362.

Horner, J., Riski, J. E., Ovelmen-Levitt, J., & Nashold, B. S. (1992). Swallowing in torticollis before and after rhizotomy. *Dysphagia, 7,* 117–125.

Horner, J., Riski, J. E., Weber, B. A., & Nashold, B. S. (1993). Swallowing, speech and brainstem auditory-evoked potentials in spasmodic torticollis. *Dysphagia, 8,* 29–34.

Hughes, C. V., Baum, B. J., Cox, P. C., Marmary, Y., Yeh, C. K., & Sonies, B. C. (1987). Oropharyngeal dysphagia: A common sequel of salivary gland dysfunction. *Dysphagia, 1,* 173–177.

Hutchins, B. (1989). Establishing a dysphagia family intervention program for head-injured patients. *Journal of Head Trauma Rehabilitation, 4,* 64–72.

Huxley, E. J., Viroslav, J., Gray, W. R., & Pierce, A. K. (1978). Pharyngeal aspiration in normal adults and patients with depressed consciousness. *American Journal of Medicine, 64,* 565–568.

The IFNB Multiple Sclerosis Study Group (1993). Interferon beta-1b is effective in relapsing-remitting multiple sclerosis. I. Clinical results of a multicenter, randomized, double-blind, placebo-controlled trial. *Neurology, 43,* 655–661.

Ivanyi, B., Phoa, S. S. K. S., & de Visser, M. (1994). Dysphagia in post-polio patients: A videofluorographic follow-up study. *Dysphagia, 9,* 96–98.

Jaradeh, S. (1994). Neurophysiology of swallowing in the aged. *Dysphagia, 9,* 218–220.

Jones, B., Buchholz, D. W., Ravich, W. J., & Donner, M. W. (1992). Swallowing dysfunction in the postpolio syndrome: A cineradiographic study. *American Journal of Roentgenology, 158,* 283–286.

Jones, B., & Donner, M. W. (1988). Examination of the patient with dysphagia. *Radiology, 167,* 319–326.

Kagel, M. C., & Leopold, N. A. (1992). Dysphagia in Huntington's disease: A 16 year retrospective. *Dysphagia, 7,* 106–114.

Kagen, L. J., Hochman, R. B., & Strong, E. W. (1985). Cricopharyngeal obstruction in inflammatory myopathy (polymyositis/dermatomyositis). *Arthritis and Rheumatism, 28,* 630–636.

Kahrilas, P. J. (1989). The anatomy and physiology of dysphagia. In D. W. Gelfard & J. E. Richter (Eds.), *Dysphagia: Diagnosis and treatment.* New York: Igaku-Shoin.

Kakigi, R., Shibasaki, H., Kuroda, Y., Shin, T., & Oona, S. (1983). Meige's syndrome associated with spasmodic dysphagia. *Journal of Neurology, Neurosurgery and Psychiatry, 46,* 589–590.

Kaplan, M. D., & Baum, B. J. (1993). The functions of saliva. *Dysphagia, 8,* 225–229.

Kenny, D. J., Koheil, R. M., Greenberg, J., Reid, D., Milner, M., Moran, R., & Judd, L. (1989). Development of a multidisciplinary feeding profile for children who are dependent feeders. *Dysphagia, 4,* 16–28.

Kiel, D. P. (1986). Oculopharyngeal muscular dystrophy as a cause of dysphagia in the elderly. *Journal of the American Gastroenterological Society, 34,* 144–147.

Kuhlemeier, K. V. (1994). Epidemiology and Dysphagia. *Dysphagia, 9,* 209–217.

Kuncl, R. W., & Wiggins, W. W. (1988). Toxic myopathies. *Neurologic Clinics, 6,* 593–619.

Lazarus, C. L. (1989). Swallowing disorders after traumatic brain injury. *Journal of Head Trauma Rehabilitation, 4,* 34–41.

Lazarus, C., & Logemann, J. (1987). Swallowing disorders in closed head trauma patients. *Archives of Physical Medicine and Rehabilitation, 68,* 79–84.

Lebo, C. P., Sang, K., & Norris, F. H. (1976). Cricopharyngeal myotomy in amyotrophic lateral sclerosis. *Laryngoscope, 86,* 862–868.

Leopold, N. A., & Kagel, M. C. (1985). Dysphagia in Huntington's disease. *Archives of Neurology, 42,* 57–60.

Levine, R., Robbins, J., & Maser, A. (1992). Periventricular white matter changes and oropharyngeal swallowing in normal individuals. *Dysphagia, 7,* 142–147.

Lieberman, A. N., Horowitz, L., Redmond, P., Pachter, L., Lieberman, I., & Liebowitz, M. (1980). Dysphagia in Parkinson's disease. *American Journal of Gastroenterology, 74,* 157–160.

Linden, P., Kuhlemeier, K. V., & Patterson, C. (1993). The probability of correctly predicting subglottic penetration from clinical observations. *Dysphagia, 8,* 170–179.

Linden, P., & Siebens, A. (1983). Dysphagia: Predicting laryngeal penetration. *Archives of Physical Medicine and Rehabilitation, 64,* 281–283.

Logemann, J. A. (1988). Dysphagia in movement disorders. In J. Jankovic & E. Tolosa (Eds.), *Advances in Neurology, 49,* 307–316.

Logemann, J. A. (1990). Effects of aging on the swallowing mechanism. *Otolaryngologic Clinics of North America, 23,* 1045–1056.

Logemann, J. A., Shanahan, T., Rademaker, A. W., Kahrilas, P. J., Lazar, R., & Halper, A. (1993). Oropharngeal swallowing after stroke in the left basal ganglion/internal capsule. *Dysphagia, 8,* 230–234.

Lueck, W., Galligan, J., & Bosma, J. F. (1952). Persistent sequelae of bulbar poliomyelitis. *Journal of Pediatrics, 41,* 549–554.

Mackay, L., & Morgan, A. S. (1993). Early swallowing disorders with severe head injuries: Relationships between RLA and the progression of oral intake. *Dysphagia, 8,* 161.

Martin, B. J. W., Corlew, M. M., Wood, H., Olson, D., Golopol, L. A., Wingo, M., & Kirmani, N. (1994). The association of swallowing dysfunction and aspiration pneumonia. *Dysphagia, 9,* 1–6.

Massengill, R., & Nashold, B. (1969). A swallowing disorder denoted in tardive dyskinesia patients. *Acta Oto-Laryngologica, 68,* 457–458.

Massey, C. E., El Gammal, T., & Brooks, B. S. (1984). Giant posterior inferior cerebellar artery aneurysm with dysphagia. *Surgical Neurology, 22,* 467–471.

McDanal, C. E. (1981). Haloperidol and laryngeal-pharyngeal dystonia. *American Journal of Psychiatry, 138,* 1262–1263.

Meadows, J. C. (1973). Dysphagia in unilateral cerebral lesions. *Journal of Neurology, Neurosurgery and Psychiatry, 36,* 853–860.

Menuck, M. (1981). Laryngeal-pharyngeal dystonia and haloperidol. *American Journal of Psychiatry, 138,* 394–395.

Metheny, J. (1978). Dermatomyositis: A vocal and swallowing disease entity. *Laryngoscope, 88,* 147–161.

Meyer, T., Logemann, J. A., & Jubelt, B. (1985). Nature of swallowing disorders in amyotrophic lateral sclerosis. *American Speech and Hearing Association, 276,* 123.

Mirrett, P. L., Riski, J. E., Glascott, J., & Johnson, V. (1994). Videofluorographic assessment of dysphagia in children with severe spastic cerebral palsy. *Dysphagia, 9,* 174–179.

Morris, S. (1982). *Program guidelines for children with feeding problems.* Edison, NJ: Childcraft.

Murray, J. P. (1962). Deglutition in myasthenia gravis. *British Journal of Radiology, 35,* 43–52.

Neumann, S., Buchholz, D., Jones, B., & Palmer, J. (1995). Pharyngeal dysfunction after lateral medullary infarction is bilateral: Review of 15 additional cases. *Dysphagia, 10,* 136.

Neumann, S., Buchholz, D., Wuttge-Hannig, A., Hannig, C., Prosiegel, M., & Schröter-Morasch, H. (1994). Bilateral pharyngeal dysfunction after lateral medullary infarction. *Dysphagia, 9,* 263.

Neumann, S., Reich, S., Buchholz, D., Purcell, L., & Jones, B. (1995). Progressive supranuclear palsy (PSP): Characteristics of dysphagia in 14 patients. Abstract presented to the 4th annual meeting of the Dysphagia Research Society.

Newton, H. B., Newton, C., Pearl, D., & Davidson, T. (1994). Swallowing assessment in primary brain tumor patients with dysphagia. *Neurology, 44,* 1927–1932.

Nilsson, H., Ekberg, O., Sjöberg, S., & Olsson, R. (1993). Pharyngeal constrictor paresis: An indicator of neurologic disease? *Dysphagia, 8,* 239–243.

Norbert, A., Norberg, B., & Bexell, G. (1980). Ethical problems in feeding patients with advanced dementia. *British Medical Journal, 281,* 847–848.

O'Connor, A., & Ardran, C. (1976). Cinefluorography in the diagnosis of pharyngeal palsies. *Journal of Laryngology and Otology, 90,* 1015–1019.

Ogg, H. L. (1975). Oral-pharyngeal development and evaluation. *Physical Therapy, 55,* 235–241.

Olivares, L., Segovia, A., & Revuelta, R. (1974). Tube feeding and lethal aspiration in neurological patients: A review of 720 autopsy cases. *Stroke, 5,* 654–656.

Ong, G. B., Lam, K. H., Lam, P. H. M., & Wong, J. (1978). Resection for carcinoma of the superior mediastinal segment of the esophagus. *World Journal of Surgery, 2,* 497–504.

Ottenbacher, K., Bundy, A., & Short, M. A. (1983). The development and treatment of oral-motor dysfunction: A review of clinical research. *Physical Occupational Therapy Pediatrics, 3,* 1–13.

Ouslander, J. G., Tymchuck, A. J., & Krynski, M. D. (1993). Decisions about enteral tube feeding among the elderly. *Journal of the American Gerontological Society, 42,* 70–77.

Palmer, J. B., & DuChane, A. S. (1991). Rehabilitation of swallowing disorders due to stroke. *Archives of Physical Medicine and Rehabilitation Clinics of North America, 2,* 529–546.

Pape, D. E., & Wigglesworth, J. S. (Eds.). (1979). Patterns of intracranial hemorrhage and ischemia in the newborn and their economic importance. In *Hemorrhage, ischemia and the perinatal brain* (pp. 1–10), Suffolk: Spastics International Medical Publications.

Riminton, D. S., Chambers, S. T., Parkin, P. J., Pollock, M., & Donaldson, I. M. (1993). Inclusion body myositis presenting solely as dysphagia. *Neurology, 43,* 1241–1243.

Riski, J. R., Horner, J., & Nashold, B. S. (1990). Swallowing function in patients with spasmodic torticollis. *Neurology, 40,* 1443–1445.

Robbins, J. (1987). Swallowing in ALS and motor neuron disorders. *Neurologic Clinics, 5,* 213–229.

Robbins, J. Hamilton, J. Lof, G., & Kempster, G. (1992a). Oropharyngeal swallowing in normal adults of different ages. *Gastroenterology, 103,* 823–829.

Robbins, J., Hamilton, J. W., Lof, G. L., & Kempster, G. B. (1992b). Oropharyngeal swallowing in normal adults of different ages. *Gastroenterology, 103,* 823–829.

Robbins, J., & Levine, R. L. (1988). Swallowing after unilateral stroke of the cerebral cortex: Preliminary evidence. *Dysphagia, 3,* 11–17.

Robbins, J., & Levine, R. L., (1993). Swallowing after lateral medullary syndrome. *Clin Comm Disord, 3*(4), 451–455.

Robbins, J. R., Levine, R. L., Maser, A. M., Rosenbek, J. R., & Kempster, G. K. (1993). Swallowing after unilateral stroke of the cerebral cortex. *Archives of Physical Medicine and Rehabilitation, 74,* 1295–1300.

Robbins, J. R., Levine, R. L., Wood, J. W., Roecker, E. R., & Luschei, E. L. (1995). Age effects on lingual pressure generation as a risk factor for dysphagia. *Gerontology, 5,* M257–262.

Robbins, J., Logemann, J. A., & Kirshner, H. S. (1986). Swallowing and speech production in Parkinson's disease. *Annals of Neurology, 19,* 283–287.

Rogers, B., Arvedson, J., Buck, G., Smart, P., & Msall, M. (1994). Characteristics of dysphagia in children with cerebral palsy. *Dysphagia, 9,* 69–73.

Rowland, L. P. (1994). Amyotrophic lateral sclerosis: Theories and therapies. *Annals of Neurology, 35,* 129–130.

Samie, M. R., Dannenhoffer, M. A., & Rozek, S. (1987). Life-threatening tardive dyskinesia caused by metoclopramide. *Movement Disorders, 2,* 125–129.

Sasaki, C. T., Suzuki, M., Horiuchi, M., & Kirchner, J. A. (1977). The effect of tracheostomy on the laryngeal closure reflex. *Laryngoscope, 87,* 1428–1433.

Schmidt, J., Holas, M., Harvorson, K., & Reding, M. (1994). Videofluoroscopic evidence of aspiration predicts pneumonia and death but not dehydration following stroke. *Dysphagia, 9,* 7–11.

Schneider, J. S., Diamond, S. G., & Markham, C. H. (1985). Deficits in orofacial sensorimotor function in Parkinson's disease. *Annals of Neurology, 19,* 275–282.

Shaker, R., & Lang, I. M. (1994). Effect of aging on the deglutitive oral, pharyngeal, and esophageal motor function. *Dysphagia, 9,* 221–228.

Sheth, N., & Diner, W. C. (1988). Swallowing problems in the elderly. *Dysphagia, 2,* 209–215.

Silbergleit, A. K., Waring, W. P., Sullivan, M. J., & Maynard, F. M. (1991). Evaluation, treatment and follow-up results of post-polio patients with dysphagia. *Otolaryngology and Head and Neck Surgery, 104,* 333–338.

Silbiger, M. L., Pikielney, R., & Donner, M. W. (1967). Neuromuscular disorders affecting the pharynx: Cineradiographic analysis. *Investigative Radiology, 2,* 442–448.

Smith, A. W., Mulder, D., & Code, C. (1957). Esophageal motility in amyotrophic lateral sclerosis. *Proceedings of the Mayo Clinic, 32,* 438.

Sonies, B. C. (1992). Swallowing and speech disturbances. In I. Litvan & Y. Agid (Eds.), *Progressive supranuclear palsy: Clinical and research approaches.* New York: Oxford University Press.

Sonies, B. C., & Dalakas, M. C. (1991). Dysphagia in patients with the post-polio syndrome. *New England Journal of Medicine, 324,* 1162–1167.

Sonies, B. C., Stone, M., & Shawker, T. (1984). Speech and swallowing in the elderly. *Gerontology, 3,* 115–123.

Speier, J. L., Owen, R. R., Knapp, M., & Canine, J. K. (1985). Occurrence of post-polio sequelae in an epidemic population. In L. S. Halstead & D. O. Wiechers (Eds.), *Late effects of poliomyelitis.* Miami: Symposia Foundation.

Straube, A., & Witt, T. N. (1990). Oculo-bulbar myasthenic symptoms as the sole sign of tumour involving or compressing the brain stem. *Journal of Neurology, 237,* 369–371.

Stroudley, J., & Walsh, M. (1991). Radiological assessment of dysphagia in Parkinson's disease. *British Journal of Radiology, 64,* 890–893.

Swick, H. M., Werlin, S. L., Doods, W. J., & Hogan, W. J. (1981). Pharyngoesophageal motor function in patients with myotonic dystrophy. *Annals of Neurology, 10,* 454–457.

Taylor, P. A., & Towey, R. M. (1971). Depression of laryngeal reflexes during ketamine anesthesia. *British Medical Journal, 2,* 688–690.

Teasell, R. W., Bach, D., & McRae, M. (1994). Prevalence and recovery of aspiration poststroke: A retrospective analysis. *Dysphagia, 9,* 35–39.

Tepid, D. C., Palmer, J. B., & Linden, P. (1987). Management of dysphagia in a patient with closed head injury: A case report. *Dysphagia, 1,* 221–226.

Tracy, J. F., Logemann, J. A., Kahrilas, P. J., Jacob, P., Kobara, M., & Krugler, C. (1989). Preliminary observations on the effects of age on oropharyngeal deglutition. *Dysphagia, 4,* 90–94.

Veis, S. L., & Logemann, J. A. (1985). Swallowing disorders in persons with cerebrovascular accident. *Archives of Physical Medicine and Rehabilitation, 66,* 372–375.

Vencovsky, J., Rehak, F., Pafko, P., Jirasek, A., Valesova, M., Alusik, S., & Trnavsky, K. (1988). Acute cricopharyngeal obstruction in dermatomyositis. *Journal of Rheumatology, 15,* 1016–1018.

Volicer, L., Seltzer, B., Rheaume, Y., Karner, J., Glennon, M., Riley, M. E., & Crino, P. (1989). Eating difficulties in patients with probable dementia of the Alzheimer type. *Journal of Geriatric Psychiatry and Neurology, 2,* 188–195.

Wade, D., & Hewer, L. (1987). Motor loss and swallowing difficulty after stroke: Frequency, recovery and prognosis. *Acta Neurologica Scandinavica, 76,* 50–54.

Weir, R. F., & Grostin, L. (1990). Decisions to abate life-sustaining treatment for non-autonomous patients. *Journal of the American Medical Association, 264,* 1846–1853.

Wilson, P. S., Bruce-Lockhart, F. J., & Johnson, A. P. (1990). Videofluoroscopy in motor neurone disease prior to cricopharyngeal myotomy. *Annals of the Royal College of Surgeons of England, 72,* 345–377.

Winstein, C. J. (1983). Neurogenic dysphagia: Frequency, progression and outcome in adults following head injury. *Physical Therapy, 63,* 1992–1997.

Wolpaw, J. R. (1985). Adaptive plasticity in the spinal stretch reflex: An accessible substrate of memory? *Cellular and Molecular Neurobiology, 5,* 147–165.

Wood, J. L., Robbins, J. A., Roecker, E. B., Robin, D. A., & Luschei, E. S. (1994). Age effects on lingual pressure generation and implications for swallowing. *Dysphagia, 9,* 270.

Wyllie, E., Wyllie, R., Cruse, R. P., Rothner, A. D., & Erenberg, G. (1986). The mechanism of nitrazepam-induced drooling and aspiration. *New England Journal of Medicine, 314,* 35–38.

Ylvisaker, M., & Logemann, J. A. (1986). Therapy for feeding and swallowing following head injury. In M. Ylvisaker (Ed.), *Management of head injured patients.* San Diego, CA: College Hill Press.

Zerhouni, E. A., Bosma, J. F., & Donner, M. W. (1987). Relationship of cervical spine disorders to dysphagia. *Dysphagia, 1,* 129–144.

12

Diseases and Operation of Head and Neck Structures Affecting Swallowing

Timothy M. McCulloch, Debra M. Jaffe, and Henry T. Hoffman

Normal individuals swallow once or twice every minute to clear saliva and mucous from the upper aerodigestive tract. When a person is unable to swallow, the ability to enjoy almost all other aspects of life is affected. Even minor, intermittent dysphagia can lead to psychological and social stresses. Episodes of choking can lead to a fear of eating that can lead to malnutrition and social withdrawal.

This chapter provides information regarding diseases of the head or neck which by themselves or secondary to defects resulting from operative therapy result in dysphagia. These conditions include congenital malformations, inflammatory, infectious, and neoplastic processes, neuromuscular disorders, and mechanical and structural abnormalities (Table 12–1). Emphasis here is placed on surgical interventions utilized to treat head and neck disease.

Oropharyngeal dysphagia is most commonly due to muscular weakness or dyscoordination, anatomic abnormalities, sensory deficits, or pain. The interdependent nature of the components of the

swallow when interrupted can lead to symptoms somewhat distant from the actual cause of dysfunction. This complexity and subordination oftentimes limits the utility of "external" treatment, forcing the physicians and therapists to rely heavily on "internal" plasticity and patient compensation to aid in improving moderate and severe dysphagia.

OROPHARYNGEAL STRUCTURES AND THEIR FUNCTION IN NORMAL SWALLOWING

The normal swallow is usually divided into stages for descriptive purposes. The oral stage of swallowing can be divided into the preparatory phase and the lingual transport phase (Baredes, 1988). The preparatory stage is composed of mastication (when appropriate) and preparation of the bolus (Logemann, 1983). These activities are dependent on the highly coordinated activities of specific orofacial muscles and an intact

343

TABLE 12–1. Major categories of oropharyngeal dysphagia.

I. Neurologic

II. Infectious

III. Tumor and malignancies

IV. Systemic disorders

V. Anatomic abnormalities

VI. Pharmacologic

VII. Idiopathic

mandible and maxilla. Salivary gland function also plays a major role in preparation of the bolus by providing adequate lubrication to the food.

The preparatory stage of the swallow begins with lip closure by the *m. obicularis oris* which is controlled by the facial nerve. With incomplete closure, drooling and loss of food may result. Once the food is within the oral cavity it is kept in contact with the teeth by the action of the buccinator muscle and tongue.

The masseter, temporalis, and pterygoid muscles (medial and lateral), which are innervated by the trigeminal nerve, are responsible for chewing. Specifically, the masseter, medial pterygoid, and portions of the temporalis are all mandibular elevators, while the posterior portion of the temporalis is a mandibular retractor and the lateral pterygoid is a mandibular depressor and protruder (Morrell, 1984). The mandible moves in patterns of inferior-superior, medial-lateral, and anterior-posterior direction to allow appropriate dental contact to crush food matter and form the bolus (Kennedy & Kent, 1988).

Primary bolus manipulation is accomplished by the anterior tongue in conjunction with an intact set of teeth and functioning buccal musculature. The tongue divides the bolus and positions it for swallowing during the pharyngeal phase, which begins once the bolus has been placed in the mid portion of the posterior tongue.

The pharyngeal stage of swallow is composed of the consecutive activity of soft palate elevation, tongue and pharyngeal wall compression, laryngeal elevation and airway closure, and cricopharyngeal opening (Kock, 1993). A coordinated brief interruption of respiration is also required as laryngeal muscles close the glottis to protect the lower airway. The pumping action of the tongue, gravity, elevation of the larynx, and sequential stripping action of the pharyngeal constrictors all assist in propelling the bolus toward the cricopharyngeal segment and upper esophagus. Cranial nerves V, VII, IX, X, and XII are involved in the pharyngeal stage of swallow (see Chapter 2).

SWALLOWING DYSFUNCTION AND SURGICAL MANAGEMENT IN INFANTS AND CHILDREN

Disorders of feeding and swallowing are not uncommon in the pediatric population. The etiologies are diverse, extending from congenital abnormalities to foreign bodies (Table 12–2). The most common abnormalities will be briefly discussed below. Treatment algorithms include surgical intervention in the majority of the these disorders. For additional information regarding dysphagia in the pediatric population, see Chapter 14.

Congenital Anatomic Abnormalities

Cleft Lip and Palate, Velopharyngeal Incompetence

Cleft palate, a common congenital defect, results from incomplete fusion of the horizontal palatal segments, while *cleft lip* results from failure of the premaxilla to fuse with the alveolus (Kaufman, 1991; Parkin, 1991). Cleft palate may present alone or in combination with cleft lip. Cleft palate may potentially impair swallowing function, as the soft palate fails to make contact with the posterior pharyngeal wall and seal the oral cavity; this dysfunction often results in nasal regurgitation. Infants with small isolated clefts of the soft palate or cleft lips alone are capable of generating

TABLE 12–2. Swallowing dysfunction in infants and children.

Congenital Anatomic Abnormalities
   Cleft lip and palate
   Laryngomalasia
   Laryngeal clefts
   Tracheo-esophageal fistula/esophageal stenosis
   Choanal atresia

Micrognathia

Vascular abnormalities
   Vascular rings
   Dysphagia lusorum

Neurologic and neuromuscular
   Cerebral palsy
   Cranial nerve palsy
   Muscular dystrophy

Prematurity and developmental delay

Inflammatory conditions

Foreign bodies

Tumors and masses

sufficient negative intraoral pressure to suckle. In contrast, infants with cleft lip and palate may have difficulties during suckling (Fisher, Painter, & Milmoe, 1981). Many infants require mechanical assistance in the form of a modified nipple or alterations in feeding positions to achieve adequate nutrition.

Cleft palates may be closed using a variety of surgical techniques. Commonly the procedure is performed when the child is about 12 months of age. The closure is accomplished by raising tissue flaps along the margins of clefts and then approximating the edges in multiple layers (Figure 12–1). The guiding principles outlined by Bardach and Salyer (1991) are:

1. complete closure of the entire palatal cleft in a single operation
2. construction of an adequately functioning soft palate
3. every attempt is made to minimize the area of exposed baseline (tissue and bone).

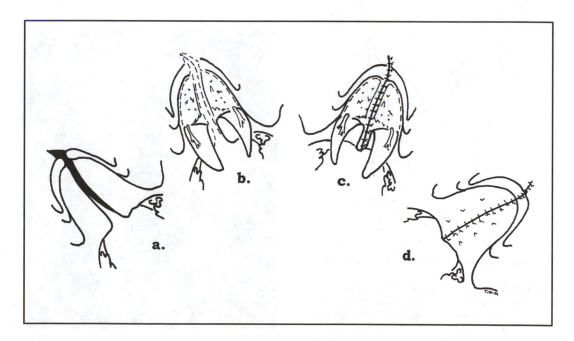

Figure 12–1. Cleft palate repair: **a.** primary cleft, **b.** mucosal flaps elevated, **c.** deep layer closure, **d.** final closure.

Velopharyngeal incompetence will remain a problem in up to 30% of patients after primary cleft palate repair (Bardach & Salyer, 1991). A second surgical procedure is often required. Velopharyngeal closure is accomplished by incorporating posterior pharyngeal mucosa into the soft palate utilizing pharyngeal flap techniques (Bardach & Salyer, 1991; Figure 12–2).

Laryngomalasia

Laryngomalasia is one of the most common causes of noisy breathing (stridor) in the infant. The stridor results from flaccid supraglottic structures prolapsing into the airway with inspiration. Clinical examination with a flexible or rigid laryngoscope reveals an omega-shaped epiglottis and hooding of the laryngeal inlet secondary to excessive tissue along the aryepiglottic folds (Figure 12–3). Most infants respond well to prone positioning; however, some develop increasing amounts of stridor during feeding efforts, resulting in failure to thrive, and cyanosis. Treatment at this point consists of epiglottoplasty (Tunckel, 1994). Usually this procedure is performed with a CO_2 laser via a transorally placed laryngoscope. The surgical goal is to remove redundant mucosa along the aryepiglottic fold to improve the supraglottic airway.

Laryngeal Clefts and Tracheoesophageal Fistula

Laryngeal clefts result from incomplete closure of the tracheoesophageal septum or cricoid cartilage or both in the sixth to seventh week of fetal life (Glossup, Smith, & Evans, 1984; Tunckel, 1994). As classified by Benjamin and Inglis (1989), poste-

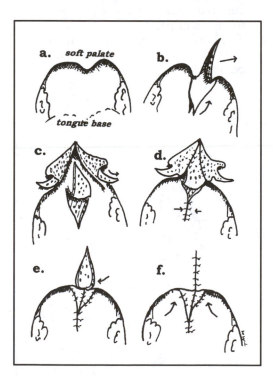

Figure 12–2. Pharyngeal flap repair: **a.** Posterior pharynx, **b.** Palate and pharyngeal incisions, **c.** Mucosal flaps rotated inferiorly off posterior palate. **d.** Pharyngeal flap sutured to posterior soft palate. **e.** Palate flap rotated and sutured medially. **f.** Final closure, arrows indicate lateral air passages.

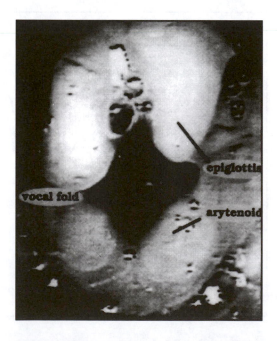

Figure 12–3. Laryngomalasia, omega-shaped epiglottis and shortened aryepiglottic folds.

rior laryngeal clefts may occur supraglottically, involving interarytenoid muscles, or may extend downward to include the cricoid cartilage (Figure 12–4). In the most severe cases cricoid and tracheal involvement coexist. Esophageal atresia may be concomitant (Tunckel, 1994). Depending on the extent of the cleft, infants may present with aspiration, cyanosis, and coughing with feeding. Diagnosis is usually made by contrast swallow study and then confirmed by direct laryngoscopy. Small clefts are usually repaired endoscopically, whereas larger ones may require open repair and laryngofissure.

Isolated tracheoesophageal fistulas may be subtle and difficult to diagnose by esophageal endoscopy. Infants present with coughing during feeding episodes and recurrent pneumonia (Tunckel, 1994). Other associated abnormalities may include tracheal stenosis, esophageal atresia, or stenosis and tracheomalacia (Tunckel, 1994). Surgical intervention consists of separation of the trachea and esophagus and reconstruction.

Choanal Atresia

Choanal atresia refers to posterior occlusion of the nasal aperture. It may be membranous (10%) or bony (90%; Cumberworth, Djazaeri, & Mackay, 1995). Although rare, when occurring bilaterally choanal atresia may present as a medical emergency (Coates, 1992). Feeding difficulties may be the first sign of choanal atresia,

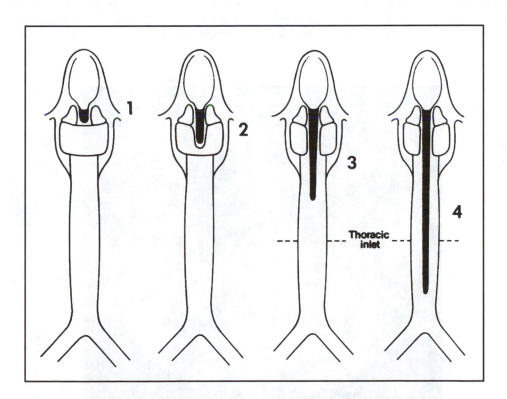

Figure 12–4. Classification of laryngeal clefts (Reprinted with permission from. Minor Congenital Laryngeal Clefts: Diagnosis and Classification. **1.** Type 1: supraglottic interarytenoid cleft. **2.** Type 2: partial cricoid cleft. **3.** Type 3: total cricoid cleft. **4.** Type 4: larygoesophageal cleft by B. Benjamin and A. Inglis, 1989. *Annals of Otology, Rhinology and Laryngology, 98,* 417–420.)

as children are obligate nasal breathers for the first 6 months of life. Feeding thus may lead to cyanotic episodes, which are relieved by crying (Brodsky & Volk, 1993). Nasopharyngoscopy with a flexible fiberscope is diagnostic (Figure 12–5). The bony extent of atresia is usually evaluated by computed tomography (CT). In bilateral cases an oral stent is placed to maintain an adequate airway. The definitive treatment requires the creation of a posterior nasal aperture utilizing laser energy, small drills, or curettes through a transantral, transseptal, or transpalatal approach (Coates, 1992).

Micrognathia

Mandibular hypoplasia, (micrognathia) may occur in isolation or be associated with congenital syndromes such as Pierre Robin syndrome and Goldenhar's syndrome. Upper airway obstruction frequently occurs in this group of patients secondary to the posterior position of the tongue superimposed upon a hypoplastic mandible. If aspiration occurs repeatedly, infants are fed through a nasogastric tube. Early in life, maintenance of a stable airway is of prime importance. As infants with this condition grow, the airway enlarges and muscle tone within the pharynx and larynx improves, allowing for a more normal airway passage (Benjamin, 1993).

Vascular Abnormalities

Vascular abnormalities of the great vessels may cause compression of the esophagus and trachea leading to feeding difficulties in children. Common causes of compressive rings include a right-sided aortic arch or double aortic arch. Dysphagia lusorum, difficulty swallowing secondary to an aberrant right subclavian

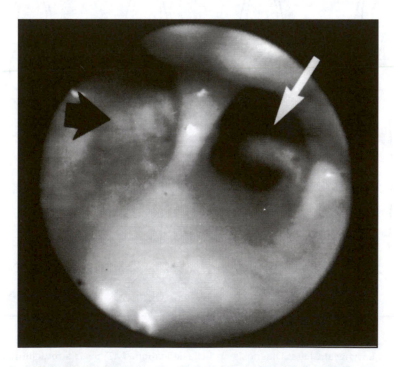

Figure 12–5. Choanal atresia, unilateral; nasopharyngeal endoscopic view, atretic nasal passage (*black arrow*), inferior turbinate (*white arrow*).

artery, can be documented in infants and children (Martin, Rudolph, Hillemeier, & Heyman, 1986). Radiologic and endoscopic evaluation are needed to diagnose and identify these lesions (Fisher et al., 1981). Surgical intervention is considered when symptoms are severe.

Neurologic and Neuromuscular Abnormalities

Many neurologic conditions are associated with feeding disorders in childhood. To determine the etiology of the disorder, a complete history, including prenatal course, and physical examination are essential.

Cerebral Palsy

Cerebral palsy is the result of a permanent deficit of the immature brain leading to movement and postural disorders (Christensen, 1989). Many of these children have some form of oral-motor dysfunction. Drooling and aspiration are common (see Chapter 14).

Cranial Nerve Palsies

Cranial nerve injuries in the pediatric population, although rare, may occur as the result of traumatic forceps delivery, congenital abnormality, basilar skull fracture, tumor, or infection. Common neural impairments include VIIth nerve injury secondary to forceps traction and Xth nerve insults due to Arnold-Chiari malformation (see Chapter 11).

Inflammatory Conditions, Infectious Etiologies

The list of inflammatory conditions causing dysphagia in the pediatric age category is extensive (tonsillitis, epiglottitis, mononucleosis, retropharyngeal abscess, and so on). Tonsillitis is perhaps the most common. Antimicrobial therapy directed against beta-hemolytic streptococcus is frequently used, although viral etiologies

are common. Epiglottitis, or acute bacterial supraglottis, is one of the more serious inflammatory conditions in the 3- to 6-year-old age group, presenting with drooling and stridor (Tunckel, 1994). A history of rapid onset, fever, drooling, and muffled voice are part of the classical clinical presentation. A lateral neck film revealing a thickened epiglottis, or "thumbprint sign" can confirm the diagnosis. Treatment requires airway management, usually with intubation, and intravenous antibiotic therapy covering *Hemophilus influenza*, the most common infectious agent.

Foreign Bodies

Ingestion or aspiration of objects in the pediatric age group is common. Swallowed foreign bodies are typically found in the 9-month to 3-year-old age category (Tunckel, 1994). A history of using the oral cavity as a receptacle for small objects is not uncommon, and bolus impaction should be suspected in a child who presents with acute onset of dysphagia. A relatively prolonged history of poor oral intake, weight loss, and airway problems may point toward an esophageal foreign body, which may go unrecognized for weeks to months. X-ray examination of the upper aerodigestive tract can be helpful diagnostically, but esophagoscopy and operative laryngoscopy are often a therapeutic necessity (Figure 12–6).

Head and Neck Tumors

In contrast to the adult population, pediatric patients have a higher percentage of benign masses as the source of swallowing disturbances. Pediatric head and neck tumors in this subcategory include lymphangiomas and capillary hemangiomas. These tumors frequently involve the tongue, which occupies a large portion of the infant oral cavity, and the floor of mouth; thus, a space-occupying lesion may lead to stridor, and airway obstruction. Treatment is difficult. Surgical resection for large lesions is usually incomplete and may leave the patient

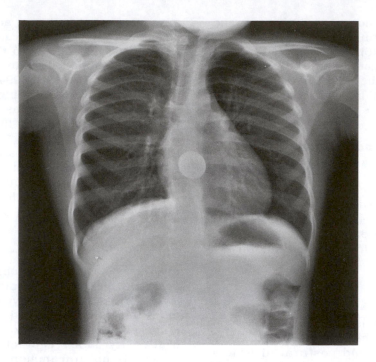

Figure 12–6. Esophageal foreign body, mid esophageal coin in 3-year-old child.

dependent on a tracheotomy and a feeding tube.

NEUROLOGIC AND NEUROMUSCULAR CAUSES OF OROPHARYNGEAL DYSPHAGIA

Neurological disorders are well-recognized origins of dysphagia. A thorough history and physical examination are essential for deducing a correct diagnosis. The most common neuropathologic entities contributing to oropharyngeal dysphagia are briefly outlined in Table 12–3. The limited role of surgical interventions is also addressed. (See Chapter 11 for additional information.)

Central Neurologic Disorders

Stroke

Stroke is perhaps the most common cause of dysphagia, usually presenting abruptly in conjunction with other neurologic findings, making the diagnosis simple and straightforward (Kuhlemeier, 1994). However, occasionally, isolated lacunar infarcts involving the corticobulbar tract may produce volitional dysphagia without affecting the reflex action of the swallow (Buchholz, 1994). Similarly, a small brain stem infarction of the nucleus ambiguus (the swallow center of the medulla) may produce isolated reflexive dysphagia with perhaps dysarthria or dysphonia (Brin, & Younger, 1988). The incidence of dysphagia in the stroke population is approximately 20% (Johnson, McKenzie, & Sievers, 1993). The most common dysfunctions identified in this group of patients are delayed initiation of the pharyngeal stage of the swallow and decreased pharyngeal transit time (Johnson et al., 1993; Veis & Logemann 1985). In videofluorographic assessments conducted on 38 stroke patients, aspiration was observed in one third of patients, and aspiration pneumonia occurred in up

TABLE 12–3. Common neurologic and neuromus-cular causes of dysphagia

Central neurologic disorders
  Stroke
  Parkinson's disease
  Bulbar palsy
  Cerebral palsy

Peripheral nerve disorders
  Vocal fold paralysis
  Bell's palsy (cranial nerve VII paralysis)
  Neurofibromatosis type II

Neuromuscular junction disorders
  Myasthenia gravis

Muscular disorders
  Cricopharyngeal dysfunction

Neuromuscular
  Amyotrophic lateral sclerosis (ALS)
  Polio and postpolio syndrome
  Multiple sclerosis

Unknown
  Spasmodic dysphonia
  Oculopharyngeal dystonia

to one half of the patients during the first year of follow-up (Johnson et al., 1993; Veis & Logemann 1985).

Early intervention in the form of blood pressure control and perhaps anticoagulation therapy (depending on the type and location of the stroke) is essential to prevent cerebrovascular extension or future cerebrovascular accidents. Most patients show improvement in swallowing function during the first year of recovery, but the extent of recovery is variable. Surgical intervention maybe helpful depending on the location and magnitude of the dysfunction. Cricopharyngeal myotomy, gastrostomy, and tracheoesophageal diversion all have a place in the treatment of this patient group (Butcher, 1982).

Parkinson's Disease

Decreased pharyngeal peristalsis, vallecular stasis, as well as esophageal dysfunction are frequently associated with Parkinson's disease (Guily et al., 1994). In a study by Bushmann et al. (1989) 20 patients with Parkinson's disease were evaluated; 15 (75%) were found to have swallowing dysfunction. The severity of the dysphagia did not coincide well with generalized parkinsonian signs; however, the swallow improved in the majority of patients after treatment with levodopa (Bushmann, Dobmeryer, Leeker, & Perlmutter, 1989). Perlman, Booth, and Grayhack (1994) found that 29% of the 21 Parkinsonian patients examined exhibited aspiration.

Huntington's Disease

Huntington's disease, a hereditary neurodegenerative disease, results from degeneration of the caudate and putamen (Kagel & Leopold, 1992). Dysphagia occurs as a result of lingual chorea, respiration-deglutition dyssynchrony, and tachyphagia (eating too quickly while large amounts of poorly masticated food remain in the mouth; Kagel & Leopold, 1992). Treatment is primarily supportive.

Cerebral Palsy

Cerebral palsy, a condition related to perinatal damage to the nervous system, presenting with progressive motor disorders, frequently incorporates deglutitive dysfunction. Patients often have poor oral competency and frequently drool. Slow oral intake and poor motor control can make feeding difficult (Guily et al., 1994). Social improvement may be achieved in this patient population through the use of salivary diversion techniques such as the Wilkey procedure, which reroutes the parotid ducts posterior to the anterior tonsillar pillar via a submucosal tunnel (Halama, 1994; Young, Chapman, & Crewe, 1992; Figure 12–7). Less commonly, chorda tympani and/or Jacobson's nerve neurectomy or ligation of the parotid duct are performed (Mathog & Fleming, 1992). Removal of submandibular glands can aid in saliva control.

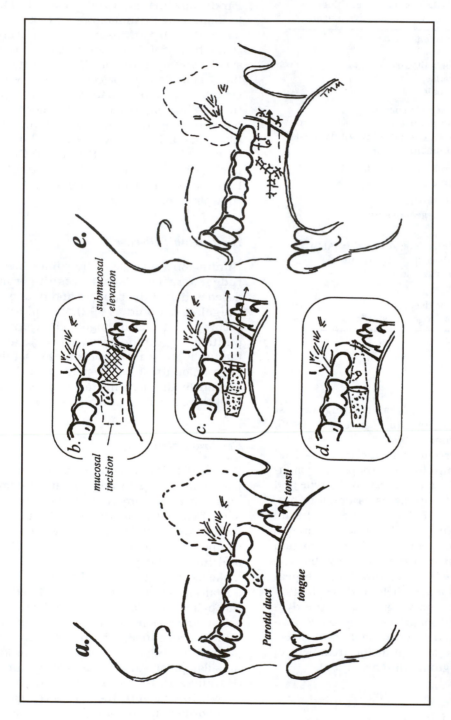

Figure 12-7. The Wilkey procedure **a.** Native state, **b.** Mucosal incisions and elevation **c.** Suture pull-through and flap rotation, **d.** Mucosal tunnel created, **a.** Final closure (arrow indicates salivary flow).

Peripheral Nerve Disorders

Cranial Nerves IX (Glossopharyngeal) and X (Vagus) Paralysis

Dysphagia associated with laryngeal paralysis may be mild to the point it largely goes unnoticed, or it may produce a life-threatening struggle for the patient to deal not only with ingested food, but also with the patient's own secretions. The degree of disability is related to the extent of injury to the vagus nerve and its branches as well as the anatomically and functionally closely related glossopharyngeal nerve. Other factors including age, coexisting swallowing deficits, and the general health of a patient influence the degree to which laryngeal paralysis affects deglutition.

The vagus nerve innervates muscles of the palate, pharynx, and larynx. Injury to the vagus nerve above its inferior ganglion (nodose ganglion), which is located immediately below the jugular foramen, will impair not only vocal fold mobility, but also the function of the pharyngeal constrictor muscles and the levator veli palatini, which aids in palatal closure (Netterville & Civantos, 1993). The nearby glossopharyngeal nerve also exits the jugular foramen and provides an important sensory branch, which passes through the middle constrictor muscle to innervate mucosa of the base of tongue and lateral pharyngeal mucosa. Loss of sensation in this region interferes with the reflexive involuntary pharyngeal stage of the swallow. Interruption of the sole motor branch of the glossopharyngeal nerve to the stylopharyngeus may also cause morbidity by impairing laryngeal elevation. Loss of sensation to the supraglottic larynx may also result from high vagal lesions affecting the superior laryngeal nerve. As with the glossopharyngeal nerve, loss of function of the sensory branch of the superior laryngeal nerve impedes swallowing by delaying or abolishing the reflexive response to the presence of material in its distribution. Tumors of the skull base and the surgery employed to treat them often result in a combined injury to both the vagus and glossopharyngeal nerves. For specific nerves insults see Table 12–4.

Compensation for loss of one component of the protective swallowing reflex often permits deglutition with little or no impairment. Incomplete glottic closure due to unilateral laryngeal paralysis may not result in aspiration if the laryngeal elevation coupled with an intact barrier of the epiglottis and aryepiglottic folds diverts material effectively from the vocal folds into the functioning pyriform sinuses.

The loss of function due to glossopharyngeal and vagal nerve sensory loss cannot be restored surgically. Conservative management to treat this deficit is employed with compensatory strategies designed to maximize remaining function. Head rotation toward the paralyzed side during a swallow helps to direct a food bolus away from the insensate side to the contralateral side where intact sensation will trigger a swallow reflex (Rasley et al., 1993). Neck flexion may help diminish exposure of the larynx to a food bolus and facilitate opening of the pharyngoesophageal segment (Castell, Castell, Schulta, & Georgeson, 1993). Modifications in food intake addressing size and consistency of the bolus are helpful. Swallowing strategies employing multiple swallows, breath holding, throat clearing, and coughing may be of benefit.

Bell's Palsy and Facial Nerve Paralysis

Facial nerve paralysis may result from trauma, infection, parotid- and skull-based tumors, or surgery. The primary manifestation related to deglutition is impaired oral closure and bolus control. Idiopathic facial nerve paralysis, or Bell's palsy, a diagnosis of exclusion, may result from viral infection (Burgess, Michaels, Bale, & Smith, 1994). Electroneurography is employed when the diagnosis is presumed in order to measure spontaneous and voluntary muscle action potentials. Treatment of facial nerve paralysis includes steroids and nerve decompression when indicated.

TABLE 12–4. Clinical results after cranial nerve injury.

Nerve Injury	Result
Facial Nerve	Slight weakness in bolus control, weak lip closure
Trigeminal Nerve (motor)	Slight weakness in mastication
Hypoglossal Nerve	Bolus control problems
	Crippled swallow if bilateral
Glossopharyngeal nerve (sensory)	Failure to trigger the pharyngeal stage of the swallow, premature spill of material from the mouth into the airway
Glossopharyngeal nerve (motor)	Deficit from loss of function not great secondary to intact function of other elevators of the larynx
Superior laryngeal nerve (sensory)	Loss of protective glottic closure and cough reflex protecting airway from material on the supraglottic larynx
Vagus nerve (motor)	Inadequate velopharyngeal closure, nasal regurgitation
	Incomplete clearing of residue in the hypopharynx, pooling of material above the level of the vocal folds, aspiration once the vocal folds open
	Inadequate glottic closure during pharyngeal transit

Neurofibromatosis

Neurofibromatosis type 2 is a rare autosomal dominant disorder that presents in early adulthood. The classical clinical presentation is hearing loss associated with bilateral acoustic neuromas. Dysphagia results from neuromas that develop on multiple cranial nerves. Skull base surgery required to treat this disease may also lead to dysphagia. Most patients eventually die of tumor-induced brain stem compression. Treatment is surgical resection of tumor masses early in the disease course and supportive in the late stages (Tees, Lofchy, & Rutka, 1992).

Neuromuscular Junction

Myasthenia Gravis

Myasthenia gravis is an immune disorder in which antibodies to acetylcholine receptors on the neuromuscular end plate are produced. This condition affects voluntary muscles, with progressive weakness during repetitive use. Most patients will present with head and neck symptoms (ptosis, diplopia, dysarthria, dysphagia). Twelve percent of patients

with myasthenia gravis will present with dysphagia symptoms, while approximately 20% of patients with myasthenia gravis have dysphagia (Carpenter, McDonald, & Howard, 1979). Muscles of mastication and pharyngeal muscles fatigue with repetitive movements as feeding progresses (Brin & Younger, 1988). Diagnosis is frequently made by detecting acetylcholine receptor antibodies in the blood or by a Tensilon challenge test, which uses a short-acting anticholinesterase to potentiate acetylcholine activity at the motor unit end plate. Anticholinesterases and immunosuppressants are used to treat this condition. Patients respond well to eating smaller, more frequent meals during the day after taking the appropriate medication.

Neuromuscular Disorders

Amyotrophic Lateral Sclerosis

Amyotrophic lateral sclerosis is characterized by degeneration of both upper and lower motor neurons in the central nervous system. Patients exhibiting only lower motor neuron signs will present with wasting and/or weakness of muscles, while patients who exhibit only upper motor neuron involvement present only with weakness (Brin & Younger, 1988). Dysphagia is often an early symptom of this disease (Guily et al., 1994). Treatment is mainly supportive. Cricopharyngeal myotomy maybe useful in the early stages of the disease when oropharyngeal motor strength is relatively intact. Once the capacity for speech is lost the role of tracheal-esophageal separation procedures increases. As the disease progresses aspiration pneumonia is common.

Polio and Postpolio Syndrome

Although polio has virtually been irradicated within the United States, patients inflicted with polio decades earlier may present in midlife with a new onset of generalized progressive weakness fatigue and pain (postpolio syndrome). It is estimated that 20 to 25% of these patients will have dysphagia (Coelho & Ferrante, 1988; Jones, Bucholz, Ravich, & Donner, 1992). Several theories have been proposed, including weakness secondary to overworked motor neurons, which survived the acute attack of polio, and age-related weakness in the context of a previous neuromuscular insult (Coelho & Ferrante, 1988; Guily et al., 1994; Jones et al., 1992).

Multiple Sclerosis

Multiple sclerosis, a demyelinating disease of the brain and spinal cord, characterized by periods of remission and exacerbation, can be associated with dysphagia in the late phase (Brin & Younger, 1988; Guily et al., 1994). Initially patients present with visual disturbances, bladder symptoms, and motor or sensory deficits (Guily et al., 1994). Diagnosis is made with the identification of plaques in the white matter of the brain on magnetic resonant imaging (MRI) examination, or by abnormal antibodies in the cerebrospinal fluid by lumbar puncture. Immunosuppressant therapy for exacer-

bations may have some limited benefit (Brin et al., 1988).

Muscular Disorders

The cricopharyngeal muscle plays an integral role in the normal swallow through its precisely timed relaxation and contraction coupled to pharyngeal constrictor activity. The cricopharyngeus, innervated by the vagopharyngeal plexus, has been reported to function in the initial propulsion of the bolus through the esophagus (Calcaterra, Kadell, & Ward, 1975). Achalasia (failure to relax), or malfunction of the cricopharyngeus secondary to a number of neuromuscular and muscular disorders (myasthenia gravis, thyrotoxicosis, muscular dystrophy, polio, stroke, Parkinson's disease, oculopharyngeal dystrophy, inclusion body myositis, and Steinert myotonic dystrophy), may lead to dysphagia and secondary aspiration (Brin & Younger, 1988; Darrow, Hoffman, Barnes, & Wiles, 1992; Guily et al., 1994).

Surgical Intervention for Neuromuscular Disorders

Surgical intervention in the treatment of dysphagia related to neurologic and neuromuscular disorders is limited. The most common procedure performed is the cricopharyngeal myotomy. Other procedures directed toward the treatment of neuromuscular diseases include closure of the velopharyngeal port and glottic restorative procedures.

Cricopharyngeal Myotomy

A cricopharyngeal myotomy diminishes the relative obstruction induced by a noncompliant or neuromuscularly impaired cricopharyngeus muscle (Figure 12–8). This procedure consists of incising the cricopharyngeal muscle down to the level of the submucosa, usually including the inferior portion of the inferior constrictor and the superior portion of the esophageal musculature, which results in

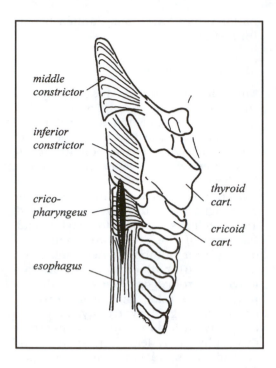

Figure 12–8. Cricopharyngeal myotomy.

permanent relaxation of the cricopharyngeus. (Bonanno, 1971; Brin & Younger, 1988; Guily et al., 1994). Success is dependent on some degree of intact pharyngeal and tongue musculature in order to generate the necessary pressure to initiate bolus transfer.

With life-threatening aspiration from dysphagia, separation of the airway and pharynx may be imperative. Tracheoesophageal diversion or laryngectomy may be necessary. The tracheoesophageal diversion first described by Lindeman (1975) completely separates the pharynx and esophagus, preventing aspiration (Figure 12–9). This procedure has the advantage over total laryngectomy in that the diversion is potentially reversible.

Closure of the Velopharyngeal Port

Inadequate function of the levator veli palatini unilaterally, with attendant nasal regurgitation, can be corrected by partial closure of the velopharyngeal port. Although the ability to pass air through the nose may be somewhat impaired, the creation of an adhesion between the palate and posterior pharyngeal wall may restore the closure during the reflexive pharyngeal phase of swallowing (Netterville & Civantos, 1993).

Restoration of Glottic Competence

Inadequate approximation of the vocal folds from laryngeal paralysis impairs swallowing because of failure of the glottis to function as a barrier. Also, inability to develop subglottic pressures results in cough ineffective in clearing aspirated material. Surgical techniques to restore glottic closure are referred to as *laryngoplastic phonosurgery*. The three basic approaches are (a) injection laryngoplasty (b) laryngeal framework surgery, and (c) arytenoid adduction (Benninger et al., 1994). Injection procedures add bulk to the vocal fold when a substance (Teflon, fat, Gelfoam) is injected into the paraglottic space either transorally or percutaneously (Figure 12–10). Laryngeal framework surgery requires a small neck incision for direct access to the laryngeal cartilage. Vocal fold medialization is accomplished by decreasing the size of the functional paraglottic space by inserting an appropriate-sized block of cartilage, silicone, or other material through a window in the cartilage adjacent to the true vocal fold (Figure 12–11). The arytenoid adduction procedure takes advantage of the ligamentous attachments of the arytenoid and cricoid cartilages. Sutures are placed through the muscular process of the arytenoid and brought out through or under the thyroid cartilage, reproducing the action of the thyroarytenoid and lateral cricoarytenoid muscles, thus closing the glottis by rotating the vocal process medially (Figure 12–12). (The arytenoid pivots on the cricoid and rotates medially.)

Miscellaneous

Spasmodic dysphonia is a neuromuscular abnormality of unclear etiology, which produces strained or tremulous speech. A small percentage of patients with this dis-

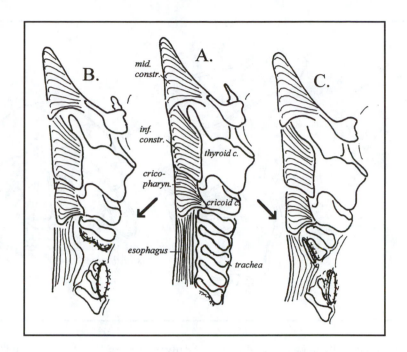

Figure 12–9. Lindeman procedure **a.** Natural state. **b.** Tracheoesophageal diversion with subglottic pouch. **c.** Tracheoesophageal diversion with tracheal stump-esophageal fistula.

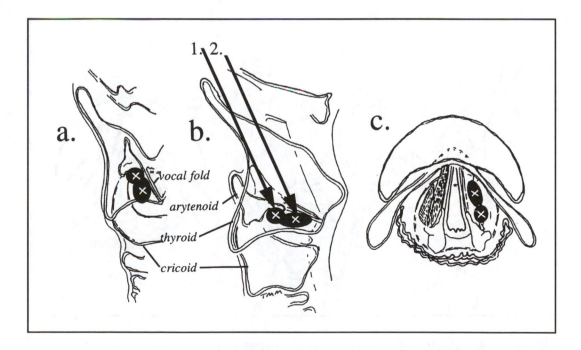

Figure 12–10. Teflon injection; needle direction and injection location: **a.** Anterior-posterior view. **b.** Lateral view. **c.** superior direct view.

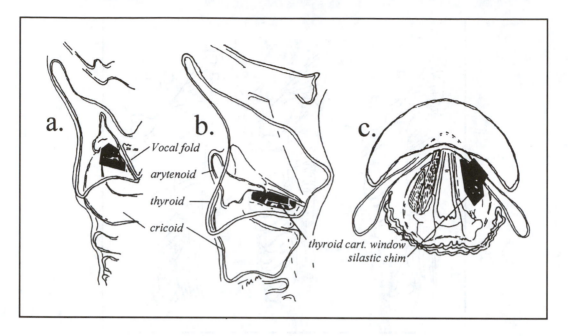

Figure 12–11. Type I Thyroplasty, vocal fold medialization utilizing silastic shim: **a.** Anterior-posterior view. **b.** Lateral view. **c.** Superior direct view.

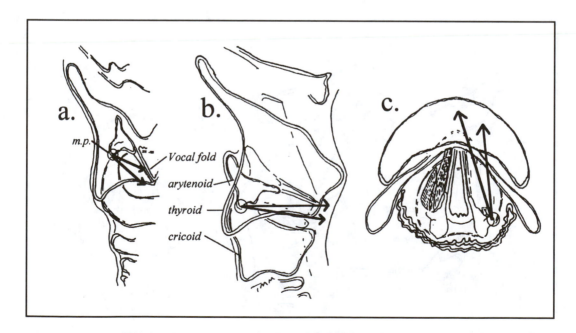

Figure 12–12. Arytenoid adduction: **a.** Anterior-posterior view. **b.** Lateral view. **c.** Superior direct view.

order will have some degree of dysphagia. A similar disease entity, *oculopharyngeal dystonia*, also produces bolus-manipulation problems. Treatment of both of these conditions consists of intramuscular botulinum toxin injections. These treatments result in muscular paralysis, which aids in the dystonia but may significantly increase the magnitude of the dysphagia for some time after the injection (Palmer et al., 1995).

Other neurologic disorders that may impair swallowing function include Eaton-Lambert syndrome, acute botulism, Guillain-Barré syndrome, porphyria, increased intracranial pressure, syringomyelia, tumor, chorea, tardive dyskinesia, and other dystonias (Brin & Younger, 1988).

INFECTIOUS DISEASES OF THE OROPHARYNX CAUSING DIFFICULTIES WITH SWALLOWING

Mucosal Inflammations and Infections

Many inflammatory conditions affect the oropharynx and lead to dysphagia and odynophagia. Although the mouth is not a sterile environment, the delicate balance of normal flora may at times be offset and serve as the catalyst in the development of oropharyngeal disease (Table 12–5).

Ludwig's Angina

Infections in the sublingual or submandibular glands occur when foreign bodies or food particles lodge in crypts in the floor of the mouth and result in soft-tissue cellulitis (Ludwig's angina). Maintenance of an adequate airway, antibiotic therapy, and exploration and drainage of infected areas should be prompt to prevent spread of infection deep into the neck and mediastinum. Antibiotics are directed at anaerobic organisms, including streptococci, staphylococci, and bacterioids, as these

TABLE 12–5. Infectious causes of oropharyngeal dysphagia.

Mucositis and cellulitis
Streptococcus
Diphtheria
Candidiasis
Epiglottitis
Herpes zoster
Ludwig's angina
Vincent's angina
Ulcer and abscess
Major apthous ulcer
Peritonsillar abscess
Retropharyngeal abscess
Buccal space abscess
Submandibular abscess
Epiglottic abscess
Tuberculosis
Systemic infections
HIV
Lyme disease
Tetanus

are the most common microorganisms in the mouth (Fritsch & Klein, 1992).

Pharyngeal Ulcers and Abscesses

Deep-space infections are serious complications of pharyngeal cellulitis. These parapharyngeal infections include peritonsillar abscess, retropharyngeal abscess, floor of mouth abscess, buccal-space abscess, and deep neck infections. The most common of these infections is the peritonsillar abscess, with its peak incidence in adolescence and young adulthood; possible serious complications include meningitis, brain abscess, and carotid hemorrhage (Garino & Ryan, 1987). Retropharyngeal and parapharyngeal abscesses occur frequently in young children secondary to suppuration of bacterial lymphadenitis in deep neck tissue planes. Buccal-space and floor of mouth infections result from dental infections and are significantly more prevalent in the adult population. Treatment is required to prevent further dissemination of infection. In all of these conditions patients present with pain, fever, and dysphagia secondary to mass effect.

Herpes Simplex Virus

Similarly herpes simplex virus (both HSV-1 and HSV-2) may present as mucosal lesions on mucous membranes in the oral cavity, vallecula, and the pyriform sinuses. Lesions may be quite painful (Barr, 1992). Acyclovir is often used to decrease viral shedding and pain especially in the immunocompromised patient.

Systemic Infections

Human Immunodeficiency Virus (HIV)

Infections with HIV may present in the form of a variety of fungal, viral, bacterial, or even neoplastic lesions that affect the head and neck region (Barr, 1992). *Candida albicans* is a common opportunistic infection afflicting these immunocompromised patients. The inflammatory response from yeast overgrowth can lead to odynophagia (see also Chapter 13.) Major apthous ulcers also occur in this group of patients, producing significant pain, and dysphagia. Treatment consists of intralesional and topical steroids as well as topical anesthetic agents.

Lyme Disease

Lyme disease is a systemic illness resulting from infection with the spirochete Borrelia burgdorferi. It may manifest itself with a variety of otolaryngologic symptoms (Moscatello, Worden, Nadelmand , Wormser, & Lucente, 1991). Specifically, facial nerve paralysis and throat pain may contribute to dysphagia. Diagnosis is made by the detection of antibody to borrelia. Treatment of choice is antibiotic therapy with tetracycline,

doxycycline, penicillin, or amoxicillin (Goldfarb & Sataloff, 1994).

Tetanus

Tetanus is the result of an anaerobic, spore-forming, gram-positive rod (*Clos-tridium tetani*; Wang & Karmody, 1985). Patients commonly present with muscle rigidity, specifically trismus and dysphagia. Diagnosis is based on clinical findings. A history of wound infection maybe helpful but frequently cannot be elicited. Treatment is supportive and includes surgical debridement of infected tissues, parenteral antibiotics, antiserum, and diazepam.

HEAD AND NECK TUMORS AND MALIGNANCIES

Almost all tumors of the head and neck will produce some degree of dysphagia. The benign masses such as lipomas or goiters may create a partial obstruction of the pharynx secondary to external compression and result in dysphagia. Other lesions such as the paragangliomas (carotid body tumors and glomus tumors) will interfere with cranial nerve function, resulting in sensory and motor deficits, thus inducing dysphagia. Dysphagia secondary to local pain occurs with mucosally based malignancies (Table 12–6).

Mucosal Malignancies

The most prevalent tumors of the head and neck are mucosal malignancies. The dysphagia induced by these tumors results from tumor mass, tumor-related tissue fixation, local inflammation, and pain. Occasionally tumors invade muscles and nerves and thus produce neuromuscular swallowing problems. Many patients continue to eat and present only after mass or pain produces marked dysphagia. Tumors arising in the tongue base and the supraglottic larynx are notorious for remaining "silent" and presenting only after nodal spread.

TABLE 12–6. Head and neck tumors and malignancies.

Mucosal malignancy
Oral cavity
Oropharynx
Larynx
Hypopharynx

Neck masses

Salivary gland tumors

Thyroid
Malignancy
Goiter
Lingual thyroid

Neuroendocrine

The treatment of these malignancies causes more dysphagia than the original tumor. Patients rarely return to their preoperative swallowing state after surgical intervention for oropharyngeal or laryngeal tumors (Logemann et al., 1993; Pauloski et al., 1994; Pauloski et al., 1993; Rademaker et al., 1993). The magnitude of the postoperative swallowing dysfunction is related to the site of the primary lesion, extent of the surgical resection, structures involved in the surgical resection (e.g., mucosa, muscle, nerve, bone), and type of reconstruction performed. Defects in structures high and lateral in the oral cavity such as the palate, upper alveolar ridge, and buccal mucosa are better compensated for than defects in the lower oral cavity and oropharynx. Prosthetic devices and rehabilitation can easily alleviate defects in static structures like the hard palate (Funk et al., 1995). The cheek and the lateral wall of the oral cavity, with their primary role of bolus retention, can be reconstructed without production of significant dysphagia. In contrast, the tongue and pharynx are dynamic structures with both sensory and motor functions crucial to normal swallowing. Surgical intervention involving these structures may cripple swallowing.

Oral and Oropharyngeal Malignancies

Floor of Mouth and Tongue

The tongue plays an integral role in bolus manipulation, bolus reduction, and propulsion of the bolus at the initiation of the pharyngeal phase of swallow. A hierarchical approach to the surgical treatment of tongue carcinoma is imperative. In 1994 Urken and colleagues presented their systematic approach to functional reconstruction after surgical intervention for tongue and oropharyngeal malignancies. These authors state, "The ultimate goal of the reconstruction of the anatomic region is to duplicate the form and function of the normal part" (p. 590). The complexities of the tongue and surrounding soft tissues make this goal beyond the reach of even the best head and neck surgeons. The preservation of normal motion, normal sensation, and normal muscular strength and bulk must be considered when contemplating tongue resection. The necessity to maintain sensation in the oral cavity and oropharyngeal mucosa is intuitively obvious. In almost all reconstructions, a significant amount of nonsensate material is added to the oral cavity. Patients with large degrees of nonsensate tissue have significant difficulty eating and swallowing primarily owing to their inability to recognize the presence of food material and, therefore, appropriately manipulate it for an effective swallow. Newer techniques such as the sensate radial forearm free flap allow the surgeon to reconstruct larger defects and provide sensation to portions of the oral cavity (Urken, Vickery, Weinberg, & Biller, 1990, Urken, & Biller, 1994).

Limited Glossectomy

When surgical resection includes one fourth to one third of the mobile tongue and a small portion of the base of tongue, the best reconstructive option is usually a skin graft placed over the raw tongue muscle (Figure 12–13). This procedure

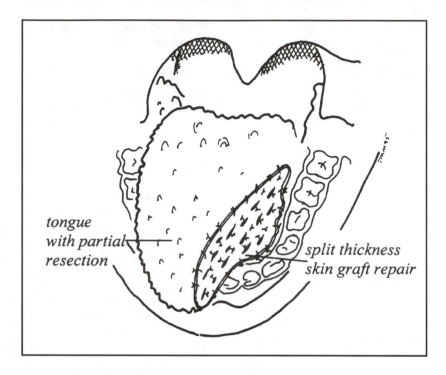

Figure 12–13. Limited glossectomy with skin graft closure.

allows for continued mobility of the remaining tongue and maintains intact proprioceptive sensation along the margins of the resection. Direct primary closure and closure by secondary intention are also options; yet limited mobility of the tongue secondary to scar contracture may result (Urken, Moscoso, Lawson, & Biller, 1994).

Small defects of the tongue base without resection of the mobile tongue are closed primarily. This procedure can be performed with posterior displacement of a portion of the mobile tongue as well as medialization of portions of pharyngeal mucosa. Once the defects extend beyond one third of the tongue base, reconstructive options are usually extended to the use of distant tissues. Independent of the reconstruction technique used, the most important factor with regard to swallowing rehabilitation is the extent of tongue resection (Hirano et al., 1992; McConnel et al., 1994).

Hemiglossectomy

The glossectomy that requires resection of one half or more of the mobile tongue or a significant portion of the base of tongue with portions of the mobile tongue requires a reconstructive procedure using distant tissues. Attempts are directed toward providing mobility of the normally innervated contralateral tongue and restoring sensation to the reconstructed area. The most useful reconstructive technique currently available is the sensate radial forearm free flap. This flap, first reported in the Chinese literature, was popularized by Urken and others during the early 1990s and has since gained wide acceptance (Urken et al., 1990; Urken, & Biller, 1994; Figure 12–14).

Other options for the repair of the hemiglossectomy include the use of skin graft or pedicle myocutaneous flaps such as the pectoralis major. The primary dis-

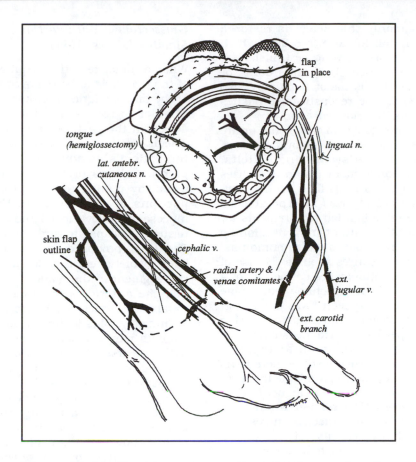

tongue
(hemiglossectomy)

lat. antebr.
cutaneous n.

skin flap
outline

cephalic v.

radial artery &
venae comitantes

flap
in place

lingual n.

ext.
jugular v.

ext. carotid
branch

Figure 12–14. Hemiglossectomy with radial forearm free flap reconstruction.

advantage of these techniques is the inability to introduce sensation. Limitations of tongue mobility and bulk may also result. (See below for surgical technique of hemiglossectomy.)

TECHNIQUES OF HEMIGLOSSECTOMY. The hemiglossectomy is utilized in the treatment of limited tongue carcinomas without mandibular involvement. The majority of these tumors range from 2–4 cm in size. Hemiglossectomy when performed with a neck dissection allows for portions of the procedure to be conducted transcervically. Anterior, superior, and lateral tongue incisions are made transorally. Lateral incision may extend through the mylohyoid and into the neck.

The posterior mucosal and muscular incisions are completed with the tongue drawn under the mandible into the cervical region. Once the resection is completed the defect is closed using transferred distant tissue.

Total Glossectomy

When glossectomy consists of total resection of the mobile tongue with the tongue base being retained, the reconstructive techniques are similar to the hemiglossectomy. Similarly, after a near total tongue base resection with retention of the mobile segment of the anterior tongue, sensation and bulk are felt to be important elements of the reconstruction.

Most commonly this defect is restored with the radial forearm free flap, which allows a sensory nerve to be transferred. Free rectus muscle, latissimus dorsi, or pedicled pectoralis major flaps may also be utilized. These reconstructive tissues provide bulk, but not sensation.

Total glossectomy, in which the entire tongue is removed, creates by far one of the most serious swallowing deficits. Reconstruction in many instances utilizes pedicled myocutaneous flaps. In the past, total laryngectomy was incorporated as one of the rehabilitation requirements for preventing the patient from developing life-threatening aspiration pneumonias. Additional procedures such as the use of extended epiglottoplasties or the use of a three-quarters laryngectomy with some preservation of speech have been suggested; however, these patients also require a permanent tracheostomy, and the lack of tongue as an articulator severely limits speech clarity. There is no reconstructive material available to reproduce the loss of the total tongue. Muscle transfers even with reinnervation have been shown to be ineffective in restoration of mobility. The use of free lateral arm flaps or lateral thigh flaps have been suggested in restoration of sensation and bulk (Urken et al., 1994). (See below for surgical technique of a total glossectomy.)

TECHNIQUES OF TOTAL GLOSSECTOMY. Total glossectomy is usually performed with concurrent neck dissection. A cervical skin flap is raised to the level of the inferior aspect of the mandible, allowing exposure of the floor of mouth musculature. Anterior incisions are made through the floor of mouth allowing the tongue to be released and visible through the neck incision. The complete glossectomy is carried out by removing tongue base musculature from the hyoid, glossopharyngeus, and styloglossus. The total glossectomy defect is reconstructed with distant tissue (pedicled pectoralis major, free rectus muscle, free latissimus muscle, free lateral arm, or radial forearm flaps).

Glossectomies With Partial Mandibular Resections

When a tumor resection requires portions of the mandible to be removed for control of the disease, a decision has to be made whether to reconstruct the mandibular defect. In the past, posterior mandibular defects were not reconstructed, allowing the patient's mandible to "swing." This practice allows primary closure of the defect by pulling together the residual portions of the tongue to the buccal mucosa and allows facial and cervical soft tissue to collapse toward the oral cavity. The defect produced by this procedure is both cosmetic and functional. The posterior segment of the mandible is deficient and the anterior segment is displaced toward the defect, leading to lower facial asymmetry. Mastication is also altered. Patients may compensate over time and with the use of glide appliances and training some degree of mastication can be restored (Figure 12–15). An advantage of this type of technique includes maintenance of sensation throughout the oral mucosa. Tongue mobility is somewhat limited; however, the decrease in size of the oral cavity allows for adequate bolus manipulation and restoration of swallow. Attempts have been made to restore posterior segmental bone defects with reconstruction bars combined with soft tissue reconstruction using a sensate radial forearm free flap. This technique has the advantage of providing better mastication as well as an improved cosmetic appearance of the posterolateral facial contours. Disadvantages of this reconstructive technique include a 6-month delay to regain sensation and, depending on the extent of the bony defect, risk of both extra-oral or intra-oral plate exposures or breakage over time.

As the size of the mandibular defect increases and as the mandibular defect moves toward the midline, bony reconstruction is indicated in almost all cases. Fibular or iliac crest free tissue transfer are principally utilized in this type of

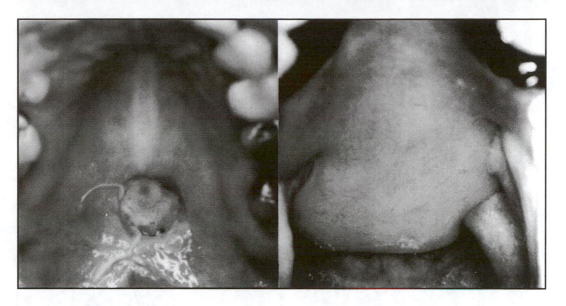

Figure 12–15. Palatal repair with obturator, (*left*) palate lesion preoperative, (*right*) obturator in place postoperative.

reconstruction. Scapular free tissue transfer is an alternative method of bone reconstruction. The advantages of the scapular and fibular free flap reconstructions include the availability of relatively loose, pliable soft tissue that can be harvested to allow for portions of the floor of mouth and tongue to be reconstructed simultaneously. The latissimus dorsi muscle, with the scapular bone and overlying skin, can be harvested and used for very large defects (Urken & Sullivan, 1995; Figure 12–16). The primary disadvantage of the scapula is its thin bone, making it less useful for dental osseointegrated implants. Other limitations to combined bone/soft tissue flaps include diminished ability to restore sensation. Oftentimes patients remain dependent on gastrostomy tubes for the maintenance of their nutrition. Over time most patients will learn to take small quantities of food and liquids transorally.

Owing to the importance of midface and mandibular contour regarding patient appearance, when the surgery extends to a near total glossectomy with mandi-bulectomy, the reconstructive goals orient toward the cosmetic result of the repair. The primary functional goals then become prevention of aspiration by anterior laryngeal suspension and achievement of adequate bulk in the oral cavity. Oftentimes these patients will also undergo postoperative radiation therapy, limiting the saliva production and perhaps thus decreasing the potential for salivary aspirations. Most of these patients do not have the option of returning to oral intake for nutritional maintenance. The enjoyment of food is lost, as the total glossectomy eliminates the ability for taste. As with total glossectomy, the addition of total laryngectomy may be indicated to prevent life-threatening aspiration.

Tonsil and Pharynx

The tonsillar fossa is a common site for squamous cell cancer as well as lymphoma. Lymphoma and small superficial squamous cell lesions are oftentimes treated with radiation therapy with good

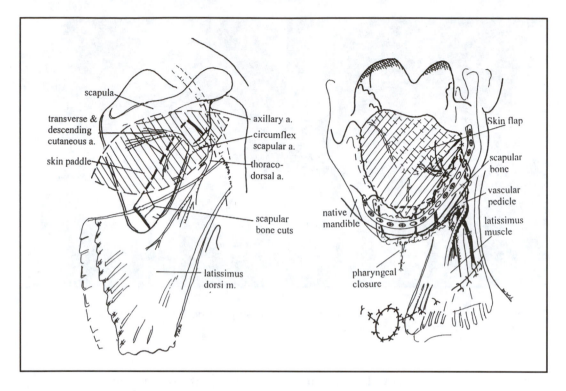

Figure 12–16. Oral cavity and neck reconstruction with free tissue transfer (latissimus dorsi with scapular bone and skin).

cure rates, whereas the larger lesions usually require surgery or combined therapy (radiation and surgery).

The extent of resection and type of closure will affect the swallow recovery (Hirano et al., 1992). Adynamic tissue in the pharynx due to denervation or reconstruction affects the clearance of the bolus from the pharynx, leaving the patient at risk for aspirating the residual material.

Larger lateral pharyngeal tumors oftentimes include portions of the tongue, tonsil, palate, and posterior pharynx. These larger defects require the implantation of distant tissue to protect the carotid artery and decrease the risk of fistula formation. Attempts at primary closure can be made if the posterior portion of the mandible is included in the resection. The most common closure materials when considering distant material are pectoral muscle and radial forearm free tissue. The advantages of the radial forearm tissue use include

the ability to better approximate the complex form of the palate, pharyngeal wall, and tongue base as well as transfer of a sensory nerve, which can be anastomosed to the glossopharyngeal, lingual, or superior laryngeal nerves. This tissue, however, still lacks the intrinsic mobility of the tissue it replaces.

Laryngeal Malignancies

Laryngeal cancers are described as supraglottic, glottic, or subglottic based on the epicenter of the lesion (Figure 12–17). Surgical treatment of laryngeal cancer includes a variety of well-described partial resection procedures in addition to total laryngectomy.

All major laryngeal procedures have some postoperative dysphagia risk associated with them. With partial laryngectomy the risk is primarily one of aspiration,

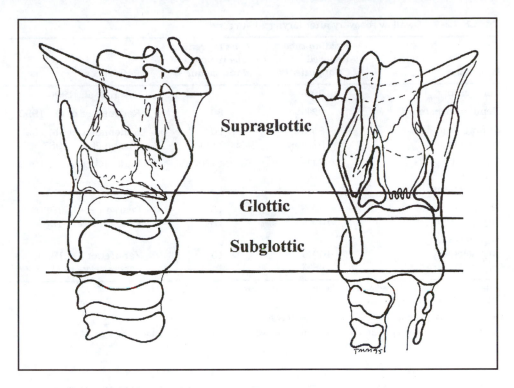

Figure 12–17. Categorization of laryngeal cancer: supraglottic (epiglottis to level of true vocal fold), glottic (true fold level and 1 cm below), and subglottic (1 cm below glottis to inferior cricoid border).

while after total laryngectomy the risk is pharyngeal stenosis (Kaplan, Dobie, & Cummings 1981; McConnel, Cerenko, & Mendelsohn, 1988). The risk increases in both cases as the magnitude of resection increases (Table 12–7).

Supraglottic Malignancies

Surgical treatment of supraglottic primary tumors of the larynx usually involves the standard supraglottic laryngectomy in which the epiglottis, the pre-epiglottic space, the aryepiglottic folds, and false vocal folds are removed (Figure 12–18). The risk of aspiration postoperatively is somewhat reduced by including laryngeal suspension as part of the closure. Aspiration risks after supraglottic laryngectomy have been reported from 50% to 67%, and aspiration pneumonia occurs in approximately 6% of patients in this group (Freeman, Marks, & Ogura, 1979; Litton & Leonard, 1969). Hirano and colleagues (1992) reported an 8% rate of secondary total laryngectomy to treat chronic aspiration. Thus, there is an important role for swallowing therapy after supraglottic laryngectomy. Patients are taught special swallowing techniques, such as the "supraglottic swallow," which encourages early stronger glottic closure and post swallow airway clearance (Logemann, 1983). Extension of the resection of the tongue base during supraglottic laryngectomy increases the aspiration risk; most reports indicate that one third of the tongue can be resected with a supraglottic laryngectomy (Rademaker et al., 1993). (See below for surgical details on standard supraglottic laryngectomy.)

Reports of laser supraglottic laryngectomy have also appeared. The primary utili-

TABLE 12–7. Swallow recovery after laryngeal surgery.

Procedure	Feeding tube removed (% of patients)	Time to feeding tube removed (days, mean)	References
Cordectomy	100%		Olsen et al., 1990[a]
Hemilaryngectomy	92%	30	Rademaker et al., 1993
Supraglottic laryngectomy	80% 92%	90 < 30 days	Rademaker et al., 1993 Hirano et al., 1987
Extended supraglottic laryngectomy	74%	150 to 335	Rademaker et al., 1993
Three-quarter laryngectomy	100% 100%	13 15	Pearson et al., 1980[b] Pearson et al., 1986[c]
Supracricoid laryngectomy	100% 98%	15 15	Zanaret et al., 1993 Laccourreye et al., 1990[d]

[a] Authors note normal swallow in patients postprocedure.

[b] Total of seven patients in study.

[c] Five out of 42 patients required revision surgery for aspiration.

[d] Authors state 25% of patients required temporary gastrostomy tubes (ranging from 1 to 24 months).

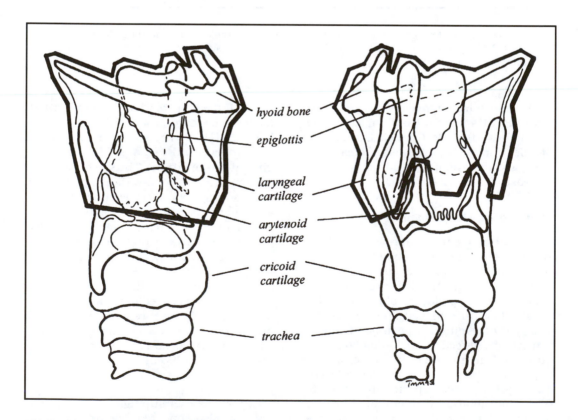

Figure 12–18. Standard supraglottic laryngectomy resection outline.

ty of this procedure is in treating small epiglottic lesions. The postoperative dysphagia has been described as minimal (Davis, Kelly, & Hayes, 1991).

Extension of the supraglottic laryngectomy (the supracricoid laryngectomy) has also been popularized. This procedure allows for additional resections of the laryngeal cartilage, anterior two thirds of the true vocal folds, and paraglottic space (Laccourreye, Laccourreye, Weinstein, Menard, & Brasnu, 1990; Figure 12–19). The patients will retain a laryngeal remnant that allows for speech and an airway. Useful swallowing is retained in 90% of patients. Swallowing rehabilitation may take up to 6 months for some patients. (See below for surgical details.)

TECHNIQUE FOR SUPRAGLOTTIC LARYNGECTOMY. The standard supraglottic laryngectomy consists of resection of laryngeal structures above the level of the true vocal folds including the superior portion of the laryngeal cartilage, the false vocal folds, the epiglottis, aryepiglottic folds, and pre-epiglottic space. A horizontal neck incision is created to expose the underlying thyroid cartilage. Strap muscles and thyroid perichondrium are deflected inferiorly, allowing direct access to the thyroid cartilage. Tongue-base musculature is excised from the hyoid, allowing entry into the pharynx at the level of the vallecula. The epiglottis is visualized and grasped, allowing direct access to the supraglottic tumor. Inferior cuts are made at the level of the mid-thyroid cartilage just above the anterior commissure. The resection is completed by making lateral cuts through the superior aspect of the pyriform mucosa and along

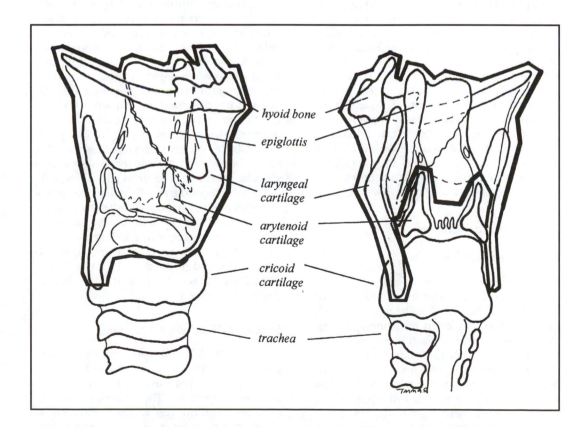

hyoid bone

epiglottis

laryngeal cartilage

arytenoid cartilage

cricoid cartilage

trachea

Figure 12–19. Supracricoid laryngectomy resection outline.

the aryepiglottic folds just above the arytenoids. The laryngeal remnant consists of the inferior portion of the thyroid cartilage, the intact true vocal folds, as well as the arytenoid cartilages. This remnant is elevated and suspended from the tongue base utilizing multiple interrupted sutures. Direct mucosal closure is only accomplished at lateral portions and over the exposed arytenoids. The supraglottic laryngectomy may be extended to include portions of the tongue base or pyriform sinus, depending on the extent tumor. A temporary tracheotomy is required during the postoperative period.

TECHNIQUE FOR THE SUPRACRICOID LARYNGECTOMY. The surgical approach for the supracricoid laryngectomy is similar to that of the supraglottic procedure. The resection includes the entire laryngeal cartilage, true and false vocal folds, preepiglottic fat, and the paraglottic space bilaterally. A portion of the epiglottis may be retained for reconstruction, which consists of inferior displacement of the epiglottis with attachment to the retained anterior cricoid ring. This technique is referred to as a *cricoepiglottopexy*. Without retention of an epiglottic remnant reconstruction consists of approximating the anterior cricoid ring to the hyoid bone and tongue base. This procedure is referred to as a *cricohyoidopexy*. A temporary tracheotomy is required in the postoperative period.

True Glottic Cancer

Partial Laryngectomy

Early true glottic cancers can be treated equally well with radiation therapy or surgery. The surgical techniques include laser cordectomy, open horizontal hemilaryngectomy, and standard hemilaryngectomy (Figure 12–20). Closure is usually accomplished with insertion of the overlying strap muscles into the larynx. Swallow recovery is similar to that with supraglottic procedures (Kronenberger & Meyers, 1994; Schoenrock, King, Everts, Schneider, &

Shumrick, 1972; Weaver & Fleming, 1978). (See below for surgical details.)

The three-quarter laryngectomy has been described to surgically treat tumor with unilateral posterior extension (Pearson, Woods, & Hartman, 1980). The surgery includes resection of a portion of the cricoid cartilage. The defect is then closed to produce a "myo-mucosal shunt" that allows for speech. The shunt is too small for use as a primary airway, thus patients require a permanent tracheostomy. The primary risk is of aspiration which occurs in 4 to 40% of patients (Netterville, 1995, personal communication; Pearson 1986). Revision surgery may alleviate the problems; however, a completion laryngectomy is required for refractory aspiration.

TECHNIQUE FOR CORDECTOMY. A cordectomy can be performed either through an open neck approach or by utilizing a rigid laryngoscope to visualize the vocal folds. The goal of this procedure is to provide complete excision of the tumor mass, including a margin of normal tissue, and obtain a specimen for pathologic review. The transoral approach requires the use of specially designed instruments and the CO_2 laser, whereas the open approach necessitates a small neck incision followed by a vertical laryngeal split. The vocal fold lesion is removed under direct visualization and the defect is allowed to granulate secondarily. The open cordectomy approach can be extended to encompass portions of the anterior commissure as well as a segment of the laryngeal cartilage. If the tumors extend onto the arytenoid cartilage or deeply invade the paraglottic space, a standard hemilaryngectomy is indicated.

Standard Hemilaryngectomy

The standard hemilaryngectomy encompasses resection of half of the laryngeal cartilage, the true and false vocal fold, and one arytenoid. The anterior commissure and one quarter of the contralateral vocal fold may be included in the resec-

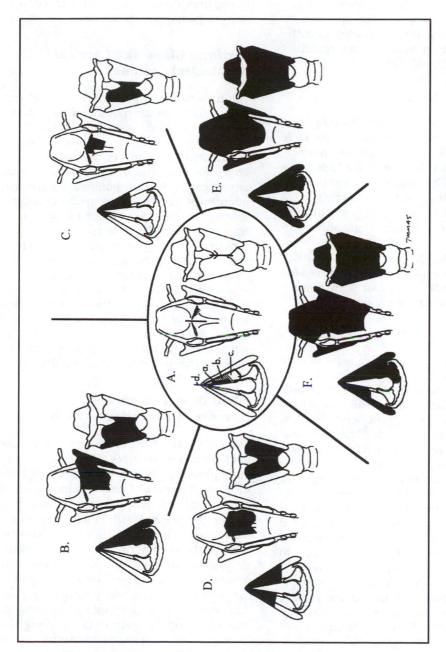

Figure 12-20. Surgical techniques utilized for true glottic cancer; extent of resection. **A.** Cordectomy. Endoscopic approach with or without CO_2 laser: (*a*) superficial excisional biopsy, (*b*) deep excisional biopsy, (*c*) complete cordectomy, (*d*) laryngofissure approach. **B.** Hemilaryngectomy. **C.** Fronto-lateral partial. **D.** Anterior partial. **E.** Anterior subtotal; **F.** Pearson's three-quarter.

tion specimen. A posterior strut of laryngeal cartilage is occasionally left in place along with the attached constrictor muscles. Reconstruction is accomplished by moving overlying strap muscles into the laryngeal lumen and closing retained laryngeal perichondrium.

Total Laryngectomy

Dysphagia after total laryngectomy has been attributed to stenosis and muscle spasm as well as to cancer recurrence. Once the latter has been excluded the treatment can be directed toward improving the swallow. Muscle spasms have been treated by secondary myotomy, myenteric plexus denervation, and botulinum toxin injection (Peterson, Hoffman, Van Demark, & Barkmeier, 1992). Mechanical stenosis requires repeated dilation or reconstruction with distant tissues. (See below for surgical details.)

Technique for Total Laryngectomy

Total laryngectomy consists of the removal of the entire cricoid and thyroid Cartilages as well as the epiglottis with the resection extending from the upper tracheal rings to the hyoid bone. Portions of the pyriform sinus and tongue base may also be included. A horizontal skin incision is placed at the level of the cricothyroid membrane and skin flaps are elevated. The hyoid bone is freed from the tongue base musculature and constrictor muscles can be released from the thyroid area. The trachea is sectioned between the second and third tracheal rings in order to create a permanent tracheostoma. The laryngeal resection is completed by performing mucosal incisions at the level of the esophageal inlet extending across the anterior portion of the pyriform sinuses up to the level of the tongue-base incision. Closure of the mucosal opening is accomplished by direct approximation of the lateral mucosal remnants with the tongue base producing a T configuration. Large laryngeal tumors and pyriform sinus malignancies require portions of the hypopharynx to be resected along with the larynx. This laryngopharyngectomy usually requires distant flap reconstruction to prevent postoperative stenosis.

Pyriform Sinus and Cervical Esophageal Lesions

The tumors of the pyriform sinus and cervical esophagus are notorious for submucosal spread of disease (Adams, 1993). To completely remove the involved tissue a total esophagectomy is necessary in the larger lesions, and in most cases a total laryngectomy is also required. The patient oftentimes presents late in the course of disease, as the early lesions may remain asymptomatic. The total esophagectomy is repaired with a gastric pull-up, in which the stomach is brought up through the chest, or with a colon interposition graft, where the left colon is utilized as a conduit from the oropharynx to the stomach. Small lesions may be removed without total esophagectomy and the repair is either accomplished with skin grafts, pedicled flaps, or free-tissue transfer techniques.

Skull Base Tumors and Tumors of Neurogenic Origin

Patients with tumors of the skull base and neural structures of the neck—glomus jugulari, glomus vagali, carotid body tumors, temporal bone carcinoma—and tumors of the infra temporal fossa will frequently present with cranial nerve dysfunction. These tumors can directly involve the cranial nerves or induce neural loss secondary to compression. The neural deficits induced by tumor growth or tumor resection will produce dysphagia secondary to paralysis of pharyngeal muscles and sensory deficits along the pharynx and supraglottic larynx. Vocal fold paralysis induced by vagal injury is also common with these lesions.

The swallowing rehabilitation in these patients usually consists of vocal fold medialization surgery, palate adhesions, and cricopharyngeal myotomy (Netterville

& Vrabec, 1994). Swallowing therapy is useful in this patient group and internal plasticity is crucial to recovery.

Salivary Gland Disease

Salivary gland disease rarely causes dysphagia. The exceptions are the deep lobe parotid tumors, which arise in the parapharyngeal space and may directly compress the pharynx. Malignant salivary gland diseases (adenoid cystic, mucoepidermoid, and acinic cell carcinoma) may involve adjacent cranial nerves and lead to dysphagia owing to directly inducing neural dysfunction or secondary to surgical resection of surrounding tissue required to adequately treat these aggressive diseases. The most common cranial nerve involved is the facial nerve; however, submandibular tumors and deep lobe parotid tumors may involve the hypoglossal, the lingual, or the glossopharyngeal nerves. Radiation therapy is usually a component of treatment in the patient group. Additional problems may occur secondary to decreased saliva production.

Thyroid Tumors

Thyroid masses like salivary disease will cause dysphagia owing to external compression and tumor induced neural dysfunction. Owing to the location of the thyroid gland, large masses can partially obstruct the movement of the bolus at the level of the cervical esophagus, most commonly occurring with massive and substernal goiters. Surgical excision is necessary to relieve these symptoms. The recurrent laryngeal nerve passes directly under the thyroid isthmus as it enters the larynx and can be invaded by tumor or injured at the time of surgery, resulting in vocal fold paralysis. Thyroid malignancies (papillary, follicular, medullary, and anaplastic) may directly invade the esophagus, producing dysphagia by obstructing the esophageal lumen. Surgical resection is the treatment of choice in most cases and includes partial esophagectomy and repair.

DISEASES AFFECTING OROPHARYNGEAL STRUCTURES OR SWALLOWING FUNCTION

Systemic diseases may have specific oropharyngeal manifestations and may affect normal swallowing function. A complete history including a thorough review of systems is essential when evaluating the dysphagic patient. Specific systemic diseases discussed in detail are presented in the list below:

Systemic Disorders

Thyroid disease

Iron deficiency

B12 deficiency

Sjögren's syndrome

Amyloidosis

Behçet's syndrome

Thyroid Disease

In the hypothyroid and hyperthyroid state the thyroid gland may become enlarged and inflamed. This goiterous thyroid may become so massive that it may compress structures in the neck such as the esophagus and trachea, resulting in dysphagia and stridor (Ingbar & Woeber, 1983).

Iron and B12 Deficiency

Vitamin deficiencies may result in considerable dysphagia. Vitamin B12 may lead to corticobulbar dysfunction and even manifest itself as dysphagia. Plummer-Vinson Syndrome is a condition likely resulting from a deficiency of iron and B12, affecting females predominantly between 40 to 70 years of age. Mucous membranes become dry and the tongue burns. Treatment includes iron, Vitamin B12, and a bland diet.

Sjögren's Syndrome

Sjögren's syndrome is an autoimmune condition characterized by insufficient production of saliva leading to xerostomia (dry mouth; Caruso, Sonies, Atkinson, & Fox, 1989). The oral transport phase is prolonged secondary to inadequate saliva production (Bubl & Schon, 1993; Caruso et al., 1989). Therapy is symptomatic.

Amyloidosis

Macroglossia may result from fibrous deposition of amyloid in the hypoglossal muscle in patients with amyloidosis. The tongue may stiffen or even obstruct the pharynx, contributing to oropharyngeal dysphagia (Deron, 1994). Treatment is supportive.

Behçet's Syndrome

Aphthous ulcers of the oral mucosa are one of the hallmarks of Behçet's syndrome. Ulceration in the esophagus has also been documented (Bubl & Schon, 1993). Therapy is directed toward the symptoms and includes topical anesthetic agents and steroids.

ANATOMIC ABNORMALITIES

The complex coordinated activity of the swallow depends directly on intact anatomic structures. Interference with normal structures secondary to the presence of a tracheotomy tube, scar formation or even the presence of a large cervical osteophyte may lead to dysphagia. Listed below are some of the major anatomic abnormalities that may lead to dysphagia.

Anatomic Abnormalities

Tracheotomy

Radiation

Fibrosis and scar

   Cervical fibrosis

   Lye ingestion

   Postsurgical scar formation

Zenker's diverticulum

Lingual thyroid

Dental abnormalities

Vascular abnormalities

Tracheotomy

The presence of a tracheotomy tube, used at times to prevent aspiration, may actually impede swallowing and provoke aspiration. Mechanical alteration of the laryngeal system from a tracheotomy tube can result in the larynx being tethered or anchored at a specific site (Bonanno, 1971). This anchoring results in a decrease in the superior and anterior displacement of the larynx. Laryngeal excursion facilitates relaxation of the cricopharyngeal muscle. Decreased excursion results in impaired cricopharyngeal opening, leading to pharyngeal residue, which could potentially be aspirated.

A three-tiered process of laryngeal closure consisting of downfolding of the epiglottis, closure of the aryepiglottic folds, and adduction of the true vocal folds, is dependent on muscular as well as passive biomechanical forces (Kock, 1993; VanDaele, Perlman, & Cassell, 1994). By anchoring the larynx the first two tiers are altered. Specifically, the epiglottis does not completely downfold, nor is there adequate closure of the aryepiglottic folds, resulting in reduced laryngeal closure (Buchwalter & Sasaki, 1984).

An inflated cuff on the tracheotomy tube also impairs normal swallowing function, as esophageal obstruction may result. Aspiration of stagnant food may occur when the cuff is deflated or when the patient inspires forcefully (Nash, 1988).

Scar and Fibrosis

Scar and fibrosis of oral cavity and pharyngeal soft tissues can occur secondary to external trauma such as caustic ingestion and burns, internal abnormalities (cervical dermoids, radiation induced fibrosis), and even as a result of surgical intervention (Figure 12–21). Treatment usually requires aggressive surgical intervention, including

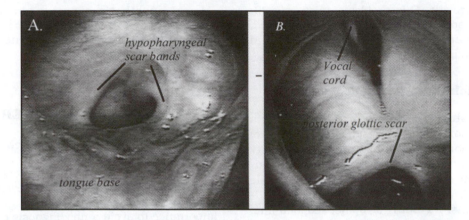

Figure 12-21. Scar and fibrosis as an etiology of dysphagia in: **a.** Tongue base area. **b.** Laryngeal level.

total pharyngectomy or pharyngoesophagectomy and secondary bypass (Chen, Tang, Shieh, Chang, & Noordhoff, 1988).

Zenker's Diverticulum

Zenker's diverticulum is a posterior outpouching of the pharynx in the pharyngoesophageal segment just proximal to the cricopharyngeus muscle. It was first described in 1764 by Ludlow. Later work by Zenker and Ziemssen (1878) provided theories as to the cause of the diverticulum. Although cricopharyngeal dysfunction has not been proven to be the cause, uniformly cricopharyngeal myotomy with or without diverticulectomy will relieve the symptoms in general and prevent recurrence.

Cervical Spine Osteophytes

Dysphagia due to cervical spine osteophytes has been recognized and reported by several authors. Dysphagia in this patient subgroup has been related primarily to large and low (C-3 and below) anterior bony lesions. The swallowing dysfunction is likely due to obstruction from external compression; however, inflammation from active joint disease has also been postulated. The lateral view of a barium swallow will illustrate the osteophyte and interruption of the barium column above the mass. Treatment can be difficult and vary from dietary management to surgical excision of the osteophyte (Brandenberg & Leibrock, 1986; Lambert, Tepperman, Jimenez, & Newman, 1981).

Vascular Anomalies

As in children, a vascular abnormality can lead to dysphagia in adults. The anomalous right subclavian artery (dysphagia lusorum) and the aortic arch have been implicated (Adkins, Maples, Graham, Witt, & Davies, 1986; Balaji, Ona, Cheeran, Paul, & Nanda, 1982).

MEDICATIONS

Medication side effects may be the most common but poorly recognized causes of oropharyngeal dysphagia. Commonly prescribed medicines or over-the-counter remedies may contribute to side effects and induce dysphagia. Specific examples are presented in further detail below.

Antibiotics

Antibiotics of almost any type can lead to secondary mucosal infections from yeast overgrowth. This problem, unless specifically sought out, diagnosed, and treated, can cause persistent mucosal pain and dysphagia.

Anticholinergic Medications

Xerostomia-inducing drugs are also a common cause of dysphagia. Dryness of the mouth as well as a decreased ability to neutralize acid in the esophagus contribute to dysphagia. Anticholinergic side effects are seen in several types of medications, including atropine, scopolamine, antihistamines, diuretics, opiates, antipsychotic drugs, and some antiarrhythmic and antihypertensive medications (Deron, 1994).

Antihypertensive Agents

Blood pressure medications include several potential problem groups. Diuretics have been discussed. Angio-tensin converting enzyme inhibitors have been linked to angioneurotic edema, which affects swallow by producing watery edematous swelling of oral cavity, pharyngeal, and laryngeal tissues.

Antipsychotic Medications

Antipsychotic medications have been a great boon to the care of patients suffering from schizophrenia. The dysphagia is related to multiple problems, anticholinergic effects producing decreased salivary flow and impaired esophageal motility, and more significantly, tardive dyskinesia, which may cause lingual and upper esophageal hyperkinesia (Sliwa & Lis, 1993).

Miscellaneous

Botulinum toxin type A, used to treat oromandibular dystonia, torticollis, and spasmodic dysphonia, may result in short-term dysphagia, and even short-term aspiration of fluids (Deron, 1994; Palmer et al., 1995).

Local anesthetic agents used in the pharynx may also lead to dysphagia and a tendency to aspirate, as afferent input is diminished (Deron, 1994).

PSYCHOGENIC SWALLOWING DISORDERS

Swallowing disorders with a psychogenic cause are rare but real. It is important to be aware of the possibility of psychogenic dysphagia when no other cause can be found. However, it is of even greater importance to avoid a misdiagnosis of psychogenic dysphagia owing to poor or inadequate diagnostic evaluation. In a review by Gilbody (1991) four subgroups of "functional" dysphagia were discussed: developmental, conditioned, primary conversion, and secondary conversion disorders.

Globus Hystericus

Globus hystericus (pharyngeus) is a common disorder in current ambulatory patient populations. It also has an ancient history, first noted by Hippocrates over two thousand years ago (Timon O'Dwyer, Cagney, & Walsh, 1991). Globus is a diagnosis of exclusion and its frequency will depend on the clinician's efforts to exclude other causes of the symptom. In the narrow sense of the term "dysphagia" globus should not be included, as this group of patients do not demonstrate a mechanical altered or abnormal swallow and tend to maintain normal weight (Timon et al., 1991).

The true etiology of globus is multifactorial. A fair number of patients with a lump in the throat sensation are found to have significant gastroesophageal reflux or esophageal dysmotility or many of the other organic causes of dysphagia (Gilbody, 1991). However, in the face of a negative extensive diagnostic workup, patient reassurance may be the most prudent course of treatment. Although patients tend to improve or remain stable with time, only a small percentage are entirely symptom-free in long-term-follow-up (Timon et al., 1991).

SUMMARY

Upon initial evaluation of the patient with oropharyngeal dysphagia a complete history and physical exam are essential. A great number of disease processes both localized and systemic can affect oropharyngeal structures and result in dysphagia. Patients who have undergone surgery in the oropharyngeal or laryngeal region may experience temporary or prolonged dysphagia. Because of the limitations of surgical reconstruction of the oral cavity, oropharynx, and larynx, patients requiring surgical treatment for head and neck malignancies continue to be a challenge for the otolaryngologist-reconstructive surgeon was well as the swallowing therapist. Advances in free-tissue transfer techniques have improved patient post-treatment swallowing, and better outcomes analysis and reporting will ensure future advancements. The complex interactive nature of the oropharyngeal swallow prevents simple treatment solutions. Surgical innovation, swallowing therapy, and patient neuromuscular plasticity are the best hope for functional restoration.

MULTIPLE CHOICE QUESTIONS

1. Which of the following medications may produce dysphagia?
   a. angiotensin-converting enzyme inhibitors
   b. diuretics
   c. antipsychotics
   d. all of the above

2. Free-tissue transfer (i.e., radial forearm, fibula) has an advantage over pedicled flap repairs primarily because of which of the following:
   a. they have more bulk
   b. they provide more activity
   c. they may provide intact sensation
   d. they are easier techniques to perform

3. After surgical treatment for oral cavity cancer, which factors will affect post-treatment swallowing?
   a. amount of tongue resected
   b. type of repair
   c. nerve resections
   d. all of the above

REFERENCES

Adams, G. L.(1993). Malignant neoplasms of the hypopharynx. In C. W. Cummings, J. M., Fredrickson, J. M. Harker, C. J. Krause, & D. E. Schuller (Eds.), *Otolaryngology—Head and neck surgery* (pp. 1955–1973). St. Louis: Mosby-Year Book.

Adkins, R. B., Maples, M. D., Graham, B. S., Witt, T. T., & Davies, J. (1986). Dysphagia associated with an aortic arch anomaly in adults. *The American Surgeon, 52,* 238–245.

Balaji, M. R., Ona, F. V., Cheeran, D., Paul, G., & Nanda, N. (1982). Dysphagia lusoria: A case report and review of diagnosis and treatment in adults. *American Journal of Gastroenterology, 77,* 899–901.

Balfe, D. M., Koehler, R. E., Setzen, M., Weyman, P. J., Baron, R. L., & Ogura, J. H. (1982). Barium examination of the esophagus after total laryngectomy. *Radiology 143,* 501–508.

Bardach, J. & Salyer, K. E. (1991) Cleft palate repair. In J. Bardach & K. E. Salyer (Eds.), *Surgical techniques in cleft lip and palate* (pp. 224–273). St. Louis: Mosby-Year Book.

Baredes, S. (1988). Surgical management of swallowing disorder. *Otolaryngologic Clinics of North America, 21*(4), 711–720.

Barr, C. E. (1992). Oral diseases in HIV-1 infection. *Dysphagia, 7,* 126–137.

Benjamin, B. (1993). Congenital disorders of the larynx. In C. W. Cummings, J. M. Fredrickson, J. M. Harker, C. J. Krause, & D. E. Schuller (Eds.), *Otolaryngology—Head and neck surgery* (pp. 1831–1853). St. Louis: Mosby-Year Book.

Benjamin, B., & Inglis, A. (1989). Minor congenital laryngeal clefts: Diagnosis and classification. *Annals of Otology, Rhinology and Laryngology, 98,* 417–420.

Benninger, M. S., Crumley, R. L., Ford, C. N., Gould, W. J., Hanson, D. G., Ossoff, R. H., Sataloff, R. T. (1994). Evaluation and treatment of the unilateral paralyzed vocal fold.

Otolaryngology—Head and Neck Surgery, 111, 497–508.

Bonanno, P. C. (1971). Swallowing dysfunction after tracheostomy. *Annals of Surgery, 174*, 29–33.

Brandenberg, S., & Leibrock L. G. (1986). Dysphagia and dysphonia secondary to anterior cervical osteophytes. *Neurosurgery, 18*(1), 90–93.

Brin, M., & Younger, D. (1988). Neurologic disorders and aspiration. *Otolaryngologic Clinics of North America, 21*(4), 691–700.

Brodsky, L. & Volk, M. (1993). The airway and swallowing. In J. C. Arvedson & L. Brodsky (Eds.), *Pediatric swallowing and feeding: Assessment and management* (pp. 93–122). San Diego, CA: Singular Publishing Group.

Bubl, R., & Schon, B. (1993). Dysphagia in dermatologic disease. *Dysphagia, 8*, 85–95.

Buchholz, D. (1994). Neurogenic dysphagia: What is the cause when the cause is not obvious. *Dysphagia, 9*, 245–255.

Buchwalter, J. A., & Sasaki, C. T. (1984). Effect of tracheotomy on laryngeal function. *Otolaryngologic Clinics of North America, 17*(1), 41–48.

Burgess, R. C., Michaels, L., Bale, J. F., & Smith, R. J. (1994). Polymerase chain reaction amplification of herpes simplex viral DNA from the geniculate ganglion of a patient with Bell's palsy. *Annals of Otology, Rhinology and Laryngology, 103*, 775–779.

Bushmann, M., Dobmeyer, S. M., Leeker, L., & Perlmutter, J. S. (1989). Swallowing abnormalities and their response to treatment in Parkinson's disease. *Neurology, 39*, 1309–1313.

Butcher, R. B. (1982). Treatment of chronic aspiration as a complication of cerebrovascular accident. *Laryngoscope, 92*, 681–685.

Calcaterra, T. C., Kadell B. M., & Ward, P. H. (1975). Dysphagia secondary to cricopharyngeal muscle dysfunction. *Archives of Otolaryngology, 101*, 726-729.

Carpenter, R., McDonald, T. J., & Howard, F. M. (1979). The otolaryngologic presentation of myasthenia gravis. *Laryngoscope, 89*, 922–927.

Caruso, A. J., Sonies, B. S., Atkinson, J. C., & Fox, P. C. (1989). Objective measures of swallowing in patients with primary Sjögren's syndrome. *Dysphagia, 4*, 101–105.

Castell, J. A., Castell, D. O. Schulta, A. R. & Georgeson, S. (1993). Effect of head position on the dynamics of the upper esophageal sphincter and pharynx. *Dysphagia, 8*, 1-6.

Chen, H., Tang, Y., Shieh, M., Chang, C., Noordhoff, M. S. (1988). Early reconstruction of pharynx and esophagus following corrosive injury with radial forearm flap in preparation for colon interposition. *Annals of Thoracic Surgery, 45*, 39-42.

Christensen, J. R. (1989). Developmental approach to pediatric neurogenic dysphagia. *Dysphagia, 3*, 131–134.

Coates, H. (1992). Nasal obstruction in the neonate and infant. *Clinical Pediatrics, 31*, 25–29.

Coelho, C. & Ferrante, R. (1988). Dysphagia in post-polio sequelae: Report of three cases. *Archives of Physical Medicine Rehabilitation, 69*, 634–636.

Cumberworth, V. L., Djazaeri, B., & Mackay, I. S. (1995). Endoscopic fenestration of choanal atresia. *The Journal of Laryngology and Otology, 109*, 31–35.

Darrow, D. H., Hoffman H. T., Barnes, G. J. & Wiley, C. A. (1992). Management of dysphagia in inclusion body myositis. *Archives of Otolaryngology—Head and Neck Surgery, 118*, 313–317.

Davis, R. K, Kelly, S. M., & Hayes, J. (1991). Endoscopic CO_2 laser excisional biopsy of early supraglottic cancer. *Laryngoscope, 101*, 680–683.

Deron, PH. (1994). Dysphagia with systemic diseases. *Acta Oto-Rhino-Laryngologica Belgica, 48*, 191–200.

Fisher, S. E., Painter, M., & Milmoe, G. (1981). Swallowing disorders in infancy. *Pediatric Clinics of North America, 28*(4), 845–853.

Freeman, R. B., Marks, J. E., & Ogura, J. H. (1979). Voice preservation in treatment of carcinoma of the pyriform sinus. *Laryngoscope, 89*, 1855.

Fritsch, D. E., & Klein, D. G. (1992). Ludwig's angina. *Heart & Lung, 21*, 39–47.

Funk, G. F., Laurenzo, J. F., Valentino, J., McCulloch, T. M., Frodel, J. L., & Hoffman, H. T. (1995). Free-tissue transfer reconstruction of midfacial and cranio-orbito-facial defects. *Archive of Otolaryngology—Head Neck Surgery, 121*, 293–303.

Garino, J. P., & Ryan, T. J. (1987). Carotid hemorrhage: A complication of peritonsillar abscess. *American Journal of Emergency Medicine, 5*, 220–223.

Gilbody, J. S. (1991). Errors of deglutition-real and imagined; or, don't forget the psyche. *The Journal of Laryngology and Otology, 105*, 807–811.

Glossop, L. P., Smith, R. J., & Evans, J. N. G. (1984). Posterior laryngeal cleft: An analysis of ten cases. *International Journal of Pediatric Otolaryngology, 7*, 133–143.

Goldfarb, D., & Sataloff, R. T. (1994). Lyme disease: A review for the otolaryngologist. *Ear Nose and Throat Journal, 73*, 824–829.

Guily, J. L., Perie, S. P., Willig, T. N., Chaussade, S. Eymard, B., & Angelard, B. (1994). Swallowing disorders in muscular diseases: Functional assessment and indication of cricopharyngeal myotomy. *Ear Nose and Throat Journal, 73*, 34–40.

Halama, A. R. (1994). Surgical treatment of oropharyngeal swallowing disorders. *Acta Oto-Rhino-Laryngologica Belgica, 48*, 217–227.

Hirano, M., Kurita, S., Tateishi, M., & Matsuoka, H. (1987). Deglutition following supraglottic horizontal laryngectomy. *Annals of Otology Rhinology and Laryngology, 96*, 7–11.

Hirano, M., Kuroiwa, Y., Tanaka, S., Matsuoka, H., Sato, K., & Yoshida, T. (1992). Dysphagia following various degrees of surgical resection for oral cancer. *Annals of Otology Rhinology and Laryngology, 101,* 138–141.

Ingbar, S. H., & Woeber K. A. (1983). Diseases of the thyroid. In R. G. Petersdorf, R. D. Adams, E. Braunwald, K. J. Isselbacher, J. B. Martin, & J. D. Wilson (Eds.), *Harrison's principles of internal medicine* (pp. 614–634). New York: McGraw-Hill.

Johnson, E., R., McKenzie, W., & Sievers, A. (1993). Aspiration pneumonia in stroke. *Archives of Physical Medicine and Rehabilitation, 74,* 973–976.

Jones, B. D., Buchholz, D. W., Ravich, W. J., & Donner, M. W. (1992). Swallowing dysfunction in the postpolio syndrome. A cinefluorographic study. *American Journal of Roentgenology, 158*(2), 283-286.

Kagel, M. C. & Leopold, N. A. (1992). Dysphagia in Huntington's disease: A 16-year retrospective. *Dysphagia, 7,* 106–114.

Kaplan, J. N., Dobie, R. A., & Cummings, C. W. (1981). The incidence of hypopharyngeal stenosis after surgery for laryngeal cancer. *Otolaryngology-Head and Neck Surgery, 89,* 956–959.

Kaufman, F. L. (1991). Managing the cleft lip and palate patients. *Pediatric Clinics of North America, 38*(5), 1127–1145.

Kennedy, J. G., & Kent, R. K.(1988). Physiological substrates of normal deglutition. *Dysphagia, 3*(1), 24–37.

Kock, W. M. (1993). Swallowing disorders. *Medical Clinics of North America, 77,* 571–582.

Kronenberger, M. B., & Meyers, A. D. (1994) Dysphagia following head and neck cancer surgery. *Dysphagia, 9,* 236–244.

Kuhlemeier, K. V. (1994). Epidemiology and dysphagia. *Dysphagia, 9,* 209–217.

Laccourreye, H., Laccourreye, O., Weinstein, G., Menard, M., & Brasnu, D. (1990). Supracricoid laryngectomy with cricohyoidopexy: A partial laryngeal procedure for selected supraglottic and transglottic carcinomas. *Laryngoscope, 100,* 735–740.

Lambert, J. R., Tepperman, P. S., Jimenez, J., & Newman, A. (1981). Cervical spine disease and dysphagia. *American Journal of Gastroenterology, 76,* 35–40.

Lindeman, R.C. (1975). Diverting the paralyzed larynx. *Laryngoscope, 85,* 157–180.

Litton, W. B., & Leonard, J. R. (1969). Aspiration after partial laryngectomy: Cinefluorographic studies. *Laryngoscope, 79,* 887–908.

Logemann, J. (1983). *Evaluation and treatment of swallowing disorders.* San Diego, CA: College-Hill Press.

Logemann, J., Pauloski, B. R., Rademaker, A. W., McConnel, F. M. S., Heiser, M. A., Cardinale, S.

Shedd, D., Stein, D., Beery, Q., Johnson, J., & Baker, T. (1993). Speech and swallow function after tonsil/base of tongue resection with primary closure. *Journal of Speech and Hearing Research, 36,* 918–926.

Ludlow, A. (1764). A case of obstructed deglutition from a preternatural dilatation of and bag formed in the pharynx. *Medical Observations and Inquiries by a Society of Physicians in London, 3,* 83–101.

Martin, G., Rudolph, C., Hillemeier, C., & Heyman, M. B. (1986). Dysphagia lusorum in children. *American Journal of Diseases of Children, 140,* 815–816.

Mathog, R. H., & Fleming, S. M. (1992). A clinical approach to dysphagia. *American Journal of Otolaryngology, 13,* 133–138.

McConnel, F. M. S., Cerenko, D., & Mendelsohn, M. S. (1988). Dysphagia after total laryngectomy. *Otolaryngologic Clinics of North America, 21,* 721–726.

McConnel, F. S., Logemann, J. A., Rademaker, A. W., Pauloski, B. R., Baker, S. R., Lewin, J., Shedd, D., Heiser, M. A., Cardinale, S., Collins, S., Graner, D., Cook, B. S., Milianti, F., & Baker, T. (1994). Surgical variables affecting postoperative swallowing efficiency in oral cancer patients: A pilot study. *Laryngoscope, 104,* 87–90.

Morrell, R. M. (1984). The neurology of swallowing. In M. E. Groher (Ed.), *Dysphagia: Diagnosis and management* (pp. 3–35). Boston: Butterworth.

Moscatello, A. L., Worden, D. L., Nadelman, R. B., Wormser, G., & Lucente, F. (1991). Otolaryngologic aspects of Lyme disease. *Laryngoscope, 101,* 592-595.

Nash, M. (1988). Swallowing problems in the tracheotomized patient. *Otolaryngology Clinics of North America, 21,* 701–709.

Netterville, J. L. & Civantos, F. J. (1993). Rehabilitation of cranial nerve deficits after neurotologic skull base surgery. *Laryngoscope, 103,* 45–54.

Netterville, J. L., & Vrabec, J. T. (1994). Unilateral palatal adhesion for paralysis after high vagal injury. *Archives of Otolaryngology—Head and Neck Surgery, 120,* 218–221.

Olsen, K. D., & DeSanto, L. W. (1990) Partial vertical laryngectomy—indications and surgical technique. *American Journal of Otolaryngology, 11,* 153–160.

Palmer, P. M., McCulloch, T. M., Lemke, J. H., Finnegan E. M., Barkmeier, J. M., & Hoffman, H. T. (1995). Analysis of magnitude and duration of swallowing disorders following treatment with botulinum toxin in patients with spasmodic dysphonia. *Dysphagia, 10,* 138.

Parkin, J. (1991). Congenital malformations of the mouth and pharynx. In C. Bluestone, S. D. Stool,

& M. D. Scheetz (Eds.), *Pediatric otolaryngology* (pp. 850–859). Philadelphia: W. B. Saunders.

Pauloski, B. R., Logemann, J. A., Rademaker, A. W., McConnel, F. M. S., Heiser, M. A. Cardinale, S., Shedd, D., Lewin, J., Baker, S. R., Graner, D., Cook, B., Milianti, R., Collin, S., & Baker, T. (1993). Speech and swallowing function after anterior tongue and floor of mouth resection with distal flap reconstruction. *Journal of Speech and Hearing Research, 36*, 267–276.

Pauloski, B. R., Logemann, J. A., Rademaker, A. W., McConnel, F. M. S., Stein, D., Beery, Q., Johnson, J., Heiser, M. A. , Cardinale, S., Shedd, D., Graner, D., Cook, B., Milianti, R., Collins, S., & Baker, T. (1994). Speech and swallowing function after oral and oropharyngeal resections: One year follow-up. *Head and Neck, 16*, 313–322.

Pearson, B. W. (1986). Near-total laryngectomy. In C.W. Cummings, J. M. Fredrickson, J. M. Krause, C. J. Krause, & D. E. Schuller (Eds.) *Otolaryngology—Head and Neck Surgery* (pp. 2117–2132) St. Louis: Mosby-Year Book.

Pearson, B. W., Woods, R. D., & Hartman, D. E. (1980). Extended hemilaryngectomy for T3 glottic carcinoma with preservation of speech and swallowing. *Laryngoscope, 90*, 1950–1961.

Perlman, A. L., Booth, B. M., & Grayhack, J. P. (1994). Videofluoroscopic predictors of aspiration in patients with oropharyngeal dysphagia. *Dysphagia, 9*, 90–95.

Peterson, K. L., Hoffman, H. T., Van Demark, D., & Barkmeier, J. M. (1992, January). *Botulinum neurotoxin A injection to the pharyngeal constrictor muscles after total laryngectomy.* Paper presented at the Southern Section of the American Laryngological, Rhinological and Otological Society, Sea Island, GA.

Rademaker, A. W., Logemann, J. A., Pauloski, B. R., Bowman, J. B., Lasarus, C. L., Sisson, G. A., Milianti, F. J., Graner, D., Cook, B. S., Collins, S. L., Stein, D. W., Beery, Q. C., Johnson, J. T., & Baker, T. M. (1993). Recovery of postoperative swallowing in patients undergoing partial laryngectomy. *Head and Neck, 15*, 325–334.

Rasley, A., Logemann, J. A., Kahrilas, P., Rademaker, A., Pauloski, B., & Dodds, W. (1993). Prevention of barium aspiration during videofluoroscopic swallowing studies: Value of change in posture. *American Journal of Roentgenology, 160*, 1005–1009.

Schoenrock, L. D., King, A. Y., Everts, E. C., Schneider, H. J., & Shumrick, D. (1972). Hemilaryngectomy: Deglutition evaluation and rehabilitation. *Transactions of the American Academy of Ophthalmology & Otolaryngology, 76*, 752–757.

Sliwa, J. A. & Lis S.(1993). Drug-induced dysphagia. *Archives of Physical Medicine and Rehabilitation, 74*, 445–447.

Tees, D., Lofchy, N., & Rutka, J. (1992). Deafness, dysphagia and a middle ear mass in a patient with neurofibromatosis type 2. *Journal of Otolaryngology, 21*, 227–229.

Timon, C., O'Dwyer, T., Cagney, D., & Walsh, M. (1991). Globus pharyngeus: Long-term follow up and prognostic factors. *Annals of Otology, Rhinology, and Laryngology, 100*, 351–354.

Tunckel, D. E. (1994). Surgical approach to diagnosis and management. In D. N. Tuchman & R. S. Walter (Eds.), *Disorders of feeding and swallowing in infants and children* (pp. 131–152). San Diego, Singular Publishing Group.

Urken, M. L., & Biller, H. F. (1994). A new design for the sensate radial forearm free flap to preserve tongue mobility following significant glossectomy. *Archives of Otolaryngology—Head and Neck Surgery, 120*, 126–131.

Urken, M. L., Moscoso, J. F., Lawson, W., & Biller, H. F. (1994). A systematic approach to functional reconstruction of the oral cavity following partial and total glossectomy. *Archives of Otolaryngology-Head and Neck Surgery, 120*, 589–601.

Urken, M. L., & Sullivan, M. J. (1995). Scapular and parascapular fasciocutaneous and osteofasciocutaneous. In M. L. Urken, M. L. Cheney, M. J. Sullivan, & H. F. Biller (Eds.), *Atlas of regional and free flaps for head and neck reconstruction.* New York: Raven Press.

Urken, M. L., Vikery, C., Weinberg, H., & Biller, H. F. (1990). The neurofasciocutaneous radial forearm flap in head and neck reconstruction: a preliminary report. *Laryngoscope, 100*, 161–173.

VanDaele, D. J., Perlman, A. L., & Cassell, M. D. (1995). Intrinsic fiber architecture and attachments of the human epiglottis and their contributions to the mechanism of deglutition. *Journal of Anatomy, 186*, 1–15.

Veis, S. L., & Logemann J. A. (1985). Swallowing disorders in persons with cerebrovascular accidents. *Archives of Physical Medicine and Rehabilitation, 66*, 372–375.

Wang, L. & Karmondy, C. S. (1985). Dysphagia as the presenting symptom of tetanus. *Archives of Otolaryngology, 111*, 342–343.

Weaver, A. W., & Fleming, S. M. (1978). Partial laryngectomy: Analysis of associated swallowing disorders. *American Journal of Surgery, 136*, 486–489.

Young, B. K., Chapman, P. J., & Crewe, T. C. (1992). Surgical management of drooling. Case report. *Australian Dental Journal, 37*, 115–117.

Zanaret, M., Giovanni, A., Gras, R., & Cannoni, M. (1993). Near total laryngectomy with epiglottic reconstruction: Long-term results in 57 patients. *American Journal of Otolaryngology, 14,* 419–425.

Zenker, F., & Ziemssen, H. V. (Eds.). (1878). Dilatations of the esophagus. *Cyclopaedia of the*

Practice of Medicine (pp. 46–68). London: Low, Marston, Searle & Rivington.

13

Esophageal Diseases

Joseph A. Murray, Satish S. C. Rao, and Konrad Schulze-Delrieu

The primary function of the esophagus is to convey food from the pharynx to the stomach. Almost any disorder affecting the esophagus can interfere with that function. Dysphagia may be the result of mechanical obstruction or of abnormal neuromuscular function or sensation. Odynophagia consists of pain during swallowing and may be due to inflammation in the mucosal lining. Other symptoms of esophageal origin include chest pain, upper back pain, heartburn, regurgitation, globus sensation, and belching.

Esophageal diseases that give rise to dysphagia can be categorized as

1. diseases primarily affecting the mucosa, including reflux esophagitis or cancer arising from the mucosal lining
2. diseases that involve the muscular wall of the esophagus or its sphincters such as achalasia and diffuse esophageal spasm
3. impacted foreign bodies
4. extrinsic diseases outside the esophagus but affecting esophageal diameter, such as compression of the esophagus by lung tumors.

The current chapter will deal with diseases unique to the smooth muscle segment of the esophagus. Diseases affecting the striated muscle portion of the esophagus and the cranial nerves are covered in Chapter 11.

DISORDERS PRIMARILY INVOLVING THE ESOPHAGEAL MUCOSA

Inflammation of the mucosa is commonly associated with dysphagia. Inflammation occurs most commonly from reflux of gastrointestinal secretions, but can be caused by ingestion of corrosives and by infection. Cancers arising in the esophageal mucosa also lead to dysphagia.

Gastroesophageal Reflux Disease

The most common esophageal problem is gastroesophageal reflux disease (GERD). This disorder is reflux of gastric contents into the esophagus, which results in esophageal or respiratory symptoms. Postprandial reflux of short duration may be seen in normal individuals. Typical symptoms of uncomplicated GERD are heartburn and acid regurgitation into the oral cavity. Gastroesophageal reflux disorder may cause dysphagia because of an inflammatory stricture or because of changes in motor function secondary to inflammation. Rarely, symptoms of GERD may be the presenting feature of scleroderma. Abnormal GER most commonly manifests as reflux esophagitis, the result of damage to the esophageal mucosa. Other problems associated with gastroesophageal reflux disorder include asthma, anginalike chest pain, laryngitis cough, earache, aspiration pneumonia, interstitial pulmonary fibrosis, and dental deterioration (Table 13–1).

Epidemiology

Estimates of the prevalence of GERD vary according to the definition used. Symptom-based population studies demonstrated that 35–44% of adult Americans complained of heartburn at least once per month. If prevalence is defined by endoscopically proven reflux esophagitis it is thought to be less than 2% (Spechler 1992).

Etiology and Pathophysiology

Gastroesophageal reflux disease is caused by a combination of factors that together result in a prolonged exposure of the esophagus to injurious gastroduodenal material. Reflux esophagitis is esophageal mucosal injury resulting from the acid exposure. With a few exceptions, gastric acid appears to be essential for the development of esophagitis. In the setting of previous gastric resection, marked bile reflux may also cause esophagitis. Other substances in the refluxate that may be injurious include pepsin, pancreatic enzymes, and bile, but these rarely cause damage in the absence of gastric acid. Esophageal damage or symptoms may be the result of failure of one or more of the several mechanisms that reduce the potential for reflux of gastric material into the esophagus. This includes:

1. *Lower esophageal sphincter (LES) dysfunction.* Between 60 and 85% of all episodes of gastroesophageal reflux are associated with an inappropriate relaxation of the LES or so-called *transient lower esophageal sphincter relaxation* (Dent, Holloway, Toouli, & Doods, 1988; Dodds et al., 1982). These are relaxations of the LES that occur without swallowing. These occur particularly after meals and can cause significant reflux into the esophagus. Diminished baseline tone of the lower esophageal sphincter is also an important contributor to the occurrence of reflux. The severity of reflux esophagitis seems to correlate inversely with the lower esophageal sphincter pressure. Patients with esophageal strictures or *Barrett's esophagus* have a lower baseline LES pressure than patients with uncomplicated GERD. However, there is considerable overlap between refluxers and normal controls. Sphincter incompetence (defined by a pressure less than 10 mmHg) may help predict those patients who may fail or recur on standard antireflux therapy. Gastric material may reflux into the esophagus freely and particularly when the intragastric pressure exceeds the intrathoracic pressure, for example, during periods of straining or recumbency. Individuals who have a greatly diminished LES tone are prone to severe reflux esophagitis and are particularly prone to reflux during supine periods.

2. *Disordered peristalsis of the esophagus.* Peristaltic activity of the esophagus is often impaired in reflux esophagitis. This may occur as a result of acid damage but in some cases it may be primary or pre-

TABLE 13–1. Pathologic manifestations of GERD.

Esophageal	*Extraesophageal*
Reflux esophagitis	Laryngitis
Barrett's esophagus	Vocal fold granulomas
Esophageal ulcer	Airways disease (bronchitis, asthma, aspiration pneumonitis, fiberotic lung disease, atelectasis)
Reflux symptoms with normal mucosa	Laryngeal cancer
Adenocarcinoma in Barrett's esophagus	Dental enamel erosion
Esophageal stricture	Halitosis

cede the damage caused by acid. The types of abnormalities seen are incomplete peristalsis in response to swallow and prolonged and often ineffective peristaltic contractions in the distal esophagus. Low-pressure peristaltic contractions that generate pressures less than 40 mmHg result in poor bolus transport (Kahrilas, Dodds, & Hogan, 1988). After a reflux episode ineffective peristalsis may result in poor or delayed clearance of acid from the esophagus.

3. *Delayed gastric emptying.* In approximately 15–25% of patients with gastroesophageal reflux a delay in gastric emptying may be a contributive factor (Shay, Eggli, McDonald, & Johnson, 1987). When gastric emptying is delayed, the stomach contents are retained for a longer period. Also the persistent gastric distension after eating may result in reflex transient lower esophageal sphincter relaxation and subsequent reflux of gastric material.

4. *Hiatal hernia.* The relationship between the presence of a hiatal hernia and the development of gastroesophageal reflux merits specific mention. Hiatal hernia is the presence of part of the stomach above the diaphragm. Although the presence of a hiatal hernia is not a prerequisite for pathologic reflux (Cohen & Harris, 1971), it can markedly exacerbate any reflux episode. The presence of a small hiatal hernia on contrast radiography is common. Its prevalence increases with age. While not by itself a predictor of reflux esophagitis, larger hiatal hernias are associated with a greater prevalence of reflux esophagitis (Ahtaridis, Snape, & Cohen, 1981; Ott, Gelfand, Chen, Wu, & Munitz, 1985; Wolf, Brahams, & Khilnani, 1959; Wright & Hurwitz, 1979). The lower esophageal sphincter resting tone tends to be diminished in this setting, probably at least in part related to the loss of augmentation of the sphincter segment by the diaphragm. By altering the anatomic relationship between the lower esophageal sphincter and the diaphragmatic pinchcock there is an increased risk of severe reflux in those patients who do have reflux. The hiatal hernia itself may act as a reservoir of gastric content above the diaphragm and increase the likelihood and volume of refluxate when a transient lower esophageal sphincter relaxation may occur.

5. *Diminished buffering capacity of saliva and of esophageal secretions.* Secretions produced by the salivary glands are essential for buffering the refluxed material. After a reflux episode, the esophageal body typically generates a secondary peristaltic wave, which clears approximately 90% of the refluxed material back into the stomach. In some conditions, such as the sicca syndrome, alcohol abuse, and ingestion of anticholinergic drugs, production of saliva is defective. The remainder of the acidic material is initially buffered by the swallowed saliva and then this material is cleared from the esophagus by successive swallows, often taking several minutes. Even small amounts of unbuffered refluxate can keep the pH quite low in the esophagus. Since pH is measured on a logarithmic scale, in order for the pH to rise by 1 unit, 90% of the volume of gastroesophageal refluxate must be cleared to the stomach if there is no buffering capacity. During sleep saliva production is diminished, with absent or infrequent swallowing, resulting in prolonged periods of esophageal acid exposure during reflux episodes. The esophagus itself has mucous glands that can produce both bicarbonate and protective mucus. This intrinsic protective activity of the esophagus may be impaired in the setting of severe acid damage. There is also some degree of local buffering capacity with an increase in mucosal blood flow in response to acidification and the presence of intercellular tight junctions to help maintain the integrity of esophageal mucosa (Orlando, 1994).

Gastroesophageal Reflux as a Primary Motility Disorder

The evidence for abnormal motility as an etiologic factor in gastroesophageal reflux is based primarily on observation of motor abnormalities in patients in whom there is already significant esophageal damage.

This includes the description as above, originally described by Cohen and Harris (1971), of a decreased resting lower esophageal sphincter pressure as the single distinguishing difference between patients with and without gastroesophageal reflux. In the studies that have compared motor function in groups of patients with gastroesophageal reflux and control subjects, the mean lower esophageal sphincter pressure is lower in patients with reflux as compared to controls. There are also several studies showing that the lower esophageal sphincter pressure correlates inversely with the severity of reflux and indeed it tends to be lower in patients who have developed Barrett's esophagus or have esophageal strictures (Cohen & Harris, 1971; Iascone, De Meester, Little, & Skinner, 1983; Kahrilas et al, 1986). Katz, Knuff, Benjamin, Castell (1986) studied 13 patients with GERD with manometry before and after healing of their esophagitis. They did not find any change in the mean LES pressure or the peristaltic amplitude (Katz et al., 1986).

The evidence is against motor abnormality being responsible for the development of reflux. Several animal studies demonstrated an effect of the infusion of acid or the production of acute injury in the esophagus interfering with motor function (Eastwood, Castell & Higgs, 1975; Shirazi, Schulze-Delrieu, Custer-Hagen, Brown, & Ren, 1989; Sinar, Fletcher, & Castell, 1980). Of course a strong supportive evidence against a primary etiologic role for motility disturbance in the setting of reflux would be evident if there was correction of motility abnormalities with healing of the esophagitis. Marshall and Gerhardt (1982) reported two cases that showed demonstrable improvement in esophageal motor function when the reflux esophagitis was healed. The efficacy of prokinetic agents metoclopramide or cisapride in healing reflux esophagitis is less than that of the potent acid suppressing agents omeprazole or dose H2 blockers. In summary it is likely that many of the peristaltic abnormalities are secondary to the acid damage. However, LES dysfunction, whether it is the original mechanism for allowing acid reflux to occur when of very low pressure, does predict relapse following healing. It is also important to heal the esophagitis before doing manometry if one is to avoid detecting acid-induced changes such as would be important when considering patients for Nissen fundoplication or to detect scleroderma.

Risks Factors

Lifestyle factors may also be involved in increasing the risk of the occurrence of gastroesophageal reflux disorders and these include

1. *Smoking.* Smoking has a dual effect on the LES competence. Nicotine usage decreases LES tone by 20–30% and this decrease can persist after the smoking. There is also an increase in intraabdominal pressure during the smoking activity itself (Kahrilas et al., 1986). It reduces the flow and bicarbonate content of saliva, with consequent delayed acid clearance (Kahrilas, 1992; Schindlbeck & Heinrich, 1987).

2. *Obesity.* The presence of obesity, particularly central obesity, results in increased abdominal pressure and an increased likelihood of reflux.

3. *Chronic alcohol ingestion.* Alcohol has a deleterious effect on lower esophageal sphincter function and on the effectiveness of esophageal clearance (Keshavarzian et al., 1991). Chronic alcoholism itself also can result in chronic parotitis and diminished saliva production.

4. *Physiologic conditions* such as pregnancy, pathologic conditions such as ascites, and ingestion of hormones such as progesterone-containing contraceptive pills may all result in an increased propensity to gastroesophageal reflux by diminishing lower esophageal sphincter tone.

5. *Dietary habits.* The ingestion of large meals, particularly those rich in fat, chocolate, caffeine, and acidic foods may particularly impair gastric emptying in the case of fats, and/or reduce lower esophageal sphincter tone, or increase the frequency for transient lower esophageal sphincter relaxations.

6. *Drugs*, including calcium channel blockers, beta agonists, and long-acting nitrates, may also impair esophageal clearance and/or lower esophageal sphincter competence.

There is frequently a family history of hiatal hernia or reflux symptoms. It is not clear whether the family risk relates to common behaviors or a genetic predisposition (Schulze-Delrieu & Anuras, 1983). Other important but rare conditions including scleroderma, nasogastric intubation, gastroparesis, or gastric acid hypersecretion such as Zollinger-Ellison syndrome may give rise to symptomatic gastroesophageal reflux.

Pathology

Excessive reflux of gastric contents may result in both esophageal and extraesophageal consequences. The earliest pathologic abnormality is reactive hyperemia of the distal esophageal mucosa. This adaptive response increases a buffering countercurrent in mucosal blood flow. However, compared to the stomach the buffering capacity of the esophagus is limited and is easily overcome. Endoscopically, reactive hyperemia manifests as congestion of the parallel epithelial blood vessels and a characteristic linear erythema in the distal esophagus. Increased turnover of the squamous mucosa in response to injury can result in squamous cell hyperplasia. This is evident as histologically increased thickness of the basal cell layer of the epithelium. The combination of loss of superficial cells and the proliferation of the basal cell layer results in an increased proportion of immature cells in the esophageal mucosa and can be readily identified in mucosal biopsy specimens. The basal layer is organized in a series of papillae, and with hyperplasia these papillae can elongate, become narrow, and even branch. By definition epithelial hyperplasia of the esophagus is present if the papillae extend more than three fourths of the way through the thickness of the squamous cell layer and if the basal cell layer occupies more than one third of the epithe-lial depth (Figure 13–1). Squamous hyperplasia may occur without endoscopically visible abnormality, hence the recommendation of obtaining biopsies when objective documentation of reflux esophagitis is required. Should the regenerative capacity of the epithelium be overcome, super-ficial areas of the epithelium are desquamated and this resulting defect in the epithelium is called an *erosion*. The pathologic changes seen here include congested blood vessels, leucocytic—particularly eosinophilic—infiltration of the epithelium and lamina propria, and the erosions covered by fibrinous exudative material, which is evident as a whitish yellow patch endoscopically (see Figure 10–2). Linear erosions often extend for several centimeters along the length of the esophagus and when severe can become confluent circum-ferentially and form large ulcers. Infiltration of the epithelium with inflammatory cells may also be seen in the absence of endoscopically visible erosions or microscopically apparent changes of ulceration.

Symptoms

GERD causes heartburn and regurgitation. Heartburn or pyrosis is a burning

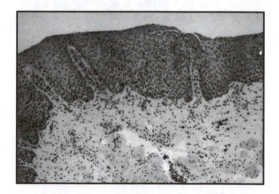

Figure 13–1. The histologic changes in the mucosa Eosinophilic infiltration of the epithelium, hyperplasia of the basal layer, and extension of the papilla to occupy more than three-fourths of the depth of the squamous cell layer (courtesy of Dr. Frank Mitros).

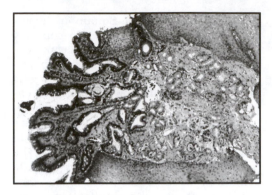

Figure 13–2. The specialized columnar epithelium of Barrett's metaplasia with adjacent squamous mucosa (courtesy of Dr. Frank Mitros).

TABLE 13–2. Symptoms of GERD.

Esophageal	*Extraesophageal*
Heartburn[a]	Hoarseness
Regurgitation	Cough
Odynophagia	Earache
Dysphagia	Wheeze
Acid reflux[a]	Globus
Belching	Water brash
	Throat clearing
	Sore throat
	Choking

[a]Pathognomic for reflux.

discomfort that ascends from the subxyphoid region retrosternally. Regurgitation is the effortless passage of gastric or esophageal contents into the esophagus and often into the pharynx and even the mouth.

In addition or instead of the classical esophageal symptoms there are many atypical or extraesophageal symptoms of GERD. Chief among these is chest pain that can often mimic anginalike pain. Indeed the majority of patients who have both coronary disease and GERD are unable to distinguish between the pains. Dysphagia may be the result of abnormal motility or mucosal damage. Odynophagia or pain on swallowing is the result of mucosal irritation. Extraesophageal manifestations include lower and upper airway symptoms, including cough, hoarseness, and wheezing (Table 13–2).

Diagnosis

The presence of GERD can usually be assumed in the setting of the classical symptoms of heartburn and regurgitation. However, GERD may cause atypical symptoms or even significant esophagitis in the absence of symptoms. The demonstration of *reflux esophagitis* on endoscopy is fairly characteristic (see Figure 10–2) of the lesion. Biopsies of involved mucosa may reveal hyperplastic or inflammatory changes described above.

Occasionally histopathologic findings of GERD may be seen in the absence of endoscopic abnormality. Other tests include 24-hr pH monitoring, which quantifies the duration of acid response in the lower esophagus (see Chapter 10) or the Bernstein test, wherein the dripping of acid into the esophagus reproduces the individual's heartburn.

Complications

GASTROESOPHAGEAL REFLUX COMPLICATED BY ESOPHAGEAL METAPLASIA (BARRETT'S ESOPHAGUS). The normal squamous epithelium is replaced with specialized columnar epithelium as a result of prolonged reflux and severe damage to the esophageal mucosa. This replacement, or metaplasia, is known as *Barrett's esophagus.* Barrett's epithelium is more resistant to the corrosive effects of acid reflux. Symptoms of reflux may abate after the development of Barrett's metaplasia. This columnar epithelium may be of different types, representing the various parts of gastric epithelium such as cardiac, fundic, body, or antral epithelium and frequently a unique specialized epithelium that mixes both gastric and intestinal metaplasia (Figure 13–2). Barrett's esophagus can be defined as a columnar epithelial lining of the tubular esophagus at least 3 cm above the LES. However, the definition will miss what is known as *short segment Barrett's* (Spechler, Zeroogian, Antonioli, Wang, & Goyal, 1994). Also in many patients with Barrett's the LES has such a low pressure that its location is difficult. The finding of a specialized columnar epithelium on a biopsy taken from the gastroesophageal junction implies the presence of Barrett's esophagus (Kim et al., 1994). Barrett's mucosa is peptic in nature and as such is prone to the development of peptic ulcers. Ulcers, unlike erosions, penetrate through the muscularis mucosae into the submucosa. These often form discrete round or oval craters within the area of Barrett's epithelium. Barrett's epithelium may be prone to malignant change, in particular, adenocarcinoma. The lifetime risk of malignant change in Barrett's esophagus has been reported up to 10% but this high incidence is probably due to bias based on selection for adenocarcinoma arising in Barrett's esophagus. The risk of malignant change increases with the length of metaplastic epithelium (Iftikhar, James, Steele, Hardcastle, & Atkinson, 1992).

Although most common in the middle aged and elderly, the condition can present at any age, including infancy. It may occur after cancer chemotherapy; however, prospective studies have not confirmed that observation (Peters, Sleijfer, van Imhoff, & Kleibeuker, 1993). Barrett's esophagus manifests itself most often as dysphagia from an esophageal stricture or, less commonly, as a bleeding esophageal ulcer. The absence of heartburn despite a highly abnormal reflux profile in many of these patients may be linked to sensory deficiencies of the metaplastic epithelium. Diagnostic studies in Barrett's esophagus reveal severe reflux and poor esophageal clearance (Iascone et al., 1983). On radiographic examination, the esophagus may be shortened, poorly distensible, and often strictured or ulcerated. Strictures are located at the junction of squamous and columnar epithelium, which is displaced proximally. Typical erosive esophagitis with

superficial ulcers is seen in the squamous mucosa proximal to the squamocolumnar junction, whereas deep peptic "Barrett's ulcers" that resemble peptic gastric ulcers occur in the metaplastic epithelium distal to the junction. A "short esophagus" (brachyesophagus) is recognized by the formation of a permanent axial (or "sliding") hiatal hernia or by transverse mucosal folds in the distal esophagus.

Endoscopy, biopsy, and cytology are essential for examination of the epithelial changes. Columnar cell metaplasia should be suspected when the esophageal mucosa is salmon-red and velvety instead of glistening smooth and pearly-pink, with proximal displacement of the squamocolumnar interface (Figure 13–2). With columnar metaplasia, there is a risk of recurrent ulceration, stricture formation, and neoplastic transformation. Effective medical or operative treatment that controls reflux is thought to halt the progression of metaplasia. Evidence is conflicting as to whether antireflux therapy can reverse the Barrett's changes or reduce the risk of adenocarcinoma development. Yearly endoscopy with multiple biopsies and cytology brushing for the early detection of dysplasia or cancer is currently recommended, although it remains to be determined whether this is cost-effective. The finding of high-grade dysplasia in Barrett's esophagus is an indication for operative resection (Pera et al., 1992; Peters et al., 1994). Survival is better with adenocarcinoma found as part of a surveillance program in an earlier stage than with adenocarcinoma in an area of previously unrecognized Barrett's esophagus. Other approaches to Barrett's esophagus included laser ablation and mucosal stripping (Overholt, Panjehpour, Tefftellar, & Rose, 1993; Wang, 1994). These are still experimental (Gray, Donnelly, & Kings-north, 1993; Streitz, Andrews, & Ellis, 1993).

Dysplastic and neoplastic change in Barrett's esophagus may be focal and not visible endoscopically. Multiple biopsies from different levels are recommended for screening. Early detection of dysplastic change may be aided by using flow cytometry (Nakamura et al., 1994). There is some evidence that oncogenic alteration in P53 may be predictive of dysplasia and cancer risk, but this awaits confirmation (Krishnadath, van Blankenstein, & Tilanus, 1995).

Dysphagia in GERD

The following mechanisms may lead to dysphagia in GERD: (a) mechanical; esophageal stricture or adenocarcinoma complicating a Barrett's esophagus and (b) motor dysfunction associated with GERD.

ESOPHAGEAL STRICTURES. Esophageal strictures complicate up to 10% of cases of reflux esophagitis. This scarring reflects long-standing mucosal injury usually in the setting of severe erosive esophagitis. These often occur at the proximal aspect of an area of Barrett's esophagus. The result is a concentric narrowing of the lumen, which tapers from above down. In cases of long-standing obstruction diverticula may form above the stricture. The stricture may vary considerably in length. The stricture is composed of scar tissue that is laid down in a circumferential pattern at the squamocolumnar junction. Typically this is internal to the muscle layer and involves the replacement of the mucosa and submucosa with scar tissue.

GERD-ASSOCIATED MOTOR DYSFUNCTION. In patients with reflux esophagitis there are well-described changes in motor function of the esophagus. There may be diminished peristaltic force. The duration of contractions in the distal esophagus may be prolonged. Many swallows may not result in peristaltic waves and effective transport of material. Much debate has centered on whether these motor effects are the cause or the result of the acid damage. There is good evidence that, when the esophagitis is healed, there may be improvement in the motor function and symptomatic improvement in dysphagia. Many patients with reflux esophagitis will complain of pain while swallowing. Cold or hot liquids may be particularly bothersome.

Treatment

Avoidance of esophageal injury is of paramount importance. Many drugs, including calcium channel blockers, theophylline, and nitrates may adversely affect the esophagus. Anticholinergic drugs may aggravate gastroesophageal reflux, since they decrease LES pressure, delay gastric emptying, and reduce salivation. Abstinence from smoking, drinking alcohol, and coffee are usually helpful.

DIETARY AND OTHER SYMPTOMATIC MEASURES. Reduction of meal size and instituting a diet low in fat, chocolate, caffeine, acidic foods, spices, and sweets provide relief in many patients with postprandial reflux symptoms. Taking fluids between rather than with meals is often advised. Avoidance of food or liquids for 2 hours before retiring at night is desirable. Weight reduction is recommended in obese patients. Antacids are often helpful in alleviating heartburn or postprandial fullness. Alginic acid preparations are also popular, but their effectiveness is not established. Smoking increases reflux and patients should be counseled to stop.

POSTURAL MEASURES. Gravity facilitates esophageal clearance during sleep. This can be accomplished by elevating the head end of the bed, by placing 4- to 6-inch blocks under the legs at the head of the bed; foam wedges long enough to elevate the entire torso can also be used. Postural measures are particularly helpful in patients with manifestations of recumbent reflux (i.e., nocturnal aspiration and cricopharyngeal spasm). Because of their inconvenience, postural measures are unlikely to be executed unless sleeping partners as well as the patients themselves understand their purpose and are told that it takes a matter of 3–4 nights to become accustomed to sleeping on a gentle incline.

DRUGS

Antisecretory Drugs

Antisecretory drugs (Histamine H$_2$-receptor antagonists or proton pump inhibitors) improve symptoms of gastroesophageal reflux and decrease the severity of esophagitis. If erosive esophagitis is documented, cimetidine (800 mg bid), famotidine (20 mg bid), or ranitidine/nizatidine (150 mg bid) should be administered for at least 3 months. Higher doses may be more effective. Omeprazole, 20–40 mg daily, or lansoprazole, 15–30 mg (proton pump inhibitors), are indicated for the treatment of severe erosive esophagitis or esophagitis refractory to other medical treatment and are the single most effective drug therapy for healing esophagitis. This efficacy is related to the greater degree and more prolonged acid suppression compared to H_2 receptor antagonists. Relapse is the rule after the drugs are discontinued unless the patient eliminated other exacerbating factors. Long-term medical treatment is indicated in patients with severe relapsing esophagitis or prominent nocturnal symptoms who are not candidates for operative treatment. Omeprazole is superior to H2 blockers in preventing relapse of GERD-related strictures (Marks et al., 1994).

Prokinetic Drugs

An adjunct to acid suppression are drugs that alter the motor activity of the upper GI tract. Three prokinetic drugs (bethanechol, metoclopramide, cisapride) increase LES pressure and improve esophageal clearance in the supine but not in the upright position (McCallum, 1990). Bethanechol and cisapride also may increase salivation. Nighttime dosing in conjunction with antisecretory or coating agents is especially indicated in conditions of nocturnal or alkaline reflux. Bethanechol, the prototype agent, is seldom used because it stimulates acid secretion and causes intestinal, bladder, and bronchial spasm. It may be gradually increased from 10 to 40 mg at bedtime if tolerated. Metoclopramide, 10 mg 4 times a day before meals, is also helpful in alleviating nausea or vomiting. However, it has very limited utility in the long-term management of reflux disease owing to central nervous system side effects, which include dystonic reactions

and tardive dyskinesia. It is probably best left to short-term or nighttime use only. Cisapride is as effective as regular dose H2 blockers in healing reflux esophagitis but its major advantage and indication is for the relief of symptoms. This it does by a combination of enhancing gastric emptying, increasing esophageal clearance and raising LES tone. It also increases salivary secretion. It is used in doses of 10–20 mg 4 times a day. It has minimal if any central CNS effects and does not produce the visceral cramps common with bethanechol or the dystonic reactions common with metoclopramide.

DILATATION OF ESOPHAGEAL STRICTURES (SEE DETAILED DISCUSSION IN CHAPTER 10). Any narrowing of the esophageal lumen may compromise nutrition and pose the risk of bolus impaction. Esophageal dilatation should be performed to the point where dysphagia resolves, which generally corresponds to a luminal diameter in excess of 14 mm. Every attempt should be made to prevent recurrent stricture formation and to dilate strictures at an early stage. There are several means by which one can dilate strictures. Commonly used are through-the-endoscope balloon dilators (see Chapter 10, Figure 10–5) which are especially useful for tight strictures. Alternatively are a series of wire guided dilators: The endoscopist places a narrow guidewire through the stricture, removes the scope, and then advances a metal (olive-shaped) or plastic Savary or Celestin dilators across the stricture. One starts with a diameter close to that of the stricture, and then gradually increases diameters to achieve relief of symptoms safely. The guidewire reduces the risk of perforation. The guidewire-directed techniques are useful for tight or rigid strictures, especially in the presence of diverticula. Fluoroscopy may aid in the orientation of dilators in complicated strictures and in caustic strictures. It is important to avoid inadvertent movement of the guidewire (Kadakia, Parker, Carrougher, & Shaffer, 1993). The third type of dilators are the mercury-weighted rubber-coated bougies.

These are swallowed by the patient and are useful for wide strictures and in some patients who need to perform repeated self-passage of these dilators.

SURGICAL TREATMENT. Several surgical techniques have been developed to treat GERD. These attempt to restore the barrier against reflux by augmenting resting LES pressure, by altering the anatomic relationship between the stomach and esophagus, and by reducing hiatal hernias. The most widely accepted operation is the *Nissen fundoplication* and its modifications. *Fundoplication* involves mobilizing the fundus of the stomach and passing it posterior to the gastroesophageal junction. It is then sutured to the anterior aspect of the gastroesophageal junction and stomach in front (Bushkin, Neustein, Parker, & Woodward, 1977). Fundoplication and similar operations can virtually eliminate gastroesophageal reflux and its symptoms. Healing of esophageal erosions and ulcerations is the rule, and strictures no longer recur. Although initial failure of the operation is rare in the hands of experienced surgeons, the likelihood of recurrent reflux increases after 5 to 10 years. Operative treatment is indicated in patients with serious complications of gastroesophageal reflux (i.e., recurrent aspiration pneumonia, peptic strictures, bleeding esophageal erosions or ulcers, and intractable symptoms) that fail to respond to rigorous medical management. Pyrosis alone may occasionally become an indication for fundoplication in patients not wishing to depend on long-term use of acid-suppressing drugs. The major complication of fundoplication is postoperative dysphagia, which was more common after the 360° wrap. The use of fundoplication is controversial in patients with scleroderma and other diseases that permanently impair esophageal motility and clearance. Many surgeons use preoperative esophageal manometry to ensure that the esophageal peristalsis is normal before the surgery, on the premise that an abnormal manometry may indicate a higher risk of postoperative dysphagia. In light of

the literature suggesting that motor function may improve after the treatment of esophagitis, it may be worthwhile to place patients on omeprazole or high-dose H_2 blockers prior to manometry. When the long-term safety of marked acid suppression is established it is likely that the necessity for surgical correction will be reduced. Occasionally, patients with scleroderma may initially present with esophageal symptoms and manometry may help to identify these patients.

The advent of laparoscopically performed *Nissen fundoplication*, which reduces morbidity of the surgery and, lessens duration of hospital stay, is awaiting the test of time to determine what the long-term results will be. Some small initial studies have shown a symptom relief rate that is as good as open fundoplication (Ferguson & Rattner, 1995; Pitcher et al., 1994).

Caustic Esophageal Injury and Dysphagia

In 1979, approximately 12,000 cases of ingestion of corrosive materials were reported in the United States (Wasserman & Ginsburg, 1985). It has been estimated that 5,000 children under 5 years are exposed to caustic injury annually (Spechler, 1990). This injury may result from accidental or deliberate ingestion of caustic agents containing alkali, acid, or other substances. Common alkaline agents include household cleansers containing ammonia and lye soaps (sodium or potassium hydroxide), strong acids such as hydrochloride, phosphoric acid, and sulfuric acid, which may be present in toilet and swimming pool cleaners, and miscellaneous substances such as bleach (5% sodium hypochlorite) and mercury-containing batteries. The severity of injury depends on the speed of transit through the esophagus, the corrosive property and the concentration of the agent, the dose consumed, and the existence of any underlying pathology. Alkaline solutions tend to cause penetrating injury, whereas acid solutions may only cause superficial damage. The alkali rapidly dissolves cell membranes, allowing rapid and deep penetration into the tissue. Tracheobronchial aspiration of these substances may lead to additional problems, including life-threatening injuries and acute dysphagia/dyspnea. Paraquat, an herbicide, while it is caustic and can present with local injury, is frequently fatal owing to delayed pulmonary/renal toxicity.

Clinical Features

The symptoms, which may be initially denied by the subject, are related to the site and degree of damage inflicted by the caustic agent. However, it is worth emphasizing that the early symptoms and signs are not reliable indicators of the severity and extent of injury, and the prognosis (Gaudreault, Parent, McGuigan, Chicone, & Lovejoy, 1983). Three phases of acute injury have been described (Johnson, 1963; Liu & Richardson, 1985). The acute phase, days 1–4, is associated with severe burning sensation in the throat and in the substernal region. This is associated with dysphagia, odynophagia, and excessive salivation. This may be associated with hoarseness of voice, stridor, and dyspnea (Kirsh & Ritter, 1976). The oropharynx and the esophageal mucosa are usually red, inflamed, and edematous, with or without superficial erosions and/or necrosis. A grayish pseudomembrane may be seen overlying the necrotic area. Pathologically, this phase is characterized by liquefactive necrosis and vascular thrombosis of the mucosa and submucosa (Fisher, Eckhauser, & Radivoyevitch, 1985).

The subacute phase, days 5–14, is classically associated with dysphagia and an inability to swallow saliva and other secretions. The esophageal wall is extremely thin and susceptible to perforation. Patients may present with dysphagia as an emergency or with fever, vomiting, pain, mediastinitis, pleural effusion, or peritonitis. Extensive mucosal sloughing may be associated with development of granulation tissue and collagen deposition. Dysphagia may be the only manifestation of the cicatrization phase, day 15 to 3 months. New onset of dysphagia indicates the development of a caustic stricture. Between 10 and 33% of patients with caustic ingestion may develop this complication (Kikendal & Johnson, 1983). Lye-induced esophageal stricture has been reported to be associated with a 1000-fold increased risk of developing squamous cell carcinoma of the esophagus, although the latent interval may range from 13 to 71 years (Appleqvist & Salmo, 1980).

Management

The management of caustic injury includes airway protection, intravenous fluids, correcting hypotension, and pain relief. Laryngeal edema may present many hours after the original ingestion and hence the patient with oropharyngeal injury must be monitored carefully. Emesis should not be induced, since this could increase the likelihood of further esophageal insult. Perforation should be immediately treated with antibiotics and surgery. Neutralization of an alkali with acid or vice versa is not effective, since they are not effective and the exothermic reaction induced by the neutralizing agent may add a thermal to the chemical injury (Rumack & Burrington, 1977). Once the patient is stabilized, an endoscopic examination may be performed to assess the severity and extent of mucosal injury. A normal endoscopy favors a good prognosis (Adam & Birck, 1982; Chung & DenBesten, 1975). A barium swallow is useful as a follow-up test for detecting esophageal strictures and in assessing the patency of any stricture following dilatation.

The use of corticosteroids in the management of acute esophageal caustic injury is controversial. Steroid use was promoted when research studies with animal models suggested that steroids could reduce the frequency of esophageal stricture formation (Spain, Molomut, & Haber, 1950), but to date no controlled study has shown the efficacy of using steroids in humans. In the face of impending complications such as perforation, sepsis, and the like, steroids should be avoided. The use of antibiotics is also controversial, but in patients with a high risk of pulmonary aspiration, sepsis, and other complications, it would seem prudent to give a course of broad spectrum antibiotics (Di Contanza, Noircleric, Jouglard, Escoffier, & Martin, 1977). Sucralfate has been used to help protect the mucosa and to promote healing, and may be a useful adjunct. Agents that inhibit maturation of collagen have also been tried in animal models (Butler, Madden, Davis, & Peacock, 1977; Gehano & Guedon, 1981), but their use in humans has not been reported. In patients with severe injuries nutritional support must be provided either via a nasogastric tube or via parenteral feeding. In the very acute situation, it may not be possible or prudent to place a nasogastric tube, at least until the danger of perforation recedes. The placement of a nasogastric tube serves many purposes; enteral feeding, maintaining patency of the esophageal lumen, and facilitating future dilation.

Esophageal stricture is the most common long-term complication and is reported to occur in 10–33% of patients with corrosive ingestion (Symbal, Vlasis, & Hatcher, 1983). This is traditionally managed with bougie dilatation. Successful endoscopic dilatation of nearly pinhole corrosive strictures suggests that many of these cases can be treated without surgery (Broor et al., 1993). Although there has been no comparison between endoscopic dilatation and surgery, in severe cases or those with complications, surgical removal of the esophagus with colon interposition may be required (Gerzic, Knezevic, Milicevis, & Jounnovic, 1990).

Pill Esophagitis

The lodging of a pill or a tablet in the esophagus may cause localized caustic damage to the mucosa (Kikendall, 1991). The pills are most often trapped in areas where the esophagus is indented by extrinsic structures such as the aortic arch, left main bronchus, diaphragmatic hiatus, or a stricture. Risk factors include preexisting esophageal disease, large size, the body posture during pill ingestion particularly in the supine position, and efforts to ingest the pill with little or no liquid to wash it down. Some pills are more harmful than others, owing to the caustic nature of their chemical composition. The most common pills that cause damage are quinidine, tetracyclines, iron, denture-cleansing pills, potassium pills, vitamin C, nonsteroidal anti-inflammatory drugs, and emepromium. The patients usually present with chest pain and/or odynophagia, often the morning after ingestion of the offending pill. The risk can be reduced by instructing the patient to take adequate liquid (3–4 oz) or even food with the medication, to avoid taking medication while recumbent, and to prescribe liquid formulations or rectal formulations where appropriate. The new onset of odynophagia in an individual taking potentially caustic medication in a high-risk manner should suggest the possibility of pill esophagitis. Endoscopy will usually reveal circumscribed ulceration, often in the proximal esophagus surrounded by normal mucosa. The treatment is symptomatic and sucralfate suspension seems to be effective in relieving symptoms. Complications such as bleeding or perforation are rare.

Sclerotherapy-Induced Stricture

An iatrogenic form of esophageal stricture may occur as the result of sclerotherapy of esophageal varices. Esophageal varices are dilated veins that occur in patients with portal hypertension most often due to liver disease. These veins tend to bleed, often massively. To stop variceal bleeding, endoscopists inject these veins with sclerosing substances that induce inflammation to obliterate the varices. Esophageal stricture is an undesirable complication of this procedure, which can result in dysphagia (Haynes, Sanowski, Foutch, & Bellapravalu, 1986). This usually occurs several weeks after sclerotherapy. Formation of strictures is more common with higher volumes or paravariceal injection of sclerosant. Usually strictures can be dilated easily without significant risk of rebleeding.

Esophageal Infections Causing Dysphagia

Bacterial, fungal, and viral infections of the esophagus are important treatable causes of acute dysphagia and odynophagia. With an increasing number of patients with immune deficiency, from HIV infection, immunosuppressive therapy, or chemotherapy for malignant conditions, the incidence of infectious esophagitis has risen steadily. Infectious esophagitis may be the first manifestation of an immunocompromised host. Many infectious diseases can cause esophagitis (Table 13–3). Rare causes include aspergillosis, histoplasmosis, blastomycosis, Varicella-Zoster virus, actinomycosis, streptococcus viridans, and treponema pallidum infections.

Candida Esophagitis

This is by far the most common infection of the esophagus. *Candida albicans* is the most frequent pathogen, but infections with *C. tropicalis*, *C. parapsilosis*, and a closely related fungus, *Torulopsis glabrata*, have all been reported. Primary infection commonly occurs in an immunocompromised host but broad spectrum antibiotic therapy and inhaled corticosteroids may also predispose to this problem particularly in the elderly.

The most common symptom is dysphagia and this is usually worse for solids than liquids. Occasionally patients may be asymptomatic or have heartburn, nausea, or vomiting. Physical examination may reveal oral plaques of candida but is generally unhelpful. A definitive diagnosis is best established with esophagoscopy (Figure 13–3). The endoscopic appearances may be graded as follows:

TABLE 13–3. Common infectious causes of esophagitis.

Cause	Endoscopic Appearance	Histologic Appearance
Candidia esophagitis	white plaques	branching hyphae
Cytomegalovirus esophagitis	large ulcers	cytoplasmic/nuclear inclusion
Herpes simplex	small ulcers	intranuclear inclusions
Tuberculosis	friable mass	acid-fast bacilli

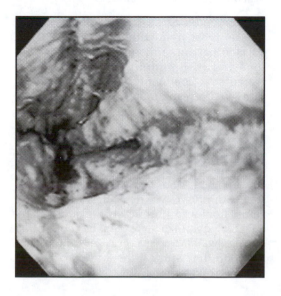

Figure 13–3. The endoscopic photograph demonstrates the white plaques of candidal esophagitis adherent to the esophageal mucosa.

Grade 1—a few raised white plaques up to 2 mm in diameter without ulceration

Grade 2—multiple plaques without ulcers

Grade 3—confluent, linear, or nodular plaques with ulceration

Grade 4—Grade 3 plus luminal narrowing.

DIAGNOSIS. The diagnosis of infections may be confirmed by histopathologic examination of the brushings or the biopsies from the plaques. Oral antifungal therapy is generally effective in the treatment of esophageal candidiasis. Oral Nystatin 400,000 units taken every 4 hours for 2–4 weeks is effective for light infection. Ketoconazole 200 mg/day is rapidly becoming the drug of choice, owing to a better compliance, a shorter duration of therapy, and less likelihood of antimicrobial resistance. These agents alter the fungal cell membrane permeability by interfering with sterol synthesis. Miconazole, fluconazole, and in resistant cases systemic amphotericin B are all suitable alternatives to ketoconazole. Candidiasis in the setting of the immunocompromised host usually requires a potent systemic antifungal. Resistance can occur especially in patients on long-term prophylaxis. *Torulopis glabrata* forms large ulcers and may require amphotericin B (Tom & Aaron, 1987). Failure of therapy in an immunocompromised patient should prompt consideration of a coexistent viral esophagitis, as it may coexist with the candida (Smith et al., 1993).

Herpes Simplex

This is the second most common esophageal infection and usually presents with a sudden onset of severe odynophagia with an inability to swallow solids and liquids. Patients may show evidence of herpes infection elsewhere such as herpes labialis. In immune-deficient patients the virus invades the mucosa, causing vesicles, which may enlarge, coalesce, and ulcerate. These lesions may bleed, perforate, or cause a tracheoesophageal fistu-

la. The diagnosis is best confirmed by endoscopy and biopsy of the mucosa. Endoscopically, discrete, stellate ulcers or diffuse shaggy esophagitis may be seen. Biopsies of the ulcer margins may reveal multinucleate squamous cells with herpes inclusion bodies. Serology for viral titers may provide additional corroborative evidence. Therapy consists of providing symptomatic relief with oral administration of 2% viscous lidocaine to help odynophagia. Specific therapy with Acyclovir, 250 mg/m^2 every 8 hours may reduce viral shedding and promote rapid healing.

Cytomegalovirus

This is a frequent cause of dysphagia in patients infected with HIV, and like other infections presents with dysphagia or odynophagia. Endoscopically small or giant ulcers may be seen, predominantly affecting the lower third of the esophagus. Pathologically, round or oval inclusion bodies may be seen in the cytoplasm of infected squamous cells. Gancyclovir is the agent of choice in treating this infection (Wilcox, Straub, & Schwartz, 1995). Foscarnet, an agent that inhibits DNA polymerase, has also been shown to be useful, but is quite toxic.

Mycobacterium Tuberculosis

In the United States tuberculous esophagitisis most frequently seen in the HIV-infected patient, although it has also been reported in nonimmune-compromised patients. It commonly affects the middle third of the esophagus and may spread from adjacent structures such as the lungs, mediastinal lymph nodes, and the larynx. In the early stages the symptoms are not readily discernible but some patients with mucosal ulceration may present with odynophagia. More frequently, patients present with progressive dysphagia from an inflammatory and fibrotic stricture. Sudden onset of dyspnea or excessive coughing during swallowing or recurrent pulmonary infection may suggest the development of a tracheoesophageal fistula.

Endoscopically the lesions vary from chronic deep ulceration to a granulomatous mass mimicking a carcinoma. Diagnosis can be established by taking brushings or biopsies from affected lesions for histopathology and by performing special stains (acid-fast or auramine staining), as well as by culturing the samples for mycobacteria. A high index of suspicion is required when examining a susceptible individual. Barium studies of the esophagus may particularly help to localize sinus tracts and fistulae and for follow-up of lesions during treatment. Standard triple or quadruple therapy with isoniazid, ethambutol, pyrazinamide, and streptomycin should be employed but, with the emergence of several resistant strains, alternative therapy with newer generation antimycobacterial agents may be required.

Rare Inflammatory Lesions of the Esophageal Mucosa

Several rare conditions affect the esophageal mucosa. As the esophagus is lined with squamous epithelium, occasionally diseases of the skin or mucous membranes may involve the esophagus. These include epidermolysis bullosa (a rare inerited blistering skin rash that heals with scarring), *pemphigus*, *Behçet's syndrome*, and dermatitis herpetiformis. Crohn's disease may occasionally cause aphthous ulceration and stricturing of the esophagus. The finding of noncaseating granulomas on biopsy or the presence of intestinal Crohn's would suggest the diagnosis.

Esophageal Rings and Webs

Cricopharyngeal Web (Plummer-Vinson Syndrome)

Plummer-Vinson syndrome (also called the Paterson-Kelly syndrome), consists of dysphagia, iron deficiency anemia, upper esophageal inflammation with web formation, angular stomatitis, and gastritis. This frequently presents in adults in their fourth or fifth decade and occurs more frequently in females than males. The etiology seems to be related to the iron deficiency. Several studies have demonstrated inflammation of the mucosa or the muscularis propria of the affected segment. Disorders related to connective tissue have also been described. Diminished force of swallowing secondary to a myopathy may be responsible for the dysphagia (Okamura, Tsutsumi, Inaki, & Mori, 1988). The web may form at the junction between the squamous mucosa of the esophagus and islands of gastric-type mucosa in the upper esophagus (Weaver, 1979). This condition may be associated with an increased risk of esophageal malignancy owing to the chronic inflammation of the esophagus. A condition similar to Plummer-Vinson syndrome occurs in artificially induced iron deficiency anemia in rabbits, in which there seems to be an alteration of the muscle fibers, due to defects in the myoglobin. A selective decrease in myoglobin was seen in the swallowing muscles of these iron-deficient animals (Tsutsumi, 1993).

DIAGNOSIS. Webs are often discovered on contrast x-ray studies and appear as a discrete indentation of the upper esophageal lumen just below the upper esophageal sphincter. Flexible endoscopy may also reveal the presence of a web. However, these webs can be missed at endoscopy since they are located immediately below the upper esophageal sphincter and are relatively wide-mouthed. The endoscope may be advanced through this area, or, the web can retard passage of the endoscope. With vigorous passage there can be bleeding, which may be brisk but usually self-limiting. On withdrawal of the scope through the upper esophagus, the torn remnants of the web may be visible. Rigid esophagoscopy, under general anesthesia, may reveal the web on careful evaluation.

TREATMENT. The primary treatment is to correct the iron deficiency. Esophageal dilatation can be performed to relieve dysphagia. The condition may recur if the iron deficiency is not corrected.

Esophageal Rings

This is a common and an incidental finding at endoscopy, with a prevalence of 14% in the population. Essentially, the condition represents a mucosal ring at the lower end of the esophagus, usually at the squamocolumnar junction (Schatzki, 1963). Most patients are asymptomatic but those with symptoms present with episodic dysphagia, usually after hurried ingestion of solid food. The dysphagia is usually transient and the patient is often successful in disimpacting the food by drinking liquids. Radiologically, this ring may appear as a symmetric invagination of the lower end of the esophagus. Endoscopically, a folded rim of mucosa that is either partially or completely occupying the esophageal lumen can be identified. The esophageal lumen is usually widely patent at the level of the ring. It may be associated with a hiatal hernia. While there is at least some connection with gastroesophageal reflux, the presence of a ring is not correlated with altered LES pressures (Chen, Ott, Donati, Wu, & Gelfand, 1994). Histologically, the ring has a squamous lining on the orad side and a columnar lining on the underside. The diagnosis can be made from the episodic history and the nonprogressive nature of the patient's symptoms. To identify the ring, the esophagus above must be well-filled with barium (or air in the case of endoscopy). If the patient is symptomatic the ring can be easily dilated either by balloon or with Savary-Gillard dilators over a guidewire.

MUSCULAR RING. Occasionally a muscular ring may be identified at the lower end of the esophagus, usually above the mucosal ring. There is thickening of the circular muscle layer with normal squamous epithelium overlying it. Both the muscular and mucosal rings may be difficult to differentiate from an annular stricture secondary to chronic reflux esophagitis. Recurrence of a ring following successful dilation suggests a reflux-related phenomenon and the need for long-term anti-reflux therapy.

CONGENITAL ESOPHAGEAL STENOSIS. This is a rare congenital defect that occurs owing to a embryogenic abnormality. It may be associated with tracheobronchial remnants. The stenosis usually presents in infancy but occasionally diagnosis is delayed until adulthood (McNally, Lemon, Goff, & Freeman, 1993). Treatment can be dilatation in the adult with surgery utilized most in the infant (Neilson, Croitoru, Guttman, Youssef, & Laberge, 1991).

Esophageal Cancers

Esophageal cancers have an incidence in the United States of 3–4/100,000. Esophageal cancers most frequently arise in the mucosa as squamous carcinoma of native squamous cells or as adenocarcinoma of the columnar lining from the so-called Barrett's metaplasia. Adenocarcinoma arising from the cardia of the stomach can also cause esophageal obstruction and seems to behave much like adenocarcinoma of the lower esophagus. Esophageal cancer of either type is more common in males than in females (3:1) and in blacks than whites (3:1). The peak ages of occurrence are over 55 in whites and over 45 in blacks (Blot, Devesa, Kneller, & Fraumeni, 1991; Wang, Antonioli, & Goldman, 1986; Yang & Davis, 1988).

Squamous Cancer

The incidence of squamous cell carcinoma varies globally with a very high incidence in locations such as the Linxian province of China, northern Iran, central Asia, and southeast Africa. Risk factors include fungal toxins from poorly stored grains, high levels of ingested nitrosoamines, and opium byproducts. The risk factors identified in the Western world are male sex, alcoholism, and smoking. Deficiencies of micronutrients such as vitamins A and C, and riboflavin, selenium, and other minerals may also increase the susceptibility. Gluten-sensitive enteropathy is associated with depletion of selenium and an increased rate of esophageal malignancy. Prior corrosive injury of the esophagus with alkaline material as well as preexisting esophageal stasis due to achalasia or stricture increases the risk for cancer. Other rare conditions such as familial hyperkeratosis of the palms and soles (tylosis) as well as the Plummer-Vinson syndrome are also associated with an increase in risk. Squamous cell carcinoma can occur in any part of the esophagus, whereas adenocarcinoma usually occurs in the lower one third.

Adenocarcinoma

Adenocarcinoma usually arises from a segment of Barrett's epithelium and probably is the result of long-standing GERD. It is less likely that some of the adenocarcinoma of the cardia actually arise in the esophagus and spread distally. The incidence of adenocarcinoma of the stomach has dramatically declined over the last 50 years, but there has been no change in the incidence of cancer arising from the cardia. The incidence of adenocarcinoma in the esophagus has risen significantly in the last 10 years in Western countries, especially in middle-aged white men (Brown, et al., 1994; Hesketh, Clapp, Doos, & Spechler, 1989; Wang, Hsieh, & Antonioli, 1994). This is in contrast to the incidence of squamous carcinoma, which is falling (Blot et al., 1991; Wang et al., 1986; Yang et al.,1988).

SYMPTOMS. Typically patients with carcinomas of the esophagus present with progressive dysphagia, more for solids than liquids, with associated weight loss. Persistent and intractable coughing may signal encroachment onto the trachea or even fistulization. Liver enlargement from metastases or palpable lymph nodes may be seen. Other tumors such as leiomyomas or Kaposi's sarcoma in AIDS may also occur as can secondary spread and especially from melanoma.

STAGING AND TREATMENT. Endoscopy with directed biopsy is the best way to diagnose esophageal carcinomas. Contrast radiography is helpful in defining the extent of the cancer. The extent of the tumor is of critical importance in planning treatment and in formulating prognosis. Imaging techniques using CT scanning and endoscopic ultrasound are especially helpful in defining the depth of penetration and whether lymph nodes are involved. In areas of the world with a high prevalence, the squamous carcinoma is often multifocal in 30% (Maeta et al., 1993).

At the time of presentation, most esophageal carcinomas have already metastasized and are therefore beyond cure. Cancers detected early at a superficial stage, through surveillance in areas of high incidence or Barrett's metaplasia, have a good prognosis. In the former category Stage O cancer 3-year survival rates of up to 100% have been described (Streitz, Ellis, Gibbs, Balogh, & Watkins, 1991). Local extension to the aorta, trachea, or other vital mediastinal structures often makes surgical resection impossible, and the operative mortality is 10 to 20%. Curative therapy is rare, with an expected mean 5-year survival of no more than 10%. Survival rates for surgical and radiation therapy are about equal, but 5-year survival rates of up to 20% have been achieved with more radical operations in patients with early or suspected localized disease. Hence, exact preoperative staging of the disease is important. In the lower esophagus, resection is preferred. Esophagectomy requires a reconstruction using a gastric tube or, less desirably, a segment of jejunum or colon. Anastomotic leaks and early recurrences are frequent complications. Radiotherapy is the treatment of choice for squamous cell carcinoma in the upper esophagus. Curative doses are often complicated by radiation esophagitis, and care must be exerted to avoid radiation injury to the heart, lungs, and spinal cord. Some reports indicate that combined radiation therapy and chemotherapy (using 5-fluorouracil and cisplatinum or mitomycin C) is advantageous before operation. It certainly can shrink the tumor and make it more amenable to surgical resection. Whether the added toxicity of the triple regimen is offset by an improvement in long-term survival is not completely established.

Palliation is directed at relieving pain, treating dysphagia, and preventing aspiration. Esophageal obstruction is relieved by dilatation, laser therapy, or electrocautery as deemed necessary. Jejunostomy may be required to maintain enteral feeding. Endoscopic placement of a prosthetic stent is the treatment of choice for fistulae between the esophagus and trachea or bronchi. Bulky intraluminal tumors may be vaporized with an endoscopically delivered laser or reduced in size with a special electrocautery device or with radiotherapy. Combined radiotherapy and chemotherapy may provide palliation for 50% of patients with advanced disease and dysphagia. Bleomycin, methotrexate, cisplatin, and other agents have some effect against esophageal cancers, but given singly, they are ineffective.

Metastatic Tumors of the Esophagus

Secondary tumors are relatively rare. The most common is spread from a pulmonary carcinoma or from the cardia of the stomach. Pharyngeal or laryngeal cancers may also spread directly into the upper esophagus. Metastatic spread occurs from breast, melanoma, Kaposi's sarcoma in immunosuppressed patients, thyroid, and lymphoma. Secondary tumors may be identified during the investigation of the primary site or may present with symptoms of GI bleeding, pain, or dysphagia. Endoscopically these may resemble a leiomyoma and are predominantly submucosal. With the exception of submucosal tumors, the majority of secondaries are readily diagnosed with biopsies and brush cytology obtained endoscopically (Kadakia, Parker, & Canales, 1992). There are several reports of successful enucleation of the submucosal tumors. The management is as for that of the primary tumor and usually entails palliative treatment of the patient's symptoms related to the esophageal lesion. Benign tumors arising from the mucosa of the stomach are rare but include embryonic cysts, and mucoceles of the duct system.

DISORDERS PRIMARILY INVOLVING THE MUSCULAR LAYER

Benign Tumors of the Esophagus

Leiomyoma of the esophagus is the most common benign neoplasm of the esophagus. Leiomyoma usually presents with dysphagia or may be an incidental finding in a patient undergoing investigation for upper GI symptoms. It originates from the smooth muscle of the lower two thirds of the esophagus. The size varies but can reach 12 cm in diameter. It usually appears as a rounded mass arising from the wall of the esophagus often with intact mucosa. Occasionally it can ulcerate or bleed. Histologically it usually consists of encapsulated whorls of smooth musclelike cells. Rarely these tumors can harbor a more malignant leiomyosarcoma.

Diagnosis

X-ray appearance may be very suggestive and endoscopy will usually demonstrate the well-rounded appearance and solid feel to these tumors, and tactile sensation will show the mucosa may move freely over the tumor. It is better not to biopsy the normal mucosa over the mass, as this may increase the risk of perforation during subsequent resection. Endoscopic ultrasound will show a characteristic appearance and facilitate an estimation of the depth of involvement (Murata et al., 1988). It may still be confused with a metastatic tumor or the very rare primary oat cell carcinoma of the esophagus.

Treatment

The treatment is usually extramucosal enucleation of the tumor via a thoracic approach, but if the lesion is located very low in the esophagus, a transabdominal approach may be required. If the latter approach is used, care should be taken not to breach the mucosa. Preservation of mucosal integrity may be easier for the surgeon if deep biopsies have not being taken prior to surgery, as this may cause tethering of the tumor to the mucosa. Smaller leiomyomas have been resected successfully via the esophagoscope with aid of ultrasound definition of the depth of the tumor. This technique uses electrocautery and ethanol injection to necrose the tumor (Eda et al., 1990; Yu, Luo, & Wang, 1992). Some feel that small (less than 2 cm) submucosal lesions in the esophageal wall may be followed conservatively if the patients are asymptomatic and there is no evidence of malignant appearance or behavior of the tumor.

Rare Tumors

Diffuse leiomyomatosis is a rare inherited condition that can be associated with Alport's syndrome (inherited renal disease and deafness). This can present with dysphagia and there are often multiple tumors involving the upper GI tract. It has even mimicked achalasia (Marshall, Diaz-Arias, Bochna, & Vogele, 1990).

There are other rare benign lesions including fibromas, lipomas, and neurofibromas often as a part of inherited neurofibromatosis syndrome. These have a similar appearance as that of the leiomyomas and are usually distinguished after surgery.

Functional Disorders of the Esophagus

Cricopharyngeal (CP) Spasm and Zenker's Diverticulum

Zenker's diverticulum is considered the end result of a repeated failure of the UES to remain open at a time when the food bolus arrives at this segment. A decrease in compliance and fibrosis of the cricopharyngeus has been identified in some of these patients (Cook, Blumbergs, Cash, Jamieson, & Shearman, 1992). It is believed that prolonged and excessive increase in intraluminal pressure at this site leads to a weakening of the muscle fibers of the pharynx at its junction with the upper esophageal sphincter. Through this weak area hypopharyngeal hernia-

tions may occur, leading to the formation of diverticula. These herniations most commonly occur on the left side, less commonly on the posterior wall and the midline, and only rarely on the right side.

The UES in cricoid achalasia is recognized radiographically as a smooth, so-called persistent *cricopharyngeal indentation bar* of the esophageal inlet. The syndrome of *cricoid achalasia* refers to the pharyngeal dysphagia and globus sensation often observed in this setting. Hypertrophy and/or fibrosis of the sphincter interferes with its compliance and hence the completeness and timing of opening during pharyngeal deglutition (Cook, Gabb, et al., 1992).

CLINICAL FEATURES. Zenker's diverticulum is commonly seen in men who are 50 years or older. Most patients describe an insidious onset of cervical dysphagia. They may regurgitate undigested food several hours or days after meals. Many patients have learned to empty the sac by manipulating their neck or performing some bodily contortion. Patients are at risk of aspiration and impaired nutrition. Careful physical examination may reveal gurgling during a test swallowing and a lump on the lateral aspect of the neck.

DIAGNOSIS. Videofluoroscopic contrast examination may reveal the diverticulum if present or a cricopharyngeal bar may be seen indenting the barium bolus. If endoscopic examination is being done great care must be taken to avoid perforating the diverticulum during insertion. Manometry recordings have demonstrated elevated pharyngeal bolus pressures.

TREATMENT. Treatment of this condition should address the underlying pathophysiology as well as the dysphagia and the associated complications. Cricopharyngeal myotomy may be undertaken alone if the sac is small, and if it is larger than 5 cm the sac should be removed. Diverticulopexy or the formation of a diverticuloesophagealostomy may also function to prevent retention and distention of the sac and cause compression and regurgitation. Large sacs that have been present for a long time may harbor a carcinoma. Sectioning of the cricopharyngeal muscle is sometimes the only treatment that may be required, especially when the diverticulum is small. Dilatation with a larger bougie also may suffice. Usually a wire-guide is used if a diverticulum is present.

Achalasia of the Esophagus

Achalasia is characterized by functional obstruction of the esophagogastric junction and retention of food in the esophagus. The functional abnormalities consist of failure or incomplete relaxation of the lower esophageal sphincter and aperistalsis of the smooth muscle, that is, the distal two thirds of the esophagus. The LES may be hypertensive, or have normal baseline tone. Achalasia is either primary idiopathic, which is common in the developed world, or secondary to Chagas disease (*Trypanosomiasis cruzei*). Primary idiopathic achalasia is associated with damage to the innervation of the smooth muscle esophagus (Kimura, 1928; Cassella, Brown, Sayre, & Ellis, 1964). The pathologic abnormalities predominantly affect the myenteric nerves of the esophagus and LES. Early autopsy studies described localized abnormalities in the vagal motor nuclei in the brain stem. Primary idiopathic achalasia is likely due to defects in the intrinsic or occasionally extrinsic vagal innervation (Cross, 1952; Hurst & Rake, 1930; Smith, 1970). There is significant muscle cell hyperplasia, which may be the result of the obstruction (Friesen, Henderson, & Hanna, 1983). The failure of relaxation of the lower esophageal sphincter is due to a loss of inhibitory innervation, probably the nitronergic inhibitory nerves that do mediate LES relaxation (Cohen, Fisher, & Tuch, 1972; Murray et al., 1995).

Derangements of other gastrointestinal and extragastrointestinal autonomic function identified in patients with achalasia suggest that the neuropathologic effects are widespread. However, these differences are usually asymptomatic (Benini et al., 1994). The cause of idiopathic achalasia is unknown. A connection to varicella-zoster infection is possible but unconfirmed (Robertson, Marti, & Atkinson, 1993). Secondary achalasia is seen commonly in South America as a delayed result of the parasitic infection with *Trypanosomiasis cruzei*, which occurs specifically in the low mountain regions of South America. Pseudoachalasia resembles achalasia in some ways. There is distal obstruction and often a dilated and aperistaltic esophagus proximal to this obstruction. However, the obstruction is usually due to infiltration and mechanical obstruction caused by a neoplasm in the cardia of the stomach or the level of the lower esophageal sphincter. Most commonly this would be caused by adenocarcinoma of the cardia of the stomach, squamous cell carcinoma of the esophagus, or a secondary metastatic tumor from pancreas, lung, or prostate among others (Parkman & Cotten, 1994). Lymphomatous or leukematous infiltration can also cause a similar pattern as can extrinsic compression from pancreatic pseudocyst, as have been reported. Primary achalasia itself may be associated with an increased risk of squamous cell neoplasia of the esophagus, probably related to cancer-inducing properties in the chronically retained esophageal residue and stasis esophagitis in the body of the esophagus (Aggestrup, Holm, & Sorensen, 1994; Meijssen, Tilanus, van Blankenstein, Hop & Ong, 1992). Case reports of adenocarcinoma have also been reported in patients who have had Barrett's metaplasia after treatment for their achalasia (Gallez, Berger, Moulinier, & Partensky, 1987; Goodman, Scott, Verani, & Berggreen, 1990).

CLINICAL FEATURES. The dysphagia is often initially intermittent and occurs for liquids and solids. There may also be symptoms of regurgitation of retained esophageal contents with aspiration. Chest pain can also occur but is rarely a solitary presenting feature. Some patients have dramatic weight loss. All ages are affected, with a predominance in the third, fourth, and fifth decades. There is a later peak, with approximately 15% of people with achalasia presenting over the age of 65.

Physical signs of achalasia are limited usually to weight loss and malnutrition, which occurs in a small number of patients, and the presence of aspiration pneumonitis or physical evidence of regurgitated material. The presence of a thoracic succussion splash has been described in patients with achalasia and may be elicited in the fasting patient by listening over the thorax, usually posteriorly, while shaking the patient vigorously. This is the result of the liquid residue in the dilated esophagus. There is usually a greatly delayed bedside swallowing test (see Chapter 5). The esophagus itself is often dilated and hypertrophied owing to the functional obstruction. In advanced cases, this becomes sigmoid-shaped and occupies a large portion of the thorax. There may be a large volume of liquid or semiliquid residual material in the esophagus. This may regurgitate, especially in the supine position, and can lead to aspiration pneumonia or, not infrequently, the discovery by the patient of regurgitated material on the pillow in the morning.

DIAGNOSIS. The diagnosis can initially be suggested by chest x-ray, which may demonstrate a dilated esophagus often with a visible air–fluid level and absence of a gastric air bubble. The lack of the air bubble is due to the fact that swallowed air is effectively prevented from escaping into the stomach owing both to the functional obstruction at the LES and often a coexisting column of water that functions as an airtight siphon valve. A barium study shows a dilated esophagus with a so-called bird beak narrowing at LES (see Chapter 6). The ingestion of gas granules or increased loading of the esophagus with barium in the upright position may result in abrupt relaxation of the LES as the weight of barium or pressure in the esophagus exceeds the resting tone of the sphincter. Endoscopic examination is required to rule out an infiltrating neoplasm affecting the cardia of the stomach or lower esophageal sphincter. Manometric

examination of esophageal motor function (see Chapter 10) will confirm the abnormalities. In long-standing achalasia barium examination and endoscopy together are usually sufficient. However, in cases without established radiographic findings, manometry will help define the abnormality and direct treatment. Autoantibodies directed against myenteric neurons have been seen in some patients (Singaram et al., 1994).

TREATMENT. As the most important and treatable functional defect in achalasia is a failure of the lower esophageal sphincter to relax appropriately, treatment efforts have been directed toward rendering this sphincter incompetent or causing it to relax at appropriate times. The pharmacologic approaches that have been tried include the use of smooth-muscle relaxants. Some act by interfering with calcium uptake in cells. Experimentally, calcium seems to be important in maintaining tone in this sphincter (Bianciani, Hillemeier, Bitar, & Makhlouf, 1987). Antianginal agents such as nitrates act as smooth-muscle relaxants via the release of nitric oxide. Both of these modalities have been found to be of limited use in idiopathic achalasia (Ghosh, Heading, & Palmer, 1994; Triadafilo-poulus, Aaronson, Sackel, & Burakoff, 1991). However, there are several South American studies suggesting that isosorbide dinitrate, a long-acting nitrate, can significantly improve dysphagia in achalasia associated with Chagas' disease (Ferreira, Lho, Patto, Froncon, & Oliveira, 1991; Figueiredo, Oliveria, Iazigi, & Matsuda, 1992). However, the nitrates properties as a muscle relaxant also cause dilation of the cranial vessels, leading to headache, often unacceptable to the patient. By and large, pharmacologic therapy is reserved for those patients who are too ill or infirm to undergo any type of procedure.

The next most common method would be an endoscopic balloon dilatation of the lower esophageal sphincter using one of a variety of balloon dilators to forcefully distend the sphincteric muscle. The basic precept is that in a sedated patient, an endoscope is passed through to first of all examine the esophagus and cardia and aspirate out any remaining residue in the esophagus. A large-diameter inflatable balloon is placed across the lower esophageal sphincter. This balloon is much larger and more rigid than the through-the-scope dilators used for esophageal strictures. Its position is verified by fluoroscopy or by direct visualization. The balloon is then inflated and this stretches and tears the muscular elements of the lower esophageal sphincter, reducing its pressure. This is an effective method for the treatment of adults with achalasia, with approximately 60–70% of patients requiring no further treatment (Reynolds & Parkman, 1989). Balloon myotomy is less efficacious in young adults and children. The reason for this difference is not known. Reports of botulinum toxin injections into the muscle layer of the lower esophageal sphincter have reported benefit in a short, uncontrolled study (Pasricha et al., 1994, 1995). However, long-term studies have not yet shown whether this is of long-term benefit. Plain bougienage using a tapered plastic dilator or mercury-filled rubber dilator is usually only of temporary benefit.

The other treatment option is the surgical approach. Here, the surgeon either through the abdominal or thoracic approach identifies the muscular elements of the lower esophageal sphincter and divides them, taking care to maintain mucosal integrity. This technique is usually highly effective in relieving the dysphagia associated with achalasia. There has been much controversy and a large body of literature addressing the necessity for incorporating an antireflux procedure into this technique, with some surgeons routinely including an antireflux procedure, most often a fundoplication, in addition to a fairly extensive myotomy. Others would emphasize the importance of a relatively short myotomy and their low long-term incidence of reflux when a short, limited myotomy is performed. These myotomies have been performed successfully, using the less-invasive technique of thorascopic or laproscopic myotomy. This surgery greatly shortens the hospital stay and reduces the postoperative morbidity. Again, the long-term efficacy of this particular surgical approach will require the test of time.

COMPLICATIONS. The complications of untreated achalasia include malnutrition, weight loss, aspiration and resultant pneumonia or pulmonary fibrosis, and rarely squamous cell carcinoma of the esophagus. The incidence of carcinoma complicating achalasia is variable. Treatment complications of balloon myotomy is associated with a small but definite risk (1–4%) for esophageal perforation. This perforation is usually evident within the first 24 hours after the procedure. Many centers perform follow-up contrast studies using hypaque to detect perforation. The usual treatment for perforation is immediate surgical repair and a definitive achalasia operation. Delayed recognition of a perforation may result in severe mediastinitis and a poor outcome. The likely success of a primary repair is inversely proportional to the delay in repair. Some minor bleeding as evidenced by some blood on the balloon postmyotomy is not unusual, but significant bleeding is unusual.

Other Motor Disorders

Although chest pain is believed to be a more common manifestation of these problems, dysphagia is an important and a frequently overlooked symptom. The features of the various esophageal motor disorders are outlined in Table 13–4. In two reports (Katz, Dalton, & Richter, 1987; Reidel & Clouse, 1985) dysphagia was observed in 40% of patients presenting with these motility disorders. Unlike achalasia, which has been well characterized clinically, functionally, radiologically, and pathologically, the other motor disorders have not been established as disease entities. They are largely manometric and/or radiologic phenomena. Furthermore, in most patients, a temporal relationship

TABLE 13–4. Manometric and clinical features of esophageal motility disorders

Entity	Dysphagia	Heartburn	Odynophagia	Chest Pain	Peristalsis	Spontaneous Contractions	LES Tone	LES Relaxation
Achalasia	++++	–	+/–	+	none	–	high or normal	no
Diffuse esophageal spasm	+++	+/–	+++	++	normal	+++	normal	yes
Nutcracker esophagus	–	–	+	?	normal high pressure	–	normal	yes
Hypertensive LES	++	–	++	+	normal	–	high	yes
Scleroderma	++	+++	–	–	low pressure	–	low	yes

between esophageal symptoms and motor abnormalities cannot be established (Richter, 1991). Hence, although one can demonstrate esophageal dysfunction, a pathologic abnormality has not been clearly identified. These disorders may be considered under the following subheadings: diffuse esophageal spasm (DES); Nutcracker esophagus; or hypertensive lower esophageal sphincter, scleroderma, and nonspecific esophageal dysmotility.

DIFFUSE ESOPHAGEAL SPASM. This condition was established as an esophageal motor abnormality in 1958 (Creamer, Donoghue, & Code, 1958). Patients usually present in their forties and there is a female preponderance (Reidel & Clouse, 1985). They may or may not have an underlying psychological dysfunction (Anderson, Dalton, Bradley, & Richter, 1989; Clouse & Lustman, 1983; Rubin, Nagler, Spiro, & Pilot, 1962; Stacher, Schmeierer, & Landgraf, 1979). Manometrically this condition is characterized by the occurrence of simultaneous contractions during dry and wet swallows, which are predominantly seen in the smooth-muscle section of the esophagus. A definitive diagnosis should only be made when at least 30% of 10–15 swallows exhibit this phenomenon (DiMarino & Cohen, 1974; Mellow, 1977). In order to make a definitive diagnosis, one should pay attention to the timing of the onset of contractions rather than to the differences between the peaks of two adjacent contractions (Richter, Blackwell, & Wu, 1987), since the onset of contraction is associated with a disturbance in the transit of esophageal bolus (Kahrilas et al., 1988; Richter et al., 1987). Simultaneous contractions disrupt the process of coordinated propulsion of a bolus through the esophagus and this could lead to dysphagia, odynophagia, or chest pain. The disturbed transit of a bolus through the esophagus is better delineated with a dynamic radiologic study such as an esophagram or a barium swallow.

DES may be caused by an abnormal neural regulation of the normal peristalsis in the esophagus, that is, a perturbation in the timing and the sequential firing of the enteric nerve ganglia. Studies have shown that a DES-like abnormality can be induced in normal subjects after intravenous infusion that binds with nitric oxide (Murray et al., 1995). This provides evidence that a disturbed synthesis or release of neurotransmitters, in particular nitric oxide or nitric oxide-like compounds may produce this phenomenon. It has been suggested that patients with DES have thickened and hypertrophic muscles (Ferguson, Woodbury, Roper, & Burford, 1969; Gillies, Nicks, & Skyring, 1967), but these pathologic findings have also been seen in asymptomatic patients at autopsy (Demian & Vargas-Cortes, 1978). Moreover, these pathologic muscle changes are not seen in all patients with DES (Ellis, Olson, Schlegel, & Code, 1964) and may be the consequence of obstruction rather than its cause.

NUTCRACKER ESOPHAGUS. This entity, which has been more recently described, consists of the occurrence of large-amplitude peristaltic contractions usually greater than 180 mmHg, and are predominantly seen in the lower third of the esophagus. Bolus transit is not affected. This is believed to be the most common motility disorder, and in one large series was seen in 485 patients with esophageal dysmotility (Katz et al., 1987). Unlike DES, these contractions are more readily observed during wet swallows than dry swallows. Wet swallows normally induce peristaltic waves with amplitudes at least 10–20% higher than dry swallows. In some individuals (30%), these contractions are associated with a prolonged duration (over 6 s), (Benjamin, Gerhardt, & Castell, 1979; Orr & Robinson, 1982). Whether this entity truly exists has been called into question as on follow-up patients may have normal amplitude contractions. The underlying mechanism for this problem is not understood. Since these patients have normal peristalsis a barium swallow is usually reported as normal.

HYPERTENSIVE LES. This is a rare condition in which the resting tone of the LES is greater than the normal upper limit (i.e. over 45 mmHg), but the LES relaxes normally and the peristalsis of the esophagus is also normal (Code, Creamer, Schegel, Olsen, & Donoghue, 1958; Waterman, et al., 1989). Although sophisticated computer techniques may reveal subtle abnormalities, the LES relaxes appropriately to swallows in most subjects. In 50% of patients this condition may be associated with high-amplitude peristaltic contractions (Richter, 1991). Barium swallow may reveal normal peristalsis with occasional stasis at the lower end of the esophagus.

Nonspecific and Miscellaneous Motility Disorders

In some patients with dysphagia, a combination of one or more of the above-mentioned patterns may be seen, without a preponderance of any one pattern. For example, a patient may show few simultaneous contractions, a few normal peristaltic contractions, and a hypertensive LES. Some authors have described manometric abnormalities in patients with unexplained dysphagia that are only evident during dry swallows. These abnormalities consist of failure to induce a contraction wave or low pressure contractions or abnormal timing of contractions (Behar & Biancani, 1993). Whether these findings reflect a true defect in bolus transport is unclear. There may be significant abnormalities seen in the setting of long-standing diabetes mellitus.

TREATMENT. To date there has been no satisfactory treatment for any of these problems. Interestingly, these motor abnormalities may not be seen in the same subjects when the studies are repeated, and only 50% show persistent abnormalities. A number of drugs such as nitrates, calcium channel blockers, and antidepressants such as Trazodone have all been tried with limited success (Richter, 1991). In a few patients the motor changes may be secondary to or associated with acid reflux, and hence aggressive antire-

flux measures together with acid suppression with H2 blockers or omeprazole may be helpful. Surgical myotomy has also been attempted for patients with DES, but so far the results are not encouraging (De Meester, 1982; Ellis, Crozier, & Shea, 1988). Esophageal dilatation has also been tried (Ebert, Ouyang, Wright, & Cohen, 1983; Winters, Artnak, & Benjamin, 1984) but the response is variable. Thus, after establishing a definitive diagnosis and excluding other pathology, a generous reassurance remains the mainstay of treatment. Some patients with psychological dysfunction may benefit with psychotherapy and/or biofeedback (Latimer, 1981).

PROGNOSIS. The long-term outcome of these patients is not known and remains to be determined.

Systemic Diseases Affecting the Esophageal Muscle Wall

Most neuromuscular diseases affect primarily the oropharyngeal apparatus and the proximal striated muscle esophagus. These are discussed in Chapter 11. Connective tissue diseases may primarily affect the smooth muscle esophagus. Examples include scleroderma, pseudo-obstruction syndromes and myotonic dystrophy.

PSEUDO-OBSTRUCTION SYNDROMES. Pseudo-obstruction is the occurrence of the features of intestinal obstruction without evidence of mechanical obstruction of the viscus. Pseudoobstruction syndromes may occur as part of a heritable condition or as sporadically occurring cases. Other visceral organs may be involved such as the bladder or ureters. The myopathic form of pseudo-obstruction may affect the smooth muscle esophagus in a manner similar to scleroderma (Rohrmann, Ricci, Krishnamurthy, & Schuffler, 1984). Esophageal manometry may demonstrate some disordered peristalsis; however, esophageal symptoms apart from reflux are rare. Usually the small intestinal symptoms predominate. Usually the symptoms of intermittent intestinal pseudo-obstruction predominate. The esophageal changes are nonspecific disorders of the propagation and the amplitude of esophageal contraction. Treatment consists of treating gastroesophageal reflux and other symptomatic treatment.

MUSCULAR DYSTROPHIES. This collection of systemic muscular disorders predominantly affects striated muscle. Myotonic dystrophy is a specific form of dystrophy characterized by increased tone and weakness in striated muscle. Characteristic features of myotonic dystrophy include, hypertonicity of muscles with often a delay in release of muscle contraction, delayed hand release with a handshake, progressive weakness of facial and limb muscles, and cataracts. The upper esophagus is frequently involved in the condition, with disordered relaxation of the upper esophageal sphincter and diminished peristaltic amplitudes in the upper and lower esophagus. Pathologic changes are most marked in the striated esophagus. Other dystrophies may affect the striated segment of the esophagus but are less likely to cause esophageal problems than myotonic dystrophy (Eckardt, Nix, Kraus, & Bohl, 1986). Treatment is symptomatic. If reflux is a problem then vigorous antireflux treatment may reduce symptoms. The outcome is determined by the progressive weakness, and pulmonary aspiration is common in the terminal stages of disease.

SCLERODERMA. Scleroderma is part of a spectrum of connective tissue disorders that cause progressive fibrosis of the dermal layer of the skin, particularly of the face, hands, and feet. It may also cause fibrosis of the lungs, kidneys, and parts of the gastrointestinal tract, including the esophagus. The spectrum of disease may extend from the limited CRST syndrome (calcinosis cutis, Raynaud's phenomena, sclerodactyly, and telangiectasia) to systemic sclerosis, a multisystem disorder. It primarily affects women in their fourth to fifth decade of life. Mortality is related primarily to renal disease.

The esophageal involvement is initially progressive fibrosis of the muscular layers. This leads to impaired peristaltic contractions and diminished and sometimes undetectable LES pressure. As a consequence of these motor changes there is an increasingly severe reflux esophagitis often complicated by strictures (Zamost et al., 1987). The syndrome, though rare, should be suspected especially in younger women. A history of Raynaud's phenomenon would be quite suggestive.

Diagnosis is dependent on identifying the clinical features. Physical exam may reveal loss of digital pulps, telangiectasia on the face or hands, hard calcium deposits in the fingers, tight pinched skin on the face, with a small mouth. Induction of vasospasm by cold immersion of the hand is unnecessary and painful. The patients historical description of the cold-induced changes should suffice. The antinuclear antibody may be positive. More specific markers include anticentromere and SCL 70. Nail fold capillaroscopy may reveal changes in the peripheral capillary beds.

The treatment of the esophageal involvement is aimed at controlling the esophagitis, usually using prokinetic agents and acid suppression. The involvement is usually progressive and higher than usual maintenance doses of H_2 antagonists or a proton pump inhibitor may be necessary. Dilatation of strictures may be required. Antireflux surgery is controversial in that some or any obstruction may lead to later problems as the peristalsis deteriorates. There is as yet no effective treatment for the underlying connective tissue disease.

RADIATION ESOPHAGITIS. The esophagus may receive significant doses of radiation during treatment for lung, breast, spinal, mediastinal, and esophageal tumors. This commonly causes esophagitis during and occasionally strictures after the radiation exposure. The patients complain of odynophagia and dysphagia. The esophagitis usually subsides after cessation of the radiation. The strictures are managed with dilatation. Treatment usually consists of pain relief, viscous lidocaine, Carafate, and acid blockers to treat any reflux problems (Soffer et al., 1994). There may also be long-term effects of the radiation on esophageal motor function, causing dysphagia (Seeman, Gates, & Traube, 1992).

Foreign Bodies Causing Dysphagia

Dysphagia associated with accidental or deliberate ingestion of foreign bodies is a medical emergency. This is one of the most frequent causes of acute dysphagia. In the United States, approximately 1,500 people die annually from ingesting foreign bodies (Schwartz & Polsky, 1975). The incidence is higher in infants (Erbes & Babbitt, 1965), psychiatric patients, and prisoners (Webb, 1992). A history of sudden onset or dysphagia after eating should alert to this possibility. In young children a history of foreign body ingestion is not always obtained, and hence one should exercise a high index of suspicion.

Types of foreign bodies that are ingested reflect only the limitations of human curiosity. Small, round-shaped objects usually traverse the esophagus without obstruction, but sharp, irregular, or larger sized objects may get impacted within the esophagus. Potentially, bolus impaction may occur at one or more of the four narrow zones within the esophagus. The most common site is the cricopharyngeal muscle, which is located between 15–17 cm from the incisor teeth. Other sites are the crossing of the aortic arch (23 cm from teeth), the impression of the left main bronchus (27 cm from teeth), and the lower esophageal sphincteric zone (40 cm from teeth). The presence of a peptic, neoplastic, or other forms of esophageal stricture, with or without a hiatal hernia, particularly a paraesophageal hiatal hernia, may increase the risk of bolus impaction, dysphagia, and perforation.

CLINICAL FEATURES. A detailed history often provides useful information regarding the nature of the ingested foreign body as well as the existence of any previous esophageal problems. Not uncommonly, patients with an esophageal stricture may present for the first time with dysphagia and a bolus impaction. Examination is usually unrevealing, except in patients with an esophageal perforation in whom subcutaneous emphysema may be detected.

DIAGNOSIS. Plain x-ray of the chest, upper abdomen, and neck may reveal the presence of a radiopaque foreign body. On the other hand, if a radiolucent object has been ingested, then a swallow with hypaque or another contrast solution along with videofluoroscopy may reveal a filling defect. Additionally this may provide information regarding an underlying pathology within the esophagus. An upper gastrointestinal endoscopy may not only confirm the presence of a foreign body but in most instances also facilitate its removal without recourse to surgery (Figure 13–4). Approximately 10–20% of foreign bodies that have been ingested may need removal, but the vast majority will pass safely through the gastrointestinal tract. However, foreign bodies that have been impacted in

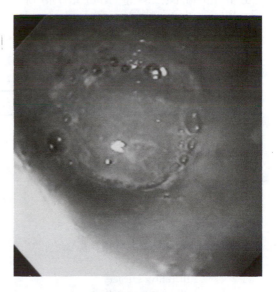

Figure 13–4. The endoscopic view reveals a green impacted foreign object in the esophagus of a 41-year-old male who presented with sudden aphagia while eating dried fruit. The offending object proved to be a piece of papaya.

the esophagus or stomach should be removed as soon as possible. The timing and need for endoscopic removal should be assessed carefully (Webb, 1992). Ingestion and/or impaction of coins, button batteries, fish bone, meat, and sharp objects require immediate removal with an endoscope, whereas cocaine bags should never be removed. Patients with cocaine ingestion must undergo immediate surgery, since perforation of the bag during endoscopic removal may lead to an overdose of the drug with a fatal outcome (Jonsson, O'Meara, & Young, 1983; Suarez, Arango, & Lester, 1977).

When removing sharp objects and button batteries it is advisable that the patient's airway be protected with endotracheal intubation or an endoscopy overtube. After successful removal, a contrast study may be required to ensure that a perforation or a fistula has not developed. In children and adults with dysphagia and complete or inadequate ventilation, the Heimlich maneuver should be used to clear the airway. Precautions: a foreign body lodged in the neck is preferably removed by an otolaryngologist, using either a rigid or a flexible endoscopic instrument. Airway protection is mandatory. When patients have experienced food bolus impaction of a serious nature, (i.e., requiring removal) or if there are repeated events then careful evaluation of swallowing should be performed. Attention should be given to the dentition and, if appropriate, neurologic status of the patient.

Extrinsic Compression of the Esophagus

There are many causes of extrinsic compression of the esophagus (Table 13–5). The most common are malignancy adjacent to the esophagus. Lung cancer, neoplastic enlargement of the lymph nodes, or mediastinal tumors all may impinge on the esophagus. Direct invasion of the esophagus is less common. Vascular structures may also press on the esophagus. These may be congenital vascular malformations of the aorta, or acquired conditions such as aneurysm of the arch of the aorta. The esophagus normally has indentations from the arch of the aorta and the left atrium of the heart. However, these do not usually impair swallowing. Ingested pills may lodge at the level of the aortic arch. There are descriptions of other structures causing esophageal obstruction, including pancreatic pseudocyst, and a large paraesophageal hernia.

TABLE 13–5. Extrinsic compression or distortion of the esophagus.

Disease	Diagnostic Tests
Congenital	
Vascular anomalies	Esophagogram, aortography
Teratomas	CT scan/MRI
Acquired	
Cancer of the lungs or mediastinum	Chest x-ray/CT scan
Tuberculosis	Chest x-ray, tuberculin skin test
Aortic aneurysm	Chest x-ray, CT scan, aortography
Enlarged lymph nodes	CT scan, mediastinoscopy
Pancreatic pseudocyst	Amylase level in aspirate
Paraesophageal hernia	Esophagogram
Iatrogenic	
Antireflux surgery	Scars, esophagogram
Right lung resection	Thoracotomy scars, chest x-ray, Esophagogram

Source: Adapted from "Uncommon Aspects of Mediastinal Teratoma" by A. Husain, J. Kernec, C. L. Rioux, & Y. Gandon, 1989. *Journal de Radiologie, 70,* 569–571.

DIAGNOSIS. Plain chest x-ray may reveal mediastinal enlargement or mass or an obvious tumor. Careful examination of the chest x-ray may reveal aortic arch enlargement. Esophagram will reveal smooth induration of the esophagus with intact mucosa. Transthoracic or transesophageal ultrasound may reveal aneurysmal dilation and the nature of the compressing mass lesion. Some masses may be biopsied via ultrasound-guided transmural biopsy. Treatment is determined by the nature of the compressing lesion.

Iatrogenic (Postsurgical Dysphagia)

Several operations may distort the esophagus or impinge upon the lumen of the esophagus. Resectional lung surgery may induce sometimes dramatic distortion of the mediastinum. The resection, particularly of the right lung usually for lung cancer, pulls the mediastinum across into the right side of the chest. The left lung hyperinflates, further pushing the mediastinum over. The distortion also twists the lower esophagus, giving further cause to block bolus distention of the esophagus. Lung cancer will occasionally invade or compress the esophagus.

The single most common surgical causes of dysphagia are the various antireflux procedures. These by their very design intend to restrict back flow through the LES. However, this increased resistance may also increase the likelihood of functional obstruction following the surgery. The most common type of antireflux surgery is the laparoscopic-placed Nissen fundoplication. In this operation the fundus of the stomach is mobilized and wrapped around the intrabdominal portion of the esophagus. If placed too tightly or if there is significantly diminished force of peristalsis, dysphagia may ensue. This most commonly occurs in the months following the surgery. Dilatation, often repeated, may be needed to give relief. Rarely will it be necessary to undo the operation, often no small feat owing to the scarring from the original operation.

Dysphagia in Sjögren's Syndrome

Sjögren's syndrome is an autoimmune condition primarily affecting the lachrymal and salivary glands, resulting in keratoconjunctivitis sicca, or dry eye syndrome, and xerostomia, dry mouth. This may occur in isolation or it may be associated with another autoimmune condition such as rheumatoid arthritis, vasculitis, or lupus. Eighty-one percent of one series of patients with Sjögren's syndrome studied complained of significant dysphagia. A smaller proportion had concomitant symptoms of heartburn or regurgitation. Motor abnormalities were only detected in a small proportion of patients with Sjögren's syndrome, suggesting that the dysphagia is likely secondary to the xerostomia, thereby illustrating the importance of lubrication in swallowing (Palma et al., 1994). However, one study revealed little correlation between the rate of salivary flow, salivary gland inflammation, and the dysphagia (Grande, Lacima, Ros, Font, & Pera, 1993).

SUMMARY

Esophageal diseases represent a distinct constituency of disorders that cause dysphagia. For many gastroenterologists they think of dysphagia as starting at the CP segment and ending at the LES, whereas for many other disciplines such as speech pathology it represents uncharted territory. The esophagus is anything but a inert tube. It is a complex conduit for food and an essential barrier to protect against the regurgitation of acid from the stomach. The coordination though not as easily appreciable as that of the oropharyngeal phase of deglutition is no less complex or interesting. The most common entity that affects esophageal function is gastroesophageal reflux disease which manifest most frequently as heartburn. It is associated with many common complications including strictures and a premalignant change called Barrett's metaplasia. The most serious esophageal disorder is cancer. This most devastating of malignancy, with in most cases a terrible outcome, has seen a dramatic increase in the incidence of adenocarcinoma. This is particularly so in white males in developed nations and represents a contrarian trend in other cancers with stable or declining incidence and mortality. The esophagus is subject to many diverse pathologic processes that belies its seemingly simple function.

MULTIPLE CHOICE QUESTIONS

1. Risk factors for esophageal cancer include all of the following except
   a. excessive alcohol ingestion
   b. Barrett's esophagus
   c. female gender
   d. geographic location

2. Risk factors for gastroesophageal reflux include all of all of the following except
   a. obesity
   b. smoking
   c. diet
   d. acne vulgaris

2. Gastroesophageal reflux episodes may result from the following except
   a. transient lower esophageal sphincter relaxations
   b. diminished lower esophageal sphincter pressure
   c. disordered tongue movements
   d. delayed gastric emptying
   e. abnormal esophageal peristalsis

3. Achalasia can result in one of the following
   a. heartburn
   b. nasal regurgitation
   c. dysphagia
   d. dysphonia

4. Caustic injury in the esophagus (pick the one true answer)
   a. is rare in children
   b. usually causes no long-term damage
   c. may be associated with an increased risk of malignancy
   d. is always associated with obvious pharyngeal irritation

5. The single most injurious substance in gastroesophageal reflux is
   a. bile
   b. gastric acid
   c. saliva
   d. mucus
   e. pepsin

5. Treatment for gastroesophageal reflux disease includes all of the following except
   a. inhibition of gastric acid secretion
   b. prokinetic drugs
   c. lifestyle alterations
   d. caffeine tablets
   e. Nissen fundoplication

6. Esophageal candidiasis is associated with each of the following except
   a. HIV infection
   b. odynophagia
   c. prior antibiotic treatment
   d. heartburn

REFERENCES

Adam, J. S. & Birck, H. G. (1982). Pediatric caustic ingestion. *Annals of Otolaryngology, Rhinology, Laryngology, 91*, 656–658.

Aggestrup, S., Holm, J. C., & Sorensen, H. R. (1994). Disponerer achalasia til esophaguscancer? [Does achalasia predispose to cancer of the esophagus?]. *Ugeskrift für Laeger, 156*, 637–639.

Ahtaridis, G., Snape, W. J., & Cohen, S. (1981). Lower esophageal sphincter pressure as an index of gastroesophageal acid reflux. *Digestive Diseases and Sciences, 26*, 993–998.

Anderson, K. O., Dalton, C. B., Bradley, L. A., & Richter, J. E. (1989). Stress: A modulator of esophageal pressures in healthy volunteers and non-cardiac chest pain patients. *Digestive Diseases and Sciences, 34*, 83.

Appleqvist, P., & Salmo, M. (1980). Lye corrosion carcinoma of the esophagus: A review of 63 cases. *Cancer, 45*, 2655–2658.

Behar, J., & Biancani, P. (1993). Pathogenesis of simultaneous esophageal contractions in patients with motility disorders. *Gastroenterology, 105*, 111–118.

Benini, L., Castellani, G., Sembenini, C., Bardelli, E., Calliari, S., Volino, C., & Vantini, I. (1994). Gastric emptying of solid meals in achalasic patients after successful pneumatic dilatation of the cardia. *Digestive Diseases and Sciences, 39,* 733–737.

Benjamin, S. B., Gerhardt, D. C., & Castell, D. O. (1979). High amplitude peristaltic esophageal contractions associated with chest pain and/or dysphagia. *Gastroenterology, 77,* 478.

Biancani, P., Hillemeier, C., Bitar, K. N., & Makhlouf, G. M. (1987). Contraction mediated by Ca2+ influx in esophageal muscle and by Ca2+ release in the LES. *American Journal of Physiology, 253,* G760–G769.

Blot, W. J., Devesa, S. S., Kneller, R. W., & Fraumeni, J. F. (1991). Rising incidence of adenocarcinoma of the esophagus and gastric cardia. Journal of the *American Medical Association, 265,* 1287–1289.

Broor, S. L., Raju, G. S., Bose, P. P., Lahoti, D., Ramesh, G. N., Kumar, A., & Sood, S. K. (1993). Long term results of endoscopic dilatation for corrosive esophageal stricture. *Gut, 34,* 1498–1501.

Brown, L. M., Silverman, D. T., Pottern, L. M., Schoenberg, J. B., Greenberg, R. S., Swanson, G.M., Liff, J. M., Schwartz, A.G., Hayes, R. B., & Blot, W. J. (1994). Adenocarcincoma of the eso-phagus and esophagogastric junction in white men in the United States: Alcohol, tobacco, and socioeconomic factors. *Cancer Causes & Control, 5,* 333–340.

Bushkin, F.L., Neustein, C.L., Parker, T.H., & Woodward, E.R. (1977). Nissen fundoplication for reflux esophagitis. *Annals of Surgery, 185,* 672.

Butler, C., Madden, J. W., Davis, W. M., & Peacock, E. E., Jr. (1977). Morphologic aspects of experimental esophageal lye strictures. II. Effect of steroid hormones, bougienage, and induced lathyrism on acute lye burns. *Surgery, 81,* 431–435.

Cassella, R. R., Brown, A. L., Sayre, G. P., & Ellis, F. H. (1964). Achalasia of the esophagus: Pathologic and etiologic considerations. *Annals of Surgery, 160,* 474–487.

Chen, M. Y. M., Ott, D. J., Donati, D. L., Wu, W. C., & Gelfand, D. W. (1994). Correlation of lower esophageal mucosal ring and lower esophageal sphincter pressure. *Digestive Diseases and Sciences, 39,* 766–769.

Chung, R. S. K., & DenBesten, L. (1975). Fiberoptic endoscopy in treatment of corrosive injury of the stomach. *Archives of Surgery, 110,* 725–728.

Clouse, R. E., & Lustman, P. J. (1983). Psychiatric illness and contraction abnormalities of the esophagus. *New England Journal of Medicine, 309,* 1337.

Code, C. F., Creamer, B., Schegel, J. P., Olsen, A. M., & Donoghue, F. E. (1958). *An atlas of esophageal motility in health and disease,* Springfield, IL: Charles C. Thomas.

Cohen, S., Fisher, R., & Tuch, A. (1972). The site of denervation in achalasia. *Gut, 13,* 556–558.

Cohen, S., & Harris, L. D. (1971). Does hiatus hernia affect competence of the gastroesophageal sphincter? *New England Journal of Medicine, 284,* 1053–1056.

Cook, I. J., Blumbergs, P., Cash, K., Jamieson, G. G., & Shearman, D.J. (1992). Structural abnormalities of the cricopharyngeus muscle in patients with pharyngeal (Zenker's) diverticulum. *Journal of Gastroenterology and Hepatology, 7,* 556–562.

Cook, I. J., Gabb, M., Panagopoulos, V., Jamieson, G. G., Dodds, W. J., Dent, J., & Shearman, D. J. (1992). Pharyngeal (Zenker's) diverticulum is a disorder of upper esophageal sphincter opening. *Gastroenterology, 103,* 1229–1335.

Creamer, B., Donoghue, F. E., & Code, C. F. (1958). Pattern of esophageal motility in diffuse spasm. *Gastroenterology, 34,* 782.

Cross, F. S. (1952). Pathologic changes in megaesophagus (esophageal dystonia). *Surgery, 31,* 647–653.

De Meester, T.R. (1982). Surgery for esophageal motor disorders. *Annals of Thoracic Surgery, 34,* 225.

Demian, S. D. E., & Vargas-Cortes, F. (1978). Idiopathic muscular hypertrophy of the esophagus. *Chest, 73,* 28.

Dent, J., Holloway, R. H., Toouli, J., & Dodds, W. J. (1988). Mechanisms of lower esophageal sphincter incompetence in patients with asymptomatic gastroesophageal reflux. *Gut, 29,* 1020.

Di Contanza, J., Noircleric, M., Jouglard, J., Escoffier, J. M., & Martin, J. (1977). New therapeutic approach to corrosive burns of the upper gastrointestinal tract. *Gut, 21,* 370.

DiMarino, J., & Cohen, S. (1974). Characteristics of lower esophageal sphincter function in symptomatic diffuse esophageal spasm. *Gastroenterology, 66,* 1.

Dodds, W. J., Dent, J., Hogan, W. J., Helm, J. F., Hauser, R., Patel, G. K., & Egide, M. S. (1982). Mechanisms of gastroesophageal reflux in patients with reflux esophagitis. *New England Journal of Medicine, 307,* 1547.

Eastwood, G. L., Castell, D. O., & Higgs, R. H. (1975). Experimenal esophagitis in cats impairs lower esophageal sphincter pressure. *Gastroenterology, 69,* 146–153.

Ebert, E. C., Ouyang, A., Wright, S. H., & Cohen, S. (1983). Pneumatic dilatation in patients with symptomatic diffuse esophageal spasm and lower esophageal sphincter dysfunction. *Digestive Disease, 28,* 481–485.

Eckardt, V. F., Nix, W., Kraus, W., & Bohl, J. (1986). Esophageal motor function in patients with muscular dystrophy. *Gastroenterology, 90,* 628–635.

Eda, Y., Asaki, S., Yamagata, L., Ohara, S., Shibuya, D., & Toyota, T. (1990). Endosocpic treatment of submucosal tumors of the esophagus: Studies in 25 patients. *Gastoenterolgia Japonica, 25,* 411–416.

Ellis, F. H., Crozier, R. E., & Shea, J. A. (1988). Long esophagomyotomy for diffuse esophageal spasm and related disorders. In J. R. Siewart & A. H. Holscher (Eds.) *Diseases of the esophagus: Pathophysiology, diagnosis, conservative and surgical treatment* (p. 913). New York: Springer-Verlag.

Ellis, F. H., Olsen, A. M., Schlegel, J. F., & Code, C. F. (1964). Surgical treatment of esophageal hypermotility disturbances. *Journal of the American Medical Association, 188,* 862–866.

Erbes, J. & Babbitt, D. P. (1965). Foreign bodies in the alimentary tract of infants and children. *Applied Therapeutics, 7,* 1103–1109.

Ferguson, C. M., & Rattner, D. W. (1995). Initial experience with laparoscopic Nissen fundoplication. *American Surgeon, 61,* 21–23.

Ferguson, T. B., Woodbury, J. D., Roper, C. L., & Burford, T. H. (1969). Giant muscular hypertrophy of the esophagus. *Annals of Thoracic Surgery, 8,* 209.

Ferreira, F., Lho, L. P., Patto, R. J., Froncon, L. E., & Oliveira, R. B. (1991). Use of isosorbide dinitrate for the sympathetic treatment of patients with Chagas' disease achalasia: A double blind crossover trial. *Brazilian Journal of Medicine & Biological Research, 24,* 1093–1098.

Figuerido, M. C., Oliveira, R. B., Iazigi, N., & Matsuda, M. M. (1992). Short report: Comparson of effects of sublingual nifedipine and isosorbide dinitrate on esophageal emptying in patients with Chagasic achalasia. *Alimentary Pharmacology and Therapeutics, 6,* 507–512.

Fisher, R. A., Eckhauser, M. L., & Radivoyevitch, M. (1985). Acid ingestion in an experimental model. *Surgical Gynecology and Obstetrics, 161,* 91–99.

Friesen, D. L., Henderson, R. D., & Hanna, W. (1983). Ultrasound of the esophageal muscle in achalasia and diffuse esophageal spasm. *American Jounal of Clinical Pathology, 79,* 319–325.

Gallez, J. F., Berger, F., Moulinier, B., & Partensky, C. (1987). Esophageal adenocarcinoma following Heller myotomy for achalasia. *Endoscopy, 19,* 76–78.

Gaudreault, P., Parent, M., McGuigan, M. A., Chicone, L., & Lovejoy, F. H. (1983). Predictability of esophageal injury from signs and symptoms: A study of caustic ingestion in 378 children. *Pediatrics, 71,* 767–770.

Gehano, P., & Guedon, C. (1981). Inhibition of experimental esophageal lye strictures by penicillamine. *Archives of Otolaryngology, 107,* 145–147.

Gerzic, Z. B., Knezevic, J. B., Milicevis, M. N., & Jounnovic, B. K. (1990). Esophagocoloplasty in the management of post corrosive strictures of the esophagus. *Annals of Surgery, 211,* 329–336.

Ghosh, S., Heading, R. C., & Palmer, K. R. (1994). Achalasia of the oesophagus in elderly patients responds poorly to conservative therapy. *Age and Aging, 23,* 280–282.

Gillies, M., Nicks, R., & Skyring, A. (1967). Clinical, manometric and pathologic studies in diffuse esophageal spasm. *British Medical Journal, 2,* 527.

Goodman, P., Scott, L. D., Verani, R. R., & Berg-green, C. C. (1990). Esophageal adenocarcinoma in a patient with surgically treated achalasia. *Digestive Diseases and Sciences, 35,* 1549–1552.

Grande, L., Lacima, G., Ros, E., Font, J., & Pera, C. (1993). Esophageal motor function in primary Sjögren's syndrome. *American Journal of Gastroenterology, 88,* 378–381.

Gray, M. R., Donnelly, R. J., & Kingsnorth, A. N. (1993). The role of smoking and alcohol in metaplasia and cancer risk in Barrett's columnar lined oesophagus. *Gut, 34,* 727–731.

Haynes, W. C., Sanowski, R. A., Foutch, P. G., & Bellapravalu, S. (1986). Strictures following endoscopic variceal sclerotherapy: Clinical course and response to therapy. *Gastrointestinal Endoscopy, 32,* 202.

Hesketh, P. J., Clapp, R. W., Doos, W. G., & Spechler, S. J. (1989). The increasing frequency of adenocarcinoma of the esophagus. *Cancer, 64,* 526–530.

Hurst, A. F. & Rake, G. W. (1930). Achalasia of the cardia. *Quarterly Journal of Medicine, 23,* 491–508.

Husain, A., Kernec, J., Rioux, C. L., & Gandon, Y. (1989). Uncommon aspects of mediastinal teratoma. CT, X-ray and MRI study, *Journal de Radiologie, 70,* 569–571.

Iascone, C., DeMeester, T. R., Little, A. G., & Skinner, D. B. (1983). Barrett's esophagus functional assessment, proposed pathogenesis, and surgical therapy. *Archives of Surgery, 118,* 543–549.

Iftikhar, S. Y., James, P. D., Steele, R. J., Hardcastle, J. D., & Atkinson, M. (1992). Length of Barrett's oesophagus: An important factor in the development of dysplasia and adenocarcinoma. *Gut, 33,* 1155–1158.

Johnson, E. E. (1963). A study of corrosive esophagitis. *Laryngoscope, 73,* 1651–1698.

Jonsson, S., O'Meara, M., & Young, J. B. (1983). Acute cocaine poisoning. *American Journal of Medicine, 75,* 1061–1064.

Kadakia, S. C., Parker, A., & Canales, L. (1992). Metastatic tumors to the upper gastrointestinal tract: Endoscopic experience. *American Journal of Gastroenterology, 87,* 1418–1423.

Kadakia, S. C., Parker, A., Carrougher, J. G., & Shaffer, R. T. (1993). Esophageal dilation with polyvinyl bougies, using a marked guidewire without the aid of fluoroscopy: An update. *American Journal of Gastroenterology, 88*, 1381–1386.

Kahrilas, P.J. (1992). Cigarette smoking and gastroesophageal reflux disease. *Digestive Disease, 1*, 61–71.

Kahrilas, P. J., Dodds, W. J., & Hogan, W. J. (1988). Effect of peristaltic dysfunction on esophageal volume clearance. *Gastroenterology, 94*, 73.

Kahrilas, P. J., Dodds, W. J., Hogan, W. J., Kern, M., Arndorfer, R. C., & Reece, A. (1986). Esophageal peristaltic dysfunction in peptic esophagitis. *Gastroenterology, 91*, 897–904.

Katz, P. O., Dalton, C. B., & Richter, J. E. (1987). Esophageal testing in patients with non-cardiac chest pain and/or dysphagia. *Annals of Internal Medicine, 106*, 593–597.

Katz, P. O., Knuff, T. E., Benjamin, S. B., & Castell, D. O. (1986). Abnormal esophageal pressures in reflux esophagitis: Cause or effect? *American Journal of Gastroenterology, 81*, 744–746.

Keshavarzian, A., Urban, G., Sedghi, S., Willson, C., Sabella, L., Sweeny, C., & Anderson, K. (1991). Effect of acute ethanol on esophageal motility in cat. *Alcoholism Clinical & Experimental Research, 15*, 116–121.

Kikendall, J. W. (1991). Pill-induced esophageal injury. *Gastroenterology Clinics of North America, 20*, 835.

Kikendall, J. W., & Johnson, L. F.(1983). Esophageal injury: Caustics and pill. In D. O. Castell & L. F. Johnson, (Eds.), *Esophageal function in health and disease* (p. 255). New York: Elsevier Science.

Kim, S. L., Waring, J. P., Spechler, S. J., Sampliner, R. E., Doos, W. G., Krol, W. F., & Williford, W. O. (1994). Diagnostic inconsistencies in Barrett's esophagus. Department of Veterans Affairs Gastroenterology Study Group. *Gastroenterology, 107*, 945–949.

Kimura, K. (1928). The nature of idiopathic esophagus dilatation. Japanese Journal of *Gastroenterology, 2*, 199–207.

Kirsch, M. M., & Ritter, F. (1976). Caustic ingestion and subsequent damage to the oropharyngeal and digestive passages. *Annals of Thoracic Surgery, 21*, 74–82.

Krishnadath, K. K., van Blankenstein, M., & Tilanus, H. W. (1995). Prognostic value of p53 in Barrett's oesophagus. *European Journal of Gastroenterology & Hepatology, 7*, 81–84.

Latimer, P. E. (1981). Biofeedback and self-regulation in the treatment of diffuse esophageal spasm: A single-case study. *Biofeedback Self Regulation, 6*, 181.

Liu, A. J. & Richardson, M. A. (1985). Effects of n-acetylcysteine on experimentally induced esophageal lye injury. *Annals Otolaryngology Rhinology Laryngology, 94*, 477–482.

Maeta, M., Kondo, A., Shibata, S., Yamashiro, H., Murakami, A., & Kaibara, N. (1993). Esophageal cancer associated with multiple cancerous lesions: Clinicopathological comparisons between multiple primary and intramural metastatic lesions. *Gastroenterologia Japonica, 28*, 187–192.

Marks, R. D., Richter, J. E., Rizzo, J., Koebler, R. E., Spenney, J. G., Mills, T. P., & Champion, G. (1994). Omeprazole versus H2-receptor antagonists in treating patients with peptic stricture and esophagitis. *Gastroenterology, 106*, 907–915.

Marshall, J. B., Diaz-Arias, A. A., Bochna, G. S., & Vogele, K. A. (1990). Achalasia due to diffuse esophageal leiomyomatosis and inherited as autosomal dominant disorder: Report of a family study. *Gastroenterology, 98*, 1358–1365.

Marshall, J. B., & Gerhardt, D. C. (1982). Improvement in esophageal motor dysfunction with the treatment of reflux esophagitis: A report of 2 cases. *American Journal of Gastroenterology, 77*, 351–354.

McCallum, R. W. (1990). Gastric emptying in esophageal reflux and the therapeutic role of prokinetic agents. *Gastroenterology Clinics of North America, 19*, 551–564.

McNally, P. R., Lemon, J. C., Goff, J. S., & Freeman, S. R. (1993). Congenital esophageal stenosis presenting as noncardiac, esophageal chest pain. *Digestive Diseases and Sciences, 38*, 369–373.

Meijssen, M. A., Tilanus, H. W., van Blankenstein, M., Hop, W. C., & Ong, G. L. (1992). Achalasia complicated by oesophageal squamous cell carcinoma: A prospective study in 195 patients. *Gut, 33*, 155–158.

Mellow, M. (1977). Symptomatic diffuse esophageal spasm. Manometric follow-up and response to cholinergic stimulation and cholinesterase inhibition. *Gastroenterology, 73*, 237.

Murata, Y., Yoshida, M., Akimoto, S., Ide, H., Suzuki, S., & Hanyu, F. (1988). Evaluation of endoscopic ultrasonography for the diagnosis of submucosal tumors of the esophagus. *Surgical Endoscopy, 2*, 51–58.

Murray, J. A., Ledlow, A., Launspach, J., Evans, D., Loveday, M., & Conklin, J. L. (1995). The effects of recombinant human hemoglobin on esophageal motor function in humans. *Gastroenterology, 109*(4):1241–8.

Nakamura, T., Nekarda, H., Hoelscher, A. H., Bollschweiler, E., Harbec, N., Becker, K., & Siewert, J. R. (1994). Prognostic value of DNA ploidy and c-erbB-2 oncoprotein overexpression in adenocarcinoma of Barrett's esophagus. *Cancer, 73*, 1785–1794.

Neilson, I. R., Croitoru, D. P., Guttman, F. M., Youssef, S., & Laberge, J. M. (1991). Distal congenital esophageal stenosis associated with esophageal atresia. *Journal of Pediatric Surgery, 26*, 478–481.

Okamura, H., Tsutsumi, S., Inaki, S., & Mori, T. (1988). Esophageal web in Plummer-Vinson syndrome. *Laryngoscope, 98*, 994–998.

Orlando, R. C. (1994). Esophageal epithelial defenses against acid injury. *American Journal of Gastroenterology, 89*, S48-S52.

Orr, W. C., & Robinson, M. G. (1982). Hypertensive peristalsis in the pathogenesis of chest pain. *American Journal of Gastroenterology, 77*, 604.

Ott, D. J., Gelfand, D.W., Chen, Y.M., Wu, W.C., & Munitz, H.A. (1985). Predictive relationship of hiatal hernia to reflux esophagitis. *Gastrointestinal Radiology, 10*, 317–320.

Overholt, B., Panjehpour, M., Tefftellar, E., & Rose, M. (1993). Photodynamic therapy for treatment of early adenocarcinoma in Barrett's esophagus. *Gastrointestinal Endoscopy, 39*, 73–76.

Palma, R., Freire, A., Freitas, J., Morbey, A., Costa, T., Saraiva, F., Queiros, F., & Carvalhinhos, A. (1994). Esophageal motility disorders in patinets with Sjögren's syndrome. *Digestive Diseases and Sciences, 39*, 758–761.

Parkman, H. P., & Cotten, S. (1994). Malignancy-induced secondary achalasia. *Dysphagia, 9*, 292–296.

Pasricha, P. J., Ravich, W. J., Hendric, T. R., Sostre, S., Jones, B., & Kalloo, A. N. (1994). Treatment of achalasia with intrasphincteric injection of Botulin toxin, a pilot trial. *Annals of Internal Medicine, 121*, 590.

Pasricha, P. J., Ravich, W. J., Hendric, T. R., Sostre, S., Jones, B., & Kalloo, A. N. (1995). Intrasphinc-teric botulinum toxin for the treatment of achalasia. *New England Journal of Medicine, 322*, 774–778.

Pera, M., Trastek, V. F., Carpenter, H. A., Allen, M. S., Deschamps, C., & Pairolero, P. C. (1992). Barrett's esophagus with high-grade dysplasia: An indication for esophagectomy? *Annals of Thoracic Surgery, 54*, 199–204.

Peters, F. T., Sleijfer, D. T., van Imhoff, G. W., & Kleibeuker, J. H. (1993). Is chemotherapy associated with development of Barrett's esophagus? *Digestive Diseases and Sciences, 38*, 923–926.

Peters, J. H., Clark, G. W., Ireland, A. P., Chandrasoma, P., Smyrk, T. C., & DeMeester, T. R. (1994). Outcome of adenocarcinoma arising in Barrett's esophagus in endoscopically surveyed and non-surveyed patients. *Journal of Thoracic & Cardiovascular Surgery, 108*, 813–821.

Pitcher, D. E., Curet, M.'J., Martin, D. T., Castillo, R. R., Gerstenberger, P. D., Vogt, D., & Zucker, K. A. (1994). Successful management of severe gastroesophageal reflux disease with laparoscopic Nissen fundoplication. *American Journal of Surgery, 168*, 547–553.

Reidel, W. L. & Clouse, R. E. (1985). Variations in clinical presentations of patients with contraction abnormalities. *Digestive Diseases and Sciences, 30*, 1065.

Reynolds, J. C., & Parkman, H. P. (1989). Achalasia. *Gastroenterology Clinics of North America, 18*, 223–255.

Richter, J. E. (1991). Motility disorders of the esophagus. In T. Yamada, D. H. Alpers, C. Owyang, D. W. Powell & F. E. Silverstein (Eds.) *Textbook of gastroenterology* (pp. 1083–1122). Philadelphia: J.B. Lippincott.

Richter, J. E., Blackwell, J. N., & Wu, W. C. (1987). Relationship of radionuclide liquid bolus transport and esophageal manometry. *Journal of Laboratory and Clinical Medicine, 109*, 217.

Robertson, C. S., Marti, B. A. B., & Atkinson, M. (1993). Varicella-zoster virus DNA in the oesophageal myenteric plexus in achalasia. *Gut, 34*, 299–302.

Rohrmann, C. A., Jr., Ricci, M. T., Krishnamurthy, S., & Schuffler, M. D. (1984). Radiologic and histologic differentiation of neuromuscular disorders of the gastrointestinal tract: Visceral myopathies, visceral neuropathies, and progressive systemic sclerosis. *American Journal of Roentgenology, 143*, 933–941.

Rubin, J., Nagler, R., Spiro, H. M., & Pilot, J. L. (1962). Measuring the effect of emotions on esophageal motility. *Psychosomatic Medicine, 24*, 170.

Rumack, B. H., & Burrington, J. D. (1977). Caustic ingestion: A rational look at diluents. *Clinical Toxicology, 11*, 27.

Schatzki, R. (1963). The lower esophageal ring. *American Journal of Roentgenology, 90*, 805.

Schindlbeck, N. E., & Heinrich, C. (1987). Influence of smoking and esophageal intubation on esophageal pHmetry. *Gastroenterology, 92*, 1994–1997.

Schulze-Delrieu, K., & Anuras, S. (1983). Chronic esophagitits in two sisters. *Digestive Diseases and Sciences, 28*, 1101–1105.

Schwartz, G. F., & Polsky, H. S. (1975). Ingested foreign bodies of the gastrointestinal tract. *American Surgeon, 42*, 236–238.

Seeman, H., Gates, J. A., & Traube, M. (1992). Esophageal motor dysfunction years after radiation therapy. *Digestive Diseases and Sciences, 37*, 303–306.

Shay, S. S., Eggli, D., McDonald, C., & Johnson, L. F. (1987). Gastric emptying of solid food in patients with gastroesophageal reflux. *Gastroenterology, 92*, 459–465.

Shirazi, S., Schulze-Delrieu, K., Custer-Hagen, T., Brown, C. K., & Ren, J. (1989). Motility changes in opossum esophagus from experimental esophagitis. *Digestive Diseases and Sciences, 34*, 1668–1676.

Sinar, D. R., Fletcher, J. R., & Castell, D. O. (1980). Acute esophagitis adversely affects esophageal peristalsis. *Clinical Research, 28*, 821A.

Singaram, C., Sweet, M. A., Belcaster, G. M., Hefle, S. L., Kalloo, A. N., & Pasricha, J. (1994). A novel autoantibody exists in patients with esophageal achalasia. *Gastroenterology, 106*, A566.

Smith, B. (1970). The neurological lesion in achalasia of the cardia. *Gut, 11*, 388–391.

Smith, P. D., Eisner, M. S., Manischewitz, J. F., Gill, V. J., Masur, H., & Fox, C. F. (1993). Esophageal disease in AIDS is associated with pathologic processes rather than mucosal human immunodeficiency virus type 1. *Journal of Infectious Disease, 167*, 547–552.

Soffer, E. E., Mitros, F., Doornbos, J. F., Friedland, J., Launspach, J., & Summers, R. W. (1994). Morphology and pathology of radiation-induced esophagitis. Double-blind study of naproxen vs placebo for prevention of radiation injury. *Digestive Diseases and Sciences, 39*, 655–660.

Spain, D. M., Molomut, N., & Haber, A. (1950). The effect of cortisone on the formation of granulation tissue in mice. *American Journal of Patho-logy, 26*, 710–711.

Spechler, S. J. (1990). Caustic ingestions. In M. B. Taylor, (Ed.) *Gastrointestinal emergencies* (pp. 13–21). Boston: Williams & Wilkins.

Spechler, S. J. (1992). Epidemiology and natural history of gastroesophageal reflux disease. *Digestion, 51* (suppl. 1), 24–291.

Spechler, S. J., Zeroogian, J. M., Antonioli, D.a., Wang, H. H., & Goyal, R. K. (1994). Prevalence of metaplasia at the gastro-oesophageal junction. *Lancet, 344*, 1533–1536.

Stacher, G., Schmeierer, C., & Landgraf, M. (1979). Tertiary esophageal contractions evoked by acoustic stimuli. *Gastroenterology, 105*, 44–49.

Streitz, J. M., Jr., Andrews, C. W., Jr., & Ellis, F. H., Jr. (1993). Endoscopic surveillance of Barrett's esophagus. Does it help? Journal of Thoracic and *Cardiovascular Surgery, 105*, 383–387.

Streitz, J. M., Jr., Ellis, F. H., Jr., Gibbs, S. P., Balogh, K., & Watkins, E., Jr. (1991). Adenocarcinoma in Barrett's esophagus. A clinicopathological study of 65 cases. *Annals of Surgery, 213*, 122–125.

Suarez, C. A., Arango, A., & Lester, J. L. (1977). Cocaine-condom ingestion: Surgical treatment. *Journal of the American Medical Association, 238*, 1391–1392.

Symbal, P. N., Vlasis, S. E., & Hatcher, C. R. (1983). Esophagitis secondary to ingestion of caustic material. *Annals of Thoracic Surgery, 36*, 73.

Tom, W., & Aaron, J. S. (1987). Esophageal ulcers caused by Torulopsis glabrata in a patient with acquired immune deficiency syndrome. *American Journal of Gastroenterology, 82*, 766–768.

Triadafilopoulas, G., Aaronson, M., Sackel, S., & Burakoff, R. (1991). Medical treatment of esophageal achalasia. Double blind crossover study with oral nifedipine, verapamil and placebo. *Digestive Diseases and Sciences, 36*, 260–267.

Tsutsumi, S. (1993). Disorders of swallowing muscles in iron deficient rabbits (Japanese). *Nippon Gibiinkoka Gakkai Kaiho, 96*, 48–57.

Wang, H. H., Antonioli, D. A., & Goldman, H. (1986). Comparative features of esophageal and gastric adenocarcinomas: Recent changes in type and frequency. *Human Pathology, 17*, 482–487.

Wang, H. H., Hsieh, C. C., & Antonioli, D. A. (1994). Rising incidence rate of esophageal adenocarcinoma and use of pharmaceutical agents that relax the lower esophageal sphincter (United States). *Cancer Causes & Control, 5*, 573–578.

Wang, K. K. (1994). Barrett's esophagus: Current and future management. *Comprehensive Therapy, 20*, 36–43.

Wasserman, R. l., & Ginsburg, C. M. (1985). Caustic substance injuries. *Journal of Pediatrics, 107*, 169–174.

Waterman, D. C., Dalton, C. B., Ott, D. J., Castell, J. A., Bradley, L. A., Castell, D. O., & Richter, J. E. (1989). Hypertensive lower esophageal sphincter: What does it mean? *Journal of Clinical Gastroenterology, 11*, 139–146.

Weaver, G. A. (1979). Upper esophageal web to a ring formed by a squamocolumnar junction with ectopic gastric mucosa (another explanation of the Paterson-Kelly, Plummer-Vinson syndrome). *Digestive Diseases and Sciences, 24*, 959–963.

Webb, W. A. (1992). Foreign bodies of the upper gastrointestinal tract. In M. B. Taylor (Ed.), *Gastrointestinal emergencies* (pp. 1–12). Baltimore: Williams & Wilkins.

Wilcox, C. M., Straub, R. F., & Schwartz, D. A. (1995). Cytomegalovirus esophagitis in AIDS: A prospective evaluation of clinical response to ganciclovir therapy, relapse rate, and long-term outcome. *American Journal of Medicine, 98*, 169–176.

Winters, C., Artnak, E. J., & Benjamin, S. B. (1984). Esophageal bougienage in symptomatic patients with the nutcracker esophagus. *Journal of the American Medical Association, 252*, 363–366.

Wolf, B. S., Brahams, S. A., & Khilnani, M. I. (1959). The incidence of hiatus hernia in routine barium meal examination. *Mt Sinai Journal of Medicine New York, 26*, 598–600.

Wright, R. A., & Hurwitz, A. L. (1979). Relationship of hiatal hernia to endoscopically proven reflux esophagitis. *Digestive Diseases and Sciences, 24*, 311–313.

Yang, P.C., & Davis, S. (1988). Incidence of cancer of the esophagus in the U.S. by histologic type. *Cancer, 61*, 612–617.

Yu, J. P., Luo, H. S., & Wang, X. Z. (1992). Endoscopic treatment of submucosal lesions of the gastrointestinal tract. *Endoscopy, 24,* 190–193.

Zamost, B. J., Hirschberg, J., Ippoliti, A. F., Furst, D. E., Clements, P. J., & Weinstein, W. M. (1987). Esophagitis in scleroderma: Prevalence and risk factors. *Gastroenterology, 92,* 421–428.

14

Swallowing and Feeding in the Pediatric Patient

Joan C. Arvedson and Brian T. Rogers

A developmental perspective forms the basis for assessment and management strategies in the pediatric population. In contrast to the normal adult's stable and mature swallow pattern, a child's growth and development are part of an ever-changing dynamic process that affects swallowing patterns. Once adequate breathing is established, the highest priority for caregivers is to meet a child's nutritional needs efficiently. An optimal nutritional status is critical for appropriate growth and for brain development, particularly in the first year of life.

Swallowing and feeding disorders in infants and children usually occur as part of a broad spectrum of complex developmental and health disorders. The swallowing and feeding problems may become evident within the first few hours of life or gradually during the first several weeks of life as airway issues or neurodevelopmental deficits are manifest. Dysphagia can also have an acute onset, as in adults, following neoplasm, traumatic brain injury, infection, asphyxia, or cerebrovascular accident (CVA). In addition, disruptions in the oral feeding process may occur as undesirable complications of central nervous system (CNS) dysgenesis and chronic cardiopulmonary disorders. Although infants and children share some similarities with adults, the developmental issues can make swallowing and feeding problems in children different from adults.

Infant feeding consists of three basic components: sucking, swallowing, and breathing. All three components must be considered in the swallowing and feeding of infants. Feeding is also a manifestation of the complex communicative and nurturing relationship between parent and child; consequently, communication problems during meals can result in feeding problems or can complicate preexisting dysphagia.

The purposes of this chapter are to review the normal development of swallowing and feeding skills, to describe some of the predominant causes of swallowing disorders in children, and to present an *inter*disciplinary team approach for the assessment and management of feeding disorders in childhood. The multifaceted nature of pediatric dysphagia mandates the involvement of multiple professional disciplines. Optimal patient care is provided when people work together for an interdisciplinary focus.

DEVELOPMENT OF FEEDING SKILLS

Swallowing and feeding disorders in children can be understood best in reference to a solid understanding of normal development of these skills. Because feeding success is dependent on the integration of function of multiple systems, development of swallowing and respiration are considered together.

Prenatal Development

The pharyngeal swallow is observed early in fetal life, by the 10th to the 11th week of gestation. Humphrey (1967) described a pharyngeal swallow in a delivered fetus at a gestational age of 12.5 weeks. True suckling begins by the 18th to 24th week (Moore, 1988). Suckling involves all oral-motor structures.

The period from 23 to 25 weeks is important in the development of the upper and lower respiratory tract (Laitman & Reidenberg, 1993). By 24 weeks, the lungs begin producing surfactant, a surface-active lipid that maintains the patency of the developing alveoli of the lungs (Crelin, 1976) and is essential for independent respiratory function. Simultaneously, structural development occurs in the oropharynx. The immature respiratory system is unable to sustain life independently at this gestational age.

Premature infants at 27 to 28 weeks' gestation make suckling movements, usually single sucks with long pauses. It is not until 32–34 weeks that the mechanisms necessary for nipple feeding become functionally coordinated (Goldson, 1987; Shaker, 1990) and some preterm infants have been found unable to nipple-feed successfully until 35 weeks (Brake, Fifer, Alfase, & Fleishman, 1988) or even over 37 weeks post-conceptual age (PCA) (Bu'Lock, Woolridge, & Baum, 1990). The linkage of suck to swallow appears well established by 32 weeks, although the linkage of suck to swallow with breathing appears to be achieved later. Breast and bottle feedings have been found to be tolerated at the same PCA by very low birth weight infants (<1500 grams) (Bier, Ferguson, Cho, Oh, & Vohr, 1993). Gradually a burst–pause pattern develops. The burst may consist of 12–15 sucks, each followed by a swallow. The young infant usually demonstrates a 1:1 ratio of sucking to swallowing, although at the end of the feeding the ratio becomes higher, with 2 to 3 sucks before swallowing (Weber, Woolridge, & Baum, 1986; Wolff, 1968). This burst is followed by an interruption (pause) of a few seconds. In some instances, the pattern is less predictable.

Further anatomic changes in the premature infant include enlargement and forward movement of the mandible. Lips and cheeks enlarge and become more firm. At term, the sucking pads (densely compacted adipose tissue within the masseter muscles) become prominent in the cheeks. These sucking pads help to stabilize the cheeks. The lips are adapted by the pars villosa, an inner ridge of specialized mucosa that consists primarily of fine villi arranged to facilitate the seal of the lips around a nipple (Bosma, 1986).

In addition, at term the infant's tongue fills the oral cavity and rests more anteriorly than in an adult. Because the tongue seems oversized for its allocated space, a relatively small mandible makes the oral cavity appear even smaller. The infant's larynx (Figure 14–1) is suspended higher in the neck than the adult larynx (Figure 14–2). The close proximity of the tongue, soft palate, and pharynx with the larynx facilitates nasal breathing during nipple feeding, although breathing ceases briefly during the pharyngeal phase of swallowing.

Suckling and Sucking

Suckling precedes *sucking*. *Suckling* is the prominent pattern from birth to about 6 months' developmental age. It is characterized by backward and forward movements of the tongue, the backward movement more pronounced (Figure 14–3). It can be most readily elicited by stroking the top of the tongue (Bosma, 1986). By 6 months of age, sucking becomes prominent. *Sucking* is characterized by strong activity of the intrinsic muscles of the tongue that raise and lower the body of the tongue. During sucking, the jaw makes a smaller vertical excursion than in suckling.

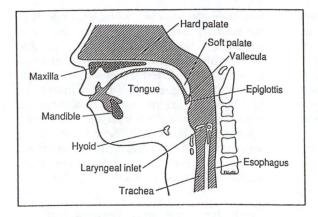

Figure 14–1. Schematic lateral view of the infant upper aerodigestive tract. Structures of the oral cavity and pharynx can be seen, as well as the laryngeal inlet, trachea, and esophagus. (From *Pediatric swallowing and feeding: Assessment and management*, by J. Arvedson, B. Rogers, & L. Brodsky, Eds., 1993, p. 6. San Diego: Singular Publishing Group. Copyright 1993 by Singular Publishing Group. Reprinted with permission.)

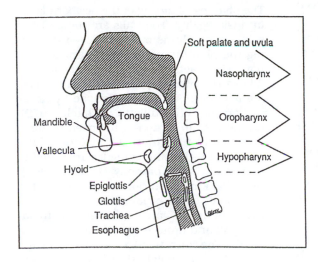

Figure 14–2. Schematic lateral view of the adult upper aerodigestive tract, demonstrating anatomical limitations of nasopharynx, oropharynx, and hypo-pharynx. (From *Pediatric swallowing and feeding: Assessment and management*, by J. Arvedson, B. Rogers, & L. Brodsky, Eds., 1993, p. 6. San Diego: Singular Publishing Group. Copyright 1993 by Singular Publishing Group. Reprinted with permission.)

Figure 14–3. Suckling and sucking comparisons of tongue and mandibular action. Suckling is characterized by in-out tongue movements and some jaw opening and closing; sucking by up–down tongue movements and less vertical jaw action. (From *Pediatric swallowing and feeding: Assessment and management*, by J. Arvedson, B. Rogers, & L. Brodsky, Eds., 1993, p. 42. San Diego: Singular Publishing Group. Copyright 1993 by Singular Publishing Group. Reprinted with permission.)

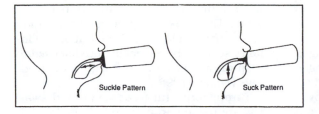

The term *sucking* is frequently used as a generic term, and will be so used in this chapter, unless there is a specific reason for distinctions between the two patterns.

Nonnutritive Sucking

Rhythmic nonnutritive sucking appears to be a prerequisite to successful nutritive sucking. Nonnutritive sucking on any object (e.g., finger, pacifier, or toy) can be carried out with no interruption of breathing (e.g., Koenig, Davies, & Thach, 1990; Mathew, Clark, & Pronske, 1985). The nonnutritive sucking rate is 2 sucks per second whereas the nutritive sucking rate is 1 suck per second. Infants on nonoral feeds who are given nonnutritive sucking experiences during nonoral supplemental feeding times have shown several positive gains: increased transcutaneous oxygen tension between 32 and 35 weeks' gestation (Paludetto, Robertson, Hack, Shivpuri, & Martin, 1984) and in healthy, crying, full-term infants (Treloar, 1994); reduced number of tube feedings prior to oral feedings (Field et al., 1982); enhanced growth and maturation (Bernbaum, Pereira, Watkins, & Peckham, 1983); improved digestion of tube feedings (Measel & Anderson, 1979); reduced amount and degree of fussing and crying during and after feeding (DiPietro, Cusson, Caughy, & Fox, 1994) and during invasive procedures, for example, heelsticks (Field & Goldson, 1984); and reduced crying and more stable heart rate in intubated infants requiring assisted mechanical ventilation (Miller & Anderson, 1993).

This skill underlying nonnutritive sucking is necessary but not sufficient to guarantee successful nutritive sucking. A swallow response does not necessarily follow nonnutritive sucking bursts. Caution is urged in interpreting nonnutritive performance as readiness for oral feeding.

Nutritive Sucking (1st 4 to 6 months)

The central element of nutritive sucking is the biphasic peristaltic action of the tongue (Bosma, Hepburn, Josell, & Baker, 1990). The central portion of the tongue moves repeatedly toward the pharynx in general sequences of negative and positive pressures (Bosma, 1992). The genioglossus muscle lowers successive sections of the median portion of the tongue downward toward the gonial process of the mandible. The transverse intrinsic lingual mus-

cles then elevate the displaced sections of the median portion upward into alignment with the lateral portions of the tongue where the styloglossus and hypoglossus muscles are inserted (Bosma et al., 1990). The whole tongue, hyoid bone, mandible, and lower lip are all moved in alternating phases downward and forward and then upward and backward. As milk is drawn and expressed from the nipple, it is moved into the pharynx by the progressing peristaltic wave (Bosma, 1992).

Suck, Swallow, and Respiration

The pharyngeal airway of the newborn lacks intrinsic rigidity. The walls are composed of soft tissues. Numerous muscles surrounding the pharynx provide mechanical support. Contraction of the tongue muscles dilates the pharyngeal airway, thus making it more resistant to collapse by negative pressure (Brouillette & Thach, 1979). An increase in flexion of the neck requires a compensatory increase in tone of the pharyngeal-dilating muscles in order to preserve airway patency (Thach, 1992). Neck flexion, posterior movement of the mandible, or external pressure over the hyoid bone all can compress the hypopharynx and limit airflow (Stark & Thach, 1976). The entrance to the larynx at the level of the aryepiglottic folds is the next most easily collapsed region (Reed, Roberts, & Thach, 1985). The feeding process places greater demands on the patency of the upper airway in infants than any other function. Sucking, swallowing, and breathing require precise coordination for infants. This need for precise coordination is also true of older children, but young infants seem to be especially predisposed to respiratory difficulties during oral feedings (Thach, 1992).

Throughout oral feeds, suck and swallow are usually in a 1:1 relationship, with respiration occurring between swallows (Koenig et al., 1990; Wilson, Thach, Brouillette, & Abu-Osba, 1981). Short periods of apnea may be noted at the beginning of a feeding run in normal newborns. Infants seem to tolerate the apnea well and resume suckling after several seconds. In contrast, the preterm infant may become hypoxic, as the alternation of breaths between swallows is the last skill to develop in the suckle feeding process.

The coordination of sucking, swallowing, and breathing during feeding is believed to be important, although difficulties in measuring ventilation during feeding have limited accurate quantification of these interactions (Mathew, 1991). Ardran and colleagues (1958) demonstrated by cineradiographic studies that infants do interrupt breathing to feed orally. More recently, measurements of nasal airflow via small flowmeters have shown that airflow is interrupted during swallowing (Koenig et al., 1990; Wilson et al., 1981). Studies do agree that minute ventilation, respiratory rate, and tidal volume decrease during continuous nutritive sucking (e.g., Durand et al., 1981; Guilleminault & Coons, 1984; Mathew, Clark, Pronske, Luna-Solarzano, & Peterson, 1985; Shivpuri, Martin, Carlo, & Fanarof, 1983; Wilson et al., 1981), even though there are methodologic and analytic differences among studies.

Initial periods of continuous sucking lasting up to 70 sec are associated with reduction in minute ventilation. This is followed by intermittent sucking periods, alternating with respiration, and recovery of minute ventilation. This recovery appears to be more robust with increasing gestational age (Mathew, Clark, Pronske et al., 1985). The etiology of this decreased ventilation remains unclear. It would appear that repeated swallowing during continuous sucking bursts seriously limits the amount of time available for ventilation. The inverse relation between swallowing and ventilation appears in large part as a secondary effect of mechanical airway closure (Mathew, 1991). The coordination of breathing, sucking, and swallowing is often imperfect in normal young infants.

Growth in the upper aerodigestive tract occurs gradually over the first several months of life, although there is relatively minimal change in proportion or form. The intraoral space increases as the mandible grows downward and forward. The oral cavity elongates in the vertical direction. The tongue has more space for the shift from suckling to sucking patterns for taking liquid. The hyoid bone and larynx shift downward so breathing and swallowing coordination becomes more similar to that of adults. The exact timing of laryngeal descent is not known. However, cineradiographic and postmortem observations indicate that by the 3rd year the larynx has lowered significantly (Laitman & Crelin, 1980).

Although the larynx remains high in the neck until the 2nd year, mouth breathing may supplement nasal breathing by 3 to 4 months of age (Curtis, Cruess, Dachman, & Maso, 1984). The sucking pads are absorbed gradually. Teeth usually begin to erupt by about 6 months of age (Moore, 1988). All 20 deciduous teeth are expected by the end of the 2nd year. Although there are several anatomic changes that prepare infants for transition feeding, the readiness for varied textures relates more directly to central nervous system maturation. For example, teeth are not necessary for munching. Children can "gum" the food in preparation for swallowing.

Transition Feeding Development

The transition from suckling to sucking over the first several months of life sets the stage for spoon feeding and cup drinking by 4 to 6 months of age. This period also may be crucial in upper respiratory/upper digestive tract activity and considerable central nervous system maturation resulting in the disappearance of some oral reflexes (e.g., rooting) and other primitive reflexes (e.g., Moro, asymmetric tonic neck reflex, tonic labyrinthine reflex, and positive support reflex). Additionally, this period may be one of relative respiratory instability due to the transition from strictly nasal breathing to a combination of nasal and mouth breathing (Laitman & Reidenberg, 1993). The upper aerodigestive tract undergoes minimal anatomic changes during this period.

When initially introduced to spoon feeding, infants essentially suck the material with lip closure around the spoon similar to that around a nipple. The peristaltic actions of the tongue that move food into the pharynx are similar to those of the suckle. The gradual change in tongue pattern used from suckling to sucking with a buildup of negative pressure in the mouth assists in readiness to take thicker food off a spoon.

The ability to maintain an upright sitting position for at least several minutes appears at a developmental age of approximately 5–7 months. This ability to maintain adequate trunk and head control underlies the ability to swallow thicker food. During this same time period, hand-to-mouth coordination gains indicate readiness toward self-feeding. Children are usually ready for cup drinking about 1 month after the introduction of spoon feeding.

Upon presentation of thicker or slightly lumpy textures that require more tongue and jaw manipulation, the child's tongue movements gradually show some lateralization along with vertical jaw action that is typical of munching. Chewable food should be introduced at about 6 to 7 months of age (Illingworth & Lister, 1964). Gradually children acquire the skills to carry out the complex act of chewing. Mature chewing involves lateral tongue action with a rotary jaw movement as the lips are maintained in a closed position. Electromyography has shown that chewing is fully mature at 3 to 6 years of age (Vitti and Basmajian, 1975). The sequential actions in chewing reflect bulbar and suprabulbar maturation.

Transitional feeding development is enhanced by diversified taste and smell experiences. The chemosensory inputs may interact with the child's perceptions of physical characteristics of food, although this interaction is not clearly identified (Bosma, 1986). Wide fluctuations in food preferences have been reported to include both texture and flavor (Davis, 1939).

The phase of transitional feeding is part of a broader developmental process that includes complex mechanisms and patterns of appetite and satiation. This evolution of transitional feeding is highly social as well as individual. The caregiver must realize that the choices of food offered to the child, the age and sensorimotor skills of the child, and the social circumstances of the mealtime are all significant factors. The child's feeding competence can be expected to diminish with fatigue, stress, or illness. The selection of food should be within the realm of the child's competence in oral-motor function, but it is not always possible to have a perfect match between a new food and the skill level. Family and cultural patterns influence the transitional feeding experiences. The dietary patterns and preferences acquired during transition feeding periods can be expected to carry over into adulthood (Bosma, 1986). These patterns and preferences in turn get passed on to succeeding generations.

Neurodevelopmental Aspects Related to Swallowing

For the first 6 months of life, infants are dependent on parents or other caregivers for feedings. During feeding, verbal and nonverbal communications between caregivers and infants are important. Maternal characteristics during feedings include affect (e.g., body posture, facial expression), sensitivity to infant cues, positioning of the infant, verbal communications, and other feeding behaviors. Infant characteristics include affect, visual communication (e.g., smiling, looking at mother as opposed to gaze aversion), vocalization, and other behaviors including consolability and general satisfaction with feedings. These infant behaviors are manifestations of both cognitive and motor development. The behaviors of infant and caregiver are interactive, resulting in changes in behavior on the part of either or both partners in the communication dyad. Thus, abnormalities of infant communication should alert the clinician to the possiblity of broader developmental impairments of children with feeding/swallowing problems (Huber, 1991). Table 14–1 outlines the neurodevelopmental milestones relevant to normal feeding skills.

TABLE 14–1. Neurodevelopmental milestones relevant to normal feeding.

Age (Months)	Cognitive/Sensory	Motor	Feeding Skills
Birth to 2	Visual fixation and tracking	Balanced flexor and extensor tone of neck and trunk	Promotion of parent–infant interaction during feeding Maintenance of semiflexed posture during feeding
3 to 4	Visual recognition of parents	Head maintained primarily in midline and aligned with trunk in supported sitting	Parents preferred for oral feedings Upright supported position to begin spoon feeding
5 to 9	Visual interest in small objects Extended reach and grasp Object permanence Stranger anxiety	Independent sitting Extended reach with pincer grasp	Feedings more frequently in upright position Initiation of finger feeding Parents preferred for feedings
18 to 24	Use of tools Increasing attention and persistence in play activities Independence from parents Parallel or imitative play	Refinement of upper extremity coordination	Use of feeding utensils Prefer to feed self over longer periods of time Imitate others during meals

Source: From Pediatric and Neurodevelopmental Evaluation by B. Rogers & J. Campbell, 1993, p. 55. In J. Arvedson & L. Brodsky (Eds.), *Pediatric Swallowing and Feeding: Assessment and Management.* San Diego: Singular Publishing Group. Copyright © 1993. Reprinted by permission.

Infants gradually become less dependent for feeding after 6 months of age as cognitive and motor development proceed. Development of visual interest in small objects (5 months), of extended reach and grasp (5 months) and of a pincer grasp (9 months) set the stage for self-feeding (Table 14–1). Refinement of self-feeding skills (e.g., use of utensils) is dependent on cognitively driven behaviors including the use of tools to obtain objects by 18 to 20 months (Bayley, 1993; Cattell, 1940). The growing independence of 2-year-olds is exemplified in their preference for their own messes rather than being fed. If these developmental trends are sup-pressed, power struggles may lead to food refusal.

Etiologies of Feeding and Swallowing Disorders in Children

Etiologies of feeding and swallowing disorders in childhood may be classified as acute or chronic conditions, the latter static or progressive (Table 14–2). Most feeding disorders are recognized on the basis of a thorough history, as are many other illnesses. In static conditions, feeding skills generally remain the same or gradually improve with age and maturation. Although feeding efficiency may vary during acute

TABLE 14-2. Etiology of dysphagia in childhood.

Site of Pathology	Acute	Chronic	
		Static	Progressive
Central nervous system	Hypoxic-ischemic encephalopathy Cerebral infarctions Intracranial hemorrhage Infections Meningitis Encephalitis Poliomyelitis Botulism Syphilis Acute bilirubin encephalopathy Metabolic encephalopathies Aminoacidopathies Disorders of carbohydrate metabolism Neonatal withdrawal syndrome (heroin, barbiturates) Traumatic encephalopathies and brain stem injuries	Arnold-Chiari malformation Genetic disorders Familial dysautonomia (Riley-Day) Mobius sequence Developmental disorders of the brain Cerebral palsy Chronic postkernicteric bilirubin encephalopathy	Arnold-Chiari malformation Intracranial malignancies Tumors Leukemia Lymphoma Degenerative white and gray matter diseases Lysosomal storage diseases Metachromatic leukodystrophy Adrenoleukodystrophy Leigh's encephalomyelopathy Neuroaxonal degeneration Zellweger's disease Wilson's disease HIV encephalopathy Rett syndrome Spinocerebellar disorders Dystonia muscluorum deformans Multiple sclerosis Amyotrophic lateral sclerosis Syringobulbia
Anterior horn cell			Infantile spinal muscular atrophy
Peripheral nervous system	Acute inflammatory polyradiculoneuropathy	Polyneuropathies	Polyneuropathies
Neuromuscular junction	Hypermagnesemia		Myasthenia gravis
Muscles	Polymyositis Dermatomyositis	Congenital myopathies Nemaline rod Myotubular Fiber type disproportion Myotonic dystrophy Congenital muscular dystrophy Infantile fascioscapulohumeral dystrophy	Metabolic myopathies Glycogen storage disease Mitochondrial Duchenne's muscular dystrophy

Respiratory tract	Otitis media	
	Sinusitis	
	Adenotonsillitis/pharyngitis	
	Severe chronic lung disease	
	Bronchopulmonary dysplasia	
	Structural anomalies of upper respiratory tract	
Cardiovascular disorders	Congenital heart disease	Congenital heart disease (may be progressive at times)
	Cyanotic	
	Congestive heart failure	
Gastrointestinal tract	Gastroesophageal reflux	Gastroesophageal reflux and esophagitis
	Peptic ulcer	Peptic ulcer
Psychological	Disorders of parent-child interaction	

Source: From Pediatric and Neurodevelopmental Evaluation by B. B. Rogers & J. Campbell, 1993, p. 58–59. In J. Arvedson & L. Brodsky (Eds.), *Pediatric Swallowing and Feeding: Assessment and Management.* San Diego: Singular Publishing Group. Copyright © 1993. Reprinted by permission.

illnesses or transition feeding periods, persistent loss of previously acquired oromotor and deglutition abilities does not occur. Regression or loss of previously acquired feeding skills is seen in both acute and progressive conditions and should prompt appropriate medical evaluation.

ASSESSMENT OF PEDIATRIC SWALLOWING/FEEDING DISORDERS

A diagnostic workup includes a thorough history, physical examination, and oral-motor/feeding examination with direct observation of feeding. In selected patients, instrumental assessments (e.g., videofluoroscopic study of the oropharyngeal swallow, pulse oximetry, airway endoscopy, upper gastrointestinal (GI) series, scintiscan, and pH monitoring) can add valuable information for optimal decision making and for monitoring of change over time.

History

Feeding History

An accurate and thorough feeding history is important and enlightening. Because perceptions of feeding problems differ with the reporter, information is best obtained from more than one caregiver or professional involved with the child. Questions must be asked in ways to delineate the feeding status as clearly as possible (Arvedson & Rogers, 1993).

1. Is the child dependent on others for feeding or is there some independent feeding? Children who have reached the developmental age for self-feeding expectations, but who are dependent on others for feeding, usually present with significant motor and/or sensory impairment, such as in cerebral palsy. Children with cerebral palsy who are also dependent feeders often demonstrate reduced oxygen saturation during feeding (Rogers, Arvedson, Msall, & Demereth, 1993). They also have shown greater probability for silent aspiration (Rogers, Arvedson, Buck, Smart, & Msall, 1994). Children who demonstrate sufficient postural support and hand-to-mouth skills to be self-feeders usually, but not always, have better coordination for safe swallow production.

2. Does the child take all feedings orally or is there some tube feeding? Most parents perceive oral feeding to be a sign of success for a child with multiple handicaps. However, there are instances in which tube feeding in multiply handicapped children allows for meeting of nutritional needs without placing undue risk on the respiratory system and/or the energy levels required for feeding orally.

3. Does the feeding problem vary by food texture, taste, temperature,or type? Aspiration and pharyngeal motility deficits may be texture-specific (Arvedson, Rogers, Buck, Smart, & Msall, 1994). Children who show incoordination in oral and pharyngeal function or show delay in producing a swallow are at greater risk for aspiration with thin liquids than with thicker textures. Some children may prefer spicy over bland food, cold vs. warm, or vice versa. All these attributes may interact and have effects on the efficiency of feeding.

4. Is the feeding problem worse at the beginning, middle, or end of meal? Awareness of the variability of feeding problems may aid in delineating the bases for the problems. For example, oral defensiveness, parent–child interaction breakdowns, poor appetite, and positioning concerns are likely to be noted before or at the beginning of a mealtime. As a mealtime progresses, children with oral-motor and swallow deficits may demonstrate fatigue, compromised cardiopulmonary function, and oropharyngeal dysphagia.

5. Does the feeding problem vary by time of day or with different feeders? Clarification of environmental factors can occur through examination of differences in methods by specific caregivers, the setting for mealtimes with possible distractions, appetite, and fatigue factors.

6. What is the child's position during mealtimes? How does it vary? Extensor arching of the trunk and extremities frequently seen during oral feeding in children with cerebral palsy is a common problem. The risk for aspiration may be increased with this posture. On the other hand, the young child with hypotonia and a "floppy" neck is at risk for aspiration with excessive flexion of the oropharynx.

7. Does the child show any indication of difficulty breathing while eating? Any change in respiratory rate and/or effort raises a big red flag and symptoms must be evaluated thoroughly so that causes can be determined.

8. Does the child have emesis? If yes, when and how much? Gastroesophageal reflux (GER) is common in children with neurogenic dysphagia. Incidences have been reported from 15% to 65% (Langer et al., 1988; Mollitt, Golladay, & Seibert, 1985; Wheatley, Wesley, Tkach, & Coran, 1991). It must be remembered that these children may have GE reflux with no evidence of emesis.

9. Does the child refuse food? If yes, under what circumstances? Food refusal may be the child's method for communicating problems with oral-motor function, airway, gastrointestinal factors, or parent–child interaction abnormalities.

10. Does the child get irritable during feeds? Or sleepy or lethargic? Irritability may signal GER, or some other gastrointestinal problem, as well as airway problems. Lethargy during meals may result from excessive fatigue, recurrent seizures, or sedating medications (e.g., anticonvulsants, muscle relaxants).

11. How many minutes does it take to feed the child? Lengthy mealtimes are of concern as feeding is a child's work, and the longer it takes to consume the required number of calories, the greater the risk for malnutrition. In general, mealtimes should take only 20 to no more than 30 minutes on a regular basis.

12. How do child and caregiver interact? Is there forced feeding? Stress by caregivers can be transmitted to a child and thus exacerbate feeding difficulties. Forced feeding is likely to lead to any number of complications (e.g., food refusal, failure to thrive, and other more global behavior maladaptions).

Medical History

The medical history should help clarify the etiology and management of feeding and swallowing disorders in childhood. Special attention should be given to the developmental history, cardiopulmonary status, and gastrointestinal health.

Most children with chronic nonprogressive dysphagia also have various developmental disabilities, most notably cerebral palsy. Both the sequelae and treatment of epilepsy, behavior disorders, and neuro-developmental disabilities can result in primary feeding problems or may complicate preexisting dysphagia. Uncontrolled or poorly controlled seizures can be a basis for altered levels of consciousness and thus interference with feeding. Anticonvulsants (barbiturates and benzodiazepames) can produce lethargy as a side effect. Some neuroleptics (e.g., chlorpromazine, thoridazine) used in the management of severe behavior disorders can result in lethargy and the development of laryngeal-pharyngeal dystonia and esophageal dysmotility (Moss & Green, 1982). Occasionally children with cerebral palsy and other central nervous system disorders are treated with benzodiazepames for spasticity. In addition to reducing spasticity, benzodiazepames have resulted in reduced pharyngeal constrictor function, cricopharyngeal incoordination, and drooling (Wyllie, Wyllie, Cruse, Rothner, & Erenberg, 1986).

Recurrent or chronic pulmonary and gastrointestinal symptoms may suggest the presence of dysphagia. Moderate to severe dysphagia commonly results in reduced fluid intake. During acute illnesses, fluid intake may dramatically be reduced with dehydration as a result. Chronically low fluid intake, particularly in patients who are nonambulatory, is likely to result in chronic constipation. Gastroesophageal reflux frequently is accompanied by vomiting, but reflux to lower esophageal levels may result in frequent belching followed by a series of swallows or apparent discomfort and no vomiting at all. The relationship of these apparent reflux episodes to respiratory symptoms such as cough, sternal retractions, noisy breathing, or cyanosis should be noted. Chronic aspiration can result in recurrent pneumonia or intractable asthma. Stridor may be caused by primary upper respiratory tract anomalies and laryngeal inflammation resulting from gastroesophageal reflux (Nielson, Heldt, & Tooley, 1990).

Physical Examination

The physical examination, guided by the feeding and medical history, will help confirm the diagnosis of dysphagia. Dysphagia is common in a number of well-known genetic syndromes. The feeding and swallowing difficulties are generally chronic and static in nature. A careful family history and dysmorphologic examination are essential for an accurate diagnosis (Table 14–3). Once a diagnosis is made, an appropriate management plan can be developed and implemented.

The physical examination should focus particularly on somatic growth, neurodevelopment, orofacial structures, and the cardiopulmonary and gastrointestinal systems. The importance of a nutritional assessment cannot be overemphasized, but will not be described in detail in this chapter. Many methods exist, because no single measure fulfills all requirements for assessing nutritional status in infants and children (e.g., Walker & Hendricks, 1985; Young, 1993).

Growth and Development

Stunted growth is common in children with dysphagia. Anthropometric measurements including weight, height, head circumference, weight for height ratio, triceps skinfold thickness, and midarm circumference are essential in assessing nutritional status. If previous growth data are limited, the interrelationships among weight, height, and head circumference measurements can still provide valuable information about the nutritional history. Signs of acute protein calorie malnutrition include reduction of weight to below the 5th percentile for age and weight-for-

height ratio less than the 10th percentile (Rossi, 1993). Chronic protein calorie malnutrition in children with neurogenic dysphagia can result in reductions of fat stores, fat-free mass (muscle area), and linear growth (Stallings, Charney, Davies, & Cronk, 1993).

Neurodevelopmental Examination

Most dysphagia in infancy and childhood results from CNS disorders. The feeding and medical history when combined (see Chapter 11) with a detailed neurologic examination will usually identify the nature of the CNS disorder. Several methods and scales can be incorporated into the examination (e.g., Capute et al., 1986; Capute & Shapiro, 1985; Rogers & Campbell, 1993).

Feeding programs should be tailored to the child's developmental status. The self-feeding skills of children and their behavior at meal times will reflect their cognitive and communication "age" and not necessarily their chronologic age. Thus, a thorough understanding of the cognitive and communication skills of each child is needed to implement any feeding program. Mental retardation and communication disorders are important risk factors in the development of behavioral food refusal and in the maintenance of maladaptive feeding behaviors after an intercurrent illness.

Orofacial Examination

Orofacial structures involved with feeding should be carefully examined. Many congenital birth syndromes can cause alterations of the orofacial structures and subsequently dysphagia. In addition, obstructive lesions of the nose, including choanal atresia or stenosis, nasal polyps, and foreign bodies may interfere with respiration. Leakage of food into the nasal cavity can result from midline defects (e.g., complete clefts of the lip and palate to subtle submucous clefts). Tonsillar and adenoidal hypertrophy in the middle childhood years can result in partial airway obstruction and mouth breathing.

TABLE 14–3. Genetic syndromes with prominent dysphagia.

Diagnoses	Anomalies	Neurodevelopmental Profile	Feeding Abnormalities
Prader-Willi Syndrome	Narrow bifrontal diameter Almond-shaped palpebral fissures Small hands and feet Obesity	Mental retardation and hypotonia	Dysphagia frequently observed in the first year
Coffin siris	Microcephaly, growth deficiency Coarse facies, full lips, wide mouth Sparse scalp hair Hypoplastic or absent fifth digit	Mental retardation and hypotonia	Difficulty sucking, swallowing, and breathing
Oculo-mandibulo-facial syndrome (Hallerman Streiff)	Short stature (proportionate) Dyscephaly, frontal bossing Mandibular and nasal cartilage hypoplasia Microstomia, glossoptosis Microphthalmia Hypotrichosis	Normal intelligence	Feeding and respiratory problems are common during infancy
Freedman-Sheldon	Masklike "Whistling facies" Hypoplastic alae nasi Club feet	Hypotonia, facial paresis, and possible myopathic arthrogryposis	Feeding problems secondary to severe microstomia
Smith-Lemli-Optiz-syndrome	Microcephaly, narrow high forehead, prominent metopic suture Hypospadia, cryptorchidism Short nose, anteverted nose, ptosis Broad maxillary-alveolar ridge Syndactyly of second and third toes	Moderate to severe mental retardation Hypotonia progressing to hypertonia	Poor suck, gastroesophageal reflux
de Lange syndrome	Hirsutism, synophrys Microcephaly Thin down-turned upper lip Micromelia, oligodactyly, or phocomelia	Mild to severe mental retardation Spasticity, motor delays	Poor suck, frequent respiratory infections
Dubowitz	Low birthweight and postnatal growth retardation Microcephaly Hoarse cry Small facies, shallow-nasal bridge, telecanthus, ptosis Micrognathia	Mild mental retardation common	Poor oral intake, frequent emesis and diarrhea during first year

(continued)

TABLE 14–3. *(continued)*

Diagnoses	Anomalies	Neurodevelopmental Profile	Feeding Abnormalities
Pierre Robin sequence	Mandibular hypoplasia Micrognathia U-shaped cleft palate	Generally normal development	Respiratory distress with feeding in infancy including coughing, grunting, and sputtering
Facio-auriculo vertebral spectrum	First and second branchial arch anomalies Microtia Maxillary and mandibular hypoplasia	Normal development	Respiratory distress with feeding in infancy
Kippel-Feil	Short neck Low hairline Fusion of cervical vertebrae	Syringomyelia may develop	Cranial nerve deficits result in dysphagia
Mobius sequence	Masklike facies at birth Cranial nerve palsies	Cognitive development usually normal	Paralysis of cranial nerves VI and VII (usually permanent) Dysphagia not usually severe unless other cranial nerves involved (CN V, IX, X, or XII)
Rubenstein-Taybi	Short stature Downward-slanting palpebral fissures Hypoplastic maxilla and narrow palate Broad thumbs and toes	Mental retardation Motor delays	Infants have a weak suck Swallowing is poorly coordinated Frequent vomiting during infancy
Beckwith-Wiedermann	Macroglossia Omphalocele Ear creases Macrosomia	Mild to moderate mental retardation has been reported Development can be normal	Feeding problems secondary to large tongue
Trisomy 18	Growth deficiency Prominent occiput Low-set ears Short sternum Congenital heart defects Micrognathia, narrow palate	Profound mental retardation Hypertonia	High-pitched cry Poor suck
Trisomy 21 (Down syndrome)	Brachycephaly with relatively flat occiput Upward-slanting palpebral fissures Small nose with flat nasal bridge Small ears Short metacarpals and phalanges Single transverse palmar crease	Hypotonia Usually moderate mental retardation	Weak suck Feeding can be further compromised by cardiovascular anomalies

Source: From Pediatric and Neurodevelopmental Evaluation by B. Rogers & J. Campbell, 1993, p. 77–80. In J. Arvedson & L. Brodsky (Eds.), *Pediatric Swallowing and Feeding: Assessment and Management.* San Diego: Singular Publishing Group. Copyright © 1993. Reprinted by permission.

Mandibular hypoplasia may disrupt the relationship between the tongue and palate and interfere with infant suckling.

Cardiopulmonary Examination

Examination of the heart and lungs may reveal important signs of chronic dysphagia and aspiration. Clinical manifestations of swallowing dysfunction in infants are primarily apnea and bradycardia during feeding (Loughlin & Lefton-Greif, 1994). Chronic and/or recurrent respiratory problems (e.g., congestion, cough, and wheezing) are also seen (Loughlin, 1989). Other symptoms include recurrent pneumonia, failure to thrive, and radiologic signs of chronic lung injury (Bauer, Figueroa-Colon, Georgeson, & Young, 1993). Diminished chest wall compliance resulting in decreased excursion can be observed in cerebral palsy and other neuromuscular conditions. Respiratory drive and respiratory rate may be elevated in the presence of aspiration (Loughlin, 1989). Wheezes or rales on auscultation of the lung fields may also indicate aspiration. Children with tracheotomy vary considerably in degree of feeding/swallow difficulties (e.g., Arvedson & Brodsky, 1992; Simon & McGowan, 1989). The degree of difficulty may relate most closely to the underlying reason(s) for the tracheotomy. Finally, primary cardiopulmonary disease may compromise oral feedings. Infants and children who are short of breath will feed poorly. Chronic lung disease and congestive heart failure are commonly characterized by progressive tachypnea or fatigue during oral feedings (Harris, 1983).

Gastrointestinal (GI) Examination

Gastroesophageal reflux (GER) is common in infants and children with feeding problems (e.g., Bagwell, 1995; Hyman, 1994; Sondheimer, 1994). GER may have a significant effect on the respiratory systems of these children. The signs of GER may be subtle, and not necessarily include emesis, particularly in children with CNS deficits (e.g., Langer et al., 1988;

Mollitt et al., 1985; Wheatley et al., 1991). Nonspecific signs of GER include, but are not limited to, irritability, stridor, postural arching, and neck hyperextension. Posturing and irritability may be symptoms of diffuse esophageal spasm (Wyllie, Wyllie, Rothner, & Morris, 1989). In some instances, GER may present only with stridor or apnea and not other symptoms (e.g., Loughlin & Lefton-Greif, 1994; Nielson et al., 1990).

Frequently infants and children with dysphagia have reduced fluid intake and thus develop severe constipation, which in turn makes them fussy and irritable during feedings. "Colic" and intermittent abdominal distension may result. On examination, stool can often be palpated or detected by dullness on percussion in the left upper and lower abdominal quadrants and in the suprapubic region. Stools testing positive for occult blood may yield the first sign of esophagitis (Antanitus, 1989).

Oral-Motor and Feeding Assessment

The oral-motor and feeding assessment consists of a prefeeding assessment, oral-motor structure and function examination, feeding observation, and in some instances, instrumental assessments. The clinical assessment is an extension of the history and physical examination previously discussed. The assessment starts with no food or liquid, and may *not* include food or liquid at all if the risks are deemed too high at that time.

There is no single test or scale that can be recommended for universal use with the pediatric population. However, there are a number of checklists and scales to assist in systematizing observations (e.g., Arvedson & Brodsky, 1993; Braun & Palmer, 1986; Case-Smith, 1988; Case-Smith, Cooper, & Scala, 1989; Chatoor, Menvielle, Getson, & O'Donnell, 1989; Cherney, 1994; Gisel & Patrick, 1988; Herman, 1991; Jelm, 1990; Kenny et al., 1989; Morris & Klein, 1987; Stratton, 1981; Tuchman & Walter, 1994; Warner, 1981).

Prefeeding Assessment

Observations are made and deviations from normal expectations are noted. These observations include the following (Arvedson & Rogers, 1993):

- Parent–child interactions
- Posture (especially head, neck, and trunk) and movement patterns
- Respiratory patterns (rate of breathing, effort, etc.)
- Affect, temperament, and overall responsiveness
- Level of alertness and ability to sustain attention to task
- Response to sensory stimulation (e.g., tactile, visual, auditory, smell)
- Ability to self-calm and self-regulate.

Oral-Motor Structure and Function Assessment

Assessment is made prior to the introduction of food and liquid. Examination includes lip and jaw position, palatal shape and height, tongue shape and movement patterns, oral reflexes, laryngeal function on the basis of vocal quality, and in infants, nonnutritive sucking. Drooling after the age of 5 years suggests the need for a comprehensive workup of drooling (Brodsky, 1993).

Feeding Assessment

In newborn infants, cardiac and respiratory status must be stable and bowel sounds should be adequate before an oral feeding assessment can be made. The feeding should be anticipated with minimal respiratory distress (Babson, Pernoll, & Benda, 1980). Infants should be observed for at least 15 to 20 minutes, as some infants may become disorganized, with signs of fatigue as the feeding progesses. Infants with cardiac abnormalities commonly present with this pattern. Infants with neurogenic dysphagia also may show increased disorganization as feeding progresses. An infant should take the necessary volume per feed within a total of 15 to 20 minutes, and no more than 30 minutes, to be a functional oral feeder.

Older infants and children are observed with a familiar feeder who simulates the typical positioning or seating system as closely as possible. Attention is paid to the child's posture, especially to the support that is provided to the child for efficient feeding.

Lip, tongue, and jaw action are observed during spoon or finger feeding. Estimates can be made for time it takes to produce a swallow, and whether multiple swallows are needed to clear a bolus of food from the oral cavity. Textures can be varied for liquids and soft food (e.g., thin vs. thick liquids via nipple or cup, smooth vs. lumpy textures for spoon feeding). Chewing and munching skills are related to expected developmental age. Children do not necessarily have to master all gradations of pureed textures to be ready for chewable food (Gisel, 1991; Gisel, Lange, & Niman, 1984). The failure to form a bolus and/or to seal the lips around a nipple or spoon, lack of tongue elevation, and delay in initiation of a swallow may all be indications of cranial nerve deficits (Table 14–4).

Instrumental Assessment

The most common instrumental assessments used with the pediatric population include the fluoroscopic oropharyngeal swallow study, ultrasonography, and pulse oximetry. Other radiographic studes and endoscopy may be useful for airway and gastroesophageal function.

The fluoroscopic study provides the most complete information about the physiology of the pharyngeal phase of the swallow (Langmore & Logemann, 1991). The oropharyngeal swallow study also may assist in optimizing position for feeding (Morton, Bonas, Fourie, & Minford, 1993).

FLUOROSCOPIC MODIFIED BARIUM SWALLOW STUDY (also commonly called the oropharyngeal swallow study or the three-phase swallow study). This study is especially useful in describing pharyngeal motility, in delineating characteristics of

TABLE 14–4. Cranial nerve function during feeding assessment.

CN	Stimulus	Normal Response	Deficit Response
V	Food on tongue	Mastication initiated	Bolus not formed
VII	Sucking Food on lower lip Smile	Lip pursing Lip closure Retraction of lips	Lack of lip seal Lack of lip movement Asymetry or lack of retraction
IX, X	Food posterior in mouth	Swallow—2 seconds Soft palate elevation	Delayed swallow Nasopharyngeal reflux
XII	Food on tongue	Tongue shape, point, and protrude	Tongue lacks thinning elevation, and has excessive thrust, atrophy

Source: From Oral-Motor and Feeding Assessment by J. Arvedson, 1993, p. 271. In J. Arvedson & L. Brodsky (Eds.), *Pediatric Swallowing and Feeding: Assessment and Management.* San Diego: Singular Publishing Group. Copyright © 1993. Reprinted by permission.

any aspiration, and in noting differences in pharyngeal motility related to food textures. Procedural descriptions can be found in several sources (e.g., Chapter 6; Benson & Lefton-Greif, 1994; Arvedson & Christensen, 1993; Logemann, 1983, 1993). Children with severe dysphagia have a high risk for medical complications during examinations. Therefore, a radiologist, and not just a radiographic technician, should be involved so medical decisions can be made promptly and appropriately when necessary. Radiographic findings (see Chapter 6) can be related to phase(s) of the swallow (Table 14–5) and, along with prior history and clinic observations, can assist in optimal decision making for management.

ULTRASONOGRAPHY. The oral phase of swallowing can be delineated well via ultrasonography, but the pharyngeal stage can only be inferred (e.g., Bosma et al., 1990; Sonies, 1987). A distinct advantage of ultrasonography is that it does not use radiation, and thus lengthy observations can be made (see Chapter 8).

PULSE OXIMETRY. One simple, noninvasive measure that can be used during clinical observations of feeding is pulse oximetry. Desaturation with oral feeding can be noted with quantification of degree and duration of desaturation. This finding can then lead to additional examina-

tions that may be needed to reach a definitive diagnosis, and thus prognosis, as well as to make management decisions (e.g., Garg, Kurzner, Bautista, & Keens, 1988; Rogers et al., 1993).

ENDOSCOPY AND RADIOGRAPHIC STUDIES FOR AIRWAY STATUS. Specific airway examination procedures include endoscopy and radiologic evaluations. Flexible endoscopy can be used to examine the upper airway from anterior nose to the supraglottic larynx (e.g., Langmore, Schatz, & Olsen, 1988) (see Chapter 7). Radiologic evaluations may include plain anteroposterior and lateral radiographs of the airway, chest x-ray, barium esophgram, and ultra-fast CT analysis (Brody, Kuhn, Seidel, & Brodsky, 1991).

STUDIES FOR GASTROINTESTINAL STATUS. The diagnosis of GER may be established by clinical evaluation, radiographic studies (upper GI and barium swallow), nu-clear medicinine studies (e.g., scintiscan), and/or esophageal pH testing (see Chapter 7). Endoscopy and biopsy of the esophagus may be useful for some children. The extended pH monitor is the most sensitive indicator of GER at present, although subjectivity does enter into the interpretation. Variables in interpretation include types of feeds, feeding volume, positioning, movements, and duration of monitoring and feeding time (Boyle, 1989). Another impor-

TABLE 14–5. Radiographic findings related to stage of swallowing.

Stage	Observed Action	Radiographic Finding
Oral Preparatory	Lack of lip closure	Food falls out of mouth
	Tongue incoordination or weakness; reduced oral sensitivity	Food stays on tongue or falls into sulci
		Lack of bolus formation
		Adherence to hard palate
	Limited mandibular movement	Piecemeal deglutition
		Aspiration *before* swallow, especially liquids and thin textures
Oral	Limited tongue action	Delayed oral transit time
	Tongue thrust	Food pushed out of mouth
		Piecemeal deglutition
	Reduced tongue elevation	Aspiration *before* swallow, especially thick textures
	Tongue incoordination	Aspiration *before* swallow, thin textures
Pharyngeal	Nasopharyngeal reflux	Velopharyngeal incoordination
	Slow swallowing	Delayed pharyngeal transit time
	Gurgly voice quality	Reduced pharyngeal peristalsis
	Coughing or gagging (Note: silent aspiration common)	Pooling in pharyngeal recesses, aspiration *before* swallow
		Residue in pharyngeal recesses, aspiration *after* swallow
	Apnea	Cricopharyngeal dysfunction
	Breathy, hoarse voice reduced laryngeal closure, reduced laryngeal elevation	Aspiration *during* swallow
Esophageal	Emesis, pain, cough, apnea, no observable symptom	Reduced esophageal peristalsis
		Gastroesophageal reflux
		Obstruction, stricture
		Tracheoesophageal fistula
		Esophagitis

Source: From Instrumental Evaluation by J. Arvedson & S. Christianson, 1993, p. 314. In J. Arvedson & L. Brodsky (Eds.), *Pediatric Swallowing and Feeding: Assessment and Management.* San Diego: Singular Publishing Group. Copyright © 1993. Reprinted by permission.

tant factor is age. Infants have more frequent reflux episodes than older children.

Behavioral Factors

Behavioral factors need to be considered, whether or not there are obvious physiologic reasons for feeding problems (e.g., Chatoor, Dickson, Schaefer, & Egan, 1986; Satter, 1990, 1992). Children with behavioral feeding problems may demonstrate motivational problems (e.g., food refusal or selectivity brought about by deficient caregiver skills or a lack of hunger/satiety cycle brought about by supplemental tube feeding) or skill deficits (e.g.,

inability to self-feed) that account for at least part of the problem. Consideration should be given to the child's learning history related to eating, feeding skills of caregivers, and child or caregiver skill deficits (Babbitt, Hoch, & Coe, 1994).

INTERDISCIPLINARY TEAM APPROACH TO ASSESSMENT AND MANAGEMENT

Expertise from varied medical and behavioral disciplines is needed for adequate diagnosis and optimal intervention. The core interdisciplinary team may include a physician, nurse, nutritionist, speech-language pathologist, and occupational therapist. The primary physician is most likely to be a developmental pediatrician, or a pediatrician with broad experience in developmental disorders. Parents or other primary caregivers are integral members of the team and should be included in assessments and in decision making. Other physician specialties may include, but are not limited to, otolaryngology, gastroenterology, pulmonology, neurology, radiology, and surgery. Other allied health specialties may include respiratory therapy, psychology, social services, education, and physical therapy. For any intervention to be successful, caregivers must be committed to the plan and be consistent in the day-to-day follow-up.

Collaborative relationships should exist between oral-motor/feeding specialists (e.g., speech-language pathologists and occupational therapists) in educational settings (e.g., early intervention or special education programs) and colleagues with expertise in pediatric swallowing and feeding disorders in medical settings. Nonphysician specialists should not evaluate feeding/swallowing problems in isolation, as the health risks are too great for fragmented assessment and therapy. Oral-motor and feeding therapy with positioning changes may be useful, but obviously this therapy will not "cure" the problem. Oral-motor therapy with a strong emphasis on oral feeding may actually place some children at higher risk for aspiration or other health-related complications. Comprehensive individualized management plans must encompass a global sensorimotor focus in light of physical, physiological, and psychological status.

MANAGEMENT OF PEDIATRIC DYSPHAGIA

Management of feeding/swallowing problems is likely to incorporate medical and/or surgical decisions, nutrition recommendations, position guidelines, and oral-motor/swallowing practice. Short-term

and long-term goals must be delineated clearly and realistically. Goals must be compatible with broad health issues. Optimal nutrition status is critical for long-term growth. Family routines are commonly disrupted when lengthy time periods each day are spent in caring for a child with special needs. In turn, all family members may be compromised. Caregivers must understand and accept the goals, as they must make a commitment to carry out the day-to-day procedures needed to meet those goals. Documentation of changes over time must be done in measurable ways.

It is not a goal of this chapter to discuss medical and surgical interventions in detail for airway and gastrointestinal problems, but rather to emphasize that in the context of a comprehensive assessment, appropriate interventions are instituted. The following section will focus on oral-motor/swallowing management. A broad-based sensory, oral-motor, and behavioral management program is advocated in an interdisciplinary team focused approach (Arvedson, 1993; Morris & Klein, 1987).

Oral-Motor and Swallowing Management

Management plans are developed from an understanding of normal oral-motor development and the observed differences in children with dysphagia. Individualized treatment plans take into account multiple interactive factors to include underlying disease state, chronologic and mental/developmental age of the child, physiologic status, and psychologic/behavioral attributes. Improvement in oral-motor function and feeding can be anticipated as the central nervous system matures, even in children with neurologic deficits. However, in some instances feeding problems will be exacerbated over time, or new feeding problems may arise. Oral feeding to meet nutritional needs is not necessarily a viable long-term goal for all children. Oral-motor stimulation is an integral part of management for children whose nutritional needs are met orally or nonorally. It is particularly important that nonnutritive oral-motor stimulation be carried out in systematic ways for children on nonoral feeds.

Nonnutritive Oral-Motor Stimulation

Nonnutritive oral-motor stimulation may be a major focus in the newborn period and also with older children. (The importance and benefits of rhythmic nonnutritive sucking as a prerequisite to successful nutritive sucking were discussed in the development section of this chapter.) Feeding difficulties are usually perceived as major problems by parents, as nearly all interactions between parent and infant relate to feeding. Nurses and parents of infants on gavage feeds by orogastric (OG) or nasogastric (NG) tubes can carry out oral stimulation techniques, with minimal training by the oral-motor/feeding specialist in most instances. A primary goal is normalization of oral-motor function, particularly nonnutritive sucking, and *not* immediate oral feeding. Another goal relates to the prevention of severe dysphagia or at least minimizing the scope of potential problems, including behavior problems. Emphasis is placed on *pleasurable, rhythmic* oral stimulation (Table 14–6).

Infants and children with severe dysphagia who are at risk for or have a history of health complications including acute and chronic lung disease, airway obstruction, and/or malnutrition are potential candidates for tube feeding. Isolated abnormalities of deglutition are rarely an indication for long-term nonoral feedings. Children whose nutritional needs must be met via nonoral means over several months or even years are usually fed through a gastrostomy tube. Oral stimulation is important for those children (e.g., Alexander, 1987; Morris, 1989). The presentation of *very* small quantities of liquid or food allows for pleasurable experiences of varied tastes, textures, odors, and temperatures. A desirable outcome of oral-motor stimulation is more frequent swallowing. It is hoped that children would then be at less risk for aspiration on their own secretions. Some children may become oral

TABLE 14–6. Nonnutritive stimulation options.

Technique	When Used	How Used
Stroking face	Initial approach with oral hypersensitivity	Palm of hand or finger rhythmically from periphery to mouth; firm, but gentle.
Stroking tongue	Infants lacking consistent sucking rhythm	Fingertip at midtongue, stroke toward front with pressure down on tongue 4 to 6 times at 1 or 2 strokes per second; hold on tongue. Repeat after several seconds.
Pacifier (or finger)	Infants with mild sucking incoordination or to encourage more sucking Reduced cheek tone	Pacifier or finger placed in mouth and held in place by caregiver if infant tends to push it out.
Cotton swab dipped in water, formula, or breast milk	Infants lacking coordinated suck/swallow/respiratory sequencing; not safe for oral feeding, but taste experiences desired	Swab placed at midtongue with downward pressure to release minimal amount of liquid, stroke as with little finger. Repeat as tolerated in pleasurable way.
Reducing sensory stimulation	Lack of ability to integrate competing sensations	Reduce noise and light levels Rocking, walking rhythmic tapping Music with regular rhythm Swaddling

Source: From Management of Swallowing Problems by J. Arvedson, 1993, p. 345. In J. Arvedson & L. Brodsky (Eds.), *Pediatric Swallowing and Feeding: Assessment and Management.* San Diego: Singular Publishing Group. Copyright © 1993. Reprinted by permission.

feeders, but others may always rely on nonoral feeding for nutritional needs.

Nutritive Oral-Motor Stimulation

Oral feeding attempts can be considered for infants of gestational age 34 to 37 weeks, and possibly even earlier in some medically stable infants of gestational age 32–33 weeks, who are easily roused and maintain alertness for at least 10–15 minutes. Respiratory stability is a prerequisite (Mathew, 1988; Mathew, Clark, & Pronske, 1985). Adequate airway protection during swallowing should be anticipated. Rhythmic suck/swallow/respiratory sequencing should be initiated readily and maintained long enough for the infant to take a full feed within 15–20 minutes.

In order to consider oral feedings in infants on tube feedings, bolus feedings should be tolerated in contrast to slow drip feedings. The presence of gastroesophageal reflux may complicate feeding attempts in some infants who would otherwise appear ready to feed orally.

With obvious sucking and swallowing problems, liquid must be introduced cautiously. The use of different nipples and containers may aid in the determination of optimal flow rates (Mathew, Belan, & Thoppil, 1992). Incoordination problems can be exacerbated with a rate that is too fast. On the other hand, the infant may become fatigued and frustrated if the flow is too slow. Guidelines are developed for individual needs: weak and dysrhythmic suck, suck and swallow incoordination, sensory problems, resistance to feeding, appetite considerations, and GE reflux (Table 14–7).

Some children with a gastrostomy tube may become oral feeders if the health problems that led to placement of the gastrostomy tube have resolved, stabilized, or been corrected (Blackman & Nelson, 1985). A shift from tube to oral feeding needs to take into account multiple factors: age of onset of nonoral alimentation, associated positive or negative social interaction with previous oral feeding attempts, the specific medical or disabling conditions, and individual temperamental characteristics (Blackman & Nelson, 1987). Blackman and Nelson (1987) reported that a brief "forced" feeding period may shorten the overall time to attain full oral feeding in carefully selected patients. Their studies have included both inpatient and outpatient programs.

Transition Feeding

By 4 to 6 months (developmental age), children who are doing at least some oral feeding should be ready for spoon feeding, with cup drinking practice initiated about 1 month after the introduction of spoon feeding. Direct oral-motor exercises have been described (e.g., Alexander, 1987; Morris, 1989; Morris & Klein, 1987). Indirect approaches include changes in position of infants being held by feeders or of older children in seating systems, changes in the physical and sensory environment, changes in food texture and temperature, adjustments of timing intervals and/or amount of food and liquid presentation, and alteration of communication signals from feeders. Children must be monitored closely for tolerance and responsiveness to various approaches. Their overall health status must also be monitored closely.

Oral-motor programs are likely to be most successful when they are part of more global early intervention programs. Emphases include maximizing oral function, enhancing communication skills, and normalizing to whatever degree possible all aspects of development and social interactions.

Medical and Surgical Management

Some aspects of pediatric dysphagia are not amenable to oral-motor intervention strategies. Certain airway anomalies require surgical management, for example, vocal fold paralysis in some instances, laryngeal clefts (Koltai, Morgan, & Evans, 1991; Myer, Cotton, Holmes, & Jackson, 1990), subglottic stenosis (Cotton & Seid, 1980; Tunkel & Zalzal, 1992; Zalzal, 1988),

TABLE 14–7. Management of sensorimotor suck and swallow problems.

Problem Area	Management Suggestions
Weak, dysrhythmic suck	Pressure to assist lip closure Tug at nipple as though pulling it out of mouth (may smooth out and strengthen the suck) Thicken liquid (rice cereal) Adjust nipple opening
Suck and swallow incoordination	Stroking hyoid musculature toward sternum Gradual introduction of liquid (finger, pacifier, cotton swab, or cheesecloth dipped in liquid and placed in mouth) Nipple changes to get optimal flow Bypassing nippling to spoon and cup

Sensory problems
  Hyposensitivity
  Hypersensitivity
	
	Firm, but gentle, stroking around mouth and on tongue
	Deep sustained pressure in and around mouth by caregiver's or infant's hand

Resistance to feeding
  Aversive
  Lethargic
 	
  Fussy
	Position change
	Prone with head supported in extension
	More upright and away from caregiver's body with back, neck, and head support
	Swaddling and holding close to caregiver's body

Appetite	Feeding when infant is hungry Demand schedule may help With tube feedings, reduce during daytime and supplement at night for some
Gastroesophageal reflux	Thickening of liquid Head elevated prone positioning (not clearly supported) Medical or surgical treatment probable

Source: From Management of Swallowing Problems by J. Arvedson, 1993, p. 351. In J. Arvedson & L. Brodsky (Eds.), *Pediatric Swallowing and Feeding: Assessment and Management.* San Diego: Singular Publishing Group. Copyright © 1993. Reprinted by permission.

vascular rings, tracheoesophageal fistula, and head and neck masses. In cases of intractable aspiration not relieved by more conservative approaches (e.g., vigorous pulmonary toilet, mechanical ventilation if needed, antibiotics, and elimination of the predisposing factors [Brodsky & Volk, 1993]), surgical management may be needed. Table 14–8 lists surgical procedures presently in use for the pediatric population.

There are several medical and/or surgical approaches to treatment of gastroesophageal reflux (discussed in Chapter 16). Conservative treatment for infants and children includes upright positioning, thickened feedings, and small, frequent feedings. There are challenges to these recommendations. The prone upright position (30° incline) has been suggested

as the most effective (Orenstein & Whitington, 1983). However, Orenstein (1990) has suggested that position changes may not make a real difference in control of GER. Frequency of emesis has been reduced with thickened feeds (1 teaspoon cereal per 1 ounce of formula) but with no reduction in episodes of reflux (Orenstein, Magill, & Brooks, 1987). Tuchman (1994) described several medications used in some cases of severe reflux. Infants with GER usually show improvement over time.

Surgical management is usually reserved for children with severe reflux who do not respond to medical management. The procedure of choice is the fundoplication, Nissen complete wrap, or Thal partial wrap (Smith, Othersen, Gogan, & Walker, 1992; Thal, 1968; van der Zee, Rövekamp, Pull ter Gunne, & Bax, 1994). The

TABLE 14–8. Management strategies for aspiration.

Technique	Advantage	Disadvantage
Endotracheal tube placement with ventilation	Reversible	Applicable in acute aspiration only
Textured foods Avoid clear liquids	Easy	Useful in only mild cases of aspiration secondary to decreased pharyngeal/laryngeal sensation
Gastrostomy/ esophagostomy	Well-tolerated Minimal maintenance Minimal change in quality of life	Requires ability to handle secretions Deprives patient of pleasure (taste, sensation) of eating
Vocal fold medialization (gel foam or Teflon injection, thyroplasty)	Retention/improvement of voice Some procedures reversible	Requires one functioning vocal fold
Tracheotomy	Straightforward procedure Reversible	Short-term solution only Provides pulmonary toilet but does not prevent aspiration Change in lifestyle
Glottic/supraglottic closures	Relatively straightforward procedure Theoretically reversible	Requires tracheotomy Surgical failure rate high
Laryngeal diversion	Straightforward procedure Theoretically reversible Low surgical failure rate	Requires tracheotomy Prevents phonation
Laryngectomy	Absolute prevention of aspiration Low surgical failure rate	Permanent Requires tracheotomy Prevents phonation

Source: From The Airway and Swallowing by L. Brodsky & M. Volk, 1993, p. 116. In J. Arvedson & L. Brodsky (Eds.), *Pediatric Swallowing and Feeding: Assessment and Management.* San Diego: Singular Publishing Group. Copyright © 1993. Reprinted by permission.

fundus of the stomach is wrapped around the distal esophagus. The fundoplication may be done with a gastrostomy tube in some children with neurologic impairment, inadequate nutritional support, and severe pharyngeal-phase swallowing deficit. Whenever a gastrostomy is considered in a child with neurologic deficits, the necessity for antireflux procedures must be questioned (e.g., Langer et al., 1988; Wheatley et al., 1991). The percutaneous approach to gastrostomy offers an attractive alternative to the open intra-abdominal technique (Kirby, Craig, Tsang, & Plotnick, 1986; Ponsky, Gauderer, Stellato, & Aszodi, 1985; Rossi, 1993). Potential postoperative complications and their management are described in other sources (e.g., Chapter 16; Low, 1994; Rossi, 1993; Tuchman, 1994).

Nutrition deficiencies may be reversed with addition of nonoral feeding, even with short-term nasogastric tube feedings (Patrick, Boland, Stoski, & Murray, 1986), as well as for longer term gastrostomy tube feedings and antireflux procedures (Rice, Seashore, & Touloukian, 1991). The same considerations in infant formula selection are made for oral and tube feedings. Because nutrient needs change throughout the first year of life, infant formulas become inadequate by 12 months of age. A commercial formula (Pediasure, Ross Laboratories, Columbus, OH) has been developed to meet the specific nutrient needs for young children 1 to 10 years of age. Unless there are needs for specialized formula because of underlying conditions, such as malabsorption, Pediasure is a satisfactory tube feeding for most children. Formulas may need to be altered by dilution and/or the addition of supplemental micronutrients (protein, vitamins, and minerals) to meet fluid and nutrient needs without excessive calories (Young, 1993). Energy needs may need to be calculated for different groups of children, for example, those with cerebral palsy (Krick, Murphy, Markham, & Shapiro, 1992).

Behavioral Feeding Problems

Management of children with predominantly, or totally, behavior-based feeding problems is usually accomplished by a combination of procedures. Babbitt and colleagues (1994) describe the use of positive (e.g., Bernal, 1972; Singer, Nofer, Benson-Szekeley, & Brooks, 1991) and negative reinforcement (e.g., Iwata, Riordan, Wohl, & Finney, 1982; Ylvisaker & Weinstein, 1989) for treatment of food refusal, extinction procedures or differential reinforcement of other behavior (e.g., Iwata et al., 1982), punishment (e.g., Blackman & Nelson, 1987; Clauser & Scibak, 1990; Starin & Fuqua, 1987), and antecedent manipulation for motivational problems (e.g., Finney, 1986; Luiselli & Gleason, 1987). Skill acquisition procedures can be used to teach new or more complex behaviors to children. The importance of parent/caregiver training cannot be underestimated. This training is necessary in order to obtain the ultimate goal of generalization and performance in the daily routines.

The interrelationships of physiologically based feeding/swallowing deficits and the behavior responses (or lack of responses) are complex. Obviously the whole child approach by an interdisciplinary team attempts to integrate all aspects of the child and the environment.

RESEARCH NEEDS

Data from adult studies cannot be extrapolated and applied directly to children with dysphagia. The normal swallow process in infants and young children needs to be defined more precisely for timing of movement through the oral, pharyngeal, and esophageal phases of the swallow. Anatomical differences between infants/young children and adults must be considered as landmarks, for events in the dynamic process of swallowing are likely to be different. Increased knowledge of the abnormal swallow will be enhanced by greater precision in measures of normal swallowing. The role of respiratory control in the development of efficient suckle feeding needs further study (Bamford, Taciak, & Gewolb, 1992). This area will continue to be of significant interest.

Tools for assessment are needed so professionals in varied settings can make observations that can be interpreted with validity and reliability by other professionals in quantifiable ways. Such tools should also be useful for measuring change over time. At present, there is a dearth of information regarding efficiency and efficacy of treatment approaches.

SUMMARY

Swallowing and feeding disorders in infants and children are most frequently part of a larger complex of neurologic, airway/pulmonary, gastrointestinal, oral-motor, and behavioral deficits. These combinations of deficits can vary significantly from one individual to the next. The deficits can also vary over time within the same individual. Because growth and maturation must be considered in assessment and management of infants and children, the issues in planning strategies for treatment and also in monitoring changes over time are different from those with adults. Thus, specialized knowledge and training are needed by professionals as they work closely in an interdisciplinary focus that includes the caregivers in all aspects of assessment and management.

MULTIPLE CHOICE QUESTIONS

1. Characteristics of newborn term infants include all except

a. the larynx is high in the neck
b. respiration is not interrupted during swallow
c. the tongue moves only in the antero-posterior direction
d. the soft palate and epiglottis are in close proximity
e. the pharyngeal airway lacks rigidity

2. Transition feeding becomes possible at about age 4–6 months primarily because of
a. anatomical growth
b. changes in relationship of anatomical structures
c. central nervous system development
d. reaching for objects beginning to occur
e. eruption of teeth

3. Behavioral feeding issues
a. usually occur apart from physiologic problems
b. should always be approached through intensive inpatient programs
c. always respond to "forced" feeding short-term programs
d. are likely to be just one part of health and developmental complexities
e. can be dealt with prior to making major nutritional decisions

4. Children with spastic quadriplegic cerebral palsy typically present with all except
a. incoordination of swallowing and respiration
b. oral-motor incoordination with oral phase swallow dysfunction
c. silent aspiration on oropharyngeal swallow study
d. nutrition problems characterized by excessive fat
e. need of specialized positioning and seating arrangements

5. Infants with bilateral choanal atresia
a. feed well at birth, then develop difficulty after several days
b. usually have no feeding difficulties as they adapt to altered anatomy
c. are likely to require a glossopexy

d. seldom have other congenital anomalies
e. are likely to have significant oral-motor incoordination in suck/swallow/respiratory coordination

6. Children who regress with oral feeding over time are most likely to have a diagnosis of
a. tracheoesophageal fistula
b. Pierre-Robin sequence
c. esophageal atresia
d. cerebral palsy
e. Prader-Willie syndrome

REFERENCES

Alexander, R. (1987). Oral-motor treatment for infants and young children with cerebral palsy. *Seminars in Speech and Language, 8*, 87–100.

Antanitus, D. (1989). Primary care physician. In I. L. Rubin & A. C. Crocer (Eds.), *Developmental disabilities: Delivery of medical care for chidren and adults* (pp. 437–438). Philadelphia: Lea and Febiger.

Ardran, G. M., Kemp, F. H., & Lind, J. (1958). A cineradiographic study of bottle feeding. *British Journal of Radiology, 31*, 11–22.

Arvedson, J. (1993). Management of swallowing problems. In J. C. Arvedson & L. Brodsky (Eds.), *Pediatric swallowing and feeding: Assessment and management* (pp. 327–387). San Diego: Singular Publishing Group.

Arvedson, J., & Brodsky, L. (1992). Pediatric tracheotomy referrals to speech-language pathology in a children's hospital. *International Journal of Pediatric Otorhinolaryngology, 23*, 237–243.

Arvedson, J., & Brodsky, L. (Eds.). (1993). *Pediatric swallowing and feeding: Assessment and management*. San Diego: Singular Publishing Group.

Arvedson, J., & Christensen, S. (1993). Instrumental evaluation. In J. C. Arvedson & L. Brodsky (Eds.), *Pediatric swallowing and feeding: Assessment and management* (pp. 293–326). San Diego: Singular Publishing Group.

Arvedson, J., & Rogers, B. (1993). Pediatric swallowing and feeding disorders. *Journal of Medical Speech-Language Pathology, 1*(4), 203–221.

Arvedson, J., Rogers, B., & Brodsky, L. (1993). Anatomy, embryology, and physiology. In J. C. Arvedson & L. Brodsky (Eds.), *Pediatric swallowing and feeding: Assessment and management* (pp. 5–51). San Diego: Singular Publishing Group.

Arvedson, J., Rogers, B., Buck, G., Smart, P., & Msall, M. (1994). Silent aspiration prominent in children with dysphagia. *International Journal of Pediatric Otorhinolaryngology, 28,* 173–181.

Babbitt, R., Hoch, T. A., & Coe, D. A. (1994). Behavioral feeding disorders. In D. N. Tuchman & R. S. Walter (Eds.), *Disorders of feeding and swallowing in infants and children: Pathophysiology, diagnosis, and treatment* (pp. 77–95). San Diego: Singular Publishing Group.

Babson, S. G., Pernoll, M. L., & Benda, G. I. (1980). Nutritional requirements and oral feeding of the low birth weight infant. In S. F. Babson, M. L. Pernoll, & G. E. Bends (Eds.), *Diagnosis and management of the fetus and neonate at risk.* St. Louis: C.V. Mosby.

Bagwell, C. E. (1995). Gastroesophageal reflux in children. [Review]. *Surgery Annual, 27,* 133–163.

Bamford, O., Taciak, V., & Gewolb, I. H. (1992). The relationship between rhythmic swallowing and breathing during suckle feeding in term neonates. *Pediatric Research, 31*(6), 619–624.

Bauer, M. L., Figueroa-Colon, R., Georgeson, K., & Young, D. W. (1993). Chronic pulmonary aspiration in children. *Southern Medical Journal, 86*(7), 789–795.

Bayley, N. (1993). *Bayley scales of infant development.* (2nd ed.). San Antonio, TX: Psychological Corporation—Harcourt-Brace Company.

Benson, J. E., & Lefton-Greif, M. A. (1994). Videofluoroscopy of swallowing in pediatric patients: A component of the total feeding evaluation. In D. N. Tuchman & R. S. Walter (Eds.), *Disorders of feeding and swallowing in infants and children: Pathophysiology, diagnosis, and treatment* (pp. 187–200). San Diego: Singular Publishing Group.

Bernal, M. E. (1972). Behavioral treatment of a child's eating problem. *Journal of Behavior Therapy and Experimental Psychiatry, 3,* 43–50.

Bernbaum, J. C., Pereira, G. R., Watkins, J. B., & Peckham, G. J. (1983). Nonnutritive sucking during gavage feeding enhances growth and maturation in premature infants. *Pediatrics, 71*(1), 41–45.

Bier, J., Ferguson, A., Cho, C., Oh, W., & Vohr, B. R. (1993). The oral motor development of low-birth-weight infants who underwent orotracheal intubation during the neonatal period. *American Journal of Diseases of Children, 147,* 858–862.

Blackman, J. A., & Nelson, C. L. A. (1985). Reinstituting oral feedings in children fed by gastrostomy tube. *Clinical Pediatrics, 24*(8), 434–438.

Blackman, J. A., & Nelson, C. L. A. (1987). Rapid introduction of oral feedings to tube-fed patients. *Journal of Developmental and Behavioral Pediatrics, 8*(2), 63–67.

Bosma, J. F. (1986). Development of feeding. *Clinical Nutrition, 5,* 210–218.

Bosma, J. F. (1992). Pharyngeal swallow: Basic mechanisms, development, and impairments.

Advances in Otolaryngology—Head and Neck Surgery, 6, 225–275.

Bosma, J. F., Hepburn, L. G., Josell, S. D., & Baker, K. (1990). Ultrasound demonstration of tongue motions during suckle feeding. *Developmental Medicine and Child Neurology, 32,* 223–229.

Boyle, J. T. (1989). Gastroesophageal reflux in the pediatric patient. *Gastroenterology Clinics of North America, 18,* 315–337.

Brake, S. C., Fifer, W. P., Alfase, G., & Fleischman, A. (1988). The first nutritive sucking responses of premature newborns. *Infant Behavior and Development, 11,* 1–19.

Braun, M. A., & Palmer, M. M. (1986). A pilot study of oral-motor dysfunction in "at-risk" infants. *Physical and Occupational Therapy in Pediatrics, 5*(4), 13–25.

Brodsky, L. (1993). Drooling in children. In J. C. Arvedson & L. Brodsky (Eds.), *Pediatric swallowing and feeding: Assessment and management* (pp. 389–416). San Diego: Singular Publishing Group.

Brodsky, L., & Volk, M. (1993). The airway and swallowing. In J. C. Arvedson & L. Brodsky (Eds.), *Pediatric swallowing and feeding: Assessment and management* (pp. 93–122). San Diego: Singular Publishing Group.

Brody, A., Kuhn, J., Seidel, F. G., & Brodsky, L. (1991). Ultrafast CT evaluation of the airway in children. *Pediatric Radiology, 178,* 181–184.

Brouillette, R. T., & Thach, B. T. (1979). A neuromuscular mechanism maintaining extra-thoracic airway patency. *Journal of Applied Physiology, 46,* 772–779.

Bu'Lock, F., Woolridge, M. W., & Baum, J. D. (1990). Development of coordination of sucking, swallowing and breathing: Ultrasound study of term and preterm infants. *Developmental Medicine and Child Neurology, 32,* 669–678.

Byrne, W. J., Campbell, M., Ascraft, E., Seibert, J. J., & Euler, A. R. (1983). A diagnostic approach to vomiting in severely retarded patients. *American Journal of Diseases of Children, 137,* 259–262.

Capute, A. J., Palmer, F. B., Shapiro, B. K., Wachtel, R. C., Schmidt, S., & Ross, A. (1986). A clinical linguistic and auditory milestone scale: Prediction of cognition in infancy. *Developmental Medicine and Child Neurology, 28,* 762–771.

Capute, A. J., & Shapiro, B. K. (1985). The motor quotient: A method for the early detection of motor delay. *American Journal of Diseases of Childhood, 139,* 940–942.

Case-Smith, J. (1988). An efficacy study of occupational therapy with high-risk neonates. *The American Journal of Occupational Therapy, 42,* 499–506.

Case-Smith, J., Cooper, P., & Scala, V. (1989). Feeding efficiency of premature neonates. *The*

American Journal of Occupational Therapy, 43, 245–250.

Cattell, P. (1940). *The measurement of intelligence of infants and young children.* New York: Johnson Reprint Corporation.

Chatoor, I., Dickson, L., Schaefer, S., & Egan, J. (1986). A developmental classification of feeding disorders associated with failure to thrive: Diagnosis and treatment. In D. Drotar (Ed.), *New directions in failure to thrive: Implications for research and practice.* New York: Plenum Press.

Chatoor, I., Menvielle, E., Getson, P., & O'Donnell, R. (1989). *Observational scale for mother-infant interaction during feeding.* Washington, DC: Children's Hospital Medical Center.

Cherney, L. R. (Ed.). (1994). *Clinical management of dysphagia in adults and children* (2nd ed.). Gaithersburg, MD: Aspen.

Clauser, B., & Scibak, J. W. (1990). Direct and generalized effects of food satiation in reducing rumination. *Research in Developmental Disabilities, 11*(1), 23–26.

Cotton, R. T., & Seid, A. B. (1980). Management of the extubation problem in the premature child: Anterior cricoid split as an alternative to tracheotomy. *Annals of Otology, Rhinology, and Laryngology, 89,* 508–511.

Crelin, E. S. (1976). Development of the upper respiratory system. *Ciba Clinical Symposium, 28*(3), 3–26.

Curtis, D. J., Cruess, D. F., Dachman, A. H., & Maso, E. (1984). Timing in the normal pharyngeal swallow. Prospective selection and evaluation of 16 normal asymptomatic patients. *Investigative Radiology, 6,* 523–529.

Davis, C. M. (1939). Results of the self-selection of diets by young children. *Canadian Medical Association Journal, 41,* 257–261.

DiPietro, J. A., Cusson, R. M., Caughy, M. A., & Fox, N. A. (1994). Behavioral and physiologic effects of nonnutritive sucking during gavage feeding in preterm infants. *Pediatric Research, 36,* 207–214.

Durand, M., Leahy, F. N., Maccallum, M., Cates, D. B., Rigato, H., & Chermick, V. (1981). Effect of feeding on the chemical control of breathing in the newborn infant. *Pediatric Research, 15,* 1509–1512.

Field, T., & Goldson, E. (1984). Pacifying effects of nonnutritive sucking on term and preterm neonates during heelsticks. *Pediatrics, 74,* 1012–1015.

Field, T., Ignatoff, E., Stringer, S., Brennan, J., Greenberg, R., Widmayer, S., & Anderson, G. C. (1982). Nonnutritive sucking during tube feedings: Effects on preterm neonates in an intensive care unit. *Pediatrics, 70,* 381–384.

Finney, J. W. (1986). Preventing common feeding problems in infants and young children. *Pediatric Clinics of North America, 33,* 775–788.

Garg, M., Kurzner, S. I., Bautista, D. B., & Keens, T. G. (1988). Clinically unsuspected hypoxia during sleep and feeding in infants with bronchopulmonary dysplasia. *Pediatrics, 81*(5), 635–642.

Gisel, E. G. (1991). Effect of food texture on the development of chewing of children between six months and two years of age. *Developmental Medicine and Child Neurology, 33,* 69–79.

Gisel, E. G., Lange, L. J., & Niman, C. W. (1984). Chewing cycles in 4- and 5-year old Down's syndrome children: A comparison of eating efficacy with normals. *American Journal of Occupational Therapy, 38,* 666–670.

Gisel, E. G., & Patrick, J. (1988). Identification of children with cerebral palsy unable to maintain a normal nutritional stage. *Lancet, 1,* 283–286.

Goldson, E. (1987). Suck and swallow in the premature infant. *Pediatrics, 43,* 96–102.

Guilleminault, C., & Coons, S. (1984). Apnea and bradycardia during feeding in infants weighing >2000 gm. *The Journal of Pediatrics, 104,* 932–935.

Harris, J. P. (1983). Heart failure. In M. Ziai (Ed.), *Bedside pediatrics: Diagnostic evluation of the child* (pp. 313–319). Boston: Little, Brown.

Herman, M. J. (1991). Comprehensive assessment of oral-motor dysfunction in failure-to-thrive infants. *Infant-Toddler Intervention, 1*(2), 109–123.

Huber, C. J. (1991). Documenting quality of parent-child interaction: Use of the NCAST scales. *Infants and Young Children, 4*(2), 63–75.

Humphrey T. (1967). Reflex activity in the oral and facial area of the human fetus. In J. F. Bosma (Ed.), *Second symposium on oral sensation and perception* (pp. 195–233). Springfield, IL: Charles C. Thomas.

Hyman, P. E. (1994). Gastroesophageal reflux: One reason why baby won't eat. *The Journal of Pediatrics, 125,* S103–S109.

Illingworth, R. S., & Lister, J. (1964). The critical or sensitive period, with special reference to certain feeding problems in infants and children. *The Journal of Pediatrics, 65,* 840–848.

Iwata, B. A., Riordan, M. M., Wohl, M. K., & Finney, J. W. (1982). Pediatric feeding disorders: Behavioral analysis and treatment. In P. J. Accardo (Ed.), *Failure to thrive in infancy and early childhood* (pp. 297–329). Baltimore: University Park Press.

Jelm, J. M. (1990). *Oral-motor/feeding rating scale.* Tucson, AZ: Therapy Skill Builders.

Kenny, D., Koheil, R., Greenberg, J., Reid, D., Milner, M., Roman, R., & Judd, P. (1989). Development of a multidisciplinary feeding profile for children who are dependent feeders. *Dysphagia, 4,* 16–28.

Kirby, D. F., Craig, R. M., Tsang, T. K., & Plotnick, B. H. (1986). Percutaneous endoscopic gastrostomies: A prospective evaluation and review of the literature. *Journal of Parenteral & Enteral Nutrition, 10,* 155–159.

Koenig, J., Davies, A. M., & Thach, B. T. (1990). Coordination of breathing, sucking and swallowing during bottle feedings in infants. *Journal of Applied Physiology, 69,* 1623–1629.

Koltai, P. J., Morgan, D., & Evans, J. N. G. (1991). Endoscopic repair of supraglottic laryngeal clefts. *Archives of Otolaryngology—Head and Neck Surgery, 117,* 273–278.

Krick, J., Murphy, P. E., Markham, J. F., & Shapiro, B. K. (1992). A proposed formula for calculating energy needs of children with cerebral palsy. *Developmental Medicine and Child Neurology, 34,* 481–487.

Laitman, J. T., & Crelin, E. S. (1980). Developmental change in the upper respiratory system of human infants. *Perinatology & Neonatology, 4,* 15–22.

Laitman, J. T., & Reidenberg, J. S. (1993). Specializations of the human upper respiratory and upper digestive systems as seen through comparative and developmental anatomy. *Dysphagia, 8,* 318–325.

Langer, J. C., Wesson, D. A., Ein, S. H., Filler, R. M., Shandling, B., Superina, R. A., & Papa, M. (1988). Feeding gastrostomy in neurologically impaired children: Is an antireflux procedure necessary? *Journal of Pediatric Gastroenterology and Nutrition, 7,* 837–841.

Langmore, S. E., & Logemann, J. A. (1991, September). After the clinical bedside swallowing examination: What next? *American Journal of Speech-Language Pathology,* 13–19.

Langmore, S. E., Schatz, K., & Olsen, N. (1988). Fiberoptic endoscopic examination of swallowing safety: A new procedure. *Dysphagia, 2,* 216–219.

Logemann, J. A. (1983). *Evaluation and treatment of swallowing disorders.* Austin, TX: Pro-Ed.

Logemann, J. A. (1993). *Manual for the videofluorographic study of swallowing.* (2nd ed.). Austin, TX: Pro-Ed.

Loughlin, G. M. (1989). Respiratory consequences of dysfunctional swallowing and aspiration. *Dysphagia, 3,* 126–130.

Loughlin, G. M., & Lefton-Greif, M. A. (1994). Dysfunctional swallowing and respiratory disease in children. *Advances in Pediatrics, 41,* 135–162.

Low, D. E. (1994). Management of the problem patient after antireflux surgery. *Gastroenterology Clinics of North America, 23,* 371–389.

Luiselli, J. K., & Gleason, D. J. (1987). Combining sensory reinforcement and texture-fading procedures to overcome chronic food refusal. *Journal of Behavior Therapy and Experimental Psychiatry, 18,* 149–155.

Mathew, O. P. (1988). Respiratory control during nipple feeding in preterm infants. *Pediatric Pulmonology, 5,* 220–224.

Mathew, O. P. (1991). Science of bottle feeding. *The Journal of Pediatrics, 119*(4), 511–519.

Mathew, O. P., Belan, M., & Thoppil, C. K. (1992). Sucking patterns of neonates during bottle feeding: Comparison of different nipple units. *American Journal of Perinatology, 9*(4), 265–269.

Mathew, O. P., Clark, M. L., & Pronske, M. H. (1985). Breathing pattern of neonates during nonnutritive sucking. *Pediatric Pulmonology, 1,* 204–206.

Mathew, O. P., Clark, M. L., Pronske, M. L., Luna-Solarzano, H. G., & Peterson, M. D. (1985). Breathing pattern and ventilation during oral feeding in term newborn infants. *Journal of Pediatrics, 106,* 810–813.

Measel, C. P., & Anderson, G. C. (1979). Nonnutritive sucking during tube feedings: Effect on clinical course in premature infants. *Journal of Obstetric, Gynecologic and Neonatal Nursing, 8,* 265–272.

Miller, H. D., & Anderson, G. C. (1993). Nonnutritive sucking: Effects on crying and heart rate in intubated infants requiring assisted mechanical ventilation. *Nursing Research, 42,* 305–307.

Mollitt, D. L., Golladay, E. S., & Seibert, J. J. (1985). Symptomatic gastroesophageal reflux following gastrostomy in neurologically impaired patients. *Pediatrics, 75,* 1124–1126.

Moore, K. L. (1988). *The developing human: Clinically oriented embryology.* (4th ed.). Philadelphia: W. B. Saunders.

Morris, S. E. (1989). Development of oral-motor skills in the neurologically impaired child receiving nonoral feedings. *Dysphagia, 3,* 135–154.

Morris, S. E., & Klein, M. D. (1987). *Pre-feeding skills: A comprehensive resource for feeding development.* Tucson, AZ: Therapy Skill Builders.

Morton, R. E., Bonas, R., Fourie, B., & Minford, J. (1993). Videofluoroscopy in the assessment of children with neurological problems. *Developmental Medicine and Child Neurology, 35,* 388–395.

Moss, H. B., & Green, A. (1982). Neuroleptic associated dysphagia confirmed by esophageal manometry. *American Journal of Psychiatry, 139,* 515–516.

Myer, C. M., Cotton, R. T., Holmes, D. K., & Jackson, R. K. (1990). Laryngeal and laryngotracheoesophageal clefts: Role of early surgical repair. *Annals of Otology, Rhinology, and Laryngology, 99,* 98–104.

Nielson, D. W., Heldt, G. P., & Tooley, W. H. (1990). Stridor and gastroesophageal reflux in infants. *Pediatrics, 85,* 1034–1039.

Orenstein, S. R. (1990). Prone positioning in infant gastroesophageal reflux: Is elevation of the head worth the trouble? *Journal of Pediatrics, 117,* 184–187.

Orenstein, S. R., Magill, H. L., & Brooks, P. (1987). Thickening of infant feedings for therapy of gastroesophageal reflux. *Journal of Pediatrics, 110,* 181–186.

Orenstein, S. R., & Whitington, P. F. (1983). Positioning for prevention of infant gastroesophageal reflux. *Journal of Pediatrics, 103*, 534–537.

Paludetto, R., Robertson, S. S., Hack, M., Shivpuri, C. R., & Martin, R. J. (1984). Transcutaneous oxygen tension during nonnutritive sucking in preterm infants. *Pediatrics, 74*, 539–542.

Patrick, J., Boland, M., Stoski, D., & Murray, G. E. (1986). Rapid correction of wasting in children with cerebral palsy. *Developmental Medicine and Child Neurology, 28*, 734–739.

Ponsky, J. L., Gauderer, M. L., Stellato, T. A., & Aszodi, A. (1985). Percutaneous approaches to enteral alimentation. *American Journal of Surgery, 149*, 102–105.

Reed, R., Roberts, J. L., & Thach, B. T. (1985). Factors influencing regional patency and configuration of the upper airway in human infants. *Journal of Applied Physiology, 58*, 635–644.

Rice, H., Seashore, J. H., & Touloukian, R. J. (1991). Evaluation of Nissen fundoplication in neurologically impaired children. *Journal of Pediatric Surgery, 26*(6), 697–701.

Rogers, B., Arvedson, J., Buck, G., Smart, P., & Msall, M. (1994). Characteristics of dysphagia in children with cerebral palsy. *Dysphagia, 9*, 69–73.

Rogers, B., Arvedson, J., Msall, M., & Demereth, R. (1993). Hypoxemia during oral feeding of children with severe cerebral palsy. *Developmental Medicine and Child Neurology, 35*, 3–10.

Rogers, B., & Campbell, J. (1993). Pediatric neurodevelopmental evaluation. In J. C. Arvedson & L. Brodsky (Eds.), *Pediatric swallowing and feeding: Assessment and management* (pp. 53–92). San Diego: Singular Publishing Group.

Rossi, T. (1993). Pediatric gastroenterology. In J. C. Arvedson & L. Brodsky (Eds.), *Pediatric swallowing and feeding: Assessment and management* (pp. 123–156). San Diego: Singular Publishing Group.

Satter, E. M. (1990). The feeding relationship: Problems and interventions. *Journal of Pediatrics, 117*(2/2), 181–189.

Satter, E. M. (1992). The feeding relationship. *Zero to Three, 12*(5), 1–9.

Shaker, C. (1990). Nipple feeding premature infants: A different perspective. *Neonatal Network, 8*, 9–17.

Shivpuri, C. R., Martin, R. J., Carlo, W. A., & Fanarof, A. A. (1983). Decreased ventilation in preterm infants during oral feeding. *Journal of Pediatrics, 103*, 285–289.

Simon, B. M., & McGowan, J. S. (1989). Tracheostomy in young children: Implications for assessment and treatment of communication and feeding disorders. *Infants and Young Children, 1*(3), 1–9.

Singer, L. T., Nofer, J. A., Benson-Szekeley, L. J., & Brooks, L. J. (1991). Behavioral assessment and management of food refusal in children with cystic fibrosis. *Developmental and Behavioral Pediatrics, 12*, 115–120.

Smith, C. D., Othersen, H. B., Jr., Gogan, N. J., & Walker, J. D. (1992). Nissen fundoplication in children with profound neurologic disability. High risks and unmet goals. *Annals of Surgery, 215*(6), 654–658.

Sondheimer, J. M. 1994). Gastroesophageal reflux in children. Clinical presentation and diagnostic evaluation. [Review]. *Gastrointestinal Endoscopy Clinics of North America, 4*, 55–74.

Sondheimer, J. M., & Morris, B. A. (1979). Gastroesophageal reflux among severely retarded children. *The Journal of Pediatrics, 94*, 710–714.

Sonies, B. (1987). Ultrasound imaging of the oral area: Clinical application and implications for rehabilitation. *Rehabilitation Report, 3*(10), 1–3.

Stallings, V. A., Charney, E. G., Davies, J. C., & Cronk, C. C. (1993). Nutritional related growth failure of children with quadriplegic cerebral palsy. *Developmental Medicine and Child Neurology, 35*, 126–138.

Starin, S. P., & Fuqua, R. W. (1987). Rumination and vomiting in the developmentally disabled: A critical review of the behavioral, medical, and psychiatric treatment research. *Research in Developmental Disabilities, 8*, 575–604.

Stark, A. R., & Thach, B. T. (1976). Mechanisms of airway obstruction leading to apnea in newborn infants. *Journal of Pediatrics, 89*, 982–985.

Stratton, M. (1981). Behavioral assessment scale of oral functions in feeding. *The American Journal of Occupational Therapy, 35*, 719–721.

Thach, B. T. (1992). Neuromuscular control of upper airway patency. *Clinics in Perinatology, 19*(4), 773–788.

Thal, A. P. (1968). A unified approach to surgical problems of the esophagogastric junction. *Annals of Surgery, 168*, 542–550.

Treloar, D. M. (1994). The effect of nonnutritive sucking on oxygenation in healthy, crying fullterm infants. *Applied Nursing Research, 7*, 52–58.

Tuchman, D. N. (1994). Gastroesophageal reflux. In D. N. Tuchman & R. S. Walter (Eds.), *Disorders of feeding and swallowing in infants and children: Pathophysiology, diagnosis, and treatment* (pp. 243–245). San Diego: Singular Publishing Group.

Tuchman, D. N., & Walter, R. S. (Eds.). (1994). *Disorders of feeding and swallowing in infants and children: Pathophysiology, diagnosis, and treatment.* San Diego: Singular Publishing Group.

Tunkel, D. E., & Zalzal, G. H. (1992). Stridor in infants and children: Ambulatory evaluation and operative diagnosis. *Clinical Pediatrics, 31*, 48–55.

van der Zee, D. C., Rövekamp, M. H., Pull ter Gunne, A. J., & Bax, N. M. A. (1994). Surgical treatment of reflux esophagitis: Nissen versus

Thal procedure. *Pediatric Surgery International, 9,* 334–337.

Vitti, M., & Basmajian, J. V. (1975). Muscles of mastication in small children: An electromyographic analysis. *American Journal of Orthodontics, 68,* 412–419.

Walker, W. A., & Hendricks, K. M. (1985). *Manual of pediatric nutrition* (p. 60). Philadelphia: W. B. Saunders.

Warner, J. (1981). *Helping the handicapped child with early feeding.* Winslow England: Winslow Press.

Weber, F., Woolridge, M. W., & Baum, J. D. (1986). An ultrasonographic study of the organization of sucking and swallowing by newborn infants. *Developmental Medicine and Child Neurology, 28,* 19–24.

Wheatley, M. J., Wesley, J. R., Tkach, D. M., & Coran, A. G. (1991). Long-term follow-up of brain-damaged children requiring feeding gastrostomy: Should an anti-reflux procedure always be performed? *Journal of Pediatric Surgery, 26,* 301–305.

Wilson, S. L, Thach, B. T., Brouillette, R. T., & Abu-Osba, Y. K. (1981). Coordination of breathing and swallowing in human infants. *Journal of Applied Physiology, 50,* 851–858.

Wolff, P. H. (1968). The serial organization of sucking in the young infant. *Pediatrics, 42,* 943–956.

Wyllie, E., Wyllie, R., Cruse, R. P., Rothner, A. D., & Erenberg, G. (1986). The mechanism of nitrazepam induced drooling and aspiration. *The New England Journal of Medicine, 314,* 35–38.

Wyllie, E., Wyllie, R., Rothnew, D., & Morris, H. H. (1989). Diffuse esophageal spasm: A cause of paroxysmal posturing and irritability in infants and mentally retarded children. *The Journal of Pediatrics, 115,* 261–263.

Ylvisaker, M., & Weinstein, M. (1989). Recovery of oral feeding after pediatric head injury. *Journal of Head Trauma Rehabilitation, 4,* 51–63.

Young, C. (1993). Nutrition. In J. C. Arvedson & L. Brodsky (Eds.), *Pediatric swallowing and feeding: Assessment and management* (pp. 157–208). San Diego: Singular Publishing Group.

Zalzal, G. H. (1988). Rib cartilage grafts for the treatment of posterior glottic and subglottic stenosis in children. *Annals of Otology, Rhinology, and Laryngology, 97,* 506–511.

15

Therapy for Oropharyngeal Swallowing Disorders

Jeri A. Logemann

Therapy for oropharyngeal dysphagia begins with the definition of the anatomy of the oropharyngeal region and the physiology of the patient's swallow. This usually involves a radiographic study of the oropharyngeal region during swallows of carefully defined bolus types (representing different viscosities and volumes, Logemann; 1993b). The clinician should differentiate radiographic symptoms from disorders. Radiographic symptoms of oropharyngeal dysphagia include residue (food remaining in the mouth, valleculae, pyriform sinuses, or on the pharyngeal walls), penetration (food or liquid entering the airway entrance), and aspiration (food or liquid entering the airway to the level of the trachea). Radiographic symptoms point toward specific swallowing disorders (Logemann, 1993b), for example, residue in the valleculae indicates reduced tongue-base movement or reduced pharyngeal wall contraction. The distinction between symptoms and disorders is critical in therapy planning. Swallowing therapy is always directed at physiologic or anatomic disorders. Symptomatic therapy would lead to such management procedures as tracheostomy or nonoral feeding for aspiration rather than swallowing therapy to normalize the patient's swallowing function and eliminate aspiration.

After defining the patient's anatomic or physiologic swallowing problems, the diagnostic radiographic study should introduce selected treatment strategies to improve the swallow, that is, to eliminate aspiration (the entry of food or liquid into the trachea below the vocal folds) or inefficient swallowing (residue remaining in the mouth or pharynx after the swallow). These treatment strategies are selected on the basis of the patient's anatomic or physiologic swallow impairments. The treatment strategies selected will also depend on the patient's medical diagnosis, including the patient's general physical condition, mental status, cognitive ability, and speech/language ability. Thus, treatment planning begins during the diagnostic procedure (Logemann, 1993a, 1993b). The report of the radiographic study should clearly identify the symptoms of the patient's swallowing disorder, the physiologic disorder, the effects of the trial therapy, and the therapy recommended.

449

COMPENSATORY TREATMENT PROCEDURES

Compensatory treatment procedures are usually introduced first during the diagnostic procedure. Compensatory treatment procedures are those that redirect or improve the flow of food and eliminate the patient's symptoms, such as aspiration, but do not necessarily change the physiology of the patient's swallow. Compensatory procedures are largely under the control of the caregiver/clinician and can, therefore, be used with patients of all ages and cognitive levels. Compensatory strategies include

1. postural changes which potentially change the dimensions of the pharynx and the direction of food flow without increasing the patient's work or effort during the swallow,
2. increasing sensory input prior to or during the swallow,
3. modifying volume and speed of food presentation,
4. changing food consistency/viscosity, and
5. introducing intraoral prosthetics.

Some of these compensatory procedures may also serve a therapy role, such as increasing sensory input.

Postural Techniques

Changing the patient's head or body posture has been reported to be effective in eliminating aspiration in 75 to 80% of dysphagic patients, including infants and children and some patients with cognitive or language impairments (Horner, Massey, Riski, Lathrop, & Chase, 1988; Logemann, 1989a, 1989b; Logemann, 1993a; Logemann, Kahrilas, Kobara, & Vakil, 1989b; Logemann, Rademaker, Pauloski, & Kahrilas, 1994; Rasley et al., 1993; Shanahan, Loge-mann, Rademaker, Pauloski, & Kahrilas, 1993; Welch, Logemann, Rademaker, & Kahrilas, 1993). However, some patients were found to be unable to use postural strategies because of cognitive disorders,

head stabilization devices, or other physical constraints.

Postural techniques redirect food flow and change pharyngeal dimensions in systematic ways. Table 15–1 presents the postures currently utilized therapeutically and their effects on specific swallowing disorders and pharyngeal dimensions. In general, postural techniques work equally well with neurologically impaired individuals and in patients who have experienced head and neck cancer resections or other structural damage, and in patients of all ages (Logemann et al., 1994; Rasley et al., 1993).

During the diagnostic radiographic procedure, the clinician should not introduce all of the postures to assess their individual effects. Rather, the clinician must select one or two postural techniques to fit the patient's physiologic or anatomic swallowing disorders identified in the earlier portion of the radiographic study (Logemann, 1993b). Then, the patient is asked to use the postural technique during swallows of the same type as those that previously exhibited aspiration or left significant residue. If the posture is effective on those swallows, increased volumes and viscosities can be introduced to define the extent of the posture's effectiveness. In this way, the effectiveness of the posture in eliminating the aspiration or reducing the residue can be defined (Logemann, 1993b).

The best measure of postural effectiveness is the judgment of the amount of aspiration with and without the posture (Horner et al., 1988; Logemann et al., 1994; Rasley et al., 1993). Postures may also improve oral and pharyngeal transit times and bolus clearance, that is, reducing residue (Logemann et al., 1989). In general, postural effects can best be observed and measured from videofluoroscopy (Shanahan et al., 1993; Welch et al., 1993). Postural effects on residue and aspiration can be observed from a videoendoscopic view of the pharynx before or after the swallow, but not during the swallow.

Postural techniques are usually used temporarily until the patient's swallow recovers or direct therapy procedures to im-

TABLE 15–1. Postural Techniques to Eliminate Aspiration or Residue.

Disorder Observed on Fluoroscopy	Posture Applied	Rationale
Inefficient oral transit (Reduced posterior propulsion of bolus by tongue)	Head back	Uses gravity to clear oral cavity
Delay in triggering the pharyngeal swallow (bolus past ramus of mandible but pharyngeal swallow is not triggered)	Chin down	Widens valleculae to prevent bolus entering airway; narrows airway entrance, reducing risk of aspiration
Reduced posterior motion of tongue-base (Residue in valleculae)	Chin down	Pushes tongue-base backward toward pharyngeal wall
Unilateral vocal fold paralysis or surgical removal (Aspiration during the swallow)	Head rotated to damaged side	Places extrinsic pressure on thyroid cartilage, improving vocal fold approximation, and directs bolus down stronger side
Reduced closure of laryngeal entrance and vocal folds (Aspiration during the swallow)	Chin down; head rotated to damaged side	Puts epiglottis in more protective position; narrows laryngeal entrance; improves vocal fold closure by applying extrinsic pressure
Reduced pharyngeal contraction (Residue spread throughout pharynx)	Lying down on one side	Eliminates gravitational effect on pharyngeal residue
Unilateral pharyngeal paresis (Residue on one side of pharynx)	Head rotated to damaged side	Eliminates damaged side of pharynx from bolus path
Unilateral oral and pharyngeal weakness on the same side (Residue in mouth and pharynx on same side)	Head tilt to stronger side	Directs bolus down stronger side by gravity
Cricopharyngeal dysfunction (Residue in pyriform sinuses)	Head rotated	Pulls cricoid cartilage away from posterior pharyngeal wall, reducing resting pressure in cricopharyngeal sphincter

prove oropharyngeal motor function take effect. Occasionally, patients with severe neurologic or structural damage must use postural techniques permanently to eliminate aspiration and ensure adequate swallow efficiency to facilitate oral intake.

Techniques to Improve Oral Sensory Awareness

Techniques to improve oral sensory awareness are generally used in patients with swallow apraxia, delayed onset of the oral swallow (which may relate to swallow apraxia), or delayed triggering of the pharyngeal swallow (Logemann, 1993b; Logemann et al., 1995). These procedures all involve providing a preliminary sensory stimulus prior to the initiation of the patient's swallow attempt (Helfrich-Miller, Rector, & Straka, 1986; Lazarus, Logemann, Rademaker, et al., 1993; Lazzara, Lazarus, & Logemann, 1986; Logemann et al., 1995; Tippett, Palmer, & Linden, 1987; Ylvisaker & Logemann, 1986). Sensory enhancement techniques include

1. increasing downward pressure of the spoon against the tongue when presenting food in the mouth;
2. presenting a sour bolus (50% lemon juice, 50% barium);
3. presenting a cold bolus;
4. presenting a bolus requiring chewing;
5. presenting a larger volume bolus (3 ml or more);
6. allowing self-feeding so that the hand-to-mouth movement provides additional sensory input;
7. thermal/tactile stimulation.

In some patients with swallow apraxia, increasing oral sensation by a preliminary stimulus such as the downward pressure of a spoon, the presentation of a bolus with increased volume, taste or temperature characteristics, or thermal/tactile stimulation may facilitate oral onset and oral transit of the swallow. Generally, presenting verbal instructions to an apraxic patient increases their difficulty. These techniques that enhance sensory input, such as bolus taste, temperature, volume, and viscosity, may also result in reduced pharyngeal delay times in some patients (Lazzara et al., 1986; Logemann et al., 1995).

Measures of the effectiveness of these procedures in increasing oral sensory input include (a) duration of time from command to swallow until initiation of the oral stage of swallow; (b) oral transit time; and (c) pharyngeal delay time (Logemann, 1993b). These can be measured from videofluoroscopy; the first two can also be measured with ultrasound. In some patients, pharyngeal delay time can be measured from videoendoscopy. However, if a patient exhibits premature spillage of a bolus because of oral abnormalities, videoendoscopy will not be capable of distinguishing premature spillage from the onset of pharyngeal delay time with the same accuracy as videofluoroscopy, since the oral stage of swallow cannot be visualized with videoendoscopy.

Modifications in Volume and Speed of Food Presentation

For some patients, a particular volume of food per swallow elicits the fastest pharyngeal swallow. In patients with a delay in pharyngeal triggering or with weakened pharyngeal swallows that require 2 to 3 swallows per bolus, taking too much food too rapidly can result in a sizable collection of food in the pharynx and aspiration. Simply taking smaller boluses at a slower rate may eliminate any risk of aspiration in these patients.

Food Consistency (Diet) Changes

Generally, elimination of certain food consistencies from the diet should be the last compensatory strategy examined (Logemann, 1993b). Eliminating certain food consistencies, such as thin liquids, from the diet can be difficult for the patient. This should only be done if other compensatory or therapy strategies are not feasible, as in a patient with a movement disorder whose posture changes continuously, who cannot follow directions and use swallow maneuvers, and for whom oral sensory procedures are inappropriate. Table 15–2 presents the easiest food consistencies and the food consistencies to be avoided for each swallow disorder.

TABLE 15–2. Food Consistencies to be Used or Avoided by Swallowing Disorder.

Swallowing Disordery	Easiest Food Consistencies	Consistencies to Avoid
Reduced range of tongue motion	Thick liquid initially, then, thin liquid	Thick foods
Reduced tongue coordination	Liquid	Thick foods
Reduced tongue strength	Thin liquid	Thick, heavy foods
Delayed pharyngeal swallow	Thick liquids and thicker foods	Thin liquids
Reduced airway closure	Pudding and thick foods	Thin liquids
Reduced laryngeal movement/ cricopharyngeal dysfunction	Thin liquid	Thicker, higher viscosity foods
Reduced pharyngeal wall contraction	Thin liquid	Thick, higher viscosity foods
Reduced tongue-base posterior movement	Thin liquid	Higher viscosity foods

Intraoral Prosthetics

Intraoral prosthetics can be an important compensatory procedure to improve swallowing in oral cancer patients with significant loss of oral tongue tissue (25% or more) or tongue movement, in neurologic patients with bilateral hypoglossal paralysis, in oral cancer patient groups with surgical ablation of part or all of the soft palate, and in neurologic patients with palatal paralysis.

A *palatal lift* prosthesis lifts the soft palate into an elevated (closed) position in patients with velar paralysis. A *palatal obturator* can be used in oral cancer patients with significant resection of the soft palate. The *palatal reshaping* prosthesis recontours the hard palate to interact with the remaining tongue, filling in the areas of the hard palate where the patient's tongue cannot make contact and enabling the patient to control and propel the bolus more efficiently (Figure 15–1). A palatal augmen-

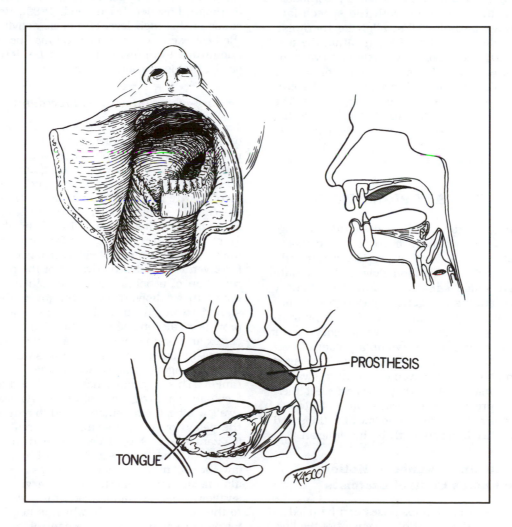

Figure 15–1. Diagram of an intraoral palatal reshaping prosthesis designed to recontour the patient's hard palate to interact with the remaining tongue.

tation or reshaping prosthesis can be extremely effective in patients with significant tongue resections or bilateral tongue paralysis (Davis, Lazarus, Logemann, & Hurst, 1987; Logemann, Kahrilas, Hurst, Davis, & Krugler, 1989). Postoperative patients often indicate that it feels as if their tongue fits their mouth again with the prosthesis in place. Without the prosthesis the patient has a large oral cavity and a very small tongue, which is incapable of controlling food in the mouth for chewing or swallowing.

These intraoral prosthetics are usually constructed by a maxillofacial prosthodontist in cooperation with the speech-language pathologist/swallowing therapist. Construction should begin within the first 4 to 6 weeks postoperatively to prevent the patient's development of poor habits for swallowing that will need to be dishabituated when they receive the prosthesis. The speech-language pathologist/swallowing therapist provides input regarding the amount of palate lowering needed and the best contour of the palate.

THERAPY PROCEDURES

Therapy procedures are designed to change swallow physiology, in contrast to compensatory strategies that are designed to redirect or improve food flow and eliminate symptoms such as aspiration. Therapy procedures are generally designed to improve range of motion of oral or pharyngeal structures, improve sensory motor integration, or take voluntary control over the timing or the coordination of selected oropharyngeal movements during swallow (Logemann, 1983). To get the best effect, therapy procedures generally, but not always, require the patient to follow directions and practice independently of the clinician.

Resistance, Range of Motion, and Bolus Control Exercises

Range of motion exercises can be used to improve the extent of movement of the lips, jaw, tongue, larynx, and vocal folds (adduc-

tion exercises; Logemann, 1983). Range of motion exercises involve extending the target structure in the desired direction until a strong stretch is felt. The structure is held in extension for 1 sec, then relaxed. Bolus control and chewing exercises can be used to improve fine motor control of the tongue. Bolus control and chewing exercises are both best done using gauze or other cloth, at least initially (Logemann, 1983). Sliding into falsetto (a very high-pitched, squeaky voice) can exercise laryngeal elevation.

There is some evidence that swallowing requires more muscle effort than other functions of the upper aerodigestive tract (Perlman, Luschei, & DuMond, 1989). Because of this high level of muscle activity, the best exercise for swallowing may be to encourage swallowing if it can be done safely, that is, without aspiration.

Sensory-motor Integration Procedures

Techniques to improve the speed of onset of the pharyngeal swallow are all designed to enhance sensory input prior to the patient's attempt to swallow (Logemann, 1983). *Thermal/tactile stimulation* and *suck-swallow* are most commonly used. Thermal/tactile stimulation involves vertically rubbing the anterior faucial arch firmly, four or five times, with a size 00 laryngeal mirror (which has been held in crushed ice for several seconds) in advance of the presentation of a bolus and the patient's attempt to swallow. This technique is designed to heighten oral awareness and provide an alerting sensory stimulus to the cortex and brain stem such that, when the patient initiates the oral stage of swallow, the pharyngeal swallow will trigger more rapidly. This technique has been found to facilitate faster triggering of the pharyngeal swallow after the stimulation and to reduce the delay for several swallows thereafter (Lazzara et al., 1986). An exaggerated suck-swallow using increased vertical tongue/jaw sucking movements with the lips closed also facilitates triggering the pharyngeal swallow. This technique also draws saliva to the back of the mouth, which is helpful for patients with poor saliva control, such as oral cancer patients.

Swallow Maneuvers: Voluntary Control Over Aspects of Pharyngeal Swallow Physiology

Swallow maneuvers are designed to place specific aspects of pharyngeal swallow physiology under voluntary control (Cook et al., 1989; Jacob, Kahrilas, Logemann, Shah, & Ha, 1989; Lazarus, Logemann, & Gibbons, 1993; Logemann, 1993a, 1993b; Logemann et al., 1992; Martin, Logemann, Shaker, & Dodds, 1993, Ohmae, Logemann, Kaiser, Hanson, & Kahrilas, 1996). Four swallow maneuvers have been developed to date (Table 15–3):

1. the supraglottic swallow—designed to close the airway at the level of the true vocal folds before and during the swallow (Logemann, 1983, Martin, Logemann, et al., 1993);
2. the super-supraglottic swallow-designed to close the airway entrance before and during the swallow (Logemann, 1993b; Martin, Logemann, et al., 1993; Ohmae et al., 1996);
3. the effortful swallow-designed to increase posterior motion of the tongue-base during the pharyngeal swallow and thus improve bolus clearance from the valleculae (Kahrilas, Lin, Logemann, Ergun, & Facchini, 1993; Kahrilas, Logemann, Lin, & Ergun, 1992; Logemann, 1993b;
4. the Mendelsohn maneuver-designed to increase the extent and duration of laryngeal elevation and thereby increase the duration and width of cricopharyngeal opening (Bartolome & Neuman, 1993; Bryant, 1991; Kahrilas, Logemann, Krugler, & Flanagan, 1991; Lazarus, Logemann, & Gibbons, 1993; Logemann & Kahrilas, 1990; Neuman, 1993; Robbins & Levine, 1993). This latter maneuver can also improve the overall coordination of the swallow (Lazarus, Logemann, & Gibbons, 1993).

The instructions for the supraglottic swallow are (Martin, Logemann, et al, 1993; Ohmae et al., 1996):

> Inhale and hold your breath. (Breath hold usually closes the vocal folds, thus closing the airway.) Swallow while holding your breath. Cough immediately after your swallow without breathing in.

Alternative instructions: Inhale and exhale a little. Hold your breath and keep hold-

TABLE 15–3. Swallow Maneuvers Designed for Particular Swallowing Disorders.

Swallow Maneuvers	Problem for which Maneuver Designed	Rationale
Supraglottic swallow	Reduced or late vocal fold closure;	Voluntary breath hold usually closes vocal folds before and during swallow (Martin , Logemann, et al., 1993)
	Delayed pharyngeal swallow	Closes vocal folds before and during delay
Super-supraglottic swallow	Reduced closure of airway entrance	Effortful breath hold tilts arytenoid forward, closing airway entrance before and during swallow (Martin, Logemann, et al., 1993; Ohmae et al., 1996)
Effortful swallow	Reduced posterior movement of the tongue-base	Effort increases posterior tongue-base movement
Mendelsohn maneuver	Reduced laryngeal movement	Laryngeal movement opens the UES; prolonging laryngeal elevation prolongs UES opening (Cook et al., 1989; Jacob et al., 1989)
	Discoordinated swallow	Normalizes timing of pharyngeal swallow events (Lazarus, Logemann, & Gibbons, 1993)

ing your breath as you swallow. After you swallow, cough.

The instructions for the super-supraglottic swallow are:

Inhale, hold your breath and bear down. The effort of bearing down usually closes the false vocal folds and tilts the arytenoids anteriorly to met the thickening base of epiglottis. After the swallow, cough to clear any leftover food.

Alternative instructions: Inhale and exhale a little. Hold your breath and bear down hard. Keep holding your breath hard as you swallow. After you swallow, cough.

The instructions for the effortful swallow are:

As you swallow, squeeze hard with all of your muscles.

Instructions for the Mendelsohn maneuver are:

Swallow your saliva several times and pay attention to your neck as you swallow. Tell me if you can feel that something (your Adam's apple or voice box) lifts and lowers as you swallow. Now, this time, when you swallow and you feel something lift as you swallow, don't let your Adam's apple drop. Hold it up with your muscles for several seconds.

Alternative instructions: Swallow your saliva several times and pay attention to the feeling in your throat as you swallow. Can you feel that in the middle of the swallow everything squeezes together at the top of your throat? Next time when you swallow, hold the squeeze for several seconds and don't let go.

All of these maneuvers can be practiced with the patient, giving the patient slow, step-by-step instructions and asking them to swallow their saliva. You do not need to use food to teach the patient these maneuvers.

During the videofluorographic study, if postural techniques and oral sensory facilitation techniques do not improve swallow physiology sufficiently to allow the patient to begin some oral intake, voluntary swallow maneuvers may be appropriate. However, these maneuvers require the ability to follow directions carefully and are not feasible in patients who have cognitive or significant language impairment. These maneuvers also require increased muscular effort and are not appropriate in patients who fatigue easily. Usually, voluntary maneuvers are utilized temporarily as the patient's swallow recovers, and are then discarded as the patient's swallow physiology returns to normal. However, there are patients who can only swallow safely and efficiently using a voluntary maneuver permanently (Kahrilas, Logemann, & Gibbons, 1992; Lazarus, Logemann, & Gibbons, 1993; Logemann & Kahrilas, 1990). For some patients, best swallow is achieved by a combination of postural changes and swallow maneuvers.

Each swallow maneuver has a specific goal to change a selected aspect of pharyngeal swallow physiology (Logemann, 1993b). Changes in these target components of the oropharyngeal swallow can be observed or measured, for example, duration and onset of closure of the airway entrance (super-supraglottic swallow), and extent and duration of laryngeal elevation (Mendelsohn maneuver) (Bartolome, & Neuman, 1993; Bryant, 1991; Cook et al., 1989; Jacob et al., 1989; Kahrilas, Logemann, Lin, & Ergun, 1992; Kahrilas et al., 1991; Kahrilas et al., 1993; Lazarus, Logemann, & Gibbons, 1993; Logemann & Kahrilas, 1990; Logemann et al., 1992; Martin, Logemann, et al., 1993; Martin, Schleicher & O'Connor, 1993; Neuman, 1993). In general, the effects of swallow maneuvers are best observed and measured using videofluoroscopy. The effects of these maneuvers on swallow safety (aspiration) and efficiency (residue) may be observed at times using videoendoscopy. However, videoendoscopy does not allow visualization of these maneuvers during the swallow, a significant limitation.

Indirect Therapy

Indirect therapy involves exercise programs or swallows of saliva but no food or liquid is given. Any of the therapy procedures described above can be done indirectly or directly. Even swallow maneuvers can be practiced with saliva only. Indirect therapy is used in patients who aspirate on all food viscosities and volumes despite introduction of compensatory strategies. Therefore, these patients are unsafe for any oral intake (Logemann, 1983; Neuman, 1993). However, indirect therapy can be combined with direct therapy.

Direct Therapy

Direct therapy is used when patients are practicing their swallow techniques with some small amounts of food or liquid. Direct therapy is used when the patient can successfully swallow at least small amounts of selected liquid or food viscosities with no aspiration (Logemann, 1983; Neuman, 1993).

Introduction of Treatment Strategies in the Diagnostic Radiographic Study

In general, the introduction of treatment strategies in the diagnostic radiographic study will begin with utilization of postural techniques, followed by introduction of techniques to increase oral sensation, when appropriate, followed by swallowing maneuvers, then combinations of these as appropriate or needed, and finally, diet (food consistency, viscosity) changes, if needed (Logemann, 1993b; Rasley et al., 1993; Logemann et al., 1994). The rationale for this sequencing of interventions is based on the muscle effort required by the patient and the ease of applying and learning the various procedures. In general, postural techniques are easily utilized by a wide range of patients, even those with reduced cognition, children, and patients with some degree of restricted physical mobility. Procedures designed to increase oral sensation can also be utilized with a wide range of patients, as they are clinician-controlled and do not require the patient to actively cooperate, other than allowing the clinician to place something into their mouth. Swallow maneuvers, on the other hand, require the ability to follow directions and voluntarily manipulate the oropharyngeal swallow as it is ongoing. Swallow maneuvers also involve increased work or muscular effort in most cases, thus increasing the patient's potential for fatigue. However, there are patients who cannot swallow successfully without swallow maneuvers (Kahrilas, Logemann, & Gibbons, 1992; Lazarus, Logemann, & Gibbons, 1993; Logemann & Kahrilas, 1990).

In some cases, introduction of therapy procedures into the diagnostic procedure can immediately enable the patient to begin eating. Introduction of these treatment strategies is particularly important because there is a growing body of literature indicating a relationship between disturbed swallowing and aspiration observed on the radiographic study and risk for aspiration pneumonia (Johnson, McKenzie, & Sievers, 1993; Martin et al., 1994; Schmidt, Holas, Halvorson, & Reding, 1994). If aspiration can be eliminated during the videofluoroscopic procedure and during subsequent oral intake, risk of pneumonia is reduced. In other cases, evaluation of the effectiveness of the therapy procedure can validate its appropriateness for use with a patient in building the neuromuscular control necessary to return to oral intake.

Not all therapy procedures can be introduced into the diagnostic setting, however; some therapy procedures take time to take effect and, therefore, do not result in immediate change. For example, resistance and range of motion exercises for the lips, tongue, and/or jaw do not have an immediate effect but, depending on the extent and severity of neuromuscular involvement, can show an effect after 2 to 3 weeks of practice. However, the clinician can still quantify the effects of range of motion exercises by measuring the patient's structural movement at each therapy session. When a second assessment is completed, change in range of motion of the target structure can be assessed by comparing the first and second studies.

The introduction of treatment techniques into the diagnostic swallowing assessment requires the clinician to interpret or "read" the radiographic study or other imaging procedure immediately and identify the physiologic dysfunction(s) so that appropriate therapy procedures can be selected and introduced. Because videofluorography involves x-ray exposure to the patient, all possible treatment techniques cannot be attempted randomly to look at their relative value in x-ray. Rather, the clinician must select those treatment techniques believed to be most appropriate for that patient's anatomy and swallow physiology. The usual limit for radiation exposure in adults is 5 minutes. It is usually possible to assess the effects of selected management/treatment procedures within that amount of exposure time.

THE INTRODUCTION OF SWALLOW THERAPY

As soon as an inpatient is medically stable and identified as dysphagic, a videofluorographic assessment of their swallow function should be accomplished by the swallow therapist and radiologist. From this assessment, an appropriate therapy plan should be initiated, with the patient seen daily in the hospital and weekly thereafter. For surgically treated head and neck cancer patients, assessment and treatment of swallow dysfunction should begin as soon as healing has progressed enough to allow them to try to swallow (usually 7–14 days postoperatively with no healing complications). If a patient is undergoing radiation therapy and begins complaining of swallowing problems, assessment and treatment should begin at that time (Lazarus,

1993). For stroke patients, assessment should take place when they are awake and alert, usually 4–7 days post ictus. Outpatients who are dysphagic should receive the same careful videofluorographic assessment and therapy as inpatients. Even if patients have been dysphagic for some time, they should receive the same type of assessment and intensive therapy (Perlman, 1993; Sonies, 1993). Patients who receive therapy months or years after the onset of their problem are still capable of achieving oral intake (Lazarus, Logemann, & Gibbons, 1993; Logemann & Kahrilas, 1990). Therapy is usually provided daily for inpatients and weekly for outpatients.

In general, tracheostomy tubes and nonoral feeding tubes are left in place during swallowing assessment and therapy, as these have not been found to significantly deter rehabilitation. However, the cuff of the tracheostomy tube should be deflated if medically feasible during the assessment and therapy. An inflated cuff can restrict laryngeal elevation and cricopharyngeal opening during the swallow. An inflated tracheostomy cuff can also cause tracheal irritation by rubbing on the tracheal walls as the larynx elevates during swallow. Therefore, it is inappropriate to feed a patient with a tracheostomy cuff inflated. If the patient is aspirating, they should not be fed orally. On occasion it may be absolutely necessary to leave the cuff inflated, such as when the patient is ventilator dependent. Many ventilators require cuff inflation.

MEDICATIONS FOR SWALLOWING DISORDERS

Currently, there are few studies of the therapeutic benefits of medications on oropharyngeal swallowing disorders. Utilization of atropine to reduce drooling (Dworkin & Nadal, 1991) has been documented. No other medications to improve specific oropharyngeal swallowing disorders have been identified.

Patients with progressive neurologic disease (e.g., Parkinson's disease, multiple sclerosis, and myasthenia gravis) sometimes experience improvement in oropharyngeal swallowing when placed on medications for their disease process. Unfortunately, detailed studies of the effects of specific medications on the oropharyngeal function of these patients have not been completed.

SUMMARY

In our experience, swallowing rehabilitation, including compensatory procedures and direct and indirect therapy can be successful in returning over 80% of oropharyngeal dysphagic patients to oral intake (Rademaker et al., 1993). It can eliminate aspiration and reduce the risk of pneumonia and other pulmonary complications, as well as improve nutritional status (Rademaker et al., 1993). Usually, the swallowing therapist is a speech-language pathologist. In some instances, another professional plays this role. The swallowing therapist participates actively in the radiographic assessment and other diagnostic procedures, as well as in designing and implementing the swallowing rehabilitation program in cooperation with the patient's attending physician, other health care professionals, the patient, and his or her family.

Acknowledgment Research reported in this manuscript funded by NIH PO1-CA40007 and RO1-NS28525

MULTIPLE CHOICE QUESTIONS

1. Indirect treatment strategies involve
   a. giving patients muscular exercises with food.
   b. giving patients muscular exercises without food.
   c. working on swallowing with food.
   d. working on swallowing without food.

2. The Mendelsohn maneuver is designed to improve
   a. airway closure.
   b. laryngeal elevation.
   c. pharyngeal peristalsis.
   d. base of tongue motion.

3. The super-supraglottic swallow is designed to
   a. close the airway at the true vocal folds.
   b. improve tongue base motion.
   c. improve cricopharyngeal opening.
   d. improve pharyngeal contraction.
   e. close the airway at its entrance.

4. The chin down posture is designed to
   a. improve airway protection.
   b. improve tongue base retraction.
   c. improve pharyngeal wall contraction.
   d. a and c above.
   e. a and b above.

5. Therapy procedures which heighten sensory awareness prior to swallowing are designed to improve
   a. pharyngeal contraction.
   b. triggering of the pharyngeal swallow.
   c. cricopharyngeal opening.
   d. laryngeal closure.
   e. velopharyngeal closure.

REFERENCES

Bartolome, G., & Neuman, D. S. (1993) Swallowing therapy in patients with neurological disorders causing cricopharyngeal dysfunction. *Dysphagia, 8*, 146–149.

Bryant, M. (1991). Biofeedback in the treatment of a selected dysphagic patient. *Dysphagia, 6*, 140–144.

Cook, I. J., Dodds, W. J., Dantas, R. O., Massey, B., Kern, M. K., Lang, I. M., Brasseur, J. G., & Hogan, W. J. (1989). Opening mechanism of the human upper esophageal sphincter. *American Journal of Physiology, 257*, G748–G759.

Davis, J., Lazarus, C., Logemann, J., & Hurst, P. (1987). Effect of a maxillary glossectomy prostheses on articulation and swallowing. *Journal of Prosthetic Dentistry, 57*(6), 715–719.

Dworkin, J. P., & Nadal, J. C. (1991). Nonsurgical treatment of drooling in a patient with closed head injury and severe dysarthria. *Dysphagia, 6*, 40–49.

Helfrich-Miller, K. R., Rector, K. L., & Straka, J. A. (1986). Dysphagia: Its treatment in the profoundly retarded patient with cerebral palsy. *Archives of Physical Medicine and Rehabilitation, 67*, 520–525.

Horner, J. Massey, E. W., Riski, J. E., Lathrop, D., & Chase, K. N. (1988). Aspiration following stroke: Clinical correlates and outcomes. *Neurology 38*, 1359–1362.

Jacob, P., Kahrilas, P. J., Logemann, J. A., Shah, V., & Ha, T. (1989). Upper esophageal sphincter opening and modulation during swallowing. *Gastroenterology, 97*, 1469–1478.

Johnson, E. R., McKenzie, S. W., & Sievers, A. (1993). Aspiration pneumonia in stroke. *Archives of Physical Medicine and Rehabilitation, 74*, 973–976.

Kahrilas, P. J., Lin, S., Logemann, J. A., Ergun, G. A., & Facchini, F. (1993). Deglutitive tongue action: Volume accommodation and bolus propulsion. *Gastroenterology, 104*, 152–162.

Kahrilas, P. J., Logemann, J. A., & Gibbons, M. S. (1992). Food intake by maneuver: An extreme compensation for impaired swallowing. *Dysphagia, 7*, 155–159.

Kahrilas, P. J., Logemann, J. A., Krugler, C., & Flanagan, E. (1991). Volitional augmentation of upper esophageal sphincter opening during swallowing. *American Journal of Physiology, 260*, G450–G456.

Kahrilas, P. J., Logemann, J. A., Lin, S., & Ergun, G. A. (1992). Pharyngeal clearance during swallow: A combined manometric and videofluoroscopic study. *Gastroenterology, 103*, 128–136.

Lazarus, C. L. (1993). Effects of radiation therapy and voluntary maneuvers on swallow functioning in head and neck cancer patients. *Clinics in Communication Disorders, 3*(4), 11–20.

Lazarus, C., Logemann, J. A., & Gibbons, P. (1993). Effects of maneuvers on swallowing function in a dysphagic oral cancer patient. *Head & Neck Surgery, 15*, 419–424.

Lazarus, C. L., Logemann, J. A., Rademaker, A. W., Kahrilas, P. J., Pajak, T., Lazar, R., & Halper, A. (1993). Effects of bolus volume, viscosity and repeated swallows in nonstroke subjects and stroke patients. *Archives of Physical Medicine and Rehabilitation, 74*, 1066–1070.

Lazzara, G., Lazarus, C., & Logemann, J. A. (1986). Impact of thermal stimulation on the triggering of the swallowing reflex. *Dysphagia 1*, 73–77.

Logemann, J. A. (1983). *Evaluation and treatment of swallowing disorders*. Austin, TX: Pro-Ed.

Logemann, J. A. (1989a). Evaluation and treatment planning for the head-injured patient with oral intake disorders. *Journal of Head Trauma Rehabilitation, 4*(4), 24–33.

Logemann, J. A. (Ed). (1989b). Swallowing disorders & rehabilitation. *Journal of Head Trauma Rehabilitation, 4*(4), Frederick, MD: Aspen.

Logemann, J. A. (1993a). The dysphagia diagnostic procedure as a treatment efficacy trial. *Clinics in Communication Disorders, 3*(4), 1–10.

Logemann, J. A. (1993b). *A manual for the videofluoroscopic evaluation of swallowing* (2nd ed.). Austin, TX: Pro-Ed.

Logemann, J., Kahrilas, P., Hurst, P., Davis, J., & Krugler, C. (1989). Effects of intraoral prosthetics on swallowing in oral cancer patients. *Dysphagia, 4*, 118–120.

Logemann, J. A., Kahrilas, P., Kobara, M., & Vakil, N. (1989). The benefit of head rotation on pharyngoesophageal dysphagia. *Archives of Physical Medicine and Rehabilitation, 70*(10), 767–771.

Logemann, J. A., & Kahrilas, P. J. (1990). Relearning to swallow post cva: Application of maneuvers and indirect biofeedback: A case study. *Neurology, 40*, 1136–1138.

Logemann, J. A., Kahrilas, P. J., Cheng, J., Pauloski, B. R., Gibbons, P. J., Rademaker, A. W., & Lin, S. (1992). Closure mechanisms of the laryngeal vestibule during swallowing. *American Journal of Physiology, 262*, G338–G344.

Logemann, J. A., Pauloski, B. R., Colangelo, L., Lazarus, C., Fujiu, M., & Kahrilas, P. J. (1995). Effects of a sour bolus on oropharyngeal swallowing measures in patients with neurogenic dysphagia. *Journal of Speech and Hearing Research, 383*, 556–563.

Logemann, J. A., Rademaker, A. W., Pauloski, B. R., & Kahrilas, P. J. (1994). Effects of postural change on aspiration in head and neck surgical patients. *Otolaryngology-Head and Neck Surgery, 110*, 222–227.

Martin, B. J. W., Schleicher, M. A., O'Connor, A. (1993). Management of dysphagia following supraglottic laryngectomy. *Clinics in Communication Disorders, 3*(4), 27–36.

Martin, B. J. W., Logemann, J. A., Shaker, R., & Dodds, W. J. (1993). Normal laryngeal valving patterns during three breath hold maneuvers: A pilot investigation. *Dysphagia, 8*, 11–20.

Martin, B. J., Corlew, M., Wood, H., Olson, D., Golopol, L., Wingo, M., & Kirmani, N. (1994). The association of swallowing dysfunction and aspiration pneumonia. *Dysphagia, 9*, 1–6.

Neuman, S. (1993). Swallowing therapy with neurologic patients: Results of direct and indirect therapy methods in 66 patients suffering from neurological disorders. *Dysphagia, 8*, 150–153.

Ohmae, Y., Logemann, J. A., Kaiser, P., Hanson, D. G., & Kahrilas, P. J. (1996). Effects of two breath holding maneuvers on oropharyngeal swallow. *Annals of Otology, Rhinology and Laryngology, 105*(2), 123–131.

Perlman, A. L. (1993). The successful treatment of challenging cases. *Clinics in Communication Disorders, 3*(4), 37–44.

Perlman, A. L., Luschei, E., & DuMond, C. (1989). Electrical activity from the superior pharyngeal constrictor during selective reflexive and non-reflexive tasks. *Journal of Speech & Hearing Research, 32*(4), 749–754.

Rademaker, A. W., Logemann, J. A., Pauloski, B. R., Bowman, J., Goepfert, H., Lazarus, C., Sisson, G., Milianti, F., Graner, D., Cook, B., Collins, S., Stein, D., & Johnson, J. (1993). Recovery of postoperative swallowing in patients undergoing partial laryngectomy. *Head and Neck Surgery, 15,* 325–334, 1993.

Rasley, A., Logemann, J. A., Kahrilas, P. J., Rademaker, A. W., Pauloski, B. R., & Dodds, W. J. (1993). Prevention of barium aspiration during videofluoroscopic swallowing studies: Value of change in posture. *American Journal of Roentgenology, 160,* 1005–1009.

Robbins, J. A., & Levine, R. (1993). Swallowing after lateral medullary syndrome plus. *Clinics in Communication Disorders, 3*(4), 45–55.

Schmidt J., Holas M., Halvorson K., & Reding, M. (1994). Videofluoroscopic evidence of aspiration predicts pneumonia and death but not dehydration following stroke. *Dysphagia, 9,* 7–11.

Shanahan, T. K., Logemann, J. A., Rademaker, A. W., Pauloski, B. R., & Kahrilas, P. J. (1993). Chin down posture effects on aspiration in dysphagic patients. *Archives of Physical Medicine and Rehabilitation, 74,* 736–739.

Sonies, B. C. (1993). Remediation challenges in treating dysphagia post head/neck cancer: A problem-oriented approach. *Clinics in Communication Disorders, 3*(4), 21–26.

Tippett, D. C., Palmer, J., & Linden, P. (1987). Management of dysphagia in a patient with closed head injury: A case report. *Dysphagia, 1,* 221–226.

Welch, M. V., Logemann, J. A., Rademaker, A. W., & Kahrilas, P. J. (1993). Changes in pharyngeal dimensions effected by chin tuck. *Archives of Physical Medicine and Rehabilitation, 74,* 178–181.

Ylvisaker, M., & Logemann, J. A. (1986). Therapy for feeding and swallowing following head injury. In M. Ylvisaker (Ed.), *Management of head injured patients.* San Diego, CA: College Hill Press.

16

Medical and Surgical Treatment Interventions in Deglutitive Dysfunction

Gulchin A. Ergun and Peter J. Kahrilas

This chapter outlines medical and surgical therapies used to treat the dysphagic patient and highlights nonoral feeding options when oral intake is no longer feasible. Although it would be desirable to include analyses of treatment outcome, cost-effectiveness, and cost-benefit, the literature regarding these is limited and simply has not been presented in this manner. While the current data is more qualitative than quantitative, we hope the future will bring reappraisal of treatment strategies, allowing more objective assessment of therapeutic options.

MEDICAL INTERVENTION

Currently, no medications have been identified as beneficial in nonspecific oropharyngeal swallowing dysfunction. Medical intervention in treating dysphagia has historically been based on recognition of the disorder underlying the swallow dysfunction, since improvement of dysphagia may occur when the underlying pathology is treated. Unfortunately many neurologic and myopathic causes of dysphagia such as multiple sclerosis or muscular dystrophy have no substantiated medical treatment, so this discussion will be necessarily limited to those diseases that are more common or have better recognized therapeutic options.

Indications for Medical Intervention

Regardless of cause certain symptoms accompanying dysphagia such as aspiration, dehydration, weight loss, and malnutrition should prompt immediate medical attention. Furthermore, treatment such as rehydration or nutritional supplementation should be initiated regardless of the underlying disease and not withheld awaiting diagnostic confirmation. Unfortunately, there is no magical drug that can alleviate all swallowing symptoms and in many instances therapy may have relatively modest goals of providing symptomatic relief such as lozenge administration in xerostomia or deliberate removal of an offending pharmacologic agent that induces xerostomia. Equally clear is that dysphagia therapy only works when applied to dysphagic symptoms, and globus sensation (feeling of a lump in the throat that is present continually and even alleviated during swallowing) should not be confused with dysphagia. The utility of swallowing therapy and behavioral management is discussed in Chapter 15.

Xerostomia

MANIFESTATIONS OF XEROSTOMIA. (See also Chapter 5.) The feeling of a dry mouth or xerostomia is a common symptom. The associated signs and symptoms include pain, burning, and soreness of the oral mucosa, especially the tongue, as well as difficulty in chewing, swallowing, and speech. Patients perceive an impairment of taste and complain of painful oral ulcers, often with increased dental caries. Patients with xerostomia who have dental prostheses have discomfort wearing dentures and all patients perceive an decreased frequency or even absolute quantity of fluid (Stuchell & Mandel, 1988). More objective facial predictors of salivary hypofunction include swollen, palpable salivary glands, dry or cracked appearance of the tongue dorsum, lipstick on upper incisors, dry buccal mucosa, and the absence of flow on parotid gland palpation. The associated dysphagia is primarily due to the absence of salivary lubrication, and drugs are the most common cause of the disorder (Hughes et al., 1987).

CAUSES OF XEROSTOMIA. (See also Chapter 5 and Table 5–6.) The most common offending agents are anorectics, anticholinergics, antidepressants, antipsychotics, sedatives, antihistamines, antihypertensives, and diuretics (Table 16–1; Atkinson & Fox, 1992). The next most frequent causes are autoimmune diseases such as Sjögren's syndrome, rheumatoid arthritis, and radiation therapy (Atkinson & Fox, 1992; Fox, 1992; Kjellen, Fransson, Lindstrom, Sokier, & Tibbling, 1986; Scully, 1986). Radiation therapy injures salivary gland parenchyma in a dose-related fashion, resulting in eventual fibrosis and secretory

gland failure. Furthermore, radiation therapy is common; head and neck cancer is diagnosed in approximately 43,000 people in the United States annually and many receive radiation therapy to the head and neck as sole or adjuvant therapy. The effects are permanent and cause salivary function decline within a matter of days. Salivary flow rates are reduced 50% after 1,000–2,000 rads and to near zero following 3,000–5,000 rads (Anderson, Izutsu, & Rice, 1981).

DIAGNOSIS OF XEROSTOMIA. The evaluation of the patient with xerostomia is generally by history and a combination of sialometry or gland imaging when clinically suggested. *Sialometry* is the evaluation of gland secretion and may be performed by examining native gland production or by stimulating the glands to measure salivary flow rates and saliva composition. Normal unstimulated salivary flow rates should be 0.3–0.5 ml/min; flow rates of less than 0.1 ml/min are consistent with xerostomia (Ship, Fox, & Baum, 1991). Should structural processes such as cysts or tumors be suspected in impairing or obstructing salivary flow, ultrasonography, computed tomography (CT), magnetic resonance imaging (MRI), contrast sialography, or dynamic Technetium-99 scintiscanning may be employed to evaluate gland parenchyma (Blitzer 1987; Markusse, Pillay, & Breedveld 1993).

TREATMENT OF XEROSTOMIA. Treatment for salivary gland hypofunction is primarily symptomatic, with frequent sips of water or fluid for hydration and meticulous oral hygiene with brushing, rinsing, and daily application of topical fluoride (Dreizen, Brown, Daly, & Drane, 1977). Although artificial salivas are broadly marketed, patients generally do not find them satisfying because they lack the natural lubrication properties of natural saliva (Duxbury, Thakker & Wastell, 1989; Kaplan & Baum, 1993).

Stimulation of Salivary Secretion. Salivary flow can be enhanced by mechanical or systemic therapy; however, the effi-

TABLE 16–1. Medications causing impaired salivary flow rates.

Drug Type	Profound Decrease	Moderate	Probable/No Effect
Antidepressants	Amitriptyline Nortriptyline Clomipramine Imipramine Desipramine Maprotiline Chlorpromazine Triflupromazine Doxepin	Dothiepin Zomelidine Nominfensin Mainserin Lofepramine Haloperidol Thioridazine	Cisflupenthixol Citalpram Transflupenthixol Lithium
Anxiolytic			Lorazepam
Antihypertensive	Clonidine		Propranolol Metoprolol Verapamil Timolol maleate
Diuretics			Bendroflumethiazide Amiloride Hydrochlorothiazide
Anticholinergic properties	Atropine Scopolamine Propantheline	L - hyoscyamine	Pirenzepine Cimetidine Ranitidine Bethanechol Metoclopramide
Antihistamines	Diphenhydramine		

Note. Adapted from J. C. Atkinson and P. C. Fox, (1992). Salivary Gland Dysfunction. *Clinics in Geriatric Medicine, 8,* 499–511.

cacy of enhancing local salivary flow is completely dependent on residual salivary function and whether the glands are capable of adequate secretory function when stimulated. If salivation is not achieved following all types of stimulation, there is no advantage to masticatory or gustatory therapy. If stimulation results in adequate salivary secretion, then treatment with either citric acid foodstuffs, sour lozenges (gustatory therapy), and/or sugarless candies and gum (masticatory therapy) should be initiated. Electrical stimulation is successful in experimentally producing salivary flow but has not proved useful clinically. It is important to recognize that any increase in saliva may benefit patients with xerostomia since it will be accompanied by the production of various beneficial constituents of saliva such as mucins, epidermal growth factor, histatis, bicarbonate, and hydrolytic enzymes (Kaplan &

Baum, 1993). Paradoxically, patients with minimal flow may derive the greatest clinical benefit from only minor increases in salivation, since patients with a greater initial salivary flow may not perceive symptomatic relief produced by an equivalent increase in volume.

Currently only one agent is licensed for the systemic therapy of xerostomia in the United States. Pilocarpine is a parasympathomimetic that functions primarily as a muscarinic agonist and causes pharmacologic stimulation of exocrine glands, resulting in diaphoresis, salivation, lacrimation, and gastric and pancreatic secretion. Pilocarpine has been used successfully in patients with Sjögren's syndrome in one open trial (Fox et al., 1991) as well as in patients with postirradiation xerostomia using 5 mg three times a day (Johnson et al., 1993) with relatively minimal side effects, mostly sweating. Anetholetrithione, a drug that increases muscarinic-cholinergic receptors, is not yet licensed in the United States but has also shown promise as an agent in relieving the symptoms of xerostomia (Fox, 1994).

Parkinson's Disease

Parkinson's disease is characterized clinically by a resting tremor, rigidity, bradykinesia, and postural instability (see also Chapter 11). Only 15–20% of patients with idiopathic Parkinson's disease complain of dysphagia, although up to 95% of patients have demonstrable abnormalities on videofluoroscopy (Lieberman et al., 1980). The defects may include both oral and pharyngeal phase swallowing problems, with impaired tongue propulsion due to lingual musculature rigidity or pharyngeal phase defects, with weak pharyngeal contractions and postdeglutitive vallecular and pyriform sinus residue (Calne, Shaw, & Spiers, 1970). With disease progression, impaired laryngeal closure may result in aspiration (Bushmann, Dobmeyer, Leeker, & Permutter, 1989).

The neuropathology of Parkinson's disease is distinctive with depigmentation of the substantia nigra and decreased production of dopamine in nigro-strial neurons. Most cases of parkinsonism are idiopathic but the Parkinsonian syndrome may accompany other degenerative neurologic diseases such olivopontocerebellar atrophy and progressive supranuclear palsy. It may also follow the use of medications affecting dopaminergic function such as phenothiazines, reserpine, or alpha-methyldopa, as well as carbon monoxide poisoning, heavy metal ingestion, or head trauma.

The resting tremor often begins in the hands then progresses to involve the legs, face, and tongue, and is suppressed by anticholinergic agents such as trihexyphenidyl hydrochloride (Artane) and benztropine mesylate (Cogentin). Although anticholinergic agents are almost universally helpful in the initial control of muscular tremors and skeletal muscle rigidity, the symptoms of bradykinesia and dysphagia may or may not improve with an anticholinergic (Hughes et al., 1993). In fact, the oral and pharyngeal phase defects may even be ex-aggerated by drug use. For example, im-paired bolus containment and poor pro-pulsion due to muscular rigidity may be aggravated by the xerostomia induced by the medication used to treat the disorder.

The mainstays of long-term therapy of Parkinson's disease are predominantly dopamine precursors (levodopa-carbidopa [Sinemet]) or dopamine receptor agonists (bromocriptine [Parlodel], pergolide mesylate [Permax]). Although some studies suggest that the use of selegiline hydrochloride (deprenyl [Eldepryl]) may delay the onset of symptoms in Parkinsonian patients, treatment with selegiline alone results in little symptomatic relief in otherwise untreated patients with Parkinson's disease. Moreover, the role of selegiline with respect to delay of onset of oral-pharyngeal symptoms is unclear (The Parkinson Study Group, 1989, 1993).

Myasthenia Gravis

Myasthenia gravis (see also Chapter 11) is caused by autoimmune destruction of acetylcholine receptors at neuromuscular junctions (Drachman, et al., 1987; Drachman, 1994). The most prominent feature is fluctuating weakness of skeletal muscles. Cranial nerves are almost always involved, particularly the ocular muscles, which accounts for the predilection of initial symptoms relating to ocular findings, such as diploplia and ptosis. Muscles of facial expression, mastication, and swallowing are the next most frequently involved, with dysphagia occurring as a prominent symptom in more than a third of cases (Osserman, 1958). Typically there is increasing muscle weakness with repetitive muscle contraction and improvement with rest. Physical findings are confined to the motor system; loss of reflexes or of sensation are not demonstrable. Radiographic abnormalities include slow tongue movement, impaired lingual bolus formation, and post-swallow residue in the valleculae and pyriform sinuses that is not cleared with repetitive swallowing.

Anticholinesterase agents remain the first line of treatment for myasthenia gravis. These drugs allow acetylcholine that is released at the neuromuscular junction to interact repetitively with the remaining acetylcholine receptors. This results in improved skeletal muscle strength and improvement of dysphagia. Unfortunately improvement is often incomplete and efficacy declines after months. Most patients require surgical thymectomy to induce remission or to reduce immunosuppressive therapy. Immunosupppressive therapy with corticosteroids, azathioprine, or cyclosporine is initiated when symptoms persist despite anticholinesterase therapy. Plasmapheresis to remove circulatory antibodies or intravenous immunoglobulins have been used as temporizing measures yet their use has not been described specifically for dysphagia. Oral administration of acetylcholine receptors to induce tolerance remains to be tested in humans, although it has been found to prevent clinical features of myasthenia gravis in a well-established rat model (Wang, Qiao, & Link, 1993).

Postpolio Dysphagia

Approximately 300,000 survivors of the last poliomyelitis epidemic in the 1950s are at risk for developing the postpolio syndrome (Munsat, 1991). This syndrome is an organic disorder resulting from new or continuing instability of previously injured motor neurons (see also Chapter 11). Typically the postpolio syndrome consists of new musculoskeletal symptoms such as weakness and atrophy in previously affected muscles. Patients become symptomatic 25–35 years after the index infection, and even muscular units that were unaffected in the original infection may develop signs of weakness. Although bulbar neuron involvement has been reported in only 15% of patients with the acute infection, studies have demonstrated that some bulbar muscle dysfunction can be demonstrated in all patients with the postpolio syndrome. Nevertheless, only 11–22% report dysphagia, suggesting that there is a slow progressive deterioration

similar to that observed in limb muscles (Halstead, Wiechers, & Rossi, 1985; Speier, Owen, Knapp, & Canine, 1987). Symptoms of dysphagia are more severe with bulbar involvement during the original infection. Abnormalities most commonly include lingual motor abnormalities with uncontrolled bolus flow into the pharynx and increased tongue-pumping gestures to initiate a swallow, as well as palatal, pharyngeal, and laryngeal weakness (Coelho & Ferrante, 1988; Sonies & Dalakas, 1991). Although pharyngeal weakness is associated with residual material remaining in the pharynx after swallowing, aspiration is infrequent (Sonies & Dalakas, 1991).

There is no specific medical treatment for the postpolio syndrome. Symptomatic patients are treated with compensatory swallowing strategies such as modifications in the swallowing position and changes in ingested food consistencies (Sonies & Dalakas, 1991; Silbergleit, Waring, Sullivan, & Maynard, 1991). The effect of compensatory swallowing strategies and of muscle strengthening exercises over long periods of time is unknown.

Chorea, Dystonia, and Dyskinesia

HUNTINGTON'S CHOREA. Dysphagia is a common complication of Huntington's disease and death usually results from respiratory complications precipitated by aspiration (Edmonds, 1966). There is no known therapy and it is important to recognize that the empiric use of neuroleptics such as phenothiazine to treat the associated choreas have not been effective in ameliorating the oropharyngeal symptoms (Leopold & Kagel, 1985). Moreover, bolus formation, swallow initiation, and transfer may even be adversely affected owing to associated xerostomia from an anticholinergic effect. Whether or not early cessation of oral intake to avoid aspiration delays death from respiratory complications has not been examined.

DYSTONIA. Dystonia is a syndrome characterized by involuntary sustained (tonic) or spasmodic (rapid or clonic) muscle contractions that frequently cause flexing or extending, twisting and squeezing movements, and/or abnormal posture. Dystonias may be primary (sporadic or genetic) or secondary. Although they can be triggered by injury to a peripheral nerve or root, central causes account for the majority of dystonias. Dystonias may be focal or segmental and task-specific (e.g., writer's cramp). Blepharospasm, cervical dystonia (spasmodic torticollis), oromandibular dystonia, and laryngeal dystonia are the most often encountered clinically. Of these, dysphagia is seen exclusively with cervical dystonia and oromandibular dystonia.

If no specifically treatable cause of dystonia can be identified, patients can be offered only symptomatic therapy. Empiric medications such as muscle relaxants and anticholinergics can ameliorate dystonic symptoms in some patients. However, the majority fail to obtain significant relief (Jankovic & Brin, 1991). Chemical denervation with botulinum toxin injection is now considered by many as the treatment of choice for cervical dystonia, blepharospasm, laryngeal dystonia, hemifacial spasm, and certain task-specific dystonias. Botulinum toxin is injected directly into the most strongly contracting muscle (with or without EMG guidance for muscle selection) and exerts its paralytic effect by binding to presynaptic cholinergic nerve terminals, ultimately inhibiting the exocytosis of acetylcholine at the motor end plate. The safety and efficacy of botulinum toxin in the treatment of cervical dystonia has now been demonstrated in several open and controlled trials (Gelb, Lowenstein, & Aminoff, 1989; Greene et al., 1990; Tsui, Eisen, Stoessl, Calne, & Calne, 1986), although a few patients do eventually tachyphylax owing to the development of blocking antibodies. Botulinum toxin injection has not been used effectively to treat the symptom of dysphagia. In fact, it should be recognized that dysphagia has also been reported as a complication of botulinum toxin therapy, particularly when administered to the sternocleidomastoid muscles. Whether this represents a complication of the site of in-jection or a dose-related phenomenon is unclear (Blackie & Lees, 1990; Stell, Thompson, & Marsden, 1988).

TARDIVE DYSKINESIA. This term is applied to an extrapyramidal syndrome characterized by involuntary choreic movements resulting from long-term exposure to neuroleptics such as phenothiazine or even metoclopramide (Miller & Janovic, 1989). Movements are stereotypical, complex, and affect the face, limbs, or trunk. The movements are considered to be secondary to dopamine receptor supersensitivity, and although symptoms can be suppressed by increasing neuroleptic dose (Greene, Shale, & Fahn, 1988), this can also exacerbate symptoms. Remission sometimes results from termination of neuroleptic use but this is unusual (Kang, Burke, & Fahn, 1986). Botulinum A toxin injection to paralyze affected muscles has been used to treat tardive dyskinesias with limited success (Blackie & Lees, 1990; Maurri & Barontini, 1990), although specific use for dysphagia has not been described.

Polymyositis

Polymyositis is an idiopathic acquired inflammatory myopathy. The chronic muscle inflammation, demonstrable histologically by muscle biopsy, is responsible for the clinical syndrome characterized by acute or subacute muscular pain, tenderness, and weakness with ultimate atrophy and fibrosis of muscles (Kagen, Hochman, & Strong, 1985; Plotz et al., 1989). The associated dysphagia may be due to impaired strength of oropharyngeal musculature or disordered pharyngoesophageal opening (Kagen et al., 1985; Plotz et al., 1989). Treatment for myositis requires immunosuppressive therapy, usually with corticosteroids or other immunosuppressive agents such as azathioprine and methotrexate. Although corticosteroids are usually chosen as first line agents there has been no demonstration of improvement in survival of steroid-treated patients (Carpenter, Bunch, Engel, & O'Brien, 1977), although patients receiving high-dose corticosteroids do have less morbidity than patients receiving no treatment (Carpenter et al., 1977). The presence of significant dysphagia has been touted as a possible marker for those patients with a worse 1-year survival (Hochberg, Feldman, & Stevens, 1986), implying a possible benefit of early recognition and treatment. However, validated and reproducible measures of oropharyngeal muscle strength and functional status as outcome variables have not been studied.

Outcomes Research

Although it would have been optimal to present the information regarding medical intervention by describing types of economic analysis of health care interventions such as cost-of-treatment, cost-effectiveness cost-utility, cost-benefit, or even cost-of-illness, the literature regarding medical or surgical therapy of dysphagia is limited and simply has not been approached in this manner. In the absence of such information more fundamental issues such as which criteria might be considered measures of effectiveness should be contemplated.

Research in the medical and surgical treatment for dysphagia has generally relied on anecdotal experience detailing improvement in the subjective sensation of dysphagia. In contrast, measures of effectiveness utilized in outcomes research would encompass symptomatic as well as objective measures of benefit. For example symptomatic benefits might include an improved sense of swallowing or ease of swallowing. Objective findings of changes in swallow function might include increased muscle strength, improved coordination, decreased number of choking or aspiration episodes, decreased nasopharyngeal regurgitation, reduced number of hospitalizations, or weight gain. These findings might be demonstrable videofluoroscopically with decreased pharyngeal residue or a reduction in swallow delay. The ultimate measures of effectiveness could range from a life saved, a life-year saved, a case of dis-

ease averted, or a quality-adjusted life-year saved reflected by reduced associated morbidities such as an improvement in weight, nutritional status, bronchopulmonary disease, or aspiration events. These variables could be assessed after any type of medical or surgical therapy, allowing, for example, evaluation of swallow function in Parkinson's disease after therapeutic use of levodopa.

The most difficult areas to assess are general items such as alertness and cognition which, if improved, might allow patients to better follow directions in improving muscle strength, range of motion, or oral sensory awareness, which would be useful in other settings such as in learning compensatory or rehabilitative swallow techniques.

SURGICAL MANAGEMENT OF IMPAIRED BOLUS TRANSIT

The common goals of both medical and surgical treatment of oropharyngeal dysphagia are to improve impaired bolus transit through the oropharynx and to minimize or prevent aspiration (Baredes, 1988; Halama, 1994). This is best accomplished by first appreciating normal swallowing physiology then defining specific dysfunction in the individual patient. Furthermore, surgery should be contemplated only in conjunction with or after attempts of swallowing rehabilitation since, in the absence of a mechanical obstruction, compensatory and indirect biofeedback therapy can return more than 80% of patients with oropharyngeal dysphagia to oral intake (Rademaker et al., 1993). Thus, surgical approaches to oropharyngeal swallowing disorders are usually not considered until all behavioral methods fail a 6-month therapeutic trial (Logemann 1994).

Oral Stage of Swallowing

The oral stage of swallowing is divided into a preparatory phase during which the bolus is manipulated by being chewed, lubricated, and held in the central groove of the tongue, and the lingual propulsion phase during which the bolus is propelled posteriorly into the pharynx. Many structural abnormalities may compromise these tasks by inhibiting manipulation and/or bolus formation and propulsion. In general, surgical treatment is aimed at reconstructing structural defects due to cancer treatment or congenital defects such as webs. Dysphagias due to oral stage problems respond best to swallowing therapy.

Pharyngeal Stage of Swallowing

Pharyngeal stage swallowing defects are some of the most difficult and distressing disorders to deal with. Bolus transport may be compromised by luminal and extraluminal causes that may be neoplastic, neuropathic, myopathic, or traumatic in origin. It is with pharyngeal stage dysfunction that laryngeal competence should also be considered because of its cardinal role in preventing aspiration. Therefore, surgical manipulations can be aimed at improving bolus transit or preventing or minimizing aspiration.

Cervical Osteophytes

It is unclear how often radiologically significant cervical osteophytes actually result in dysphagia. Estimates in the literature describe symptomatic hypertrophic cervical osteophytes of the anterior cervical vertebrae occurring in up to 6–22% of the elderly population (Bone, Namum, & Harris, 1990; Saffouri & Ward, 1974). Dysphagia is felt to be mechanical in origin either as a result of extrinsic compression of the pharynx or from periesophageal inflammation by pharyngoesphageal motion over the cervical exostoses predominantly at the C3-C6 vertebral locations (Papandoulos et al., 1989). Development of osteophytes may be related to DISH (diffuse idiopathic skeletal hyperostosis ankylosing spondylosis), infectious spondylosis, previous surgical fusion of the cervical vertebrae, local trauma, as well as be idiopathic in origin (Halama, 1994). Surgical treatment remains controversial. Objective criteria have not been consistently used to assess surgical results; moreover, short-term results have been used to assess long-term outcome without longitudinal follow-up. In view of these limitations, most feel surgery should be performed only for those with severe dysphagia in whom conservative treatment has failed (Halama, 1994).

Essentially three surgical approaches are used to remove hypertrophic cervical osteophytes (Halama, 1994). The most common is the anterolateral extrapharyngeal approach. The left side is preferentially chosen and cervical vertebrae C2–C7 can be approached with good exposure. The second approach is posterior and extrapharyngeal; this approach is used for access to the cervical spine above C3. The third approach is transorally and is successful in providing exposure to the C1–C4 vertebrae. Complications include vocal fold paralysis or paresis. Rarer problems include vertebral disc prolapse, fistula, hematoma, infection, aspiration, and Horner's syndrome (Welsh, Welsh, & Chinnici, 1987).

Cricopharyngeal Myotomy

The most common and best understood use of cricopharyngeal myotomy has been in the treatment of hypopharyngeal diverticula (symptomatic outpouching through the muscular pharyngeal wall above the cricopharyngeus muscle). Diverticula can occur throughout the hypopharynx but when hypopharyngeal diverticula are located posteriorly between the intersection of the transverse fibers of the cricopharyngeus and obliquely oriented fibers of the inferior pharyngeal constrictors (Killian's dehiscence), they are called *Zenker's diverticula*, in recognition of the German pathologist Friedrich Albert von Zenker (Figure 16–1). Although Zenker felt that the pathogenesis of hypopharyngeal herniation was due to abnormally high hypopharyngeal pressures caused by defective coordination of the upper

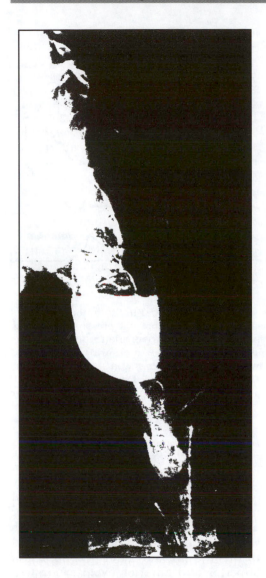

Figure 16–1. Radiograph of a Zenker's diverticulum. (With permission from G. A. Ergun and P. J. Kahrilas, (1993). Oropharyngeal dysphagia in the elderly. *Practical Gastroenterology, 17,* 9–16.)

esophageal sphincter (UES) relaxation during pharyngeal bolus propulsion, demonstration of this incoordination was never conclusively proven.

PATHOPHYSIOLOGY OF ZENKER'S DIVERTICULA. This pathophysiology of Zenker's diverticula has been clarified by Cook and colleagues using simultaneous videoradiography and manometry to study pharyngeal coordination, UES opening, and flow pressures during swallowing in 14 patients with symptomatic Zenker's diverticula (Cook, Gabb, et al., 1992). These investigators found normal timings of sphincter relaxation, opening, and closure, signifying normal coordination of the actions between the pharynx and the sphincter. The extent of hyoid bone and laryngeal movement, both contributing to the anterior traction forces that pull open the UES, were normal but hypopharyngeal intrabolus pressures were abnormally increased (Figure 16–2). This suggests that although the sphincter relaxed normally, it opened incompletely. This suggests that the disorder is caused by poor sphincter compliance rather than pharyngeal-sphincter incoordination, impaired opening forces on the sphincter, or cricopharyngeal spasm (Cook, 1993), favoring a primary morphologic abnormality of the cricopharyngeus muscle increasing resistance to bolus passage. Examination of cricopharyngeal muscle specimens excised from patients undergoing myotomy for Zenker's diverticulum supported this concept, showing pathologic atrophy and fibrosis. Moreover, in vitro contractility studies of these specimens showed slower and weaker contraction curves compared to normal muscle (Cook, Blumbergs, Cash, Jamieson, & Shearman, 1992; Lerut, van Raemdonck, Guelinckx, Dom, & Gebaes, 1992).

TREATMENT OF ZENKER'S DIVERTICULUM. This is predominantly surgical, consisting of a cricopharyngeal myotomy (see Chapter 12) coupled with either excision of the diverticulum or diverticulopexy. Most surgeons traditionally perform an external diverticulectomy combined with a myotomy through a left cervical incision with good to excellent relief of symptoms in 90% of operated patients and an operative mortality of approximately 1% (Feussner, Kauer, & Siewert, 1993; Lindgren & Ekberg, 1990). Endoscopic treatment with permucosal myotomy without diverticulopexy or diverticulum

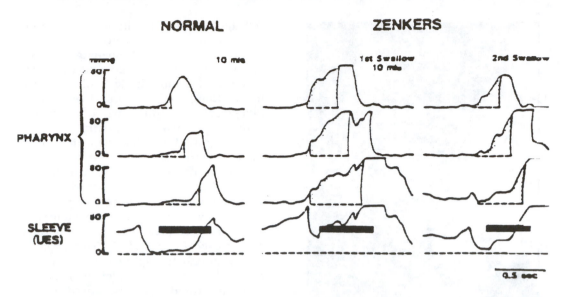

Figure 16–2. Manometric tracing during a swallow with 10 ml liquid barium in a normal control and a patient with Zenker's diverticulum. The values on the *y* axis represent pressure in mmHg, with the top three panels showing tracings at three locations in the pharynx and the lowest tracing in the UES. Note that the tracing in Zenker's has much higher intrabolus pressure waves (stippled areas) than those in the normals and that UES opening duration (solid bars) was shorter. (With permission from I. J. Cook, M. Gabb, V. Panagopoulos, G. G. Jamieson, W. J. Dodds, J. Dent, & D. J. Shearman, 1992. Pharyngeal [Zenker's] diverticulum is a disorder of upper esophageal sphincter opening. *Gastroenterology. 103*, 1229–1235.)

excision has been described in a large Dutch series (Wouters & van Overbeek, 1992) but this has not been performed extensively in the United States or Europe. Most surgeons still prefer external diverticulectomy combined with myotomy (Halama, 1994). The prevalence, etiology, and recurrence rate of the myopathy (after myotomy) is unknown.

Cricopharyngeal Myotomy for Dysfunctions of the Pharyngoesophageal Junction

MECHANISMS RESPONSIBLE FOR DYS-FUNCTION OF THE PHARYNGOESO-PHAGEAL JUNCTION. Myotomy has also been performed to treat pharyngoesophagel dysfunction due to other causes. The biomechanical determinants of UES opening and laryngeal elevation are largely dependent on anterior traction via the hyoid axis. Thus, although UES relaxation occurs during the swallow-associat-ed laryngeal elevation, UES opening occurs later, resulting from traction on the anterior sphincter wall caused by contraction of the supra- and infrahyoid musculature. Sphincter opening diameter and duration increase with larger bolus volumes and are related to increased intrabolus pressure and persistence of superior and anterior hyoid excursion, respectively. Consequently, pharyngoesophageal segment dysfunction may occur when any aspect of this mechanism is impaired, be it laryngeal elevation, sphincter opening, or hyoid excursion. This, too, should explain why the term *cricopharyngeal achalasia* is a misnomer. The cricopharyngeus is a striated muscle, which is dependent on tonic excitation to maintain contractility. If innervation to the cricopharyngeus is lost, the sphincter becomes flaccid, not contracted. Therefore, impaired opening results from failure of traction, or pulling open, rather than a failure of relaxation.

CRICOPHARYNGEAL BAR. This term refers to an impingement of the lumen of the pharyngoesophageal junction as seen radiographically during swallowing studies. It is important to recognize both that the pharyngoesophageal segment may be obstructive to bolus transit *without* the presence of a hypopharyngeal diverticulum and that the presence of a cricopharyngeal bar may very well confuse the picture in a dysphagic patient. This confusion persists because the functional significance of a cricopharyngeal bar is variable and the role of the cricopharyngeal bar in dysphagia is not easily ascertained. The incidence of cricopharyngeal bar increases with age, being reported in approximately 5% of elderly nondysphagic subjects (Ekberg & Nylander, 1982). Retrospective reviews of radiologic studies report a prevalence of 5–11%, with dysphagia reported in only 15% of these (Ekberg & Nylander, 1982). Thus it appears that the cricopharyngeal bar contributes to dysphagia in only a minority of cases in which it is identified. However, the relative contribution of a cricopharyngeal bar to the symptom of dysphagia increases in the presence of coexisting abnormalities of pharyngeal function. Cricopharyngeal myotomy is indicated in the dysphagic patient with a cricopharyngeal bar in whom the bar has been documented to be obstructive to bolus flow, with increased intrabolus pressures and decreased transphincteric flow rate evident during manometry and fluoroscopy. Whether the cricopharyngeal bar shares the myopathy observed with Zenker's diverticula and whether obstructive symptoms respond to passive dilatation (e.g., bougienage) remains unanswered.

Cricopharyngeal myotomies have also been performed in order to relieve dysphagia due to cricopharyngeal dysfunction associated with cervical esophageal stenosis, neurologic diseases (CNS or peripheral), muscular diseases, and Parkinson's disease. To date, there has been no definitive analysis of the efficacy of a myotomy under these circumstances. However, in one review of cricopharyngeal myotomy performed on 60 patients suf-

fering from cervical dysphagia of varied cause, division of the muscle created a symptom-free interval in all patients for 2 to 10 years postoperatively (Lindgren & Ekberg, 1990). Of interest, close to two thirds (37) of these patients had a Zenker's diverticulum, which one would expect to respond favorably to the surgery. Similarly, in 10 patients, myotomy was used to treat an obstructive problem due to cervical esophageal web and postcricoid stenosis, with the expected relief. The remaining 13 patients were subdivided into neuromuscular disease (9 patients) and cricopharyngeal achalasia (4 patients). The results were extremely disappointing in patients with neuromuscular disease, with only temporary improvement of dysphagia before progression of the underlying disease. Of the patients labeled with "cricopharyngeal achalasia," 2 had cricopharyngeal bars and only those 2 responded to myotomy. This literature suggests that cricopharyngeal myotomy only results in improvement of oropharyngeal dysphagia if it interrupts a primary process affecting sphincter opening or if it relieves obstruction to bolus flow. An example of the former is cricopharyngeal myopathy in conjunction with hypopharyngeal diverticula. Possible examples of the latter are impaired hypopharyngeal opening due to paralysis, or fibrosis of the suprahyoid muscles due to dermatomyositis or radiation, or impaired elevation of the larynx after laryngectomy. Those usages for myotomy, however, have not been subject to critical analysis. Cricopharyngeal myotomy is not generally a treatment for aspiration attributable to neurologic causes. Patients with difficulty in all phases of swallowing due to neurologic impairment receive little or no benefit from cricopharyngeal myotomy (Blitzer, 1990).

RISKS OF CRICOPHARYNGEAL MYOTOMY. Cricopharyngeal myotomy as a treatment for dysphagia also has inherent limitations that must be considered. For example, if there is absence of laryngeal elevation, cricopharyngeal myotomy will not improve opening. Furthermore, the eradication of normal cricopharyngeal function effectively removes the only natural barrier for aspiration of gastric contents should reflux to the proximal esophagus occur. In fact, if there is impaired laryngeal competence, a cricopharyngeal myotomy could be disastrous in a patient with vigorous gastroesophageal reflux such that a concomitant fundoplication may be necessary to eradicate reflux. How often pharyngeal regurgitation and aspiration occurs as a result of cricopharyngeal myotomy is unknown.

Operations for Deglutitive Aspiration

Chronic aspiration is a life-threatening and debilitating aspect of deglutitive dysfunction. Aspiration may occur as a result of an impaired swallow, allowing ingesta to overwhelm a competent larynx, or it may occur as a result of a normal swallow in the presence of an incompetent laryngeal closure mechanism. Consequently, swallowing therapists have focused on behavioral strategies to modify an abnormal swallow to augment protective airway mechanisms. Surgical solutions have similarly focused on ways to augment protective airway mechanisms or circumvent dysfunction. Surgeons have struggled to define the optimal surgical design. Sasaki defines the *optimal* surgery as a "simple, reliable, and potentially reversible procedure to restore normal speech and swallowing" (Sasaki, Milmoe, & Yanagisawa, 1990, p. 422.). Surgical alternatives in the oropharynx can be categorized as *conservative* if preserving both speech and swallowing function, and as radical if permanently separating the deglutitive conduit from the airway.

Conservative Procedures

VOCAL FOLD AUGMENTATION OR MEDIALIZATION. Mild cases of aspiration due to impaired vocal fold movement may be amenable to treatment with vocal fold augmentation (see Chapter 12). Vocal fold augmentation is advocated for a sympto-

matic open glottis due to mechanical impairment or neuromuscular disability that prevents contralateral fold adduction. If vocal fold medialization is necessary for a relatively short period of time, as with recovery from neurologic insult, an absorbable item such as gelfoam, collagen, fat, or glycerine may be injected directly into the vocal fold. Should there be no hope of functional improvement, then either medialization can be performed (see Chapter 12) or Teflon, which is not absorbed and not easily removed from the larynx, may be injected into the vocal fold via direct laryngoscopy under local anesthesia (Figure 16–3) (Ward, Hanson, & Abemayor, 1985). Generally, surgery is avoided for at least 6 months after the initial injury unless it is absolutely certain that the recurrent laryngeal nerve or vagus was severed during surgery. In patients with larger laryngeal defects where Teflon may not be adequate, more permanent augmentations may be performed using auto-genous costochondral, nasal septal, thyroid cartilage, or silastic block implants (Blitzer, Krespi, Oppenheimer, & Levine, 1988).

Justification for these procedures derives from the attempt to preserve speech. Unfortunately, there have been no controlled studies of the efficacy of vocal fold augmentation or medialization in controlling aspiration or in improving glottic closure using radiologic or endoscopic examinations.

LARYNGEAL SUSPENSION PROCEDURES. Disruption of the normal relationship between the base of the tongue, pharynx, and larynx after ablative head and neck surgery, neoplasm, or trauma can prevent normal laryngeal function during swallowing, with aspiration resulting from compromised airway protection. Patients with this type of aspiration may benefit from a laryngeal suspension procedure. A midline anteriorly based suspension has been advocated by Calcaterra (1971). In this suspension a nonabsorbable suture is placed from the mandible or other anterior structure and is sewn to the thyroid lamina anteriorly, tilting and raising the larynx to a position

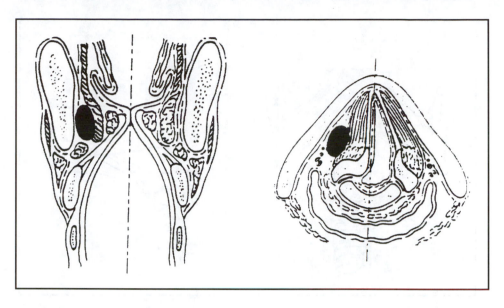

Figure 16–3. Teflon injection for unilateral vocal fold paralysis. The left figure (coronal view) demonstrates a Teflon bolus injection (black oval) pushing the entire vocalis muscle mass medially. On the right is the horizontal view. (With permission from B. J. Bailey, and H. F. Biller, H. F., (Eds.), 1985. *Surgery of the Larynx.* Philadelphia: W. B. Saunders.)

under the base of the tongue removed from the bolus path to avoid aspiration during swallowing (Figure 16–4) (Calcaterra, 1971; Edgerton & Duncan, 1959; Hillel & Goode, 1983). Variations on this procedure have been reported in which a lateral suspension from the mandibular condyle is intended to increase pharyngeal opening and thereby further increase laryngeal protection (Hillel & Goode, 1983). Lastly, Kashima (1986) described a correction for impaired laryngeal elevation by suturing the digastric sling to the strap muscles below the line of the pharyngomyotomy. He suggested that the laryngeal elevation would be enhanced by partial division or denervation of the infrahyoid strap muscles. There have been no controlled studies comparing these procedures at present.

NOVEL THERAPIES INCLUDING EPIGLOT-TOPLASTY AND PARTIAL CRICOID RESEC-TION. The repertoire of surgical procedures for treating aspiration that preserve both speech and swallowing function is limited. Novel therapies directed at extra-

glottic causes of aspiration have been attempted using videofluoroscopy to guide to specific surgery (Mendelsohn, 1993). For example, in one report of two patients, detailed preoperative barium examination, in one case, demonstrated a loss of bolus control during the oral stage with spillage over the epiglottis into the larynx before the pharyngeal stage was triggered. In the second case, videofluoroscopy revealed severe hypopharyngeal residue, with aspiration in conjunction with impaired laryngeal elevation and bolus obstruction at the pharyngoesophageal segment. In the first case, epiglottoplasty was performed to create a protective roof over the airway, and in the second case, a translaryngeal resection of the cricoid lamina with cricopharyngeal myotomy was performed to control the aspiration of hypopharyngeal residue. Both patients were able to resume oral feeding (Mendel-sohn, 1993).

Radical Procedures

Radical procedures to alleviate deglutitive aspiration are defined as those that per-

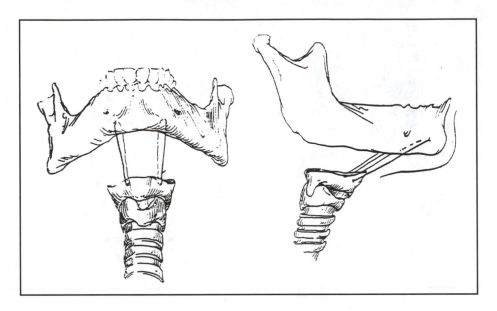

Figure 16–4. Laryngeal suspension. The larynx is repositioned anteriorly and superiorly via suspension sutures from the mandible. (With permission from B. J. Bailey, and H. F. Biller, (Eds.), 1985. *Surgery of the Larynx.* Philadelphia: W. B. Saunders.)

manently divert the deglutitive stream from the airway and include glottic prostheses, laryngeal closure (glottic and supraglottic closure) with tracheotomy, laryngeal diversion, or laryngectomy. None of these procedures preserve glottic function so all result in tracheotomies with impairment or complete elimination of normal speech.

GLOTTIC STENTS. Glottic stents are custom-made prostheses that are placed in the larynx endoscopically and held in place with percutaneous sutures (Weisberger & Huesbsch, 1982). Stents were designed to separate food and air passage without the need of an inflated cuffed tracheotomy tube (Figure 16–5). A modification described by Eliachar and Miller (1994) further allows for phonation and simplified tube placement. With this modification, the patient has a tracheotomy for an airway and the silicon stent is inserted through the tracheotomy below the glottis and extends through the vocal folds. At the superior end of the stent is a dome with a slit in it which, in theory,

occludes the larynx to prevent aspiration but allows phonation through the slit. Use of laryngeal stents has not become widespread. Use has been primarily for a short-term basis (months) in patients in whom laryngeal function is expected to return.

The complications of laryngeal stent placement are related to local discomfort, laryngeal inflammation with subsequent scarring, leakage around the prosthesis due to poor sealing, and the patients' inability to phonate. Although laryngeal stenting has been attractive to surgeons because of the low morbidity, they have not achieved the kind of popularity or predictable result associated with radical surgeries.

LARYNGEAL CLOSURES. Laryngeal closures procedures were devised to create an adequate division of food and air passages while attempting to avoid the tracheal damage that accompanies a constantly inflated cuffed tracheotomy tube. They were also designed as potentially reversible procedures that could be done electively after tracheotomy and patient stabilization.

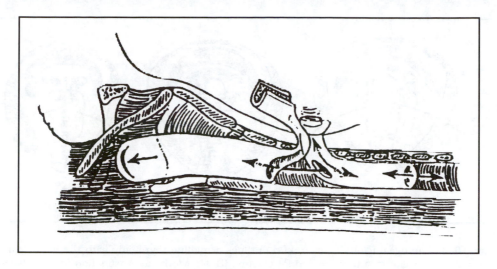

Figure 16–5. Glottic stent. (Adapted from C. W. Cummings [Ed.], 1993. *Otolaryngology–Head and Neck Surgery* [2nd ed]. St. Louis: Mosby-Year Book.)

Laryngeal closures may be categorized anatomically as closures performed at supraglottic, glottic, and subglottic levels. Habal reported a potentially reversible horizontal closure of the supraglottis utilizing an epiglottic flap. In this procedure, via pharyngotomy, the glossoepiglottic ligaments are cut, the lateral margins of the epiglottis, aryepiglottic folds, and arytenoids are denuded of mucosa, and the epiglottis is tilted over the arytenoids and sutured posteriorly to the aryepiglottic folds and arytenoid (Habal & Murray, 1972). In a second layer, the mucosa of the pyriform sinus is distributed over the epiglottis and patients breathe through a noncuffed tracheotomy tube. This was accompanied by a cricopharyngeal myotomy and anterior laryngeal suspension. Vertical supraglottic closure in which a small opening is left at the level of the tip of the epiglottis, allowing phonation in some patients but avoiding aspiration, was reported 11 years later (Biller, Lawson, & Baek, 1983). Although touted as a reversible procedure, only one reversal has been reported for this particular procedure. The most common problem with this type of surgery is separation of the epiglottis from the larynx postoperatively, such that success is reported in only

slightly more than half of patients examined (Eisele, 1991).

Kitahara reported successful laryngeal closure at the level of the false folds through a laryngofissure. In this procedure suture material is sewn along an incised line made on the convexities of the false fold and continued across the posterior commissure. Fast-hardening glue is then applied along the lines of suture to close the larynx. The authors reported successful laryngeal reopening 6 months after primary surgery, without aspiration and with adequate phonation (Kitahara et al., 1993).

The glottic closure procedure was initially described by Montgomery (1975). In this procedure the vocal folds are denuded of mucosa bilaterally and the glottis is closed via a figure-of-eight suture positioned such that fibrosis with union of the vocal folds ensues (Figure 16–6). Unfortunately, although described as potentially reversible, the laryngeal webs that invariably develop are difficult to remove and the vocal folds do not function properly upon removal of the suture, owing to scarring. Moreover, if the vocal folds were functional preoperatively, the union or seal often pulls apart before healing, with resultant posterior leaking. These compli-

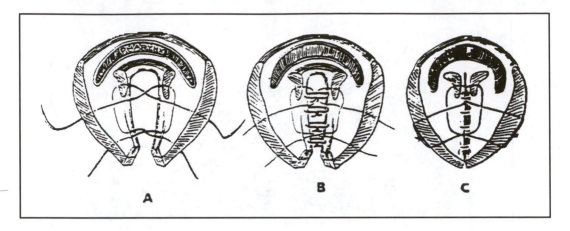

Figure 16–6. Laryngeal (glottic) closure. (A) outlines a midline thyrotomy with the glottic mucosa removed and transglottic sutures placed for closure. (B) shows the approximation of the false vocal folds. (C) depicts the closed glottis. (With permission from C. W. Cummings [Ed.], 1993. *Otolaryngology–Head and Neck Surgery* [2nd ed.]. St. Louis: Mosby-Year Book.)

cations have prompted modifications utilizing a sternocleidomastoid muscle flap interposed into the subglottic region to improve sealing (Sasaki et al., 1990) but this made reversibility more difficult. Thus glottic closure is recommended in patients in whom laryngeal function is not expected to return. Success rates in eliminating deglutitive aspiration of up to 93% have been reported (Eisele, 1991).

Subglottic closures or laryngeal diversion procedures are highly successful in eliminating aspiration but leave the patient without a voice and with a permanent tracheostoma. The procedures are designed to separate the lower respiratory tract from the upper digestive tract without affecting the glottic and supraglottic parts of the larynx (also see Chapter 12). The two basic surgical procedures are the tracheoesophageal diversion and laryngotracheal separation. Tracheoesophageal separation was first described by Lindeman in 1975 (Yaring-ton, Lindeman, & Sutton, 1976; Figure 16–7). In this surgery the subglottic trachea is severed at the third or fourth ring and the distal portion is brought out and sewn to the skin of the neck as a tracheotomy. A small hole is made in the esophagus at the level of the proximal tracheal stump and the edges of

the esophageal aperture are sutured to the proximal trachea, creating an end-to-side anastomosis. This method allows all saliva or ingesta entering the larynx to exit into the esophagus while allowing for complete separation of the airway. Unfortunately, there can be no phonation with this procedure. However, if the patient recovers enough deglutitive function, the procedure is reversible and several successful reversals have been reported (Lindeman, 1975).

Laryngotracheal separation was designed for patients with very proximal tracheotomies (preventing the tracheoesophageal anastomosis) and persistent aspiration. In this procedure the laryngotracheal separation is done by dividing the trachea horizontally at the level of the second or third tracheal ring or at the level of the tracheotomy. The proximal tracheal segment is then closed, left as a blind pouch, and the distal portion is extruded through the skin as a stoma (Figure 16–8). Secretion accumulation within the blind pouch was not found to be problematic.

Several alternative separation and diversion procedures have marked the literature since the original one described by Lindeman, each incorporating some modification to make the technique either easi-

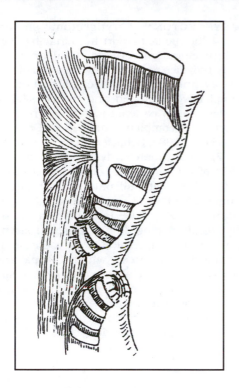

Figure 16–7. Tracheoesophageal diversion. (With permission from C. W. Cummings [Ed.], 1993. *Otolaryngology—Head and Neck Surgery* [2nd ed.]. St. Louis: Mosby-Year Book.)

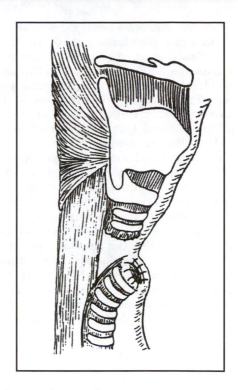

Figure 16–8. Laryngotracheal separation. Note how the proximal edges of the trachea are closed as a blind pouch. (With permission from C. W. Cummings [Ed.], 1993. *Otolaryngology—Head and Neck Surgery* [2nd ed.]. St. Louis: Mosby-Year Book.)

er to perform, or less complicated (based on site of tracheotomy), thereby utilizing less surgical time while maintaining adequate diversion (Baron & Dedo, 1908; Krespi & Sisson, 1985; McIlwain, Bryce, Gilbert, & Grace, 1991). Favorable results in controlling aspiration have been reported with these modifications such that most patients are able to tolerate oral diets after surgery (Eisele, 1991). Nonetheless, the laryngotracheal separation is preferred over the tracheo-esophageal separation because the technically difficult aspect of performing the additional tracheoesophageal anastomosis is avoided.

TRACHEOTOMY. The most common procedure performed for controlling aspiration is still a tracheotomy with a cuffed tube, and

many would argue that this is still the procedure of choice in treating chronic aspiration (see related discussions in Chapters 4 and 5). Tracheotomy does partially protect the lower respiratory tract from material that passes the laryngeal sphincter and permits adequate pulmonary toilet in patients with compromised pulmonary function. However, its effectiveness decreases as the volume of aspirated material increases. In fact, the major swallowing disorder associated with tracheotomy is aspiration. Although many physicians perceive tracheotomy as a solution to long-term aspiration, in reality, it may pose more problems with posttracheotomy aspiration than it actually solves (Nash, 1988). Tracheotomy potentially increases aspiration by limiting laryngeal elevation during swallow, compromises laryngeal sensitivity with loss of a coordinated glottic closure reflex (Sasaki et al., 1977), and decreases the patient's ability to generate adequate subglottic pressure to produce an effective cough (Figure 16–9). Prolonged use of an inflated cuff may cause tracheal stenosis and the inflated tracheotomy cuff may interfere with swallowing by compressing the esophagus. Additionally, accumulated secretions and saliva retained above the cuff result in eventual leakage especially when the cuff is periodically deflated. Thus, the tracheotomy may not necessarily control aspiration and has the extreme potential for aggravating the situation. Finally, the tracheotomy usually does not permit the patient with severe aspiration to resume oral feeding. In view of these limitations, the use of tracheotomy as a treatment of aspiration should be discouraged (Halama, 1994).

LARYNGECTOMY. Laryngectomy should always be the last resort in managing deglutitive aspiration. Although total laryngectomy provides a complete separation of the airway and food passage, phonation is completely eliminated and the possibility for reversal in patients who might recover function is completely abolished (Cannon & McLean, 1982; Schaefer, Close, & Reisch, 1987). Unfortunately, dysphagia is a side effect of the procedure, occurring 10–58% of the time, with all patients exhibiting altered swallowing mechanisms (Jung & Adams, 1980). The lack of pharyngoesphageal opening due to impaired laryngeal elevation necessitates an increase in tongue driving forces, which the patient may or may not be able to compensate for. Furthermore, overall morbidity is increased with extensive resections.

In summary, structural anomalies preventing normal swallowing can usually be

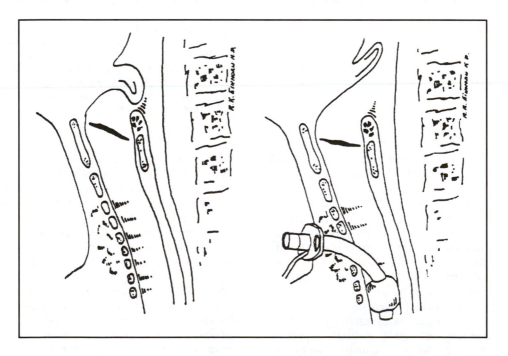

Figure 16–9. Mechanical restriction of laryngeal elevation due to the presence of a tracheotomy tube. The figure on the left shows the normal elevation of the larynx during swallowing, while the figure on the right shows the impaired laryngeal excursion. (With permission from M. Nash, 1988. Swallowing Problems in the Tracheotomized Patient. *Otolaryngologic Clinics of North America, 21,* 701–709.)

compensated for surgically, but neuro-muscular diseases causing significant aspiration are much more difficult to treat surgically. Surgical therapy should be based on a complete understanding of the normal sequence of swallowing and surgery should be designed to address the specific dysfunction identified by a thorough evaluation. If the surgical goal is not clearly identified, the result is often disappointing, merely achieving the irreversible mechanical separation between air and foodway but without predictable functional gain. This can result in situations where the consequences of treatment may be as difficult for the patient to tolerate as the underlying disease itself.

Future approaches to the management of deglutitive aspiration may include artificial dynamic control of the incompetent larynx. Implantable pressure sensors and nerve stimulators offer the potential of allowing the vocal folds to close during swallowing and remain open during inspiratory effort. Preliminary canine experiments have demonstrated that pharyngeal pressure could be detected by prosthetic surfaces implanted in situ and used to trigger vocal fold closure by the coordinated stimulation of the recurrent laryngeal nerve (Broniatowski et al., 1987; Broniatowski, Iiyes, Jacobs, Nose, & Tucker, 1988; Broniatowski et al., 1990). Thus, although not yet tested in the humans, exciting research looms on the horizon as a potential solution for chronic aspiration without ablative surgery.

NUTRITIONAL SUPPORT BYPASSING OROPHARYNGEAL SWALLOWING

Indications for Cessation of Oral Intake

In dysphagia, one must determine the adequacy of oral intake. Nutritional support is needed to alleviate inadequate fluid or caloric intake as well as to enhance chances for recovery from coexistent ill-nesses. Yet attempts to decrease morbidity or mortality may conflict with quality of life.

Termination of oral intake is never easy in a conscious patient. However, it is a decision that is easier to make if the patient is dysphagic and is unable to maintain adequate oral intake despite behavioral, medical, or conservative surgical treatments for the underlying condition. Similarly, the choice is simplified if there are associated complications related to oral intake such as aspiration pneumonia making oral intake unacceptable. It is harder to recommend the cessation of oral intake if symptoms are infrequent, unpredictable, unverified by functional studies, and if nutritional status is seemingly maintained. All in all, although difficult, the decision for nonoral feeding must be made by weighing the risks and the benefits of all approaches with patients and their families.

Nonoral Feeding Options

The delivery of nutrients into the gastrointestinal tract through a feeding tube is the preferred method of feeding patients unable to ingest an adequate quantity of nutrients or calories by mouth but who have a functional digestive tract. In addition to being less expensive (Table 16–2), enteral nutrition provides important nutrients not present in total parenteral nutrition, including glutamine and short-chain fatty acids. Furthermore, there is better preservation of both intestinal absorptive and immune function.

Delivery of nutrients to the gastrointestinal tract can be performed in a variety of manners, via either nasogastric tubes, or endoscopically or surgically placed gastrostomy or jejunostomy feeding tubes (Kirby, DeLegge, & Fleming, 1995). Modern, small-diameter, flexible feeding tubes have eliminated much of the discomfort associated with the larger bore catheters used in the past. Because of the discomfort, larger tubes can only be left in place for brief periods without causing tissue irritation or pressure necrosis. Small diameter tubes, however,

TABLE 16–2. Comparative costs for enteral and parenteral feeding.

Drug Type	Enteral Feeding	Parenteral Feeding
First week nursing visits	$402	$670
Subsequent week nursing	—	$134
Week of feeding solutions	$425	$4306
First month therapy	$2102	$18,430

work well in providing temporary nutritional supplementation in patients who can eat, but require supplementation, or in temporarily debilitated patients (e.g., unconsciousness or on tracheal intubation) with a completely functional gastrointestinal tract. A gastrostomy tube is indicated when transnasal passage of a tube is impossible or when long-term feeding is anticipated.

Gastrostomies

The standard surgical gastrostomy was first successfully performed in 1876 and provided feeding access through a large bore (24–30 French) catheter. Placement of gastrostomies requires laparotomy usually with general anesthesia, thereby placing debilitated patients at increased risk. The reported complication rates of surgical gastrostomy have not changed much in the pediatric or adult literature since the late 1940s, with major and minor complication rates varying from 4 to 35% (Dye & Paterson, 1984); the overwhelming majority report less than 9% for both.

The development of an endoscopic procedure for gastrostomy tube placement (percutaneous endoscopic (PEG) tube) has effectively replaced the traditional surgical gastrostomy and is considered the procedure of choice in most patients (Table 16–3). The technique has become a bedside procedure, does not require general anesthesia, is relatively safe, and is easy to perform. Percutaneous gastrostomy is well-tolerated, and in most patients, feedings can commence within 24 hours of tube placement. Usually the patient's diet can be advanced to the appropriate caloric intake within 1 week.

There are two methods of percutaneous gastrostomy tube placement; the "pull" and "push" techniques. The Ponsky-Gauderer technique is the most widely used pull-through method (Gauderer, Ponsky, & Izant, 1980; Gauderer & Pinsky, 1981). The patient is fasted 8–12 hours before placement and the procedure may be performed under conscious sedation. An endoscope is passed into the stomach. The stomach is then insufflated with the endoscope and the site for gastrostomy placement is selected at a point of bright transillumination through the anterior abdominal wall. The skin is punctured at this site with a large-gauge catheter and the catheter is identified within the stomach endoscopically. A silk suture or plastic line is passed through the plastic cannula into the stomach, grasped with a biopsy forceps, and withdrawn from the patient along with the endoscope. The suture is then attached to the PEG tube, which is pulled through the mouth, esophagus, and the anterior abdominal wall, leaving the tubing assembly exiting the abdominal wall and the mushroom bumper internally positioned against the gastric wall. An external bumper or fixation disk is then applied to the external tubing assembly (Figure 16–10).

The Sach-Vine technique is an example of the push-through PEG technique. The initial portion of the procedure is identical to the Ponsky-Gauderer technique but a needle with stylet is inserted into the stomach and, instead of suture material, a flexible tip guidewire is inserted through the needle into the stomach where it is ensnared and removed orally

TABLE 16–3. Comparison of surgically and endoscopically placed gastrostomies.

Surgical Gastrostomy	Percutaneous Endoscopic Gastrostomy
Performed by surgeons	Performed predominantly by gastroenterologists, sometimes radiologists and surgeons
Performed in the operating room	Performed in GI lab or bedside
Requires general anesthesia	Conscious sedation
Feeding starts 1–3 days after placement	Feeding starts within 24 hrs. of placement
Expensive	Less expensive than the cost of a surgical gastrostomy

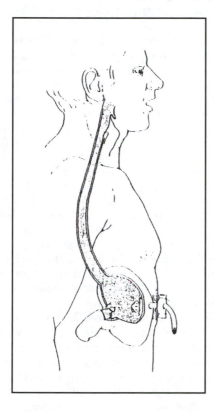

Figure 16–10. Patient with successful placement of a percutaneous endoscopic gastrostomy. Note that the gastrostomy has been placed through the abdominal wall into the anterior wall of the stomach. (With permission from from M. V. Sivak [Ed.], 1987. *Gastroenterologic Endoscopy* Philadelphia: W. B. Saunders Co.)

together with the endoscope. Over this guidewire a Sachs-Vine feeding tube with an advancing tapered tip is pushed through the mouth and into the stomach and then through the anterior abdominal wall. Once the tube penetrates the skin surface of the anterior abdominal wall, it is pulled out the rest of the way. The two techniques (push vs. pull) are comparable with respect to time of insertion and complication rate and choice is usually based on endoscopist preference and kit availability (Hogan et al., 1986).

A feeding jejunostomy has several advantages over a gastrostomy, making it ideal in specific circumstances such as in patients with obstructing carcinomas, patients in whom gastric resection is anticipated, or in those patients with ileus. Jejunostomies are believed to be associated with a reduced risk of aspiration because feedings are delivered distal to the pylorus, although aspiration of oral secretions is not addressed. Modification of the PEG technique for tube placement permits placement of jejunostomy tubes endoscopically. In this case, the gastrostomy tube is used as a conduit for a jejunal feeding tube, which is passed manually through the PEG tube. Once in the gastric lumen the jejunal tube is endoscopically grasped and guided into the jejunum. Using this technique, a preexisting surgically placed gastrostomy can be similarly converted to a jejunostomy (Strodel et al., 1984).

Among the many benefits of the endoscopic techniques over the surgical placement of gastrostomies or jejunostomies is the cost effectiveness and decreased length of hospital stay. In general, patients are not hospitalized specifically for PEG placement; it is usually performed during the management of other coincident problems during an ongoing hospitalization. Moreover, without anesthesia and operating room costs, PEG placement costs approximately one third of what a surgical gastrostomy costs. Furthermore, the placement of a tube for enteral nutrition does not obviate oral intake. Patients can still eat around the tube. Also, should the cause of dysphagia resolve (e.g., mucositis secondary to chemotherapy or reversible neurological damage after a head trauma), then the tube can be simply removed by pulling it out.

Complications from PEG placement occur approximately 6–10% of the time and are usually minor (Larson et al., 1987; Ponsky & Aszodi, 1984). The most common complication is infection at the site of insertion, manifested by local tenderness and erythema within a few days of tube placement. The administration of a single dose of intravenous antibiotics preoperatively and postoperatively minimizes infectious complications as does adequate skin care of the gastrostomy site after (Kozarek, Ball, & Patterson, 1986). It is common to see exudate or granulation tissue around the tube and this too is minimized by swabbing the site with hydrogen peroxide and leaving the site open to air. Occlusive dressings should be avoided. Other complications include tube dislodgement, stomal leak, pneumoperitoneum (of no consequence in the absence of peritoneal signs), and, less often, peritonitis, or bleeding. Although complications such as ileus, leakage of feedings into the peritoneal cavity, omental hematomas, and gastrocolic fistula have been reported, they are rare (Mamel, 1989).

Percutaneous endoscopic gastrostomies are contraindicated only when technical reasons make placement hazardous. Examples include esophageal obstruction (when an endoscope cannot be passed into the stomach), failure to transilluminate (making it impossible to know if there is an absence of intervening organs), ascites (inability to adequately appose/adhese the stomach to the abdominal wall), intestinal tract obstruction, tumor infiltration of the stomach, as well as intrabdominal sepsis. Previous abdominal surgeries do not preclude placement of PEG, although this does increase the risk of placement.

Indications for Parenteral Nutrition

Total parenteral nutrition (TPN) is indicated for those patients who cannot meet their nutritional needs for a prolonged period of time via the gastrointestinal tract. Although the most common indications are related to intestinal failure such as massive small bowel resection or mucosal intestinal disease-limiting absorption such as sprue or amyloidosis, diseases of the central nervous system compromising swallowing function are also a frequent indication when tube feeding cannot be used. Vascular access for TPN can be via a peripheral vein or via central intravenous access. Since there are few patients for whom the peripheral route provides optimum nutrition long term we will limit our discussion to central parenteral nutrition.

Total parenteral nutrition is delivered into a vein with a high blood flow rate, usually the superior vena cava. Large veins are selected to avoid the risk of phlebitis from the hypertonic fluid. Although the middle to inferior part of the superior vena cava is preferable, the left subclavian is the next best choice, and the internal jugular veins may be used if subclavian access is not feasible. There are substantial risks associated with central line placement including pneumothorax, arterial bleeding, brachial plexus injury, air embolism, hemothorax, and catheter infection. Successful TPN requires that central venous access be maintained long term. Infection, occlusion, and accidental removal are the most frequent reasons for catheter loss.

The complications related to total parenteral nutrition are not limited to just those associated with catheter placement. Complications may also be mechanical, metabolic, or septic. Metabolic complications occur commonly in patients on TPN, and high or low serum concentrations of virtually any component present in TPN have been described. The most frequent problems are those of hyperglycemia, hypophosphatemia, and hypokalemia. Hypomagnesemia is most likely to occur in patients who are chronic alcoholics, severely malnourished, or those receiving diuretics. Fluid overload should be monitored by frequent assessment of weight and total intake and output. Finally, hypoglycemia occurs if central TPN infusion is stopped abruptly, and this risk is increased if there is insulin in the TPN or if the infusion rate is high.

The occurrence of sepsis due to central TPN has been greatly reduced with the current methods for preparing the TPN components and strict adherence to protocols for aseptic catheter insertion and inspection/care. It is always worrisome for the patient with a central line when fever and leukocytosis develop; however, it is seldom necessary to remove the catheter immediately. In general the site must be examined, the dressing changed, and the patient must be evaluated for any other potential site of infection. Blood cultures should be obtained through the catheter as well as through peripheral veins. In the following 24 hours more directed therapy can be provided based on this initial evaluation.

Patients who require parenteral nutrition but who are otherwise stable enough to leave the hospital should be evaluated for nutritional support at home or in a nonacute facility. Guidelines have been published regarding standards for home nutrition support for the use of home TPN. When lifelong hospitalization is the only alternative to home TPN it is usually in the patient's best interest to go home on TPN. Under these circumstances, every effort must be made to maximize the safety and efficacy in performing this supplementation at home.

SUMMARY

The mainstays of therapy for the dysphagic patient are usually in the hands of a multidisciplinary team, which includes gastroenterologists, speech pathologists, and head and neck surgeons. Proper treatment of most disorders is contingent on correctly diagnosing the underlying abnormality; unfortunately, many causes of oropharyngeal dysphagia have no substantiated medical treatments. Surgical treatment is best reserved for those with specific swallowing dysfunction failing swallowing rehabilitation. If it is agreed upon that there is no potential for rehabilitation and no utility of compensatory maneuvers to increase swallowing efficiency and decrease aspiration risk then other nutritional options such as feeding tubes, gastrostomies, or even total parenteral nutrition may be considered.

MULTIPLE CHOICE QUESTIONS

1. Which of the following statements regarding Zenker's diverticulum are true?
   a. This disorder is caused by poor coordination between the pharynx and the upper esophageal sphincter.
   b. This disorder is characterized by increased hypopharyngeal intrabolus pressures and increased resistance to bolus passage.
   c. Examination of the cricopharyngeus muscle in patients with Zenker's diverticulum shows pathologic atrophy and fibrosis.

2. Which of the following statements regarding postpolio syndrome are correct?
   a. Postpolio syndrome consists of new musculoskeletal symptoms such as

weakness in muscles previously affected during the first attack of poliomyelitis.

   b. Dysphagia is a common symptom in patients with postpolio syndrome.

   c. Anticholinesterase agents are the first line of treatment for postpolio syndrome.

3. Which of the following statements regarding deglutitive aspiration are true?

   a. Injection of Teflon into the vocal fold is advocated as a treatment option if there is a symptomatic open glottis and permanently impaired vocal fold movement.

   b. Laryngectomy is the last resort in managing deglutitive aspiration.

   c. Total parenteral nutrition is the preferred method of feeding patients with a functional digestive tract who are unable to ingest an adequate quantity of nutrients.

4. Which of the following statements regarding tracheotomy are true?

   a. Aspiration is the most common swallowing disorder associated with tracheotomy.

   b. Tracheotomy may potentially increase aspiration by limiting laryngeal elevation during swallowing.

   c. Prolonged use of an inflated cuff may cause tracheal stenosis.

   d. All of the above are true.

5. A 45-year-old woman with depression is also diagnosed as having Sjögren's syndrome and complains of burning and soreness of her mouth (especially tongue) and difficulty in chewing and swallowing. Her oral exam shows dry buccal mucosa and absence of salivary flow on parotid gland palpation. Which of the following statements are likely to be true?

   a. Sjögren's syndrome is the most common cause of xerostomia.

   b. Xerostomia is most likely to be due to the antidepressant she is on.

   c. Treatment should begin with a prescription for artificial saliva.

   d. Salivary flow can be enhanced by mechanical therapy such as chewing gum.

6. Describe the complications that can be observed during total parenteral nutrition.

REFERENCES

Anderson, M. W., Izutsu, K. T., Rice, J. C. (1981). Parotid gland pathophysiology after mixed gamma and neutron irradiation of cancer patients. *Oral Surgery, 52,* 495–500.

Atkinson, J. C., & Fox, P. C. (1992). Salivary gland dysfunction. *Clinics in Geriatric Medicine, 8,* 499–511.

Bailey, B. J., & Biller, H. F. (Eds.). (1985). *Surgery of the larynx.* Philadelphia: W. B. Saunders.

Baredes, S. (1988). Surgical management of swallowing disorders. *Otolaryngologic Clinics of North America, 21,* 711–726.

Baron, B. C., & Dedo, H. H. (1980). Separation of the larynx and trachea for intractable aspiration. *Laryngoscope, 90,* 1927–1932.

Biller, H. F., Lawson, W., & Baek, S. M. (1983). Total glossectomy: A technique of reconstruction eliminating laryngectomy. *Archives of Otolaryngology, 109,* 69–73.

Blackie, J. D., & Lees, A. J. (1990). Botulinum toxin treatment in spasmodic torticollis. *Journal of Neurology, Neurosurgery & Psychiatry, 53,* 640–643.

Blitzer, A. (1987). Inflammatory and obstructive disorders of salivary glands. *Journal of Dental Research, 66,* 675–679.

Blitzer, A. (1990). Approaches to the patient with aspiration and swallowing disabilities. *Dysphagia, 5,* 129–137.

Blitzer, A., Krespi, Y. P., Oppenheimer, R. W., & Levine, T. M. (1988). Surgical management of aspiration. *Otolaryngologic Clinics of North America, 21,* 743–750.

Bone, R. C., Namum, A. M., & Harris, A. S. (1990). Evaluation and correction of dysphagia producing cervical osteophytosis. *Laryngoscope, 84,* 2045–2050.

Broniatowski, M., Davies, C. R., Jacobs, G. B., Jasso, J., Gerrity, R.G., Nose, Y., & Tucker, H. M. (1990). Artificial restoration of voice. I: Experiments in phonatory control of the reinnervated larynx. *Laryngoscope, 100,* 1219–1224.

Broniatowski, M., Ilyes, L. A., Jacobs, G. B., Nose, Y., & Tucker, H. M. (1988). Artificial reflex arc: A potential solution for chronic aspiration. II: A canine study based on a laryngeal prosthesis. *Laryngoscope, 98,* 235–237.

Broniatowski, M., Ilyes, L. A., Jacobs, G. B., Stepnick, W. I., Nose, Y., & Tucker, H. M. (1987). Artificial reflex arc: A potential solution for chronic aspiration. I: Cutaneous biologic sensors in the neck triggering strap muscle contraction in the canine. *Laryngoscope, 97,* 331–333.

Bushmann, M., Dobmeyer, S. M., Leeker, L., & Permutter, J. S. (1989). Swallowing abnormalities and their response to treatment in Parkinson's disease. *Neurology, 39,* 1309–1314.

Calcaterra, T. C. (1971). Laryngeal suspension after supraglottic laryngectomy. *Archives of Otolaryngology, 94,* 306–309.

Calne, D. B. , Shaw, D. G., & Spiers, A. S. D. (1970). Swallowing in Parkinsonism. *British Journal of Radiology, 43,* 456–457.

Cannon, C. R., & McLean, W. C. (1982). Laryngectomy for chronic aspiration. *American Journal of Otolaryngology, 3,* 145–149.

Carpenter, J. R., Bunch, T. W., Engel, A. G., & O'Brien, P. C. (1977). Survival in polymyositis: Corticosteroids and risk factors. *Annals of Internal Medicine, 111,* 143–157.

Coelho, C. A., & Ferrante, R. (1988). Dysphagia in postpolio sequelae: Report of three cases. *Archives of Physical Medicine and Rehabilitation, 69,* 634–636.

Cook, I. J. (1993). Cricopharyngeal function and dysfunction. *Dysphagia , 8,* 244–251.

Cook, I. J., Blumbergs, P., Cash, K., Jamieson, G. G., & Shearman, D. J. (1992). Structural abnormalities of the cricopharyngeus muscle in patients with pharyngeal (Zenker's) diverticulum. *Journal of Gastroenterology Hepatology, 7,* 556–562.

Cook, I. J., Gabb, M., Panagopoulos, V., Jamieson, G.G., Dodds, W. J., Dent, J., & Shearman, D. J. (1992). Pharyngeal (Zenker's) diverticulum is a disorder of upper esophageal sphincter opening. *Gastroenterology, 103,* 1229–1235.

Cummings, C. W. (Ed.). (1993). Tracheoesophageal diversion. In *Otolaryngology—Head and Neck Surgery.* (2nd ed.). St. Louis: Mosby-Year Book.

Drachman, D. B., De Silva, S., Ramsay, D., & Pestronk, A. (1987). Humoral pathogenesis of myasthenia gravis. *Annals of the New York Academy of Sciences, 505,* 90–105.

Drachman, D. B. (1994). Myasthenia gravis. *New England Journal of Medicine, 330,* 1797–1810.

Dreizen, S., Brown, L. R., Daly, T. E., & Drane, J. B. (1977). Prevention of xerostomia-related dental caries in irradiated cancer patients. *Journal of Dental Research, 56,* 99–104.

Duxbury, A. J., Thakker, N. S., & Wastell, D. G. (1989). A double-blind cross-over trial of a mucin-containing artificial saliva. *British Dental Journal, 166,* 115–120.

Dye, K., & Paterson, P. (1984). A comparison between percutaneous endoscopic gastrostomy (PEG) and surgical gastrostomy. *American Journal of Gastroenterology, 79,* 811.

Edgerton, M. T., & Duncan, M. M. (1959). Reconstruction with loss of the hyomandibular complex in excision of large cancers. *Archives of Surgery, 78,* 425–436.

Edmonds, C. (1966). Huntington's chorea, dysphagia and death. *Medical Journal of Australia, 2,* 273–274.

Eisele, D. W. (1991). Surgical approaches to aspiration. *Dysphagia, 6,* 71–78.

Ekberg, O., & Nylander, G. (1982). Dysfunction of the cricopharyngeal muscle. A cineradiographic study of patients with dysphagia. *Radiology, 143,* 481–486.

Eliachar, I., & Miller, F. R. (1994). Aspiration. In G. A. Gates (Ed.), *Current therapy in otolaryngology, head and neck surgery* (pp. 462–466) St. Louis: C. V. Mosby.

Ergun, G. A., & Kahrilas, P. J. (1993). Oropharyngeal dysphagia in the elderly. *Practical Gastroenterology, 17,* 9–16

Feussner, H., Kauer, W., & Siewert, J. R. (1993). The surgical management of motility disorders. *Dysphagia, 8,* 135-145.

Fox, R. I. (Ed.). (1992). Sjögren's syndrome. *Rheumatic Disease Clinics of North America, 18,* 507–717.

Fox, P. C. (1994). Pilocarpine–A treatment for dry mouth. *The Moisture Seekers Newsletter, 12,* 1–3.

Fox, P. C., Atkinson, J. C., Macynski, A. A., Wolff, A., Kung, D. S., Valdez, I. H., Jackson, W., Delapenha, R. A., Shiroky, J., & Baum, B. J. (1991). Pilocarpine treatment of salivary gland hypofunction and dry mouth (xerostomia). *Archives of Internal Medicine, 151,* 1149–1152.

Gauderer, M. W., & Ponsky, J. L. (1981). A simplified technique for constructing a tube feeding gastrostomy. *Surgery Gynecology Obstetrics, 152,* 83–85.

Gauderer, M. W., Ponsky, J. L., & Izant, R. J. (1980). Gastrostomy without laparoscopy: A percutaneous endoscopic technique. *Journal of Pediatric Surgery, 15,* 872–875.

Gelb, D. J., Lowenstein, D. H., & Aminoff, M. J. (1989). Controlled trial of botulinum toxin injections in the treatment of spasmodic torticollis. *Neurology, 39,* 80–84.

Greene, P., Kang, U., Fahn, S., Brin, M. F., Moskowitz, C., & Flaster, E. (1990). Double-blind, placebo-controlled trial of botulinum toxin injections for the treatment of spasmodic torticollis. *Neurology, 40,* 1213–1218.

Greene, P. E., Shale, H., & Fahn, S. (1988). Analysis of open-label trials in torsion dystonia using high dosages of anticholinergics and other drugs. *Movement Disorders, 3,* 46–60.

Habal, M. B., & Murray, J. E. (1972). Surgical treatment of life-endangering chronic aspiration pneumonia. *Plastic and Reconstructive Surgery, 49,* 305–311.

Halama, A. R. (1994). Surgical treatment of oropharyngeal swallowing disorders. *Acta Oto-Rhino-Laryngologica Belgica, 48,* 217–227.

Halstead, L. S., Wiechers, D. O., & Rossi, C. D. (1985). Late effects of poliomyelitis: A national survey. In L. S. Haltead, D. O. Wiechers (Eds.), *Late effects of poliomyelitis* (pp. 11–31). Miami: Symposia Foundation.

Hillel, A. D., & Goode, R. L. (1983). Lateral laryngeal suspension: A new procedure to minimize swallowing disorders followng tongue base resection. *Laryngoscope, 93,* 26–31.

Hochberg, M. C., Feldman, D., & Stevens, M. B. (1986). Adult onset polymyositis/dermatomyositis: An analysis of clinical and laboratory features and survival in 76 patients with a review of the literature. *Seminars in Arthritis and Rheumatism, 15,* 168–178.

Hogan, R. B., Demarco, D. C., Hamilton, J. K., Walker, C. O., & Polter, D. E. (1986). Percutaneous endoscopic gastrostomy: To push or pull: A prospective randomized trial. *Gastrointestinal Endoscopy, 32*(4), 253–258.

Hughes, A. J., Daniel, S. E., Blankson, S., & Lees, A. J. (1993). A clinicopathologic study of 100 cases of Parkinson's disease. *Archives of Neurology, 50*(2), 140–148.

Hughes, C. V., Baum, B. J., Fox, P. C., Marmary, Y., Yeh, C-K, & Sonies, B. C. (1987). Oral-pharyngeal dysphagia: A common sequela of salivary gland dysfunction. *Dysphagia, 1,* 173–177.

Jankovic, J. & Brin, MF. (1991). Therapeutic uses of botulinum toxin. *New England Journal of Medicine, 324,* 1186–1194.

Johnson, J. T., Ferretti, G. A., Nethery, W. J., Valdez, I. H., Fox, P. C., Ng, D., Muscoplat, C. G., & Gallagher, S. C. (1993). Oral pilocarpine for post-irradiation xerostomia in patients with head and neck cancer. *New England Journal of Medicine, 329,* 390–395.

Jung, T. T. & Adams, G. L. (1980). Dysphagia in laryngectomized patients. *Otolaryngology Head and Neck Surgery, 88,* 25–33.

Kagen, L. J., Hochman, R. B., & Strong. E. W. (1985). Cricopharyngeal obstruction in inflammatory myopathy (polymyositis/dermatomyosisitis). *Arthritis and Rheumatism, 28,* 630–636.

Kang, U. J., Burke, R. E., & Fahn, S. (1986). Natural history and treatment of tardive dystonia. *Movement Disorders, 1,* 193–208.

Kaplan, M. D., & Baum, B. J. (1993). The functions of saliva. *Dysphagia, 8,* 225–229.

Kashima, H. K. (1986) Postoperative dysphagia. In B. C. Gates, (Ed.), *Complications in Otolaryngology Head Neck Surgery* (pp. 21–27), Philadelphia: B. C. Decker.

Kirby, D. L., DeLegge, M. H., & Fleming, C. R. (1995). American Gastroenterological Association technical review on tube feeding for enteral nutrition. *Gastroenterology, 108,* 1282–1301.

Kitahara, S., Ikeda, M., Ohmae, Y., Nakanoboh, M., Inoye, T., & Healy, G. B. (1993). Laryngeal closure at the level of the false cord for the treatment of aspiration. *Journal of Laryngology and Otology, 107,* 826–828.

Kjellen, G., Fransson, S. G., Lindstrom, F., Sokjer, H., & Tibbling, L. (1986). Esophageal function, radiography, and dysphagia in Sjögren's syndrome. *Digestive Diseases and Sciences, 31,* 225–229.

Kozarek, R. A., Ball, T. J., & Patterson, D. J. (1986). Prophylactic antibiotics in percutaneous endoscopic gastrostomy: Need or nuisance? *Gastrointestinal Endoscopy, 32,* 147–148.

Krespi, Y. P., & Sisson, G. (1985). Management of chronic aspiration by subtotal and submucosal cricoid resection. *Annals of Otology Rhinology and Laryngology, 94,* 580–583.

Larson, D. E, Burton, D. D., Schroeder, K. W., & DiMagno, E. P. (1987). Percutaneous endoscopic gastrostomy: Indications, success, complications and mortality in 314 consecutive patients. *Gastrotenterology, 93,* 48–52.

Leopold, N. A., & Kagel, M. C. (1985). Dysphagia in Huntington's disease. *Archives of Neurology, 42,* 57–60.

Lerut, T., van Raemdonck, D., Guelinckx, P., Dom R, & Geboes, K. (1992). Zenker's diverticulum: Is a myotomy of the cricopharyngeus useful? How long should it be? *Hepatology-Gastroenterology, 39,* 127–131.

Lieberman, A. N., Horowitz, L., Redmond, P., Pachter, L., Lieberman, I., & Leibowitz, M. (1980). Dysphagia in Parkinson's disease. *American Journal of Gastroenterology, 74,* 157–160.

Lindeman, R. C. (1975). Diverting the paralyzed larynx. *Laryngoscope, 85,* 157–180.

Lindgren, S., & Ekberg, O. (1990). Cricopharyngeal myotomy in the treatment of dysphagia. *Clinical Otolaryngology, 15,* 221–227.

Logemann, J. A. (1994). Rehabilitation of oropharyngeal swallowing disorders. *Acta Oto-Rhino-Laryngologica Belgica, 48,* 207–215.

Mamel, J. J. (1989). Percutaneous endoscopic gastrostomy. *American Journal of Gastroenterology, 84,* 703–710.

Markusse, H. M., Pillay, M., & Breedveld, F. C. (1993). The diagnostic value of salivary gland scintigraphy in patients suspected of primary Sjögren's syndrome. *British Journal of Rheumatology, 32,* 231–235.

Maurri, S., & Barontini, F. (1990). Responsiveness of idiopathic spasmodic torticollis to botulinum A toxin injection. A critical evaluation of five cases.

Clinical in Neurology and Neurosurgery, 92, 165–168.

McIlwain, J.C., Bryce, D. P., Gilbert, R., & Grace, A. (1991). Subglottic laryngeal closure for aspiration. *Clinics in Otolaryngology, 16,* 33–38.

Mendelsohn, M. (1993). A guided approach to surgery for aspiration: Two case reports. *The Journal of Laryngology and Otology , 107,* 121–126.

Miller, L. G., & Janovic, J. (1989). Metoclopramide-induced movement disorders. *Archives of Internal Medicine, 149,* 2486–2492.

Montgomery, W. W. (1975). Surgical laryngeal closure to eliminate chronic aspiration. *New England Journal of Medicine, 292,* 1390–1391.

Munsat, T. L. (1991). Poliomyelitis—New problems with an old disease. *New England Journal of Medicine, 324,* 1206–1207.

Nash, M. (1988). Swallowing problems in the tracheotomized patient. *Otolaryngologic Clinics of North America, 21,* 701–709.

Osserman, K.E.. (1958). *Myasthenia gravis.* New York: Grune & Stratton.

The Parkinson Study Group. (1989). Effect of deprenyl on the progression of disability in early Parkinson's disease. *New England Journal of Medicine, 321,* 1364 -1371.

Papandoulos, S. M., Chen, J. C., Fledenzer, J. A., Bucci, M. N., & McGillicuddy, J. E. (1989). Anterior cervical osteophtes as a cause of progressive dysphagia. *Acta Neurochirurgica, 101,* 63–65.

The Parkinson Study Group. (1993). Effects of tocopherol and deprenyl on the progression of disability in early Parkinson's disease. *New England Journal of Medicine, 328,* 176–183.

Plotz, P. H., Dalakas, M., Leff, R. L., Love, L. A., Miller, F. W., & Cronin, M. E. (1989). Current concepts in the idiopathic inflammatory myopathies: Polymyositis, dermatomyositis, and related disorders. *Annals of Internal Medicine, 111,* 143–157.

Ponsky, J. L., & Aszodi, A. A. (1984). Percutaneous endoscopic jejunosotomy. *American Journal of Gastroenterology, 79,* 113–116.

Rademaker, A. W., Logemann, J. A., Pauloski, B. R., Bowman, J., Goepfert, H., Lazarus, C., Sisson, G., Milianti, F., Graner, D., Cook, B., Collins, S., Stein, D., & Johnson, J. (1993). Recovery of postoperative swallowing in patients undergoing partial laryngectomy. *Head & Neck, 15,* 325–334.

Saffouri, M. H., & Ward, P. H. (1974). Surgical correction of dysphagia due to cervical osteophytes. *Annals of Otology Rhinology Laryngology, 83,* 65–70.

Sasaki, C. T., Milmoe, G., & Yanagisawa, E. (1990). Surgical closure of the larynx for intractable aspiration. *Archives of Otolaryngology, 106,* 422–423.

Sasaki, C. T., Suzuki, M., Horiuchi, M., & Kirchner, J. A. (1977). The effect of tracheostomy on the laryngeal closure reflex. *Laryngoscope, 87,* 1428–1433.

Schaefer, S., Close, L. G., & Reisch, J. S. (1987). Conservation of the hypopharyngeal mucous membrane in total laryngectomy. *Archives of Otolaryngology and Head and Neck Surgery, 113,* 491–495.

Scully, C. (1986). Sjögren's syndrome: clinical and laboratory features, immunopathogenesis and management. *Oral Surgery Oral Medicine Oral Pathology, 62,* 510–523.

Ship, J. A., Fox, P. C., & Baum, B. J. (1991). How much saliva is enough? 'Normal' function defined. *Journal of the American Dental Association, 122,* 63–69.

Silbergleit, A. K., Waring, W. P, Sullivan, M. .J, & Maynard, F. M. (1991). Evaluation, treatment, and follow-up results of post polio patients with dysphagia. *Otolaryngology—Head and Neck Surgery, 104,* 333–338.

Sivak, M. V. (Ed.). (1987). *Gastroenterologic endoscopy.* Philadelphia: W. B. Saunders Co.

Sonies, B. C., & Dalakas, M. C. (1991). Dysphagia in patients with the post-polio syndrome. *New England Journal of Medicine, 324,* 1162–1167.

Speier, J. L., Owen, R. R., Knapp, M., & Canine, J. K. (1987). Occurrence of post-polio sequelae in an epidemic population. In L. S. Halstead, D. O. Wiechers (Eds.), Occurrence of post-polio sequelae in an epidemic population. *Birth Defects: Original Article Series.* 23(4), 39–48.

Stell, R., Thompson, P. D., & Marsden, C. D. (1988). Botulinum toxin in spasmodic torticollis. *Journal of Neurology Neurosurgery Psychiatry, 51,* 920–923.

Strodel, W. E., Eckhauser, F. E., Dent, T. L., & Lemmer, J. Q. (1984). Gastrostomy to jejunostomy conversion. *Gastrointestinal Endoscopy, 30,* 35–36.

Stuchell, R. N., & Mandel, I. D. (1988). Salivary gland dysfunction and swallowing disorders. *Otolaryngologic Clinics of North America, 21,* 649-661.

Tsui, J., Eisen, A., Stoessl, A., Calne, S., & Calne, D. (1986). Double-blind study of botulinum toxin in spasmodic torticollis. *Lancet, 2,* 245–247.

Wang, Z. Y., Qiao, J., & Link, H. (1993). Suppression of experimental autoimmune myasthenia gravis by oral administration of acetylcholine receptor. *Annals of the New York Academy of Sciences, 44,* 209–214.

Ward, P. H., Hanson, D. G., & Abemayor, E. (1985). Transcutaneous Teflon injection of the paralyzed vocal cord: A new technique. *Laryngoscope, 95,* 644–649.

Weisberger, E. C., & Huesbsch, S. A. (1982). Endoscopic treatment of aspiration using a laryngeal stent. *Otolaryngology—Head and Neck Surgery, 90,* 215–922.

Welsh, L. W., Welsh, J. J., & Chinnici, J. C. (1987). Dysphagia due to cervical spine injury. *Annals of Otololoy, Rhinology, and Laryngology, 96*, 112–115.

Wouters, B., & van Overbeek, J. J. M. (1992). Endoscopic treatment of the hypopharyngeal (Zenker's) diverticulum. *Hepatology-Gastroenterology, 39*, 105–108.

Yarington, C.T., Lindeman, R. C., & Sutton, D. (1976). Clinical experience with the tracheoesophageal anastomosis for intractable aspiration. *Annals of Otology, Rhinology, and Laryngology, 85*, 609–612.

Glossary

abscess: A localized collection of pus caused by infection.

acetylcholine, also Ach: A common central and peripheral neurotransmitter released at synapses of some pre- and postganglionic parasympathetic neurons, preganglionic sympathetic neurons, somatic neurons, and some central neuron synapses. Postsynaptic receptors are designated as muscarinic or nicotinic according to whether the drugs muscarine or nicotine mimic their response to Ach.

achalasia: Dysfunction of the esophagus, consisting of failure or incomplete relaxation of the lower esophageal sphincter and absent peristalsis of the esophagus, often leading to dilation of the esophagus.

action potential: Electrical event associated with longitudinally propagated change of potential across a cell membrane, reflecting activation of excitable cells such as nerve or muscle.

acute upper airway obstruction: Occlusion of the route for passage of air into and out of the lungs, most commonly due to foreign bodies lodging in or around the larynx.

adrenergic innervation: Characterized by synapses that secrete epinephrine or norepinephrine as the neurotransmitter and are found particularly in the sympathetic division of the autonomic nervous system.

adult respiratory distress syndrome: A symptom complex of acute respiratory failure, characterized by hypoxemia and diffuse infiltrates on chest radiographs and associated with diffuse injury to the pulmonary alveoli.

afferent: Neurons that carry input toward the central nervous system.

alveolus: The distal saccular airspaces of the lungs, across whose lining gas exchanges occurs.

amyloidosis: Condition resulting from deposition of amyloid in various tissues throughout the body.

amyotrophic lateral sclerosis: Neuromuscular disorder characterized by degeneration of both upper and lower motor neurons in the central nervous system.

anaerobic infections: Infections caused by anaerobic bacteria, that is, those which do not require (and in most cases cannot tolerate) the presence of oxygen.

anatomic dead space: The area of conducting airways (nose, mouth, pharynx, larynx, trachea, bronchi, nonrespiratory bronchioles) which do not participate in gas exchange.

anticholinesterase agents: Drugs that allow acetylcholine, which is released at the neuromuscular junction, to interact repetitively with the remaining acetylcholine receptors. Pyridostignine (Mestinon) is the most widely used anticholinesterase agent in the United States.

antigen: A substance that can be recognized as foreign by the immune system because it reacts with specific receptors on lymphocytes.

apnea: Cessation of respiratory airflow of any duration.

apraxia: Inability to voluntarily execute a learned sequence of motor actions. The function may remain intact on an involuntary basis. In the context of swallowing, patients seem to have forgotten how to feed or how to initiate swallowing. This occurs primarily with unilateral lesions of the cerebral cortex, such as hemispheric infarcts, or with dementias.

artifical saliva: An artifical, manufactured preparation of saliva containing glycoproteins and mucin.

aspiration: The penetration of secretions or ingesta below the level of the true vocal folds. This can interfere with effective air exchange (and lead to asphixiation, for instance) or cause pulmonary inflammation and infection (so-called aspiration pneumonia). Aspiration may occur prior to the actual swallow through an unguarded larynx, during the pharyngeal stage of swallowing from overflow of residue contained in the pharyngeal re-cesses, or from reflux of gastric contents.

aspiration pneumonia: Infection of the lung following aspiration.

aspiration pneumonitis: Inflammation (not necessarily due to infection) of the lung following aspiration.

asthma: See **obstructive lung disease**.

atelectasis: Literally, collapse of an area of lung; refers to microscopic collapse of individual alveoli as well as to larger lung units such as lung lobes.

autonomic innervation: The nervous system that innervates the visceral organs. It has two divisions, the sympathetic and parasympathetic.

auxiliary respiratory muscles: These are the accessory muscles of breathing that serve to assist in the expansion or compression of the rib cage by fixing, elevating, or depressing the ribs. They include muscles of the thoracic cavity, abdominal wall, and back. Contraction may allow for deep inhalation, forced exhalation, or performance of a Valsalva maneuver.

axial: Refers to slices taken at 90° to the long axis of the body, the same axis as slices through a loaf of bread.

axial tomograms: Refers to radiographic slices taken at 90° to the long axis of the body.

band-reject filter: Electrical device which attentuates signal frequencies within a specified frequency band between high and low extremes.

Barrett's esophagus: Columnar metaplasia of the esophagus. The normal squamous epithelium is replaced with specialized columnar epithelium as a result of prolonged reflux and severe damage to the esophageal mucosa. This is associated with chronic reflux esophagitis and is considered a premalignant lesion that can lead to adenocarcinoma.

Behçet's syndrome: Condition characterized by aphthous ulcers on various mucosal surfaces.

Bell's palsy: Idiopathic facial nerve palsy.

Bernstein test: A test whereby acid is dripped into the distal esophagus through a nasogastric tube and the patient's symptoms are recorded. Used in the past to help determine whether a patient has gastroesophageal reflux.

biopsy: Removal of tissue from living body and its examination for diagnostic purposes.

biphasic: Referring to a time-limited event or signal (including action potentials) possessing two distinct portions (e.g., one negative, another positive), as opposed to monophasic, triphasic, or polyphasic.

bipolar electrode: Electrode or electrode pair that measures electrical events (action potentials) at two distinct points; in electrophysiology, the resulting signals are usually supplied one to an inverting input, the other to a noninverting input of a differential amplifier.

bolus pressure, also luminal pressure: The presure recorded within a liquid bolus within a free lumen. During pharyngeal and esophageal peristalsis, bolus pressure is typically much lower than squeeze pressure.

botulinum toxin: One of the most lethal biologic toxins, which exerts its parlytic effect by binding to presynaptic cholinergic nerve terminals.

bradycardia: Slowed heart rate. For full-term neonates heart rate (HR) typically falls between 120 and 140 BPM, with rates from 70 to 170 BPM acceptable under conditions (e.g., Crane, 1986). Premature infants have higher HR, not uncommon to range 160 to 180 BPM. Individual infants have less variability within themselves. During work, such as feeding, it is common to see the HR increase 10 BPM over the baseline value.

brain stem: The region of the central nervous system immediately above the spinal cord and below the forebrain. It contains the cranial nuclei, extensive reticular formation, and three divisions, the medulla, pons, and midbrain.

breathing-swallowing coordination: Apnea which usually interrupts expiration in normal subjects, with resumption of expiration after deglutition.

bronchiectasis: Chronic dilatation of the bronchi characterized by excessive sputum production and generally due to previous inflammation or infection of the airways.

bronchospasm: Reflex constriction of the airways in response to a variety of stimuli, often associated with cough, wheezing, and mucus production.

bulbar palsy: A clinical syndrome characterized by dysphagia, dysphonia, and/or dysarthria resulting from disease of the motor unit (i.e., including lower motor neurons [brain stem nuclei], cranial nerves, neuromuscular junctions, or muscles). Findings often include muscle atrophy and decreased reflexes of the face, tongue, and throat.

cachexia: Profound weight loss.

café coronary syndrome: Clinical syndrome of choking, facial cyanosis, and eventual collapse due to acute upper airway obstruction, generally caused by a bolus of meat.

calcitonin gene-related peptide (CGRP): A peptide that can serve as a transmitter within the CNS and is also present in the gastrointestinal tract.

capacitance: The ratio between the electrical charge given a conductive body and the potential difference between it and another adjacent charged body (unit: farad).

capillary hemangioma: Congenital vascular lesion, usually flat but may have elevated portions.

catecholamines: A group of transmitters released by neurons and the adrenal gland; includes dopamine, norepinephrine, and epinephrine.

central grooving: Movement of the tongue to form a central depressed area where the food bolus is gathered and shaped into a globular mass before it is propelled posteriorly.

central nervous system (CNS): The brain and spinal cord.

cerebral palsy: Static encephalopathy related to perinatal brain injury.

cervical osteophyte: Bony outgrowth of the cervical vertebra.

chemical pneumonitis: Lung inflammation due to aspiration of irritating chemicals.

chemical shift artifact: An artifact in fast MR scanning caused by a change in the resonant frequency of protons in different environments. For example, protons in fat may have different elements surrounding them than those in fluid or soft tissue. This produces slightly different spin frequencies when the two tissues are exposed to the same magnetic field. Because of this, there may be spatial misregistration between these two types of tissues.

chemosensitive sensory fibers: Sensory fibers with receptors on the membranes of their terminals that respond to specific chemicals like NH_4Cl.

choanal atresia: Failure of the oronasal membrane to rupture (at about 6 weeks gestation) preventing the separation of nasal cavity from oral cavity. Thus breathing is accomplished through the mouth, not the nose. Bilateral choanal atresia makes it impossible for an infant to suck, swallow, and breathe in a coordinated way. Thus oral feeding is usually impossible.

cholecystokinin: A peptide hormone secreted by the duodenum that regulates gastric motility and secretion, gall bladder contraction, and pancreatic enzyme secretion. It is also thought to be a neurotransmitter.

cholinergic: Working through the release of acetylcholine: See also **acetylcholine**.

cholinergic neurons: Neurons that secrete acetylcholine (ACh) at their terminals and include neurons within the central nervous system, including all of the alpha motoneurons that innervate skeletal muscle fibers, neurons within autonomic nervous system between pre- and postganglionic nerve fibers, and some postganglionic neurons that innervate cardiac and smooth muscle. Although ACh is released at all cholinergic synapses, the receptor on the postsynaptic membrane will differ for the type of synapse (i.e., muscaric and nicotinic).

cleft lip: A congenital defect resulting from failure of the premaxilla to fuse with the alveolus.

cleft palate: A congenital defect resulting from incomplete fusion of the horizontal palatal segments.

chronic aspiration: Repeated or intractable episodes of aspiration.

chronic bronchitis: Clinical syndrome of sputum production for at least 3 months in each of 2 successive years in a patient in whom other causes of chronic cough have been excluded.

chronic obstructive pulmonary disease (COPD): A group of clinical diagnoses in which airflow is deranged owing to excessive bronchial secretions (chronic bronchitis, cystic fibrosis), increases in airway muscle tone (asthma), or destruction of the structural elements that normally maintain

airway patency (emphysema, bronchiectasis). One or more of these conditions may exist in an individual patient. All are associated with varying degrees of shortness of breath and cough.

ciliary defects: Dysfunction of the hairlike processes on airway cells that are normally responsible for propulsion of airway secretions, owing either to deficiency in the number or function of cilia.

cold spots: Receptive fields of sensory nerve fibers that discharge in response to temperatures in a specific way. Stimulating this receptive field with a warm probe will elicit the perception of cold.

common mode rejection ratio (CMRR): The ratio (often in dB) between the amplitude of the output of a differential amplifier, when a signal is fed to only one input, with the other input shorted to ground, and the amplifier output when the same signal is supplied to both inputs of a differential amplifier.

common mode signal: A signal or component thereof that is presented to both inputs in a bipolar EMG electrode array, or to both inputs of a differential amplifier.

compensation: Lessening of a swallowing (or other) problem by learned behavior, increased use of alternative mechanisms, or the inherent plasticity of the nervous system and of swallowing functions. Compensation may occur through use of postures that change pharyngeal dimensions and redirect bolus flow, through adaptations in bolus volume, bolus delivery or consistency, or through the use of sensory reinforcements or prostheses.

computed tomography (CT): Term referring to a specialized x-ray examination that produces thin (usually 10-mm thick) cross-sectional reconstructions of the body using computer back-projection techniques.

cordectomy: Removal of a portion of the vocal fold secondary to suspicious lesion.

cost-effectiveness analysis: A type of comparative analysis typically conducted when a new intervention is found to be more expensive, but also more effective, than standard care. Measures of effectiveness may be in monetary or nonmonetary terms such as lives saved.

cough: The sudden and forceful expulsion of air from the lungs.

cranial motor nuclei: The numerous well-organized motoneuron pools within the brain stem that innervate muscles of the head and oropharynx.

cricopharyngeal bar: Posterior impingement of the pharyngoesophageal junction lumen as seen during radiographic studies. Symptomatic primarily in context of Zenker's diverticulum (see **diverticulum**) and pharyngeal paralysis.

cystic fibrosis: An inherited disease caused by mutation in a membrane chloride channel and characterized by excessive production of tenacious mucus and repeated respiratory infection. An autosomal dominant disorder which is the most common lethal genetic disease involving caucasian children (approximately 1:2000 live births).

dead space ventilation: The volume of inhaled gas that does not come in contact with alveoli and hence does not contribute to gas exchange.

decerebrate preparation: Complete separation of the cortex and subcortical tissue from the brain stem and spinal cord so that ascending and descending pathways no longer conduct. The level of decerebration varies but minimally includes the spinal cord and medulla. Such an animal preparation can be studied without using an anesthetic and actually, if properly maintained and supported, can live in a chronic condition.

degenerative neurologic diseases: A wide variety of chronic disorders of the nervous system, generally associated with progressive loss of neurologic function and most frequently resulting from inborn errors of metabolism.

deglutition: The act of swallowing.

denervation: removal of nervous input to a tissue. Cooling of nerve fibers, for example, temporarily interrupts nervous input. Cutting fibers or disease leads to more permanent denervation. Regeneration and repair typically follow denervation.

depolarization: A transient electrical change that occurs across the membrane of muscle and neurons in which the inside of the membrane becomes more positive in charge (moves from a negative level toward zero). It occurs naturally with the movement of positive ions into the muscle cell or neuron, or with negative ions moving out. Depolarization occurs due to ionic channels opening briefly for specific ions like sodium which will normally move into the muscle or neuron and carry a positive charge.

derivative: A function that is the result of differentiation of another function, and thus corresponds to the slope of the original function.

differential amplifier: An amplifier that removes common mode components from two signals, for example, by inverting one input and then summing the two.

differential recording: The electrophysiologic technique based on the recording of action potentials from a limited spatial region by use of bipolar electrodes connected to a differential amplifier.

diffuse esophageal spasm: An esophageal motor abnormality characterized by the occurrence of simultaneous contractions during dry and wet swallows, which are predominantly seen in the smooth-muscle section of the esophagus. It commonly causes chest pain and dysphagia.

direct therapy: Therapy during which patients practice their swallow techniques with some small amounts of food or liquid.

discharge: Electrical signals defined and recorded as action potentials or spikes by electrical recording micropipettes placed within the cell or near and outside the cell. Neurons and muscles have distinct membranes with channels which will transiently open to allow specific ions to move across the membrane into or out of the cell. The movement of ions creates a current which can be measured as a voltage, the action potential. Discharge is the number of action potentials that a neuron or muscle fiber will produce.

disease of the neuromuscular junction: Disorders resulting in muscular weakness owing to inhibition of neurotransmitter delivery, usually a consequence of poisoning or autoimmunity.

diverticulum: A saccular deformation of an organ wall. In some diverticula, only the mucosal lining herniates through a dehiscence in the wall. In others, all layers of the wall form a permanent bulge. Diverticulae are named primarily for their sites: Zenker's diverticula form in the hypopharynx just above the UES. When large, undigeseted food may collect and putrify in them. Midesophageal traction diverticula occur over the tracheal bifurcation, epinephric or pulsion diverticula in the distal esophagus.

dopamine: A transmitter and hormone within the central and peripheral nervous system released at the synapse of neurons. It is the precursor to norepinephrine and epinephrine.

dorsal motor nucleus: A pool of preganglionic parasympathetic neurons which innervate several internal organs including the gastrointestinal tract. Some of its neurons innervate the smooth muscle of the esophagus sending their axons through the vagus nerve (X).

drowning: Suffocation and death resulting from filling of the lungs with water or other fluids.

dyskinesia: An involuntary movement disorder (e.g., tardive dyskinesia, a condition associated with chronic neuroleptic treatment and characterized by involuntary movements around the mouth).

dysphagia: Impaired swallowing. Can occur anywhere from the mouth to the stomach.

dysphasia lusorum: Difficulty swallowing secondary to an aberrant right subclavian artery.

dyspnea: Subjective difficulty or distress in breathing; frequently rapid breathing.

dystonia: Sustained involuntary movements, such as spasmodic torticollis (turning of the neck).

echo-planar imaging: An imaging technique using magnetic resonance imaging methods and specialized pulse sequences to allow rapid image acquisition.

edema, edematous: Swelling; an accumulation of an excessive amount of fluid in cells, tissues, or serous cavities.

efferent: The neurons that proceed from the central nervous system and innervate a peripheral target organ like skeletal muscles, smooth muscles, or cardiac muscle. Efferent includes motor neurons innervating their target organs.

eicosanoids: A general term for modified fatty acids which are products of arachidonic acid and function as paracrine or autocrine agents.

electrical stimulation: The membranes of muscle and neurons have ionic channels which are sensitive to changes in electrical voltage. A transient change in voltage across a membrane of these two types of cells results in a progressive and transient change in ionic channels across the cells. Electrical stimulation is an experimental method to depolarize neurons and muscle cells using these ionic channels.

electrode: A terminal in an electrical circuit that transfers current in either direction between a conventional conductor and gas or an electrolyte, or a patient body or instrument. It may be a recording electrode or stimulating electrode. Electrodes can be pipettes with specific chemical concentrations or metal with titanium, silver, and stainless steel commonly used. Electrodes can vary in size from a pipette with a tip of 1-2 microns to a large wire 1-2 mm in diameter. Electrodes can be of surface or penetrating type,.

electromyogram: Record of muscle action potentials sensed by electrodes over a limited time period.

electromyography: The technique of recording electromyograms and the associated physiological and electrodiagnostic disciplines.

EMG: Electromyography.

emphysema: Pathologic accumulation of air within the lungs due to permanent enlargement of the airspaces distal to the terminal bronchioles, accompanied by destruction of the alveolar walls without fibrosis.

empyema: Infection of the pleural space, frequently by anaerobic bacteria.

endolarynx: Structures within the laryngeal vestibule.

endoplasmic reticulum: An internal cell organelle where proteins are assembled.

endoscopic debridement: Removal of foreign material or devitalized or contaminated tissues using an endoscope.

erythema: Redness of skin; inflammation.

esophageal dilatation: Stretching of the walls of the esophagus to recover the lumen at the site of strictures. Devices used for dilatation include mercury-filled bougies, inflatable balloons, metal olives, and firm plastic rods of graded sizes.

esophageal spasm, also segmental or diffuse esophageal spasm: An abnormality characterized by the occurrence of simultaneous powerful contractions predominantly in the smooth muscle segment of the esophagus. Commonly causes chest pain and dysphagia.

esophageal strictures: Narrowing of the esophageal lumen which leads to mechanical obstruction of the bolus passage. Strictures may be caused by webs (see **Plummer-Vinson; Schatze's rings**), by cancers (malignant strictures), or extrinsic compression (enlarged blood vessels, pulmonary tumors, goiters). Ingestion of lye may lead to formation of tight and tortuous fibrotic strictures. Peptic strictures are those occurring in reflux esophagitis; peptic strictures are short and concentric. Treatment of strictures aims to recover the full size of the lumen, primarily through esophageal dilatation.

esophagitis: Inflammation of the esophagus, most commonly caused by gastroesophageal reflux ("reflux esophagitis"), ingestion of corrosives (e.g., "pill esophagitis") and infections (e.g., "fungal or viral esophagitis"). Mucosal lesions of typical esophagitis include erosions, exudate, or ulcerations which may lead to heartburn, chest pain, dysphagia, and odynophagia. Severe or chronic esophagitis may be complicated by formation of esophageal strictures or by mucosal metaplasia (see **Barrett's esophagus**).

extrapyramidal syndrome: Symptoms referable to the central nervous system outside the pyramidal tracts.

fast adapting sensory fiber: Some sensory fibers discharge action potentials when the stimulus is placed or removed and will cease discharging while the stimulus remains on the receptive field. These sensory fibers indicate when a stimulus has arrived and been removed.

fast CT scanning: Synonymous with ultrafast CT scanning.

fiberoptic bronchoscope: A type of small diameter (typically 3–6 mm) flexible endoscope used to examine the bronchi.

fiberoptics: The conduction of light from a source through a bundle of glass or plastic fibers; in wide use for illumination of endoscopic systems.

fiberscope: A glass-fiber viewing instrument with complete flexibility of shaft and improved light transmission.

filter: A device (often electrical) that attenuates some frequency band or bands of a signal, leaving others relatively unchanged.

frequency response: A function or functions which specify the relation between amplitude response and frequency characteristics, showing the manner in which the gain and phase of a system vary with the frequency of a stimulus.

functional residual capacity (FRC): The amount of air remaining in the chest at end-expiration.

GABA (gamma-amino butyric acid): The major neurotransmitter responsible for synaptic inhibition at supraspinal levels. The GABA$_A$ receptor subtype represents a ligand-gated chloride channel, the activity of which is inhibited by bicuculline and picrotoxin.

gamma camera: Imaging device composed of a sheet of thallium-activated sodium iodide crystal that fluoresces when radiation from a radionuclide strikes its surface. This instrument is placed near the patient to locate the area of the body that has collected radionuclide.

gap junction: Protein channels that, like the cytoplasm of adjacent cells, allow ions and small molecules to move between cells.

gastroesophageal reflux: Retrograde flow of gastric or biliary secretions from the stomach into the esophagus (and possibly into the upper airway).

gastroesophageal reflux disorder: Reflux of gastric contents into the esophagus, resulting in damage or symptoms.

gestational age: Age computed from first day of last menstrual period to any point thereafter, usually not calculated beyond the first few months of life after birth.

globus hystericus: A condition in which the sensation of a lump in the throat persists despite a normal physical examination.

glossopharyngeal nerve: One of the 12 cranial nerves that carry sensory, motor, and autonomic nerve fibers.

glutamate: The amionic form of glutamic acid and a major excitatory transmitter in the CNS. There are two major excitatory amino acid receptor types:

> **Ionotropic excitatory amino acid receptor:** A ligand-gated channel at which glutamate, aspartate, and certain glutamatelike agonists act to increase membrane conductance (open the channel) to produce membrane depolarization.

metabotropic glutamate receptor: A G-protein coupled receptor that activates signal transduction via second messengers.

goiter: An increased size of the thyroid gland. Goiters are rarely of the size to cause mechanical obstruction of the bolus passage. However, thyroid disease is associated with various neuromuscular diseases, including myasthenia gravis.

ground: Electrical conductor connected to the electrical return in a power system, for example, earth, or to a large conductor conventionally used as a reference potential (zero), for example, the steel frame of a car.

H$_2$ receptor blocker: Histamine mediates its effects through several different receptors. Acid secreton by gastric mucosa is mediated by H$_2$, the type 2 histamine receptors. Drugs like cimetidine and rantidine block H$_2$ receptors and thereby reduce gastric acid secretion.

helical CT: The latest generation of computed tomography scanners that produce scans by moving the patient at a constrant rate through the bore of a CT scanner while the scanning tube is rotated around the patient. This produces a true volumetric data set.

hiatus hernia: Protrusion of part of the stomach through the diaphragm into the thorax. This is an anatomical term and should not necessarily be equated with symptoms or a diseased state, although it is commonly associated with gastroesophageal reflux.

histochemical: Relating to the branch of histology that applies chemical techniques to identify components of cells and tissues.

human immunodeficiency virus 1 (HIV-1): A retrovirus that is the causative agent of the acquired immunodeficiency syndrome (AIDS).

Huntington's disease: An inherited disease of the central nervous system characterized by progressive dementia and involuntary choreic movements, resulting from degeneration of the caudate and putamen nuclei.

hypercapnia: Excessive CO_2 in the blood, produced by inadequate ventilation of alveoli.

hyperpolarization: An electrical charge across the membrane of a neuron or muscle cell in which the inside of the membrane becomes more negative. It makes the cell less able to depolarize and decreases the likelihood that action potentials will be generated.

hypoglossal nucleus: One of the cranial motor nuclei with motoneurons that innervate the extrinsic and intrinsic muscles of the tongue. Only one muscle protrudes the tongue so that most motoneurons innervate muscles that retract the tongue or alter its shape.

hypopharyngeal diverticula: Outpouching of the muscular pharyngeal wall above the cricopharyngeus muscle.

hypoplasia: Underdevelopment of structures.

hypoxia: Deficiency of oxygen reaching tissues of the body.

iatrogenic: This refers to an illness or adverse affect resulting from a medical or surgical test or treatment.

immotile cilia syndromes: A clinical syndrome of recurrent sinusitis and respiratory infections associated with immotile cilia and owing to lack of inner and outer dynein arms of cilia.

impedance: A system function consisting of the ratio between a velocitylike quantity (e.g., electric current), which constitutes the denominator of the ratio, and a forcelike quantity (e.g., electric voltage), which consitutes the numerator of the ratio.

incidence: The rate of new occurrences of a disease or condition within a defined population at risk during a specified time span.

indirect therapy: Exercise programs or swallows of saliva during which no food or liquid is given.

inflammatory neuropathies: Disorders of peripheral nerves mediated by cellular and humoral products of inflammation, typically triggered by autoimmunity.

input impedance: The impedance presented by an electric circuit to its signal source, for example, the reactance of the differential amplifier input capacitance considered in parallel with the amplifier input resistance.

integration: The process or technique of finding a mathematical function (integral) of a given variable, of which a given function is the derivative with respect to the same variable.

interference pattern: Record of action potentials summing the simultaneous electrical activity of several different signal sources, for example, of different motor units in electromyography.

interference signal: Extraneous signal superimposed on a signal of interest, for example, in EMG of a given muscle it may be a 60 Hz (or its integral multiple) signal, or the electrocardiogram, or a signal from a distant muscle.

interneurons: Neurons with their cell bodies and axons entirely within the CNS that relay from one part of the CNS to another. They relay inputs from sensory neurons and motor outputs to motoneurons.

interstitial pulmonary fibrosis: Scarring and abnormal deposition of collagen within alveolar walls, leading to increased stiffness of lungs and impaired oxygenation. May be caused by autoimmunity, drug hypersensitivity, infection, irradiation, or occupational exposures.

intrinsic laryngeal musculature: The cricothyroid, lateral cricoarytenoid, transverse and oblique arytenoid, posterior cricoarytenoid, thyroarytenoid muscles, which control the area of the glottic aperture.

ionizing radiation: Radiation that produces ion pairs along its path through a substance and therefore has the potential to damage the body tissues. It is produced when radiation from radionuclides or x-rays passes through the body.

Karagener's syndrome: A subset of the immotile cilia syndrome, characterized by the triad of bronchiectasis, nasal polyps or sinusitis, and situs inversus totalis.

laryngeal cleft: A cleft in the larynx that may present with cough during feeding. Stridor may be present at rest or increased with feeds; an anatomic abnormality resulting from incomplete closure of the tracheo-esophageal septum or cricoid cartilage or both in the sixth to seventh week of fetal life.

laryngeal diversion procedures: Also known as subglottic closures, designed to separate the lower respiratory tract from the upper digestive tract without affecting the glottic or supraglottic parts of the larynx.

laryngeal suspension: The elevation of suspension of the larynx to a position under the tongue where it is removed from the bolus path to avoid aspiration during swallowing.

laryngeal vestibule: The structures comprising the endolarynx, bounded by the rim of the epiglottis, superior edge of the aryepiglottic folds, tips of the arytenoid cartilages, and superior edge of the interarytenoid space.

laryngomalacia: Anatomic abnormality in which flaccid supraglottic structures prolapse into the airway, with inspiration leading to stridor, and even failure to thrive.

laryngospasm: A spasmodic closure of the glottic aperture; an exaggeration of the laryngeal adductory response in response to an aversive stimulus.

laryngotracheal separation: A type of subglottic closure where the trachea is brought to the skin as a tracheotomy but the proximal segment is left closed as a blind pouch.

latency: The time period intervening between a triggering event (e.g., electrical stimulation) and the onset of the response to that event (e.g., action potentials, or muscle contraction).

leiomyoma: A tumor (usually benign) originating from the smooth muscle. Histologically, it usually consists of encapsulated whorls of smooth musclelike cells.

lingual nerve: One of the branches of the trigeminal nerve that innervates the anterior portion of the tongue and carries input of sensory fibers responding to taste, touch, and pressure.

lower esophageal sphincter (LES): Specialized muscle that closes the gastroesophageal junction and prevents gastroesophageal reflux by its tonic contraction; relaxes in response to swallowing. Transient LES relaxations in the absence of swallowing or TLESRs. A high-pressure zone in the distal esophagus that relaxes with swallowing.

Ludwig's angina: Soft-tissue infection of the floor of the mouth.

lyme disease: A systemic illness resulting from infection with the spirochete *Borrelia burgdorferi.*

lymphangioma: A congenital endothelial-lined swelling of lymphatic origin.

lymphatics: The vessels found in most organs which collect lymph and return it to the bloodstream via the thoracic duct.

lymphocytes: A type of nonphagocytic mononuclear leucocyte which comprise T cells, B cells, and natural killer (NK) cells. Individual lymphocytes recognize antigens and orchestrate virtually all components of the immune response.

macrophages: A type of mononuclear phagocytic leukocyte that has differentiated within a tissue.

magnetic resonance imaging (MRI): A scanning technique that allows visualization of the soft tissues of the body by imaging the signal produced by the protons of soft tissues after a magnetic field in which the patient is placed has been perturbed by a second magnetic pulse. Allows scanning and reconstruction much like CT scanning but with no ionizing radiation.

major histocompatibility complex (MHC): A complex of cell-surface proteins essential for presentation of antigens to lymphocytes. They consist of two major classes of molecules: class I, which are found on all cells, and class II, which are usually found on certain subsets of immune cells, but which are inducible.

mandibular hypoplasia: Underdevelopment of the mandible as seen in some children with craniofacial anomalies (e.g., Pierre Robin sequence, hemifacial microsomias, Treacher Collins).

marginated: Pertaining to leukocytes that have adhered to the epithelium.

medulla: The lowest part of the brain stem situated immediately rostral to the spinal cord. It contains several important neuronal pathways controlling respiration, blood pressure, and swallowing.

medullary respiratory center: A group of nuclei in the lower medulla of the brain stem that are the integrative center for inspiration and expiration.

membrane channel: A protein or glycoprotein that spans the lipid bylayer of the cell membrane and forms a channel between the intracellular and extracellular space. Channels are selective, allowing the passage of particular ionic species. They may be opened or closed by changes in membrane potential, hormones, neurotransmitters, or changes in the ionic milieu of the cytoplasm.

micrognathia: Mandibular hypoplasia.

midface hypoplasia: Underdevelopment of the midface as in Crouzon and Apert syndromes.

milk scan: A radionuclide test for aspiration where small amounts of radionuclide are placed in milk and ingested by an infant.

minute ventilation (Ve): Expired volume per unit time per kilogram of body weight (Timms et al., 1993). Oral feeding results in an impairment of ventilation during continuous sucking. The subsequent recovery during intermittent sucking depends on postconceptional age (Shivpuri et al., 1983). The recovery or increase may be a complex phenomenon that begins with respiratory inhibition caused by frequent sucking and swallowing, followed by an increase in Ve as arterial CO_2 rises and the frequency of sucking and swallowing decreases.

monoamine oxidase: An enzyme that inactivates catecholamine transmitters and serotonin.

motilin: A polypeptide secreted by cells within the duodenum which causes contraction of intestinal smooth muscle.

monopolar electrode: Electrode used in a derivation for recording of bioelectric signals, in which the voltage input to the amplifier is measured between a single electrode and a reference electrode.

motoneuron pool: Alpha motoneurons which innervate one muscle are located close together and define a pool of neurons which innervate that muscle. A nucleus (i.e., motor trigeminal nucleus) will have several motoneuron pools innervating different muscles.

motoneurons: The neurons that innervate muscles. The motoneurons innervating skeletal muscle have their cell bodies within the central nervous system and are designated alpha motoneurons. Gamma motoneurons innervate sensory receptors in muscles, labeled muscle spindles, and bias their discharge: They do not directly excite working muscle fibers. The autonomic nervous system has motoneurons that innervate visceral smooth muscle.

motor trigeminal nucleus: A cranial motor nucleus with motoneurons which innervate several muscles of the mandible such as the jaw-closing muscles (i.e., masseter) and a jaw-opening muscle (i.e., anterior digastric) as well as muscles of the floor of the mouth.

motor unit: Unit of the neuromuscular system composed of a lower motor neuron, its axon, and the muscle fibers which it innervates.

mucociliary action: The process by which hygroscopic glycoproteins secreted by airway secretory cells are driven towards the mouth by the beating of cilia on airway cells.

mucociliary escalator: Term for bulk transport mechanism by which tracheobronchial secretions continuously move proximately for elimination.

muscaric receptor: Refers to a type of acetylcholine receptor that is activated by the mushroom poison, muscarine. This receptor is located on smooth muscle, cardiac muscle, some glands, and some neurons.

muscle unit: Group of muscle fibers innervated as part of a given motor unit.

myasthenia gravis: An autoimmune disease characterized by muscle weakness and progressive fatigue. It is due to a functional decrease in the amount of acetylcholine at the neuromuscular junction, causing failure in inducing normal muscle contraction.

myelinated fiber: Neurons either have a sheath of myelin around their axons or exist without this additional covering. Sensory and motor neurons with myelin conduct action potentials much faster than unmyelinated neurons because depolarization does not occur along adjacent membrane but actually leaps from node to node. A node is a periodic break in the myelin along the axon of the neuron. Myelinated fibers are larger than unmyelinated fibers.

myenteric plexus: A nerve cell network between circular and longitudinal muscles in the esophagus, stomach, and intestinal walls.

myogenic: Originating in muscle.

myoglobin: Small protein molecule, analogous to hemoglobin, that stores oxygen and transports it from the muscle capillaries into muscle fibers, facilitating oxygen diffusion.

myology: The scientific study of muscles and of their pathology and disease.

myopathies: A generic term for disease of the muscles.

myosin: A complex protein within muscle cells that participates in the contractile process by its cyclical interaction with actin.

myosin ATPase: An enzyme located on part of the protein myosin. It hydrolyzes adenosine triphosphate (ADP), splitting it into ADP and inorganic phosphate, which provides the energy for muscle contraction.

myotonias: Diseases of muscles associated with tonic spasm and irritability, usually due to a genetic disorder.

near drowning: Nonfatal lung injury resulting from filling of the lungs with water or other fluids.

neurofibromatosis: Rare autosomal dominant disorder of neuromas developing on multiple cranial nerves.

neuropeptides: Polypeptides which serve hormonal transmitter or other signaling functions in various tissues and are released by many nerves and by specialized (APUD) cells within the mucosa of the gastrointestinal tract (see **Secretin**, for example). Other important neuropeptides include gastrin which stimulates gastric acid secretion after being released into the bloodstream by the atrial mucosa; cholecystokinin which contracts the gallbladder after being released into the blood from duodenal cells. Others are vasoactive intestinal peptide (VIP), substance P, etc., which act as neurotransmitters or modulate the effects of other neurotransmitters in postganglionic autonomic synapses of the myenteric plexus.

neurotransmitter: The chemical or chemicals secreted at nerve terminals that change the activity of its target neurons or muscle cells. Neurotransmitters include various amino acids, catecholamines, acetylcholine, certain peptides, and nitric oxide.

neutrophils: A type of multinucleated leukocyte (white blood cell) essential for defense against bacteria and fungi. Neutrophils are short-lived cells that have no capacity to divide; therefore, during ongoing infection, they must be replenished continuously from the bloodstream.

nicotinic: Refers to a type of acetylcholine receptor that is activated by nicotine. The receptors to this type of ACh are located on motor end plates of alpha motoneurons innervating skeletal muscle and on ganglionic autonomic neurons.

Nissen fundoplication: Surgical procedure used to treat gastroesophageal reflux. The fundoplication involves wrapping of the fundus of the stomach around the gastroesophageal junction.

nitric oxide: A neurotransmitter that is released from neurons of the CNS, enteric and peripheral nervous systems and is not contained in vesicles. It inhibits gastrointestinal motor function.

nodose ganglion: The inferior ganglion of the vagus nerve, containing cell bodies concerned with special visceral sensation and general visceral afferents from the viscera.

norepinephrine (also noradrenaline): A catecholamine neurotransmitter released at most sympathetic postganglionic endings, from the adrenal medulla, and in many CNS regions.

nosocomial: Hospital-acquired; term usually used to refer to infections.

nosocomial pneumonias: Pneumonias, chiefly caused by gram-negative organisms, acquired in the hospital, especially in association with endotracheal intubation and mechanical ventilation.

notch filter: A filter that attenuates a given frequency band of the input signal. Also known as a band-reject filter.

nucleus ambiguus: One of the cranial motor nuclei of the brain stem with motoneurons that innervate laryngeal, pharyngeal, and esophageal muscles.

nucleus of the tractus solitarius: One of the cranial sensory nuclei of the brain stem which receives sensory input from the oral, pharyngeal, and laryngeal regions. Some of the sensory input is involved with taste. Interneurons within discrete subdivisions of the nucleus serve multiple functions, including controlling blood pressure, respiratory rhythmicity, swallowing, and taste.

obstructive lung disease: A syndrome in which airflow out of the lungs is impeded by narrowing of the small or medium-sized airways due to spasm, inflammation, or scarring. Overinflation of the lung, prolongation of expiration, air hunger, dyspnea, and respiratory insufficiency may result.

odynophagia: Pain on swallowing.

off-contraction, also off-response: A contraction that occurs with a latency period following the end of the stimulus. The off-contraction of esophageal smooth muscle,

for example, is associated with depolarization of the muscle cells and the generation of spike potentials.

opsonization: The process of coating a bacteria or other particulate antigen with substances (including complement components, immunoglobulins, surfactant proteins) which increases the rate of their phagocytosis by macrophages or granulocytic leukocytes.

oral preparatory stage: Stage of swallowing in which the tongue gathers the food bolus and forms it into a centrally located globular mass ready to be propelled over the back of the tongue.

oral intake: Intake of nutrition by mouth.

oral secretions: The mixture of saliva and organisms residing in the mouth.

oral stage of swallowing: The voluntary first stage of swallowing in which a bolus is formed and propelled toward the pharynx through repeated contractions of the tongue.

oropharyngeal transit time: The time taken between the beginning of swallowing and the time where the bolus passes out of the oropharynx.

oxygen saturation: The amount of oxygen present in the blood and available for exchange at the tissue level, typically measured in capillary blood flow by a pulse oximeter with external sensor. The levels are expressed as a percentage of 100. Normal infant has oxygen saturation above 95% in most conditions. Premature infants may be considered to have acceptable saturation levels above 90%. Below 90% some degree of hypoxia is indicated.

papilloma: A circumscribed benign epithelial tumor projecting from the surrounding surface.

parasympathetic: One of the two divisions of the autonomic nervous system. It is defined anatomically by postganglionic fibers that arise from ganglia close to the organ they innervate. Acetylcholine is the neurotransmitter released from parasympathetic neurons.

parenchyma: The essential substance of an organ. In the case of the lungs, the distal airspaces.

parenchymal cells: Cells which normally reside in the distal airspaces of the lungs, including alveolar type I and type II epithelial cells, alveolar endothelial cells, alveolar macrophages, fibroblasts, and pericytes.

patch clamp: A technique in which a tiny membrane patch is sucked into a pipette so that single or a few membrane channels can be studied by changing ions and current levels.

penetration: Entry of oropharyngeal contents into the larynx above the true vocal folds. Some authors define penetration as entry through the larynx and into the trachea. It is important for authors to define their use of the term.

peptide: A short polypeptide chain with less than 50 amino acids.

percutaneous endoscopic gastrostomy (PEG): Feeding tube placed directly into the stomach from the skin, utilizing an endoscope for guidance.

peristalsis: A coordinated propulsive contraction of the esophagus which occludes the esophageal lumen to propel the bolus through the esophagus and into the stomach. When the contraction follows a pharyngeal swallow and begins at the cricopharyngeal level, it is a *primary* peristalsis. If the contraction is stimulated by residual bolus that has been left behind, or by distension (e.g., from reflux), it is called *secondary* peristalsis.

phagocytosis: The process whereby foreign particles (bacteria, aspirated food) are ingested by macrophages or neutrophils.

phrenic nerve: A general motor and sensory nerve that arises from the cervical plexus (C3-C5) and which innervates the diaphragm, pericardium, peritoneum, and sympathetic plexes.

phrenoesophageal ligament or membrane: An extension of the fascia of the diaphragm which anchors the gastroesophageal junction in the hiatus of the diaphragm. The ligament contains collagen and elastic fibers which allow the gastroesophageal junction to move up into the hiatus on swallowing and then move back down to its resting position. Degeneration and laxity of the membrane is a feature of hiatus hernias.

pill esophagitis: Inflammation caused by the corrosive effects of medications that become lodged in the esophagus.

pleura: Paired layers of connective tissue covering the lung (visceral pleura) and lining the inner chest wall (parietal pleura). Between these two layers a potential space (the pleural space) can become filled with fluid (pleural effusion) or pus (empyema).

plexus: Anatomical network of nerves, veins, or lymphatic vessels.

Plummer-Vinson syndrome (also described as the Paterson-Kelly syndrome): Dysphagia, iron-deficiency anemia, upper esophageal inflammation with web formation, angular stomatitis, and atrophic gastritis. Predominantly affects females between the ages of 40 and 70.

pneumomediastinum: Presence of air within the mediastinum, generally as a result of rupture of the alveoli or esophagus. A potential complication of positive pressure mechanical ventilation or of the Heimlich maneuver.

polymyositis: Inflammatory disease of skeletal muscle, characterized by weakness.

polyposis: Presence of several polyps.

pons: The more rostral region of the brain stem above the medulla in which sensory and motor nuclei are surrounded by ascending and descending pathways and netlike arrangements of neurons defined as the *reticular formation.*

positive end expiratory pressure: The application of a small amount (typically 5–20 cm H_2O) of positive airway pressure during mechanical ventilation to minimiza alveolar collapse.

postconceptual age: Number of weeks following conception, approximately 2 weeks less than gestational age.

postganglionic neuron: The axons of the autonomic nervous system that are innervated by neurons from the CNS and that innervate visceral organs. The postganglionic axons originate from cell bodies within ganglionic tissues that are situated outside the central nervous system. Ganglionic neurons within the sympathetic system have long axons to innervate their target organ, whereas those of the parasympathetic system are short as their ganglia are close to or within their target tissue.

postpolio syndrome: A clinical syndrome consisting of progressive fatigue, weakness, and pain occurring in patients with a remote history of poliomyelitis.

postsynaptic inhibition: An input to nerve or muscle cells which decreases their chance of opening their membrane channels and conducting action potentials by hyperpolarizing them (see also **hyperpolarization**).

postprandial aspiration: Aspiration in relationship to a meal.

postural strategies: Changing of the patient's head or body posture (to eliminate aspiration) which changes the dimension of the pharynx and the direction of food flow without increasing the patient's work or effort during swallow.

potassium ion: Exists in high concentrations inside cells, and determines largely the membrane potential of muscle and nerve cells. Opening of potassium channels in the membrane moves potassium out of the cell and renders the inside of the cell more negative.

preganglionic neuron: The neurons of the autonomic nervous system that innervate the ganglionic cells. The cell bodies of preganglionic neurons are situated within the central nervous system and send their axons to ganglia. The sympathetic nervous system has short preganglionic fibers as most ganglia are close to the spinal cord. The parasympathetic nervous system has long preganglionic fibers which reach ganglia close to the target organ.

prevalence: The proportion of a defined population which has a disease or condition at a specified time.

primitive reflexes: Considered normal in the newborn period: Descriptions are from Rogers & Campbell (1993).

> **Asymmetric tonic neck reflex (ATNR):** Can be elicited by turning an infant's head laterally in a supine position. Visible evidence includes extension of the extremities on the chin side or flexion on the occiput side. The ATNR is commonly persistent in children with severe motor deficits related to cerebral palsy.

> **Moro reflex:** Elicited with infant in supine position. The head is allowed to drop back suddenly from at least 3 cm off a padded surface. On extension of the neck, there is a quick symmetrical abduction and upward movement of the arms followed by opening of the hands. Adduction and flexion of the arms can then be noted.

> **Positive support reflex:** Can be elicited by suspending the infant around the trunk or axillae with the head in neutral or midline flexed position. The infant is bounced five times on the balls of his feet. The balls of the feet are then brought into contact with the table surface. Co-contraction of opposing muscle groups of the legs occurs, resulting in a position capable of supporting weight.

> **Tonic labyrinthine reflex:** Can be evaluated in supine or prone position. In supine, infant's head is extended 45° below the horizontal and then flexed 45° above the horizontal. While the neck is extended 45°, the limbs extend. With the neck flexed 45°, the limbs flex.

prostaglandins: One of a group of modified unsaturated fatty acids called eicosanoids that function mainly as paracrine or autocrine substances.

pseudobulbar palsy: A clinical syndrome characterized by dysphagia, dysphonia, and/or dysarthria resulting from disease above the level of brainstem nuclei (i.e., including the cerebral hemispheres and corticobulbar tracts). Findings often include upper motor neuron signs (increased reflexes and incoordination) and emotional lability.

ptosis: Drooping of the upper eyelid from paralysis or weakness.

pulse sequence: Series of electromagnetic pulses used to excite the spins of body protons and generate the signal used to construct the magnetic resonance image.

pyriform sinuses: Spaces created by the ways in which the inferior pharyngeal constrictors attach to the outside of the larynx. The pyriform sinuses are part of the natural pathway of food into the esophagus.

radiation absorbed dose (RAD): A unit of absorbed dose of ionizing radiation equal to 100 ergs per gram of absorbing material. This is a measure of the radiation dose a patient receives with X-rays or radionuclides.

radiographic study/modified barium swallow: A moving X-ray of oropharyngeal swallow on designated boluses.

radiolabel: A compound that has a radionuclide attached to it and can be imaged with a gamma camera after ingestion of injection of the compound into the body.

radionuclides: Isotopes of elements with unstable nuclei that emit radiation at a known rate of decay.

radiopharmaceutical: A compound suitable for injection into the body that is labeled with a radionuclide.

real-time ultrasound: Ultrasound images can be reconstructed rapidly, which allows the operator to view the movement of the structures imaged as if viewing a movie. That is, one seeing the movement of tissues with no distortion of time relationships.

receptive field: The region of the body which, when receiving a particular stimulus, will excite a sensory fiber to discharge action potentials toward the cell body.

receptors: Molecular structures embeded in the plasma membrane that interact with and are activated by particular stimuli such as neurotransmitters, hormones, NaCl, or H_2O. Activation of a receptor may change a variety of cellular processes. It may alter the activity of ionic channels or change biochemicals processed in within the cell.

recurrent laryngeal nerve: A branch of the vagus nerve which provides partial sensory innervation to the larynx and motor innervation to the thyroarytenoid, lateral cricoarytenoid, interarytenoids, and posterior cricoarytenoid muscles.

reflux esophagitis: Inflammation of the esophageal mucosa, resulting from reflux of gastric contents into the esophagus; a syndrome that can present clinically as heartburn, chest pain, or dysphagia. Endoscopically the mucosal appearance can range from normal, a single or few erosions in the distal esophagus, to extensive ulcerative tissues. Histologically, it shows changes in the architecture of the epithelium and infiltration by inflammatory cells. Chronic reflux can be complicated by the development of stricture or Barrett's esophagus.

reserpine: A drug which depletes serotonin and catecholamines.

residual volume: The amount of gas remaining in the lungs after maximal voluntary expiration. This volume, which does not contribute to effective gas exchange, is increased in patients with obstructive lung diseases.

residue: Material left in the oral, pharyngeal, or laryngeal cavity after the swallow.

respiratory muscles: Any of the muscles involved in inhalation or exhalation. Include the diaphragm, the muscles of the rib cage (parasternal, internal and external intercostals, and scalene); the abdominal muscles (internal and external obliques, transversus abdominis, and rectus abdominis), and muscles of the upper airways, which are essential to maintain airway patency.

resistance: Quantity or property of opposition to electron movement (current) through a conductor (unit: ohm). Resistance is the real part of complex impedance.

resting membrane potential: The potential difference across the plasma membrane when the ionic movements across the plasma membrane are in equilibrium. At rest the interior of the cell is negative to its exterior.

restrictive ventilatory defect: Classification of respiratory pathology in which the patient's ability to fully inflate the lungs is diminished. May be due to neuromuscular diseases (causing respiratory muscle weakness), to defects in the thoracic spine, ribs, or pleura (causing a mechanical obstruction to lung inflation), or to fibrosis or surgical removal of the lungs.

reticular formation: A region of the brain stem characterized by unorganized nerve cells and fibers appearing histologically as a network of intertwining cells and fibers. Different regions of the reticular formation are separated functionally. Some of the interneurons in this region function in the swallowing pathway.

retrograde: The direction of movement of an electrical signal (i.e., action potential) or chemicals in the reverse direction from the normal conduction of action potentials of the neuron. For a motor fiber, retrograde conduction would be movement of an action potential or chemical toward the cell body.

rhinosinusitis: Inflammation of the lining membrane of one of the paranasal sinuses.

rigid bronchoscopes: A type of metal endoscope used to examine the bronchi. They are of larger diameter than flexible bronchoscopes and thus are preferred for surgery or removal of foreign bodies.

salivagram: Radionuclide study where a small amount of saline with a high concentration radionuclide is placed on the child's tongue following by scanning of the lungs with a gamma camera to look for radionuclide activity, suggestive of aspiration.

salivary flow: Normal flow of saliva from the parotid gland. Normal salivary flow is about 0.3–0.5 ml/min.

Schatzki's ring: Also known as *B ring*. A mucosal ring at the lower end of the esophagus, usually at the squamocolumnar junction. The upper surface of the ring is lined by squamous, esophageal epithelium, while the lower surface is lined by columnar gastric epithelium. It is typically seen in the setting of chronic gastroesophageal reflux and may be associated with a hiatal hernia.

scintigraphy: Images produced by a gamma camera recording the emissions of radionuclide energy from a patient.

scleroderma and progressive systemic sclerosis: A connective tissue disorder which leads to progressive fibrosis of the dermal layer of the skin, of smooth muscle, or other visceral tissues.

sclerotherapy: see **varices**.

sclerodoma: Part of a spectrum of connective tissue disorders that causes progressive fibrosis of the dermal layer of the skin, particularly of the face, hands, and feet.

secretin: A polypeptide that functions as a hormone secreted by the duodenum to affect the pancreas and as a neurotransmitter in many regions of the CNS and enteric nervous system.

sensitivity: The fraction of subjects with a condition that test positive for that condition; also known as the true positive rate.

sensory neuron (fiber): A neuron that consists of a long dendritic process that extends from the cell body to its target organ and an axon that synapses on an interneuron within the central nervous system. The cell body of the neuron usually resides within central nervous system locations like the dorsal horn of the spinal cord, the nucleus tractus solitarius, or the trigeminal sensory nuclei. The sensory fiber can end directly within the target organ or synapse and innervate a receptor organ (i.e., muscle spindle) within the tissue.

serotonin: A biogenic amine neurotransmitter (i.e., 5-hydroxytryptamine).

sialometry: Evaluation of salivary gland secretion.

sicca syndrome, Sjögren syndrome: Dryness of the mucous membrane in head and neck from destruction of gland. Tongue may be sore, coated, and fissured. Inability to produce tears leads to conjunctivitis, inability to produce saliva leads to inability to swallow dry food. Sjögren's syndrome refers to gland destruction by autoimmune disease, including rheumatoid arthritis and lupus. Gland destruction or malfunction also occurs from radiation, exision, dehydration, and drugs.

silent period: The temporary cessation of ongoing bioelectric (most often EMG) activity, for example, as a reflex inhibitory effect.

sleep apnea: A periodic cessation of breathing during sleep, often related to airway collapse from weakness of pharyngeal muscles. Symptoms include irregular breathing and loud snoring during sleep and excessive daytime sleepiness.

slow adapting sensory fiber: Sensory fibers that discharge action potentials during the entire period the stimulus is applied to the receptive field of the sensory neuron (in contrast to fast adapting fibers). Slow adapting fibers vary their discharge with the intensity of the stimulus. See also **fast adapting fiber**.

smooth muscle: Muscle type found in viscera and the walls of the gastrointestinal tract. Unlike in skeletal muscle, contractiile proteins are not arranged into "striated" units; membrane ion channels provide for longer action potentials; control of contractions through autonomic innervation, in esophageal and gastrointestinal smooth muscle through myenteric plexus neurons.

sodium ion: The membranes of nerve and muscle cells at rest keep sodium out of the cell. When channels within the membrane open shortly to sodium ions, the current of positive ions moving into the cell leads to an action potential across the membrane.

spasmodic dysphonia: A neuromuscular abnormality of unclear etiology that produces strained or tremulous speech.

specificity: The fraction of subjects without a condition that test negative for that condition; also known as the *true negative rate*.

spike potential: Brief electrical voltage changes which occur in certain smooth muscle and are related to ionic channels like calcium.

spillage: Material that has spilled into the pharynx before the pharyngeal swallow response has begun.

spiral CT: Synonymous with helical computed tomography scanning.

squamocolumnar junction (SJC): Also referred to as *ora serrate* or *Z Line*, an anatomical landmark that defines, in a normal condition, the transition zone in the distal esophagus between the gastric and esophageal-type epithelium. The area is located approoximately 40 cm from the incisors in adults, and normally close to the gastroesophageal junction (the zone where the tubular esophagus joins the saccular stomach), to the diaphragmatic hiatus, and to the LES. A proximally displaced SCJ is typical is typical of Barrett's esophagus. A prominent luminal indentation at the SCJ is known as Schatzke's ring. See also **Barrett's esophagus** and **Schatzke's ring**.

squeeze pressure, also contact pressure: Pressure exerted on a sensor as the lumen is cleared of contents and obliterated. During peristalsis of the pharynx and the esophagus, squeeze pressures typically follow and exceed bolus pressures (see also **bolus pressures**).

standard hemilaryngectomy: Resection of half of the laryngeal cartilage, the true and false vocal fold, and one arytenoid.

stenosis: A narrowing or constriction.

striated muscle: Muscle whose contractile proteins are arranged into specific "striated" units; most skeletal muscles (those attached to the bones of the body), but also the pharynx, larynx, and the esophagus, contain striated muscles.

stridor: An upper airway noise that indicates turbulent flow through a narrow airway, usually on inspiration, but can be on expiration. Stridor is not a diagnosis itself but rather an indication of airway abnormality.

stroke: A neurologic deficit resulting from either hemorrhage into brain parenchyma or infarction of brain tissue.

subglottic stenosis: Narrowing in the trachea below the level of the glottis that may result in airway obstruction, and thus can interfere with feeding.

symptomatic benefits: Benefits received only as an improvement of symptoms associated with a disease.

substance P: A neuropeptide transmitter released by sensory neurons and in other synapses.

sucking and suckling: In sucking, the body of the tongue is moved up and down by the activity of its muscles; suckling is a form of sucking present in the first few months of life in which backward movements of the tongue are pronounced.

superior laryngeal nerve: (SLN): One of the branches of the vagus nerve that innervates the laryngeal (cricothyroid) and hypopharyngeal region. It is composed of predominantly sensory fibers with a small component of motor fibers supplying the cricothyroid and upper esophageal striated muscle.

supracricoid laryngectomy: Resection of the entire laryngeal cartilage, true and false vocal folds, preepiglottic fat, and the paraglottic space bilaterally; a portion of the epiglottis may or may not be preserved.

supraglottic laryngectomy: Resection of laryngeal structures above the level of the true vocal folds, including the superior portion of the laryngeal cartilage, the false vocal folds, the epiglottis, aryepiglottic folds, and preepiglottic space.

surfactant: A complex mixture of phospholipids (chiefly lecithin and sphingomyelin) secreted by alveolar type II cells that reduce the surface tension of the pulmonary alveoli and thus reduce the tendency of the alveoli to collapse.

swallow apnea: The normal interruption of the respiratory cycle during expiration induced by a swallow.

swallow maneuver: Designed to place specific aspects of swallow physiology under voluntary control Four swallow maneuvers have been developed to date: (a) the supraglottic swallow, (b) the super-supraglottic swallow, (c) the effortful swallow, and (d) the Mendelsohn maneuver.

sympathetic: One of the divisions of the autonomic nervous system. It is defined anatomically by preganglionic fibers that originate from the thoracic and lumbar levels of the spinal cord and by postganglionic fibers that originate in a chain of ganglia close to the vertebral column. The main neural neurotransmitter released by the postganglionic fibers is norepinephrine.

synapse: A commection between two neurons or between a neuron and muscle at which signals are relayed. In chemical-type synapses, the presynaptic neuron releases a transmitter like acetylcholine into the open cleft which separates it from the postsynaptic neuron or muscle. The transmitter interacts with receptors to initiate specific responses. See also synaptic transmitter and neurotransmitter. Another type of synapse is called electrical.

synaptic transmitter: The chemical messenger released by the presynaptic terminal of a neuron upon arrival of an action potential. Transmitter is released as packets which move across the synaptic cleft to link with receptors on the postsynaptic membrane. More than one type of transmitter can be released from one neuron, and more than one type of postsynaptic receptor will combine with the transmitter.

syncope: Temporary loss of consciousness due to transient cerebral hypoperfusion, which in turn may result from either rapid or slow cardiac arrhythmias (bradycardia and tachycardia, respectively).

tardive dyskinesia: An extrapyramidal syndrome characterized by involuntary choreic movements resulting from long-term exposure to neuroleptics such as phenothiazine.

taste receptor: Specialized chemoreceptors which respond to substances dissolved in oral fluids. The different substances activate different types of membrane channels or transmembrane receptors. The receptor is located in a complex organ (taste bud) with other types of cells and synaptically excites the sensory fibers innervating it.

technetium 99m: A radionuclide commonly used for evaluation of the gastrointestinal tract. It may be linked to food or other ligands for injection in the body to be taken up by various organs.

technetium 99m sulfur colloid: A radiopharmaceutical consisting of technetium bound to sulfur colloid particles which may be used to evaluate the gastrointestinal transit or uptake of the tracer by the reticuloendothelial system.

tertiary contractions: Simultaneous, nonpropulsive contractions that occur at any level of the esophagus.

tetrodotoxin: A toxin from the Japanese puffer fish which blocks sodium channels in the neuronal membrane from the outside with or without the channel opening so that depolarization cannot occur.

therapy procedure/exercise: Designed to change swallow physiology and requires a cooperative effort from the patient, often over a period of time.

threshold: The membrane potential at which neurons and muscle cells generate potentials.

thyrotropin releasing factor (TRF): TRF is primarily a hypothalamic hormone and stimulates release of thyrotropin and prolactin from the anterior pituitary.

tidal volume: The volume of air inspired in a single breath.

time-activity curves: A graph over time of the amount of radioactivity in a certain organ or in the blood. Such curves allow the quantification of physiologic events using radionuclides.

total parenteral nutrition (TPN): Nutritional needs provided exclusively through intravenous access and not the gastrointestinal tract.

tongue pumping: Repeated rockinglike motion of the tongue preceding swallowing.

topical anesthetic: Anesthetics applied to a local region through injection, direct application by touch or spraying. The anesthetic is not given systemically and has a direct effect on specific neurons, depending on its dose and concentration as well as the local blood supply.

total glossectomy: Resection of the entire tongue, including removal of the tonge-base musculature from the hyoid, glossopharyngeus, and styloglossus.

total laryngectomy: Removal of the entire cricoid and thyroid cartilages as well as the epiglottis, with resection extending from the upper tracheal rings to hyoid bone.

toxic aspirations: Inhalation of substances such as strong acids, strong bases, or petrochemicals which lead to rapid, direct injury to the airspaces.

tracheal intubation: Placement of a tube into the trachea, either translaryngeally or via a tracheostomy.

tracheoesophageal fistula (TEF): Abnormal communication between the trachea and the esophagus, occurring during the 4th week of development because of incomplete division of the cranial part of the foregut into respiratory and digestive portions. Incidence is 1 in 2,500 births, with majority in males. TEF is the most common malformation of the respiratory tract in infancy.

tracheoesophageal separation: A type of subglottic closure where the subglottic trachea is brought to the skin as a tracheotomy but the supraglottic portion of the trachea is attached to the esophagus so that all ingesta entering the larynx can exit into the esophagus.

tracheomalacia: Pathologic softening of the tracheal cartilages, often the result of tracheal ischemia during endotracheal intubation.

tracheostomy: A surgically created opening into the trachea through the anterior neck.

transcutaneous oxygen tension (TcPO$_2$): Measure of oxygenation. Nonnutritive sucking in preterm infants has been shown to be beneficial in increasing TcPO$_2$ (e.g., Paludetto et al., 1984).

transient lower esophageal sphincter relaxation (TLESR): Relaxations of the lower esophageal sphincter that occur without associated swallowing activity. These events account for 60–80% of gastroesophageal reflux events.

treatment strategies/interventions: During the diagnostic radiographic study, management strategies to improve the swallow should be introduced, beginning with **postural techniques**, followed by introduction of **techniques to increase oral sensation** (when appropriate), and finally, **diet** (food consistency, viscosity) **changes**, if needed.

trigeminal nerve: One of the major cranial nerves with three major divisions and one motor division. It innervates the head and oral cavity.

trigeminal sensory nuclei: A collection of three sensory nuclei in the brain stem with the mesencephalic, main sensory, and spinal trigeminal the three components. Most of the sensory input from the head and neck synapses within these nuclei with the nucleus of the tractus solitarius, a second sensory nucleus.

tubal feeding: Alimentation using liquid formulation passed into the enteral tract via tubes, which may be placed through the mouth or nose (e.g., Dobhoff feeding tubes) or percutaneously.

ultrafast computed tomography: Synonymous with fast CT scanning. A technique of CT scanning in which the x-ray rapidly scans the patient in several planes; fast enough to freeze rapid motions such as occur in the oropharynx during swallowing.

ultrafast MRI: A scanning technique using certain sequences of magnetic pulses allowing rapid magnetic resonance imaging scans to be performed.

ultrasound imaging: A method of evaluating the soft tissues where imaging is done using high-frequency sound waves. Tissue contrast is provided by the differences in each tissue's ability to reflect sound.

ultrasound transducer: A portion of the ultrasound machine that is placed in contact with the patient's skin, which sends and receives high-frequency sound waves in a manner that allows the reflected sound to be reconstructed into real-time images of soft tissues.

upper esophageal sphincter (UES): Formed by the cricopharyngeus muscle, which by its tonic contraction closes the lumen between the pharynx and the esophagus. Swallowing shortly relaxes the cricopharyngeus. Opening of the UES segment is enhanced by the pull from the hyoid ascent and the pressure exerted by the luminal bolus.

vagotomy: The transection of at least one vagus nerve, usually by sectioning. Transient vagotomy can occur with cooling temperatures applied by a temperature probe directly to the nerve. Depending on the level of the section, certain organs will remain innervated.

vagus nerve: The tenth cranial nerve, which arises from the lateral side of the medulla oblongata and innervates a wide variety of visceral organs, including the tongue (sensory), pharynx (sensory and motor), larynx (sensory and motor), lungs and heart (parasympathetic and visceral afferent).

valleculae: The space between the base of the tongue and the epiglottis. Residue in the valliculae indicates a problem in movement of the tongue base.

Valsalva maneuver: Produced by forceful expiration against the closed glottis.

variceal sclerotherapy: Injections of sclerosant agents into dilated veins (varices) in the esophagus to stop or prevent bleeding.

varices: Veins that are grossly enlarged because of increased outflow resistance. Varices at the gastroesophageal junction are common in chronic liver disease, and prone to torrential bleeding. Injection of sclerosants into the varices can stop bleeding by obliteration of the venous lumen.

varicosities: Swollen regions of an axon containing neurotransmitter vesicles so that it is similar to presynaptic terminals. Evident with smooth muscle innervation.

vasoactive intestinal polypeptide (VIP): A polypeptide which can serve as a neurotransmitter in the autonomic nervous system.

vasopressin: A peptide hormone synthesized in the hypothalamus and primarily released from the posterior pituitary.

vasovagal response: fainting.

vasovagal syndrome: A paroxysmal condition marked by a slow pulse and fall in blood pressure, due to stimulation of the vagus nerve, mediated through the carotid sinus.

VFE (videofluoroscopic examination): Examination of oral and pharyngeal swallowing function. Also called *dysphagia diagnostic study* (DSS), *functional assessment of swallowing* (FAS), *videofluoroscopic swallow study* (VSS), *cookie swallow test, and modified barium swallow* (MBS). The primary purpose of this examination to to determine the cause(s) of dysfunction of the oral and/or pharyngeal stages.

videofluorographic study/modified barium swallow: a moving x-ray of oral and pharyngeal stages of the swallow with designated bolnses.

vocal fold augmentation: The injection of an absorbable or nonabsorbable substance to achieve vocal fold closure and prevent aspiraton related to vocal fold paralysis.

volume conduction: Passive conduction of a current from a potential source through tissue or body fluid, not limited to a plane such as a membrane surface but through a bulk conductor.

warm spots: Receptive fields of sensory nerve fibers which discharge when a stimulus increasing temperature across a specific range is placed within its receptive field.

xerostomia: Dry mouth due to salivary gland dysfunction. Can occur as a result of medication, disease, or radiation therapy.

Zenker's diverticulum: Herniation of the pharyngeal mucosa at the level of the upper esophageal sphincter. The diverticulum usually protrudes between the fibers of the cricopharyngeus and inferior constrictor muscles. These herniations most commonly occur on the left side, less commonly on the posterior wall and the midline, and only rarely on the right side.

Answers to Multiple Choice Questions

CHAPTER 1

1. b and c
2. a and c
3. c
4. a and d

CHAPTER 2

1. b
2. d
3. b
4. a, b, and c

CHAPTER 3

No questions

CHAPTER 4

1. e
2. a
3. c
4. d
5. c

CHAPTER 5

1. d
2. a
3. e

CHAPTER 6

1. a, b, and c
2. b
3. d
4. a, b, and c

CHAPTER 7

1. c
2. a

3. e
4. e
5. b

CHAPTER 8

1. a, b, and c
2. b and c
3. a

CHAPTER 9

1. e
2. e
3. d
4. d
5. c
6. f

CHAPTER 10

1. b, c, and d
2. c
3. b
4. b
5. a
6. a

CHAPTER 11

1. c
2. a
3. b
4. d

CHAPTER 12

1. d
2. a and c
3. d

CHAPTER 13

1. c
2. d
3. c
4. c
5. b
6. d
7. d

CHAPTER 14

1. b
2. c
3. d
4. d
5. e
6. d

CHAPTER 15

1. b and d
2. b
3. e
4. e
5. b

CHAPTER 16

1. b and c
2. a
3. a and b
4. d
5. b and d
6. Electrolyte disturbances, such as hypokalemia, infection such as line sepsis, or bacteremia, phlebitis or thrombosis, fluid overload, vitamin or mineral deficiency.

Index